American Pharmacy

*An Introduction to Pharmaceutical Techniques
and Dosage Forms*

Contributors

L. L. AUGSBURGER, PH.D.
*Assistant Professor of Pharmacy,
University of Maryland
School of Pharmacy*

GILBERT S. BANKER, PH.D.
*Professor of Industrial Pharmacy
and Head, Industrial and Physical
Pharmacy Department, School of
Pharmacy and Pharmacal Sciences,
Purdue University, Indiana*

SEYMOUR M. BLAUG, PH.D.
*Professor of Pharmacy, College of
Pharmacy, University of Iowa*

E. A. BRECHT, PH.D.
*Professor of Pharmaceutics,
School of Pharmacy,
Northeast Louisiana University*

PATRICK P. DELUCA, PH.D.
*Assistant Dean and Associate
Professor of Pharmacy, College of
Pharmacy, University of Kentucky
Medical Center*

LEWIS W. DITTERT, PH.D.
*Professor of Pharmacy, College of
Pharmacy, University of Kentucky
Medical Center*

RODNEY D. ICE, PH.D.
*Director, Radiopharmaceutical
Services and Associate Professor
of Pharmacy, College of Pharmacy,
University of Michigan*

NICHOLAS G. LORDI, PH.D.
*Professor of Pharmacy, College of
Pharmacy, Rutgers, The State
University, New Jersey*

ALFRED N. MARTIN, PH.D.
*Professor and Director, Drug Dynamics
Institute, University of Texas,
College of Pharmacy*

ELMER M. PLEIN, PH.D.
*Coordinator of Pharmaceutical Services
and Professor of Pharmacy,
University of Washington*

THOMAS DUDLEY ROWE, PH.D.
*Dean and Professor of Pharmacy,
University of Michigan College
of Pharmacy*

HANS SCHOTT, PH.D.
*Professor of Physical and Colloid
Chemistry, Temple University School
of Pharmacy, Philadelphia, Pennsylvania*

T. WERNER SCHWARZ, PH.D.
*Associate Professor of Pharmacy and
Pharmaceutical Chemistry, School of
Pharmacy, University of California,
San Francisco Medical Center*

JOSEPH B. SPROWLS, PH.D.
*Late Dean, College of Pharmacy,
University of Texas*

MITCHELL JOHN STOKLOSA, SC.D.
*Dean of Students and Professor of
Pharmacy, Massachusetts College
of Pharmacy*

JAMES SWARBRICK, D.SC., PH.D.
*Director of Product Development,
Sterling-Winthrop Research
Institute, Rensselaer, New York*

GEORGE ZOGRAFI, PH.D.
*Professor of Pharmaceutics, University
of Wisconsin School of Pharmacy*

LOUIS C. ZOPF, D.SC.
*Dean Emeritus, College of Pharmacy,
University of Iowa*

Sprowls' American Pharmacy

An Introduction to Pharmaceutical Techniques and Dosage Forms

Edited by

LEWIS W. DITTERT, Ph.D.

Professor of Pharmacy, College of Pharmacy
University of Kentucky Medical Center

SEVENTH EDITION

J. B. Lippincott Company

Philadelphia • Toronto

The use of portions of the text of the *United States Pharmacopeia, Eighteenth Revision*, official September 1, 1970, is by permission received from the Board of Trustees of the United States Pharmacopeial Convention. The said Convention is not responsible for any inaccuracy of quotation or for any false or misleading implications that may arise by reason of separation of excerpts from the original context.

Permission to use portions of the text of The *National Formulary, Thirteenth Edition*, official September 1, 1970, has been granted by the American Pharmaceutical Association. The American Pharmaceutical Association is not responsible for any inaccuracy of quotation or for false implications that may arise by reason of the separation of excerpts from the original context.

The use in this volume of certain portions of the text of AMA Drug Evaluations, 1971, is by virtue of permission received from the American Medical Association. The said Association is not responsible for the accuracy of transpositions or excerpts taken from texts under its authority, or for false implications that may arise by reason of the separation of excerpts from the original context.

ISBN-0-397-52058-1

Library of Congress Catalog Card No. 73-20013

Printed in the United States of America

3   5   4

Library of Congress Cataloging in Publication Data

Sprowls, Joseph Barnett, ed.
   Sprowls' American pharmacy.

   Previous editions edited by R. A. Lyman.
   Includes bibliographies.
   1. Pharmacy. I. Dittert, Lewis W., ed.
II. Lyman, Rufus Ashley, 1875–1957, ed. III. Title.
IV. Title: American pharmacy. [DNLM: 1. Pharmacy.
QV704 D613a 1974]
RS91.S76   1974   615'.4   73-20013
ISBN 0-397-52058-1
                                       Rev.

Dedicated to the Memory of
RUFUS ASHLEY LYMAN, M.D.,
GEORGE URDANG, Ph.G., D. Sc. Nat., Sc.D. (h.c.),
and
JOSEPH B. SPROWLS, Ph.D.,
without whose pioneering efforts the present edition
would never have come into being

Preface

The practice of pharmacy and emphasis in pharmaceutical education have changed considerably since the first volume of *American Pharmacy* appeared in 1945. In that volume, the attempt was made to distill the essence of the science and art of pharmaceutical compounding. The format of the early volumes was to first review scientific principles, and then discuss the step-by-step manipulations involved in formulating and preparing pharmaceutical dosage forms. Heavy emphasis was placed on preparations appearing in the official compendia which illustrated various formulation and compounding techniques. During that period, pharmaceutical education and practice also emphasized the compounding and dispensing roles of the pharmacist.

With the sixth edition, a change in format appeared. The scientific review section was dissolved, and much of its material was incorporated into the chapters dealing with the various dosage forms. This change was possible because most pharmacy students had completed courses in chemistry, biology, physics, and mathematics before their studies of pharmaceutical techniques began, and it was possible to present the scientific aspects on a higher level than previously.

The sixth edition also placed more emphasis on the large-scale manufacturing of dosage forms, and discussions of aspects of their in-vivo performance began to appear. These and other features of the sixth edition led its Editor-in-Chief, Dr. Joseph B. Sprowls, to refer to it as a "treatise on dosage forms" which endeavored to deal with all aspects of the subject—from fundamental scientific principles through extemporaneous compounding and large-scale manufacturing to their ultimate in-vivo performance in patients. This approach recognized the decreasing role of the pharmacist as a practitioner of extemporaneous compounding and the increasing use of premanufactured pharmaceuticals during the 1960's. Today, this evolutionary process is, for practical purposes, complete. Less than 2 percent of all prescriptions filled in the United States are compounded extemporaneously, and, in fact, a rapidly growing number of pharmaceuticals are not even repackaged by the pharmacist. Unit doses and prepackaged courses of therapy are becoming the order of the day.

The seventh edition of *American Pharmacy* has attempted to move with this trend. In this edition, less emphasis has been placed upon compendial preparations and extemporaneous compounding techniques, and more space has been devoted to the complex scientific aspects and the large-scale manufacturing techniques involved in the formulation and production of modern pharmaceuticals. Notable examples of these changes are found in the chapters on colloids, coarse dispersions, and radioactive dosage forms which deal at length with the many complex scientific principles involved in those pharmaceutical systems. Similarly, the chapters on powdered dosage forms, tablets, and sterile products have been thoroughly revised and now deal predominantly with manipulative techniques that are carried out with the aid of complex manufacturing machinery. Finally, all chapters include some discussion of the in-vivo performance (or biopharmaceutics) of the dosage forms under consideration, and this aspect is covered particularly well in the chapters on ointments and suppositories.

These changes have been made because the trend in pharmaceutical education is to prepare the pharmacist to play a key role on the health care team as the expert on drug products and their usage. Several states have already given pharmacists the option of selecting the product containing the drug substance called for by the physician. And in certain types of practice, pharmacists are monitoring drug response in patients and adjusting dosage regimens to produce the safest, most beneficial results in therapy. For these roles, it is not necessary that the pharmacist be able to actually prepare tablets, for example. But he certainly must understand all the scientific and technical aspects involved in their manufacture, and, in particular, he must thoroughly understand all the factors affecting their in-vivo performance. This edition of *American Pharmacy* does not pretend to cover all of these aspects in complete detail, but it should give the student a solid introduction to the principles that will be developed in his more advanced courses. It certainly should provide him with the information he will need concerning pharmaceutical product formulation.

It would be impossible to thank, specifically, all those who contributed to the preparation of this edition of *American Pharmacy*. Besides the authors, many pharmaceutical manufacturers, scientific supply companies, and other industrial concerns contributed information and/or pictures and illustrations, and many scientists from both the academic and industrial communities supplied information or critically reviewed material presented in this volume. I would like to express my gratitude specifically to the authors who were diligent in meeting their deadlines and gracious in accepting editorial suggestions and who achieved a high degree of excellence in their writings. I would also like to thank Mr. J. Stuart Freeman, Jr., Medical Editor of J. B. Lippincott Co., and Ms. Naomi Coplin for their expert guidance and particularly for their understanding and patience.

I could not consider this preface to be complete without paying a personal tribute to the man who, among his many other duties, served as Editor-in-Chief of both the 5th and the 6th editions. Joseph B. Sprowls was a great educator, a great writer, a great professional leader—but most of all, he was a great human being. He gave all he had to his profession, and it was a bountiful gift. He will be sorely missed.

LEWIS W. DITTERT, Editor

Contents

American Pharmacy

*An Introduction to Pharmaceutical Techniques
and Dosage Forms*

1

Joseph B. Sprowls, Ph.D.
Late Dean, College of Pharmacy, University of Texas

An Introduction to Dosage Forms

The term *dosage form* is of very recent coinage, so recent, in fact, that its definition may not be found in a standard dictionary. Nevertheless, the term is so completely descriptive that one immediately understands its intent; therefore, it promises to have considerable usage in the future. *Dosage* is defined in *Stedman's Medical Dictionary** as "the giving of medicine or other therapeutic agent in prescribed amounts." The *dosage form,* therefore is *a preparation devised to make possible the administration of medications in measured, or prescribed, amounts.* The term *pharmaceutical* has sometimes been used as a noun to denote preparations of such nature, but simultaneous use of the word in an adjectival form with a much broader connotation has prevented its having a precise meaning. In using the term dosage form, one must bear in mind that not all medications are administered internally and that many are applied to external membranes or to the skin. In such instances, the dosage is controlled not through the volume or weight of preparation administered but by adjusting the concentration of active ingredients contained in the finished product. In all instances, the primary objective is to present the active constituent in the form and the concentration or amount that are capable of effecting a beneficial response in the average instance of use. Procedures required for achieving this objective have at times become highly elaborate.

Although the use of modern drugs may be said to be based on the most elaborate research and investigation, the form in which medicines are administered, like so many objects that trace their origin to an-

tiquity, represent not so much the result of scientific study as a combination of tradition, empiricism and inventiveness. Only recently has it been possible to apply scientific methodology to the preparation of therapeutic forms. The time is quickly coming when it will be possible to administer drugs to a variety of patients in forms and on regimens scientifically or mathematically designed to produce and maintain a planned effect in each particular patient. Such an approach to therapy is now employed routinely in some hospitals for potentially hazardous drugs such as digoxin and kanamycin. The span of time that elapses between discovery and implementation of a concept grows shorter continually and the development of pharmacy has been phenomenal during the past three decades. Furthermore, the ability of the pharmacist to serve as an expert in the therapeutic use of drugs has been developing very rapidly; and, if the trend continues, it is quite possible that the age of scientific medication will have arrived before this text ceases to be useful.

The origin of medicines is lost in antiquity. Of the early writings which have been discovered to date, many give evidence of an already developed practice of medicine involving the use of drugs. Sir William Osler once wrote that "the desire to take medicines is perhaps the greatest feature which distinguishes man from the animals." A description of medications used by the ancient Mesopotamians or Egyptians is surprising in its similarity to modern dosage forms, yet the coincidence can be ascribed largely to circumstance. After all, the ancients were faced with the same avenues of ingress to the body, the same barriers to penetration

* Stedman's Medical Dictionary. ed. 21. Williams & Wilkins, 1966.

and the same physiologic defenses that we face today.

The first volume of *Medicine and Pharmacy, an Informal History** begins as follows:

A bellyache feels the same in a cave or a penthouse. It hurts, and the immediate reaction of its unhappy victim is to try to find a wiser man than himself to drive the hurt away.

Such may be the first reaction, but the second is to seek something which may be swallowed or administered to relieve the pain. One can perhaps imagine a prehistoric man searching wildly for anything which might relieve the distress of acute indigestion— trying barks, leaves and roots, perhaps dying from the poison of one which proved not a boon but a bane. Likewise, one can picture such a one, having suffered a bruised shin, applying embrocations of leaves and mud to ease the soreness. Through crude experiments such as these, some valuable drugs were discovered and many useful dosage forms devised, while at the same time a great many follies and foolish notions emerged. In their earliest forms, the practices of pharmacy and medicine were indistinguishable and were accommodated to a presupposition of magic and supernatural intervention. In the course of time, these beliefs were abandoned and the practices were separated. The preparation and the perfection of dosage forms became the responsibility of the pharmacist, while the functions of diagnosing and prescribing rested on the physician. The search for new remedies and the invention of new dosage forms has involved the collaborative effort of pharmacists and physicians, and the record of these investigations extends back for more than 4,000 years.

Although physical forms of medication have not changed dramatically, the attitude of the public toward accepting medicines and the purposes for which medicines are administered have changed with the passage of time. Whereas drugs were once looked on as substances to be used for the relief of acute illness, they are employed presently as much for prevention as for the treatment of disease or its consequences. For

many persons, the constant use of drugs is essential for life; for example, in diabetes the administration of insulin may be a process extending throughout the life of the individual. In other circumstances, drugs may be taken routinely for the purpose of maintaining good physical and mental health. Vitamins and tranquilizers are examples of drugs which, respectively, serve such purposes. The use of drugs to sustain life and to ease suffering during periods of acute illness remain as important applications.

These widely accepted and important functions have elevated pharmaceuticals to a position of significance in our society. Their impact is reflected in every set of vital statistics published, in the volumes of laws that have been passed for their standardization and regulation, in the size of the industry that has developed for their production and distribution, even through such insignificant trivia as ornamented cases which are sold in large numbers for the carrying of one's personal supply of medication. As the use of contraceptive medication has become widely accepted and acceptable, even the world's birth rate is reflecting the impact of the modern science of pharmacy.

It was said above that the basic dosage forms have changed little in physical form since earlier times, yet it is a fact that the industrial revolution brought a number of advances. Dosage forms whose production requires the use of intricate machines were beyond man's realization until his mechanical skills had progressed sufficiently and such machines could be fabricated. Among products that awaited such development are compressed tablets, encased powders (capsules), and sterile injectables (ampuls and multiple-dose vials). The onrush of modern technology has made possible even more dramatic concepts such as the sustained-release capsule, tablet, or liquid and the aerosols. Even the remarkable property of radioactivity has been harnessed and made useful in forms suitable for diagnostic and therapeutic purposes. New perspectives, coupled with the spirit of science and invention which is alive in our society today, give promise of a constant flow of improved dosage forms that will surpass in effectiveness and physical pre-

---

* Schering Corporation, Bloomfield, N. J., 1955.

cision the products available to any previous generation.

THE HISTORY OF DOSAGE FORMS*

Many records of ancient pharmacy have been made available to us through the research of archeologists and through chance discoveries of ancient documents. These indicate that practically all historic cultures had well-developed procedures for the treatment of disease and the production of dosage forms. All of these made use of drugs, even though in many instances the physical substances administered were thought to be effective only because of some accompanying ritual or religious practice. The following may be mentioned as being the most significant ancient records containing extensive pharmaceutical material:

The Sumerian Pharmacological Tablet. This small clay tablet—only 3¾ by 6½ inches—has inscribed on it 15 prescriptions and instructions to the pharmacist for proper preparation of them in dosage forms. This tablet is in the Museum of the University of Pennsylvania, and it was written in Nippur in Mesoptamia about 2200 B.C.[5]

The Egyptian Medical Papyri. The two most important of these are: The Edwin Smith Surgical Papyrus and the Ebers Papyrus. The Edwin Smith Papyrus contains, along with operative instructions to physicians, recipes and directions for the compounding of the requisite medicines and dosage forms. The papyrus which was written about 1650 B.C., contains material from the era 2500 B.C.[2] The Ebers Papyrus, which contains about 875 recipes for medicines, was written about 1550 B.C.[9]

The Assyrian Medico-Pharmaceutical Tablets. These texts were copies of Babylonian texts from about 1,000 B.C. which were kept in the library of Assurbanipal in Nineveh (668–627 B.C.). Three of these tablets form a bilingual pharmacopoeia which gives the Sumerian and the Assyro-

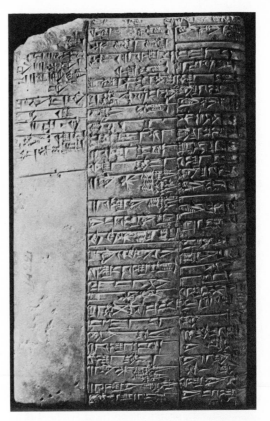

Fig. 1-1. The earliest pharmacopoeia. A Sumerian medical tablet. (From the University of Pennsylvania Museum)

Babylonian names for drugs and medicinal materials in parallel columns. Other texts of this type were found and proved to be the "catalogues" of ancient pharmacies.[26]

The Old Testament. Numerous passages in the Bible mentioned drugs and present formulas for the preparation of some, along with descriptions of their usage.[12]

Several other papyri have not been mentioned here because they are primarily devoted to surgical procedures or gynecology. For a more complete listing the student may consult references given at the end of this chapter.

The Ancient Period.† Samuel Noah Kramer[14] refers to the Sumerian Pharmacological tablet mentioned above as "the first

---

* This presentation is not intended to serve as a review of the history of pharmacy. The intent is to focus on those factors that have contributed to the evolution of our major forms of dosage. In several instances this record is augmented by discussions elsewhere in the text.

† The author wishes to acknowledge the aid of Wm. White, Jr., Ancient Historian of Temple University, in the preparation of this section.

pharmacopoeia," and well it may be. The tablet records the practices of an ancient Sumerian physician and describes both drugs and preparations which were used by him in the treatment of his patients. Present are both internal and external preparations, the latter including salves and filtrates. The salves were made by powdering one or more simple drugs, infusing the powder with wine and adding both common tree oil and cedar oil to the mixture. As described, this is more in the nature of an embrocation or liniment than an ointment as we know it. The absence of animal fat is notable, since the Egyptians and the Babylonians at a slightly later period made much use of animal fats in their external preparations. On the other hand, we must recognize that the tablet probably represents a very small portion of the scope of pharmaceuticals as used by the Sumerians. In addition to this is the fact that many of the later Babylonian texts use Sumerian words for descriptions not yet found in any of the known Sumerian texts but which must have existed. As more translations become available, it will be possible to construct a more complete interpretation of medical practice and pharmaceutical method during these early civilizations.

Another prescription was made by kneading river clay and other simple drugs in water and honey, then "sea" oil was spread over the mixture. Terms such as sea oil are meaningless, as it is not known whether such designations are literal or are folk-names such as *foxglove* and *lady's slipper,* which, when applied to botanical materials, have nothing to do with the actual components of the plant. In later years, the practice of rubbing an insoluble powder with a liquid ingredient for the purpose of reducing the size of the particles and producing a smooth mixture came to be called *levigation,* a term still in use in our day (see Chap. 8, Ointments). The Sumerians used water and honey for this purpose in the prescription noted; today it would more likely be liquid petrolatum, a substance which was unknown until the 19th century.

The process of decoction, i.e., boiling in water, was used in preparing some of the Sumerian prescriptions. Alkali and salts were added while boiling, perhaps to increase the concentration of extracted material. Filtration is also mentioned, as is decantation, and their use in other preparations is assumed by the writer of the prescription.

Internal liquids were prepared from simple drugs by infusion, generally using beer, wine or possibly milk as the solvent. Solutions were made by grinding drugs to a powder and dissolving them in wine or beer. It is notable that Thompson, in his translations of the tablets from the library of Assurbanipal,[27] describes a similar method of extraction in which wine is used as the solvent. The mixture of drugs with solvent was allowed to stand overnight, and the supernatant liquid was decanted and drunk the following morning for its medicinal effect.

Thompson's translations of the Assyrian pharmaceutical texts reveal that the *poultice* was an ancient form of external preparation. An early form of such was a concoction of rotten grain and water. Another contained powdered "siklu"—a kind of garlic or onion —kneaded with cassia juice, while a third consisted of mashed turnips kneaded with milk to produce a soft paste. These soft mixtures usually were applied directly to the skin and held in place by a bandage, although in at least one instance the patient was instructed to sit in a poultice for the relief of sore muscles. The use of hot baths and steam for sore muscles also was advised. The early practice of fashioning a poultice from simple household materials has survived to modern times and has its parallel in the common mustard poultice (or plaster) which is prepared by moistening powdered mustard or a mixture of flour and mustard, spreading on cloth, and applying. Plasters also are referred to in the Assyrian tablets and were made by spreading a moistened mixture of drugs on cloth or leather to make a compress.

Lotions for the eyes are mentioned, which were made by dissolving alkaline salts in water. In later times, such preparations came to be known among the Greeks and Romans as *collyria,* from the Greek word Kōlla meaning *glue, wheat-paste* and, by extension, *eye-salve.*

The following prescription from Thompson* demonstrates a preparation used in treating an eye disease:

. . . thou shalt beat leaves of tamarisk, steep them in strong vinegar, leave them out under the stars; in the morning thou shalt squeeze them in a helmet; white alum, storax, Akkadian salt, fat, cornflour, nigella, gum of copper, separately thou shalt bray [pound or rub]; thou shalt take equal part of them, put them together, pour them into the helmet in which thou hast squeezed the tamarisk; in curd and sinus-mineral thou shalt knead it, and open his eyelids with a finger and put it in his eyes. While his eyes contain dimness, his eyes thou shalt smear, and for nine days thou shalt do this.

The reader will note once more the practice of permitting the preparations to stand overnight, this time "under the stars." The probability is that the ancient pharmacist attached much significance to the presence of astral bodies, since the supernatural played a very strong part in all phases of medical practice. Sigerist[21] makes the statement that "Mesopotamian medicine was psychosomatic in all its aspects."

The use of injections, such as *Enemata* or *clysters,* was known in Sumero-Babylonian medical practice, and in Egypt ancient catheters have been found. The use of *inhalations* (aromatic powders to be burned and the smoke or fumes inhaled) was as much based on ritual as medical usage. Mixtures of drugs with honey and sweet tree sap were common. These might represent an early type of the preparations called *theriacs, electuaries,* or *confections* in later periods. The development of this type of preparation will be deferred for later discussion.

Methods used for administering drugs during the Babylonian period are of some interest. Liquid potions frequently were drunk through a tube. Medicaments to be administered to the nose, the ear or the urethra usually were blown through a tube, the same method as used in administering the enema.

As further examples of preparations and dosage forms probably invented before re-

corded history, we may mention the ointments, the confections and the perfumes described in the Old Testament and inhalations and enemas used by the ancient Hindus.† An interesting description of a holy anointing ointment may be found in Chapter 30 of the book of Exodus. The ointment contains myrrh, sweet cinnamon (canella), sweet calamus, and cassia made into an ointment with olive oil as base.

Although records indicate that China had a well-developed literature on pharmacology by the 5th century B.C., it is doubtful if this had an appreciable influence on the development of medicine and pharmacy in the Western world, with the exception of a few innovations which came by way of commerce through India and Arabia in Roman times.

The most complete record of Egyptian pharmacology extant is the Ebers Papyrus, which, like the Assyro-Babylonian material, is the embodiment of long-standing tradition. The papyrus mentions all of the dosage forms that were known to the Babylonians and includes as well some additional ones which either were African in origin or arose after the Babylonian corpus had been compiled. Preparations mentioned in the Ebers Papyrus but not previously described here are the following: fumigations, embrocations, gargles, eye salves, pills, boluses (large pills), lozenges, cakes, plugs for the anus, and suppositories.

A famous preparation from the Ebers Papyrus which was used until recent times is Hiera Picra or *sacred bitters.* This powder contained aloe and canella and was the prototype of bitter powders used through many succeeding generations and bearing the general title *hiera.* Aloe was always the principal ingredient, with various aromatic substances added to soften the irritant effect and mask some of the bitter taste. A powder of Aloe and Canella was carried in the early pharmacopoeias of this country and last

---

* Thompson, R. C.: Assyrian Medical Texts. Proc. Roy. Soc. Med. [Sect. Hist. Med.], *17*:28–29, 1924.

† Jürgen Thorwald (*Science and Secrets of Early Medicine,* Harcourt Brace, New York, 1963) suggests that a medical practice existed in India as early as the second millenium B.C. and that many Egyptian or Greek concepts were borrowed from this source.

recognized in the Third Edition of the *National Formulary* (official until 1926). Thus, this single combination of drugs persisted as the basis for many formulas for at least 3,500 years of recorded time.

A number of the early hieras were prepared later in pill form for more convenient administration. Thus, the pills of Rufus (later Pilulae Pestilentiales) was originally a hiera which was made into pill form by the Arabs and popularized in this form by the Arabian authority Avicenna. Pills of Aloe and Mastic (the basis for the Rufus formula) were last official in the United States in the Eighth Edition of the *National Formulary*.

Kramer[14] takes note of the fact that Sumerian prescriptions make no mention of proportions of ingredients to be used in compounding the formulas as given. He speculates that the quantities to be used were known to the ancient physicians and used by them on the basis of experience; however, it may be that the necessity for care in dosage had not yet been recognized. The Assyrians, likewise, rarely mention the amounts of drugs to be used, and this is difficult to explain because their technology was well advanced and they did make some use of poisonous drugs. The basis for this unusual omission has not yet been adequately explained. Certainly, an appreciation of the need for measured dosage had been developed by the Egyptians, else there would be little reason for their use of divided dosage forms such as pills, boluses and lozenges. Furthermore, Egyptian prescriptions, as represented in the Ebers Papyrus, carry designations of the quantity of drug to be used in each instance. Leake[15] has pointed out that the Egyptians particularly noted the quantities to be used when the drugs were poisonous or expensive.

Prescriptions in the Ebers Papyrus are preceded by an indication of the disease condition in which they are to be used. In addition, they often indicate the incantation or song to be rendered as the prescription is administered and, sometimes, the dress which the physician is to wear. This clearly indicates the extent to which theurgic concepts influenced the medical practice of the

Egyptians. In his discussion of this period, Sigerist[21] says

The art of medicine consisted in selecting the right drugs, preparing them in the magically correct way, and speaking the appropriate words over them.*

The Ebers Papyrus lists more than 700 drugs in more than 800 prescriptions. Included are drugs from every category of substances which is used today, with the exception of purified chemicals: fruits and berries, vegetables, woods or gums, roots and mineral drugs. One category of agents, not used today, was sometimes referred to as "disgusting drugs"—the excrement of animals, blood of animals, skins of animals (particularly reptiles)—even the excrement of flies.† Internal remedies were given usually as potions, using beer, sweet beer, wine (prepared from either grapes or dates) or milk as the solvent. The milk might be human or obtained from the cow or ass. Cakes were formed by mixing drugs with honey or grease and shaping. Sometimes cakes containing honey were baked. The preparation of ointments utilized vegetable oils such as olive and castor, while stiffer ointments were prepared with the fat of various animals.

The administration of medications differed little from procedures used by the Babylonians. Internally used liquids were common, but many other forms were used. Enemas were common and used not only for flushing the rectum but also for the administration of drugs. Fumigations were used for treating disease conditions of the anus and the vagina. The Ebers Papyrus suggests that an eye remedy be instilled by means of a vulture's feather.

The following prescription from the Ebers Papyrus suggests a suppositorylike preparation which would be medicating as well as supportive:

For dislocation in the hinder part, myrrh, frankincense, rushnut from the garden, *nhtt*‡

---

* Sigerist, H.: A History of Medicine. vol. 1, New York, Oxford University Press, 1955.
† An extensive list of individual drugs is presented by Sigerist.
‡ Possibly a fig or bud of the sycamore.

from the shore, celery, coriander, oil, salt, are boiled together, applied in seed wool and put in the hinder part.

Awareness existed of the discomfort which cold liquids can produce, a fact which is indicated by the number of times indications are given that preparations should be eaten or drunk "warm" or at an "agreeable warmth." Most preparations were administered for four days, presumably because of some magical significance associated with the number 4.

For obvious reasons, the development of pharmaceuticals has been dependent partially on the availability of suitable tools for the apothecary's art. Egyptian pharmacists were well prepared to carry out the simple procedures required, since they possessed mortars of stone and wood and containers of pottery or glass.

Greco-Roman Period. By the time of the Greek period (ca. 600 B.C.) the art of pharmacy was practiced by groups of specialists. There was the *pharmacopolos* who sold drugs in public places, the *rhizotomos* who collected roots and herbs and expressed juices for medicinal purposes and the *pharmacopoios,* who was a maker of remedies. Greek apothecaries used vessels of clay, alabaster and lead to contain solid substances and of silver, glass, horn or nonporous earthenware for liquids.

The Greeks contributed little that was new in terms of dosage forms, although they greatly increased the breadth of man's knowledge in regard to the value of known drugs. This they did as a result of their critical evaluation of cause and effect, which itself was made possible by the relative freedom of natural "sciences" from supernatural domination. The most notable of such observers was Hippocrates, who described nearly 400 simples and a large number of preparations. Hippocrates made use of those dosage forms which by then were well established: poultices and fomentations, ointments and cerates, oils, collyria, lohochs, pills and troches, inhalations, potions and enemas. One of the notable preparations used by Hippocrates—and, perhaps originated by him—was *Oxymel of Squill* (from

the Greek *oxys,* sharp and *mel,* honey). This preparation consists of an extract of squill containing vinegar and honey and has been used as an expectorant until modern times. The *N.F. X* (last official in 1959) recognized Vinegar of Squill and directed its use in preparing Syrup of Squill.

Serapion of Alexander (ca. 150 B.C.) selected the most revolting and unpleasant drugs then in use and passed them on for use by later generations. His influence gave rise to the long-existent feeling in European medicine that the value of drugs could be measured in terms of their disagreeable nature. By way of contrast, the Arabian school of medicine produced a number of pleasant-tasting products which will be described later. It was not until the latter half of the 18th century that Western concepts were changed sufficiently to permit the general acceptance of agreeably flavored medications.

The reader must bear in mind that the interval of time during which Greek authority prevailed in medicine extended for approximately 600 years and that unprecedented advances took place during the interval. Therefore, it should not be surprising that some comparatively simple concepts which existed at the beginning of the period became complicated with the passage of time. So it was with pharmaceuticals. Medicines as used by Hippocrates were simple admixtures; however, before the Greek period had drawn to a close, pharmaceuticals containing large numbers of ingredients were commonplace. An example of this may be followed in the history of *Confectio Mithridates,* which has been known variously as a confection or a theriac. The term *theriac* was first used by Nicander of Colophon, the celebrated physician and poet c.125 B.C., who wrote two volumes in verse on the subject of antidotes to poisons. One work dealt with *theriaca,* preparations used in the treatment of bites by venomous serpents and animals; the other dealt with *alexipharmacs,* or antidotes to poisons which have been swallowed. For a time, the two types of preparations were treated as distinct classes; however, in time, only the theriacs survived, and they were regarded as general antidotes or panaceas to all disease. Since these often contained honey or sweet fruits, they frequently were classified as *confections*. Mithridates VI Eupator (132–63 B.C.), King of Pontus, lived in constant fear of poisoning and did much experimentation with possible antidotes. During his lifetime, it was believed that he had discovered an antidote to poisons, and Pompey, finding such a formula in his papers, published it with the claim that it had such powers. The formula was called *Confectio Mithridates*. The recipe is said to have called for 20 leaves of rue, a pinch of salt, 2 nuts and 2 dried figs.

Andromaches, physician to Nero, elaborated on the formula and called his preparation a theriac. Among the ingredients that he added was viper's flesh, which was supposed to have a magical effect in the prevention of poisoning, particularly as related to the bite of serpents. This concept (which obviously is a manifestation of a much earlier concept of the healing power of serpents) became so firmly entrenched that viper's flesh was included as an ingredient of most theriacs for some nineteen centuries. During the Greco-Roman period the formulas progressed from the simple formula of Nicander to complex mixtures containing as many as 50 or 60 ingredients. These usually were called confections or electuaries.

Wooton[30] indicates that the most common forms of medicine used by Greek pharmacists were confections or electuaries. The former were mixtures of powders with fruits or honey and were made by triturating the ingredients together in a mortar until a soft mass was formed. The mass was stored in pots or jars and removed with a spatula when needed. These most often were administered by forming a portion of the mass into a small round ball. The Greeks called these small portions *katapotia,* meaning "things to be swallowed," although at some point the word *pilula* came into use, for Pliny mentions the word *pilula* in referring to a small globular form of medication. The term *pill* eventually became predominant for this particular form of medication.

The *electuary* was a somewhat thinner form of confection which was consumed by licking from a spoon or other implement. In later years it was commonly smeared on a piece of wood or a licorice root. The word

electuary is a corruption of the Greek *ekleikton,* meaning "something to be licked." With the passage of centuries, the terms electuary, confection, and theriac were used more or less interchangeably, much to the dismay of such commentators as Moses Charas[3] of the 17th century (*see* p. 20). The effect of such preparations on the proliferation of formulas and ingredients (polypharmacy) can scarcely be exaggerated.

The writings of Cornelius Celsus (ca. 25 to 50 B.C.) give considerable information regarding the practice of pharmacy by the Romans. Among the new preparations that he mentions are cataplasms (which he called *malagma*) and troches. Cataplasms were made by boiling flour in water to make a stiff paste which then was admixed with melted gums or wax. More recently cataplasms have been prepared by rubbing together glycerin and a dry powder (such as kaloin) to make a very firm mixture. Cataplasm of Kaolin was last official in *N.F. IX.* Troches (from the Greek *trochos,* wheel) were molded and dried forms of medication made by rubbing dry ingredients together, moistening with wine or vinegar to make a mass, molding into the desired shape (usually flat and round) and drying until firm. The term *pastilla* was applied to these preparations by the Romans. Although these techniques were undoubtedly refined by Roman apothecaries, it is evident that the dosage form does not differ in any essential way from some forms that were available in earlier periods. It is notable that both words, troche and pastille, have modern pharmaceutical usage. Other preparations described by Celsus are vaginal suppositories, catapotia, conserves, collyria and cerates.

The art of pharmacy was given great impetus by Claudius Galen (ca. 131–201 A.D.), who strove to improve dosage forms and served not only as a compiler of formulas but also as a classifier and an inventor of dosage forms. He introduced a number of prescriptions and medical concepts which dominated European medicine and pharmacy for centuries. It will be impossible in this brief history to do more than mention some of his most significant or lasting contributions. Certainly, among these must be mentioned the invention of "cold cream," an ointment prepared from borax and animal fat, which was known as *unguentum* or *ceratum refrigerans.*

The use of clays was encouraged by Galen, both in internal preparations (theriacs) and in external preparations such as poultices. These natural earths had been in use among the Greeks, and the most famous was *terra sigillata* from the island of Lemnos. This was a yellow or yellowish-red clay that was later mined under monopoly of the Sultan of Turkey and was believed to protect the user against poisons. Galen therefore made much of its potential value in protecting against poisons. The clay was marketed in small molded blocks bearing the impress of the Sultan's seal, thus indicating its authenticity. The use of such a seal is believed to represent one of the earliest examples of a trademark.

Galen made use of diachylon plaster and ensured its popularity for centuries to come, although his diachylon was not the "lead plaster" of later centuries but a mixture of vegetable juices with lead acetate and vegetable oil.

Among the specific types of preparations mentioned by Galen are fomentations, poultices, gargles, pessaries, catapotias (katapotias), ointments, oils, cerates, collyria, looches (or lohochs), tablets and inhalations. Galen is believed to have been the first to mention the use of rectal suppositories made with soap.* A collyrium used in Galen's time and called "Attalian" contained castor, aloes, saffron, myrrh, lycium, prepared cadmia, antimony and acacia juice. Only the saffron and acacia have been associated with collyria in recent times. Saffron is still used as a coloring matter in some commercial eye drops. It is listed as an ingredient of Yellow Astringent Eye Wash, which appeared in the Pharmaceutical Recipe Book of 1936.[20]

Mineral drugs were rejected by Galen, a fact which for several centuries inhibited investigation of the medicinal value of inorganic substances.

The Greco-Roman period taken as a whole added little in the way of original dosage forms; however, the preparation of dosage forms emerged as a distinct art which seemed to warrant attention for its own sake. In Europe these advances were submerged by the period commonly referred to as "the dark ages," but they quickly sprang to life in that culture which we refer to as "Arabian."

Arabian Period. During the Middle Ages, the people of the Near East, under the Arabian culture, made significant progress in the science of pharmacy. This resulted from their particular interest in health, a fervent interest in science of mathematics (which led them to offer protective custody to captured or refugee scholars from various nations) and their genius for organization. Wooton[30] credits the Arabians with having raised pharmacy to its proper dignity, an accomplishment which resulted largely from their recognition of pharmacy as a distinct area of practice. The evolution by them of elaborate procedures for the preparation of dosage forms encouraged this distinction.

Alchemy, which attracted the attention of many Arabian physicians and pharmacists, produced several advances which ultimately had significant effect on the nature of dosage forms. Whereas Greek and Roman medicine had dealt almost exclusively with vegetable drugs, chemical discoveries made by the alchemists led to a new interest in the use of inorganic substances in medicine. Specifically introduced by Arabian physicians and pharmacists after production by Arabian alchemists were corrosive sublimate, red precipitate and silver nitrate. Ointment of mercury was first used by the physician Rhazes (865–925) in the treatment of skin diseases, and this early use led to its later adoption by Paracelsus in the treatment of syphilis.

Perhaps the greatest contribution of Arabian pharmacists was the refinement of dosage forms and an emphasis on elegance in their preparation. Previously, little attention had been given to the attractiveness or the acceptability of pharmaceuticals. As a matter of fact, it was generally accepted that medicines were by nature disagreeable. The Arabians developed the first pleasantly flavored preparations in the form of juleps and syrups. The word *julep* was applied by the Arabians to clear, sweetened liquids.* It is said to have been derived from the Persian *gul* (rose) and *ap* (water). Syrup is a more recent form of the Arabic *sharab* or *shureb*. Sugar, which the Arabians obtained from India, was often used in the making of these preparations. In his Minhâj al-dukkân, Kôhên al Attâr (1259) lists 156 recipes for syrups.[18]

A similar type of preparation introduced during the period was the *conserve*. This was made by covering fresh drugs with a layer of sugar and permitting them to stand until a soft mass was produced. Later these were made by beating fresh vegetable substances with sugar until the whole was converted to a uniform soft mass. Unlike the confections, which were made with honey, conserves usually became hardened due to evaporation of water.

Rhazes placed great emphasis on the determination of the most effective as well as the most acceptable methods of administering drugs. He favored pills because of the ease with which they may be taken. He is said also to have made the first mention of a distilled liquor similar to brandy or arrack. Mesuë (777–857) condemned the use of harsh cathartics and suggested the use of mild laxatives, such as senna, cassia fistula, tamarind and jujube. These drugs were used in preparing electuaries which, because of their mildness, were called *lenitive* electuaries. Various preparations known as Lenitive Confection and containing senna as a major ingredient remained in use as late as the 19th century.

The Persian Avicenna (980–1037) originated the concept of silvering and gilding pills. While this originally was done in the belief that it would improve effectiveness, in time it was utilized purely for esthetic purposes.

In appraising the effect of the Arabian period on the development of European pharmacology in later years, we must not overlook developments in the Western caliphate. In Spain, particularly, authorities such as Albucasis (d. 1013) were developing a type of medical practice which leaned heavily on surgery and alchemy. The writings of these authorities unquestionably assisted in bringing about the ultimate acceptance of chemical substances into European pharmacy.

The establishment of hospitals, as originated by the Arabians, furthered the development of pharmacy as a field of specialization, because preparation of a large volume of pharmaceuticals necessitated the attention of persons who could devote their full time to this function. The following excerpt from the foundation deed of the Mûristân (hospital) of the Mameluke sultan, Qualâûn, in Cairo (from Meyerhof[18]) demonstrates not only the extent to which pharmacy had become a distinct practice but also the recognition which was given to the need for pleasant beverages. It also lists some of the preparations in common use:

The director of the foundation is to defray the expenses for the sugar and the fruit for electuaries and refreshing drinks, as well as for the yeast that is required for the preparation of beverages, furthermore for all other medicaments, herbs, and salves, eye medicines, powders, balsams, theriacs, pastilles, beverages, and other things that the hospital needs. Each medicament should be prepared in good time and stored in special containers. The director is to replace the medicaments that have been handed out from the income of the foundation. Each patient is to receive only the requisite quantity of medicine and no more . . . .†

According to Meyerhof, these articles were prepared between the years of 1285 and 1287.

Besides being practiced in the hospital, pharmacy was usually practiced in small shops called *saidanani* or *saidalani* (the latter term still denotes a qualified pharmacist in Arabia). Legal recognition of the pharmacist and his practice came about near the end of the Arabian period of influence (ca. 1240) through the well-known

---

* Although no longer used in pharmacy, the term julep has been used in this country to describe a sweetened, flavored alcoholic beverage (as a mint julep).

† Meyerhof, M.: Pharmacology during the Golden Age of Arabian medicine. Ciba Symp., *6:* 1866, 1944.

edict of Frederick II of Sicily. In summarizing the effects of the Arabian period, Stubb and Bleigh[24] state: "With the Arabs began the real craft of the apothecaries."

Medieval Pharmacy. In Medieval Europe neither pharmacy nor medicine made appreciable progress. Pharmacy existed primarily in the monasteries, where gardens of medicinal herbs were cultivated and medical advice was freely dispensed by the monks, although members of the official orders were prohibited from practicing medicine. It was during this period that many of our common plant and drug names came into use, for example, rosemary, St. John's-wort, and others. The influence of herbs introduced through the monastery gardens may still be found in folk medicine and in the assortment of herbs used in the kitchens of the Western world. The religious fervor of the period had its influence on the preparations and the techniques which were used. This is well exemplified by the preparation *Ointment of the Twelve Apostles,* which not only contained 12 ingredients but was prepared to the accompaniment of a recitation of prayers or psalms. It is believed that the incantations were used as a means of measuring the appropriate time of trituration for each combination of ingredients.

The record of medieval pharmacy comes to us largely through a number of publications called herbals or "leech books," which are mostly of unknown authorship. Examples are the *Book of the Bald,* which was circulated during the 9th and the 10th centuries, the *Herbarum Apuleii Platonici,* known in a Saxon edition of the 10th century, and the *Lacnunga* of similar date. Collectively, these books indicate a heavy reliance on vegetable drugs, often administered in simple form such as infusions or decoctions, and an almost complete absence of rationale in the preparation or administration of dosage forms. The *Hortus Sanitatus,* published in Strasburg about 1507, is perhaps the best known of all herbals because it was the first to be set in type after the invention of printing.

The conditions that existed in Europe from the fall of Rome until the 12th cen-

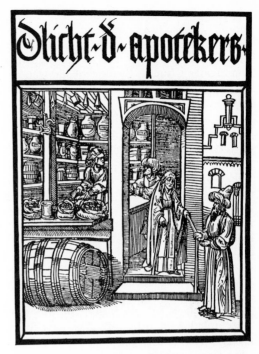

FIG. 1-2. "Light of the Pharmacist," the title of this woodcut, implied the illumination provided by learning when, later, it was used to ornament the 1515 edition of Quiricus de Augustis' *Lumen Apothecariorum,* a kind of pharmaceutical textbook that may be considered as one of the earliest precursors of *American Pharmacy.* (From the American Institute of the History of Pharmacy)

tury were not conducive to the development of an art as elaborate as the preparation of dosage forms, and no new forms can be attributed to this period. However, it would appear that some additions were made to the list of vegetable drugs in common use; furthermore, various formulations which were popularized through the leech books may be found in authoritative medical texts and pharmacopoeias of later centuries.

A great deal of progress was made by European pharmacists during the 13th and 14th centuries, resulting in developments that influenced dosage forms. This is the period during which the knowledge of the ancients began to be rediscovered by Europeans, through the return of crusaders from Arabian countries. It was also the period when great plagues swept over Europe, calling forth the concerted effort of pharmacists and physicians. The practice of alchemy was rampant and brought with it its share of valuable discoveries as well as the perpetration of many frauds. Significant innovations resulted from the widespread application of distillation.

The alchemists literally distilled "everything in sight" and by this means produced the first alcohol. This product is described in the writings of both Albertus Magnus (1193–1280), who called it *aqua ardens,* and Raymond Lully (1235–1315) , who called it both *aqua vitae* and *aqua ardens.** Lully discovered the art of concentrating alcohol by both distillation and dehydration and was the first to use the solvent in the extraction of drugs, thereby producing the type of solutions we know as tinctures. A contemporary, Arnold of Villanova, used alcohol (which he called *spirit of wine*) in the extraction of drugs. It may have been his use which caused the word *spirit* eventually to be associated with alcoholic preparations, even though for several centuries the title was attached to preparations rather indiscriminately. Usually, but not always, these were volatile products obtained by distillation.

The introduction of concentrated alcohol as a menstruum for the extraction of drugs marks one of the turning points in the development of dosage forms. From this application derived the classes of preparations known as fluidextracts, extracts, and resins. Further refinement of the extraction process revealed the alkaloids and other plant principles of importance. One has only to consider the number of preparations in use today that contain some proportion of al-

cohol or depend on an alcoholic extraction for their potency to recognize the impact that the discovery of alcohol has had on the nature of dosage forms.

A demonstration of the bridge between Arabian pharmacy and pharmacy as it developed in Europe following the Crusades is found in the writings of Mesuë Junior. For a long time these manuscripts were attributed to an Arabian authority who was believed to have lived during the 10th century. More recently it has been concluded that the manuscripts were prepared by an Italian writer of the 13th century who drew on Arabian Byzantine authors for his formulas. Compilations such as the 15th century manuscripts represented in Figure 1-3 had great influence upon the pharmacopoeias published in Europe during the same period.

The invention of printing made possible the wide distribution of books of formulas, thus providing an opportunity for pharmacists in various parts of the world to exchange information. Furthermore, a means was presented for standardization of products through the publication of formulas adopted by authoritative groups. One of the earliest of these is the *Dispensatorium* of Val-

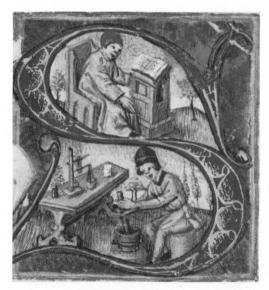

FIG. 1-3.   Miniature from a 15th century manuscript of the Antidotary attributed to Johannes Mesuë, Jr. (From the American Institute of the History of Pharmacy)

---

* It is difficult to determine exactly when distilled beverages were first known and used. The process of distillation was known to the ancients; however, there is no indication that it was used to produce an alcoholic beverage. There are some indications that the Arabs may have produced a spirit from wine, and the inhabitants of Ireland used a product called "uisgea-beatha" (from which the word whiskey derives) as early as the 12th century. According to *A History of Technology,* Clarendon Press, Oxford, 1957, alcohol was probably produced in Italy about 1100 A.D. at the University of Salerno. The first recorded isolation of pure alcohol appears to be as recorded above.

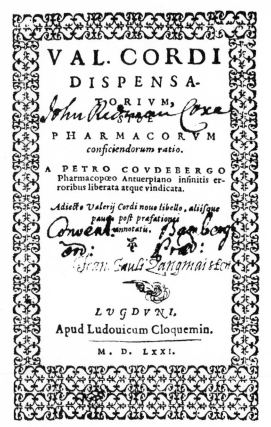

VAL. CORDI
DISPENSA-
TORIVM,
PHARMACORVM
conficiendorum ratio.

A PETRO COVDEBERGO
Pharmacopœo Antuerpiano infinitis er-
roribus liberata atque vindicata.

Adiecto Valerij Cordi nouo libello, aliisque
paucis post prefationes
annotatu.

LVGDVNI,
Apud Ludouicum Cloquemin.
M. D. LXXI.

FIG. 1-4. Title page of the Dispensatory of Valerius Cordus, as revised and annotated by Petro Couderbergo in Lugdunum (Lyons) in 1571. This copy, which is in the Library of Temple University, bears the signature of John Redman Coxe.

erius Cordus, which was officially adopted by the City of Nuremberg in 1546.* Some attention is given here to the contents of this book because Cordus had made a special study of formularies in use in European cities; therefore, his compilation probably represents a good cross section of dosage forms used at that time. The list of preparations is as follows: Aromatic confections, opiate confections, syrups (including oxysaccharins and juleps), condita (jellies), conserves, robs, lohochs, lenitives and solu-

tions, pills, troches, oils, ointments, cerates, plasters and miscellaneous simple preparations. The 48 confections are often exceedingly complex. One formula lists 82 ingredients, some of which are already compounded. The 25 Opiate Confections usually contain opium in some form, although in a few instances the term appears to be loosely applied. *Robs* consisted of fruit juices thickened by evaporation and mixed with honey or sugar. *Lohoch* is another name for a type of thickened preparation intended to be licked from a spoon. These are known also as *leeches* and *linctuses*.

In general, procedures described by Cordus differ little from those used by the Greeks and the Romans, except for the process of distillation which is directed for the preparation of some of the oils and represents a technique little used in pharmacy until the Arabian period.

The Arabian influence is quite evident in the formulas listed in the Dispensatory. Preparations such as robs, syrups, and juleps are clearly Arabic in origin. The chapter titled Syrups includes a total of 60 formulas. Close examination of the prescriptions reveals a number of drugs introduced first into Arabian pharmacology through sources in India and China. Occurring in the titles of preparations are such names as Rhazes, Mesuë, Avicenna and Nicolaus, as well as the older names Galen, Andromachus and Damocrates. The arrangement of sections in the book reflects dependence on the pattern established by Persian or Arabian authors.

The Dispensatory of Valerius Cordus served as the basis for a number of pharmacopeias published in the various cities of Europe in succeeding years.

The great medical iconoclast of the 15th century, Paracelsus (1493–1541), made dramatic suggestions which were contrary to all accepted medical and pharmaceutical authority of his time and ultimately led to significant changes in the nature of dosage forms. One of these was a sweeping condemnation of polypharmacy. It was Paracelsus' contention that the process of disease would yield most easily to a single specific drug or a combination of a few drugs. He also suggested the possibility of extracting active components from drugs, a concept

* The first pharmacopoeia to be adopted by an organized group was the *Nuovo Receptario* adopted by the guild of physicians and pharmacists of the City of Florence in 1498; however, Sonnedecker acknowledges the Nuremberg dispensatory as the first to have governmental sanction and support.[22]

which came to fruition with the isolation of morphine from opium some three centuries later. He restored the internal use of inorganic chemicals to a position of respectability among European physicians. Paracelsus' promotion of iatrochemistry (chemistry of healing) was one of the early movements that laid the foundations for the modern science of medicinal chemistry. Among the dosage forms popularized by Paracelsus were tinctures and extracts. Among the drugs he helped to popularize were opium (used in a preparation that he called laudanum) and mercury.*

Modern Pharmacy. Modern pharmacy as we know it began largely during the 17th and 18th centuries. During this period many new drugs were introduced as well as a number of preparations still in common use or only recently abandoned. Among the chemicals introduced were calomel, Glauber's salt, Rochelle salt, ammonium chloride and carbonate, magnesia, potassium acetate, phosphorus, boric acid and milk sugar. Some of the newly introduced vegetables drugs were Peru balsam, tolu balsam, cinchona, coca, ipecac, tea, coffee, chocolate and tobacco. New preparations included the tinctures of benzoin and tolu, Gregory's powder (compound licorice powder), infusion of digitalis, Black Draught (infusion of senna), Godfrey's cordial (compound tincture of senna), and paregoric (camphorated tincture of opium). The discovery of the fixed oil from cocoa beans about 1700 went practically unnoticed; however, this substance was destined to be recognized by Antoine Baumé late in the 18th century as a suppository base and to serve for at least a century as the most popular choice for this purpose.

During the 17th century the first patents were issued for specific combinations of drugs. These patents were issued under the English Statute of Monopolies of 1624 and gave rise to a practice now often followed by the inventors of therapeutic agents or devices, that is, the establishment of proprietary claim under patent laws which have almost universal acceptance. The first medicinal patent was for Epsom salts in 1698.[22]

Many pharmacopeias were published during the 17th century, and this movement resulted in a general standardization of formulations. The one destined to have the greatest influence on American national standards was the *Pharmacopoeia Londonensis,* first published in 1618.† The contents of the London Pharmacopoeia were as follows: 213 distilled waters (178 simple, 35 compound), 151 oils, 115 candies and conserves, 90 syrups, 58 electuaries, 53 ointments, 51 plasters and cerates, 45 lozenges, 43 powders or species, 36 pills, 18 mels and oxymels, 18 juices and linctuses, 10 medicated vinegars, 8 decoctions, 3 medicated wines, 1 vulnery potion, 17 chemicals.

The influence of the alchemist on dosage forms is immediately obvious from the list of products prepared by distillation. These are not limited to the 213 waters but also include a number of oils. That polypharmacy was still rampant is indicated by the recipe for a preparation titled *Antidotus magnus Mattiole.* The formula calls for 130 ingredients, some of which already contain a number of ingredients. The list of chemicals (17 in all) is small by comparison with a modern pharmacopeia; however, it represents a trend toward the acceptance of chemicals as therapeutic agents. Although no tinctures appear in the list, such preparations were coming into considerable use, and the revision of 1650 listed 7 such preparations.

Pill tiles made their first appearance during the 17th century, and the pill cutter and divider appeared about a century later. Introduction of these tools gives evidence that this form of medication was extensively used during the period.

The introduction and the widespread sale of proprietary remedies during the 18th century created a new demand for small bottles. Many of these were blown in special

---

* Any attempt to summarize the total contribution of Paracelsus must fail because his influence was exerted in so many directions. The reader is urged to consult such references as Stillman, J. M.: *Paracelsus.* Chicago, 1920, or Pachter, H. M.: Paracelsus: Magic into Science. N. Y., Abelard, 1951.

† A facsimile reproduction of the Pharmacopoeia with comments was published by Urdang through the sponsorship of the State Historical Society of Wisconsin, 1944.

Table 1-1

Preparation	Proprietary Name	Earliest Recognition
Compound Tincture of Gentian	Stoughton's Great Cordial Elixir	Patented, 1712
Compound Tincture of Lavender	Palsy Drops	P. L. 1721
Compound Tincture of Opium and Gambir	Bateman's Pectoral Drops	Introduced 1726
Compound Tincture of Benzoin	Traumatic Balsam	P. L. 1746
Compound Ticture of Cinchona	Huxham's Tincture	P. L. 1788
Compound Tincture of Senna	Duffy's Elixir	Introduced ca. 1810

shapes for purposes of enhancing the salability of the medication. Some of these products became common household remedies and their sale unquestionably encouraged the development of the modern prescription bottle. In this connection, it must be recognized that throughout earlier history medications usually had been dispensed in single dose units. It was common practice for the pharmacist to deliver each dose to the patient's home or for the patient to obtain each dose from the pharmacy as needed. This practice largely persisted until the middle of the 19th century, by which time the advantage of prescribing multiple doses for an illness had become generally recognized. Flat prescription bottles of the type used today did not come into common use until the beginning of the 19th century.

It is not possible to list here all of the new preparations introduced by pharmacists during the 17th and the 18th centuries, many of which will be mentioned in the historical sections of chapters to follow. It will be sufficient at this point to indicate the general nature of the newer forms.

As previously noted, tinctures were coming into use. These were made by the infusion of vegetable drugs with alcohol or by solution of chemical substances in alcohol or an alcoholic extract of vegetable drugs. Many of these came into use as proprietary forms and were adopted later by pharmacopeias, as may be seen from the list in Table 1-1.

All of these preparations have been recognized at some time by the *United States Pharmacopeia,* with the exception of Compound Tincture of Opium and Gambir (which was recognized by the First Edition of the *National Formulary*) and Compound

Tincture of Senna. The latter was recognized by several editions of the British Pharmacopoeia. Compound Tincture of Benzoin is still listed in the *U.S.P.,* while Compound Tincture of Gentian survived through the *National Formulary,* Eleventh Edition.

Not all preparations introduced during the period depended on a base of alcohol, as the following examples demonstrate. Compound Decoction of Sarsaparilla was introduced through the P.L. of 1788, and Infusion of Digitalis came into use through the writings of Withering in 1785. Both of these were aqueous preparations. Vinegar of Opium was introduced as a proprietary known as Black Drop. As given by Wootton[30] the original formula contained no vinegar, but this is present in the recipes which became official in the Edinburgh and other pharmacopeias. Fowler's Drops, an aqueous solution of arsenic, was introduced in 1786 and was recognized as recently as the *N.F. XI* under the title Solution of Potassium Arsenite. Spirit of Mindererus, a solution of ammonium acetate, was popularized early in the 18th century.

Aromatic Ammonia Spirit was introduced by the P.L. of 1711 under the title Spiritus Sal Volatilis Oleosus. This preparation is still officially recognized under its modern name and is widely used as a home remedy.

While these preparations are mostly liquid in form and, therefore, not radically different from some earlier dosage forms, they do reflect three trends that eventually became predominant in liquid dosage forms and may be enumerated as (1) greatly simplified formulas, (2) increasing use of chemicals (even in combination with vegetable extracts) and (3) increased emphasis on alcohol as a solvent.

With the 19th century a new spirit of science and inventiveness was ushered in. Chemistry had been established as a scientific discipline, and its followers were beginning to make significant contributions. The pioneering work of Lavoisier had revealed the relationship of hydrogen and oxygen in the composition of water and had overthrown the fallacious phlogiston theory. In 1804 Serturner isolated morphine from opium, although he did not publish his results until 1815. This was quickly followed by the isolation of emetine in 1817, strychnine in 1818 and quinine in 1819. Such discoveries were destined to alter concepts of materia medica and to affect greatly the nature of dosage forms. The interest of pharmacists began to shift from crude drugs to their active components, and the polypharmacal preparations of an earlier day gave way to simple extractives or products formed through chemical synthesis. One senses a development of a therapeutic rationale in many of the preparations which were introduced—for example, the recommendation of iron salts for anemia, bitters for improvement of appetite, freshly prepared sulfur ointment in the treatment of scabies, etc. Empiricism was still the guiding force in most therapy, as it is in a great many instances today.

The influence that a single drug may have on the nature of dosage forms may be seen in the influence of the drug morphine on the development of hypodermic medication. It is said that Sir Christopher Wren developed a technique for making intravenous injections while serving as professor of anatomy at Oxford[16]; however, the use of modern methods began with Alexander Wood of Edinburgh and Francis Rynd of Dublin. Both men employed solutions of morphine in their experiments, Rynd using trocar and cannula and Wood a type of syringe made for him by a Mr. Ferguson of London in 1853. Wood's results were published in 1855 and the method quickly came into popular use. Morphine was the drug administered by this method most frequently for several years, because it had been discovered that morphine had greater effectiveness when given by this means. Demonstration of the biologic role of bac-

teria and consequent recognition of the need for a container suitable for maintaining sterility led to the invention of the ampul by Limousin in 1886. Through these two discoveries, the modern period of injectable medicine had its beginning.*

Percolation came into pharmaceutical use in 1825 as a result of application by the Boullays (father and son) of a procedure which had been introduced in Paris for the preparation of coffee.[6] The process was made official by the French *Codex* of 1837, the *Edinburgh Pharmacopoeia* of 1838 and the *United States Pharmacopoeia* of 1842. The process of percolation is primarily significant because it simplified the process of drug extraction and had much to do with the development of preparations known as fluidextracts. The last mentioned term was first used by Ellis in 1835,[10] and it gradually came into common use through its application by Procter and others to liquid alcoholic or hydroalcoholic extracts of vegetable drugs. The phenomenal rise and fall of fluidextracts is revealed in the following summary. They were first recognized by the Pharmacopoeia of 1850, which included 7 such concentrates. In the Pharmacopoeia of 1890 the number officially recognized had risen to 88. The present pharmacopeia (1970) recognizes only two. A further discussion of these preparations may be found in Chapter 5.

Fluidglycerates may be mentioned appropriately here, even though they were introduced a century later. First suggested by Beringer[1] in 1908, they resemble fluidextracts except that they are made by extracting drugs with a menstruum of glycerin and water instead of alcohol. They have never found wide acceptance, even though theoretically glycerin solutions are more stable than are solutions made with alcohol.

Application of ether to the extraction of drugs led to the introduction of the oleoresins early in the century. The word oleoresin was first used by Peschier in 1828.

The use of heavy machinery in pharmacy began with drug milling as carried out by

---

* An excellent review of the development of hypodermic medication has been prepared by P. H. Van Itallie. See Pulse of Pharmacy, *19*:3–16, 1965.

of a simple cylinder or bottom die into which was fitted a compression tool. Powders were forced into tablet shape by striking the compression tool with a mallet (see Fig. 1-6). By the end of the century, greatly improved machines were available, and the tablet was rapidly gaining in acceptance both in the United States and in Europe.

Tablet triturates were introduced in 1878 by Dr. R. M. Fuller of New York. While originally intended as a palatable and convenient dosage form for the administration of small doses of potent drugs by mouth, they served the purposes of the homeopath quite well and unquestionably helped to further the use of homeopathic doses. The method of preparation is more expensive than the compression procedure and has not been able to compete except as a means of preparing hypodermic tablets.

Additional examples of mechanical processes introduced to pharmacy during the 19th century are the following:

1. The machine-spreading of plasters
2. The use of metal moulds for the shaping of suppositories
3. Preparation of pills by machine
4. Manufacture and filling of capsules by machine.

Plasters are among the most ancient of pharmaceuticals, and Galen developed a number of practical formulas and procedures for their preparation which endured for centuries. The spreading of the plaster mass always presented a difficult problem for the pharmacist, since it was necessary to keep the mass warm in order for it to be malleable. Plaster irons of numerous types were invented for this purpose during the 19th century. Mather of England patented in 1852 a method of spreading plasters on leather by the use of heated rollers. This made it possible to produce plasters which were thinner and more uniform. Two years later Tomlinson patented a plaster that consisted of a plain woven material coated on one side with a waterproofing material. This procedure, coupled with the use of gum rubber, completed the requirements for the modern adhesive plaster—the only preparation of this group with significant use today, except for the common corn plaster which

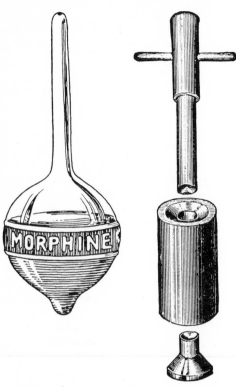

(*Left*). FIG. 1-5.   Ampul as first described by Limousin. This illustration is redrawn from his article appearing in Arch. de Pharmacie, 1886. (From Wyeth Laboratories, Philadelphia)

(*Right*). FIG. 1-6.   Early tablet machine. This one, attributed to Joseph Remington, is somewhat more elaborate than earlier machines, since the lower punch may be removed from the base of the compression cylinder to permit easy removal of the finished tablet.

Hagner of Philadelphia in 1841. It may have been the consequent availability of a ready supply of finely powdered material which led Dunton of Philadelphia to begin the compression of tablets during the 1860's. Invention of the compressed tablet machine is credited to William Brockedon of England in 1843; however, acceptance of the dosage form in England must be credited largely to the American pharmacists S. M. Burroughs and Henry Wellcome. In the United States the firms of John Wyeth and Brother of Philadelphia and Sharp and Dohme of Baltimore pioneered the development. The earliest tablet machines consisted

is recognized by the *U.S.P. XVIII* as Salicylic Acid Plaster.

Throughout the ages, suppositories were shaped by hand in much the same manner as pills. Even though Antoine Baumé had described in 1766 the use of a suppository mold into which liquefied cocoa butter could be poured, the value of this procedure did not gain popular recognition until the 19th century. In 1852 Alfred B. Taylor[25] described a method of molding suppositories by pouring a melted mass into paper cones placed in sand in order to "preserve their position." Metal molds consisting of a metal block into which holes had been bored were first made by Bullock and Cranshaw in 1867. During the next decade, a number of such fusion molds were patented. The first compression mold was invented by Heyl in 1879 and was introduced under the name of its assignor as the Archbald mold. The Whitall Tatum machine which is still in use was patented by Charles A. Tatum in 1895.

The invention of these simple and rapid procedures for the preparation of suppositories coupled with the desirable physical properties of coca butter helped to popularize this form of medication and to bring into common use this single unit dosage form.

Mention has been made of the development during the 18th century of a machine with which the pill pipe could be divided into uniform lengths for rolling into pills. During the 19th century various pill machines were invented. These consisted of two sets of corrugated brass plates which were rubbed together over the pill pipe in such a way that the pills were cut into equal lengths and also rounded in a single operation. Such machines were patented by Wirz of Philadelphia in 1867 and Cooper of Philadelphia in 1872. A machine patented by J. C. Ayer and Company in 1867 was said to be capable of producing a "barrel of pills per day." According to Griffenhagen,[13] some 150 patents for pill machines were issued by the United States Patent Office during the period 1857 to 1891. The type of machine used by industry today—capable of producing pills by the hundred thousands per day—came into use at the end of the

century. At this time pills were the most popular individualized dosage form.

Nineteenth century pharmacists were concerned with means for disguising the taste of drugs. From these efforts came the invention of wafers, cachets, konseals and capsules. The first three named represent uses of containers made of rice flour. Wafers were made by folding a dose of drug inside a moistened rice wafer. Both konseals and cachets are molded containers made of rice flour. They differ only in shape and come in two pieces (top and bottom) which are moistened and pressed together after a measured dose of drug has been placed in the bottom half. The finished konseals are of various shapes but resemble two tiny hats pressed together at the brims, while the cachets resemble two tiny bowls joined at the rims (Fig. 1-7). The cachet was invented by Limousin in 1873. These forms have been replaced by the hard gelatin capsule.

Capsules are so well known that they require no description. As first invented by Mather and Dublanc in 1833–34, they were soft gelatin and presented many difficulties. The hard gelatin capsule invented by Murdock in 1848 presented so many advantages that it quickly replaced the other form. In very recent years there has been a revival of interest in the soft gelatin capsule as a result of inventions that made possible a continuous flow operation in which a film of gelatin is molded, or pressed, about a measured dose of powders. A more complete discussion will be found in Chapter 10.

The introduction of elixirs during the latter half of the 19th century was also the result of attempts by pharmacists to disguise the taste of drugs. The American pharmacist

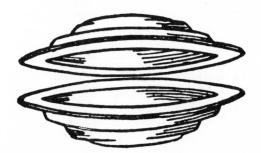

Fig. 1-7.　Cachet.

John Uri Lloyd was primarily responsible for the development of these sweetened, flavored hydroalcoholic preparations which have become so popular in the United States. At the peak of their popularity, the *National Formulary* recognized 61 separate elixirs. The present *National Formulary* recognizes 15 formulas, two of which occur under the single title Iso-Alcoholic Elixir.

The 20th century has seen the introduction of two totally new methods for administering drugs. Both of these may be classified as mists or sprays. The *Hypospray** is a device which administers drugs hypodermically by utilizing a blast of compressed air to force a very fine spray through the skin. Aerosols are applied topically by spraying a propellant-borne mist of drug or solution of drug over an area of skin or mucous membrane. These are described in Chapter 12. The sustained release dosage forms, which are of recent invention, involve novel applications of well-known procedures to provide continuous or controlled release of dosage over a period of time. Thus, their development represents a significant step toward the perfection of the pharmaceutic art (see Chap. 11).

The most significant advancement in dosage forms during this century has been the perfection of single-unit forms. Compressed tablets are produced in great numbers yet with a negligible variance in weight, dose-content, and appearance. Capsules, because of the procedures involved, are slightly less accurate. Details of color, taste, size, shape and characteristic markings are carefully evaluated before a new product is introduced. Every detail of formulation is investigated in order to ensure optimum release of active ingredients. For the first time in history it has been possible to relate biomedical research to the technology of pharmacy, thereby developing a new area of study which is currently referred to as biopharmaceutics or biopharmacy. Through this scientific approach to the design of dosage forms, pharmacy has made a significant contribution to the science (in contrast to the art) of therapeutics. The application

of mechanical devices and quality control procedures has made possible a degree of uniformity of product which, though taken for granted, is a marvel of our age.

The emphasis on products that can be carefully standardized and justified on the basis of reliable scientific data has led to virtual abandonment of several dosage forms in recent decades. While not a completely reliable index, the disappearance of products from both the *United States Pharmacopeia* and the *National Formulary* may be taken as good evidence that a product has declined in use to the point at which it is no longer of great significance. Such a fate has overcome infusions and decoctions. Decoctions were last official in the *U.S.P. XII,* at which time a general procedure was presented for the preparation of these products. The last formula for infusions appeared in the *N.F. IX,* which contained general directions for their extemporaneous production. The last cataplasm to appear in the official books was Cataplasm of Kaolin of the *N.F. X.* These products still enjoy limited use in the form of proprietary products.

STANDARDIZATION OF DOSAGE FORMS

To those familiar with the potency of modern pharmaceuticals, the casual attention given in earlier periods to such matters as standards of strength and accuracy in dosage may be startling. In the historical section it was noted that some early prescriptions make no mention of quantity of ingredients. In later periods, the quantities of ingredients were always specified; however, specific directions regarding dosage were much less common. Where instructions for dosage did occur, they were often quite indefinite. For example, electuaries were commonly prescribed to be taken in a portion "the size of a nut." Pills were frequently directed to be "the size of a pea." Formulas for pill masses were presented with no direction concerning the number of pills to be formed; thus, the pharmacist used his own judgment in deciding on the size of pills to be made.

* Trademark R. P. Scherer Corporation.

A common procedure in the administering of extractive matter from vegetable drugs was to permit the drug to steep overnight in water, beer or wine and to drink the supernatant liquid on the following morning. Obviously, wide variations in the potency of dangerous drugs could lead to fatal consequences under such conditions of use. Yet the extent of knowledge in existence at the time permitted no reliable controls. Pharmacists selected their drugs on the basis of color, odor, appearance and time of collection, and such requirements constituted the only controls.

Accuracy in the preparation of dosage forms was often impossible because of insufficient knowledge of potent ingredients or because the nature of the dosage form prevented accurate formulation. The latter problem is well demonstrated by this translation from the writings of Charas,[3] in which he is discussing opiates, electuaries and confections:

It is very difficult to describe [designate] each one of the proportions exactly, the amount of pulp, powders, and sugars and honey which enter into the composition of opiates or the liquid or solid electuaries. It is not possible to give a general rule for the amount of fluid necessary in order to enclose or incorporate the quality of various medicaments which one is to make by decoction or infusion in order to cook the syrup or the honey because the dose of one or the other may be increased or diminished according to the nature of the medicament, the intent of the physician, the period of illness, the seriousness of it, and the skill of the pharmacist.

Probably their very complexity kept most products from being more toxic. With as many as 100 drugs present in a preparation, the quantity of any one ingredient would not be appreciable, even in a mass the size of a walnut. Nevertheless, accidental poisonings did occur, and at various periods the law has provided punishment for the physician adjudged guilty of administering a toxic dose. One of the thousand and one tales of the Arabian Nights relates an episode in which an unqualified physician is put to death because he made such a mistake.[11]

Frederick II, in his significant code of law

PHARMACOPEE
ROYALE
GALENIQUE
ET
CHYMIQUE.

Par MOYSE CHARAS, Docteur en Medecine, ci-devant Démonstrateur de l'une & de l'autre Pharmacie au Jardin Royal des Plantes.

NOUVELLE EDITION,

Reveüe, corrigée & augmentée par l'Auteur, avec les Formules Latines & Françoises.

A LYON,
Chez ANISSON & POSÜEL.

M. DCCXVII.
AVEC PRIVILEGE DU ROY.

Fig. 1-8. Title page of the *Pharmacopée Royale* of Moses Charas, 1717. (From the Library, Temple University School of Pharmacy)

(1240) which first gave legal definition to the practice of pharmacy, required physicians to swear that they would give information of such fact if an apothecary sold adulterated drugs. Apothecaries were instructed to keep all regular drugs and simples for no longer than 1 year from the date of purchase and to store and use them properly. Frederick's edicts, which were generally adopted throughout Europe, led to the practice of placing the inspection of drugs under the supervision of physicians. An Act of Henry VIII in 1540 instructed the physicians and surgeons of London to appoint a committee of four to "search, view, and see" apothecary wares, drugs and stuffs in their houses. It was common practice by that time for the pharmacists of a city to prepare theriac in a public ceremony under the watchful eyes of the master apothecary and the prominent physicians of the city. After the formation of apothecary guilds, the supervision of the quality of drugs gradually passed to these groups. This gave precedence to the system commonly used in America of placing control of drug standards under boards of pharmacy which enforce requirements established by legislative statute in the respective states.

The standardization of formulas was difficult in earlier periods because of the absence of uniform weights and measures. Adoption of such uniform standards began in Europe during the 13th and the 14th centuries (see Chap. 2).* Although worldwide agreement has not been reached on systems of weights and measures for common use, the metric system has provided a means of transposing values from one common system to another. This system was standardized in 1889.

The publication of pharmacopeias provided a means for the widespread adoption of standard formulas, and this possibility quickly became a reality. The *Nuovo Receptario Compositum* was such a book of standards, published in 1498 and accepted as authoritative by the physicians and the apothecaries of the city of Florence.[28] The issue of 1498 indicates that it was compiled by the "Most Renowned College of the Distinguished Doctors of Art and Medicine" at the request of the "executive officers of the guild of the apothecaries."[28] The *Dispensatorium Pharmacopolarum* of Valerius Cordus (previously mentioned) became a legal authority by action of the Senate of Nuremberg. This body passed an edict directing all pharmacists to prepare their medications in accordance with the formulas as prescribed by Cordus. The *Pharmacopoeia Londonensis* was sponsored by the London College of Physicians, but it derived its authority from an edict of James I which commanded all apothecaries within the "Realme of England" to compound their medicines as set down in the book. It thereby became the first set of standards to prevail at a national level.

By such actions, various formularies were established as authoritative throughout the

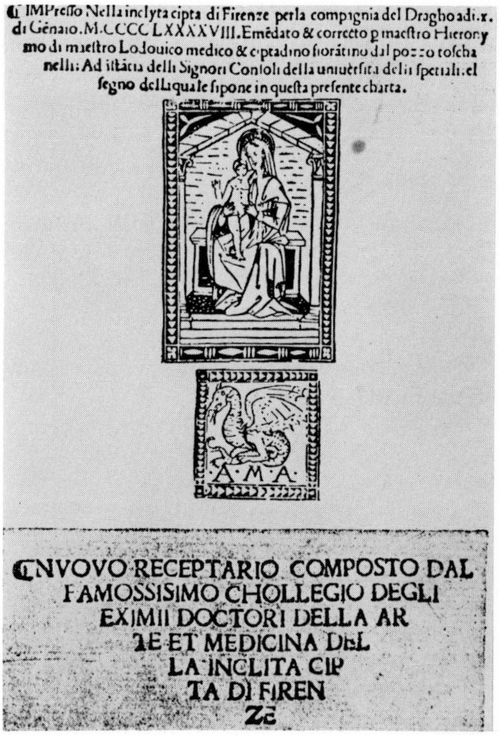

FIG. 1-9. Colophon and title page of *Nuovo Receptario,* Florence, 1498. (From the American Institute of the History of Pharmacy)

municipalities and the countries of Europe. Thus, the custom of establishing legal or quasilegal standards for drugs and pharmaceuticals was well established long before the American colonies carried the seed of a nation yet to be born. It is not surprising, therefore, that the United States had been in existence for less than 50 years when its first book of national standards for pharmaceuticals was adopted.

It was in 1820 that the *United States Pharmacopoeia* made its appearance under the sponsorship of the Medical Societies and Colleges. This writing was stimulated largely by Dr. Lyman Spalding who had begun his efforts for a national convention 3 years earlier. A second revision appeared in 1830 under the same authority. Pharmacists were included for the first time in the revision of 1842 and have participated in each subsequent revision. Pharmacopeial conventions were repeated at 10-year intervals from 1820 to 1950, and revisions were provided

---

* See also an Excellent Review of English Systems by Matthews.[16]

more frequently through authority granted to the Committee on Revision to issue supplements. Since 1950, the *U.S.P.* has been revised at 5-year intervals in recognition of the very rapid progress being made in pharmaceutics and medicine in modern times.

In 1888 the American Pharmaceutical Association prepared a second book of standards for products which enjoyed popular use but were not recognized by the Pharmacopeia. This compilation, called the *National Formulary,* has undergone continuous revision by a committee of the American Pharmaceutical Association.

With the passage of the Federal Food and Drugs Act of 1906, both the *United States Pharmacopeia* and the *National Formulary* became legal standards for all pharmaceuticals exchange in interstate commerce. It is notable that, in adopting the Federal Food and Drugs Act of 1906, the Congress placed its stamp of approval on the propriety of accepting a set of standards developed by pharmacists and physicians for their own guidance. This was in accordance with the practice long used in countries of Europe, and our Supreme Court has upheld the privilege of the Congress to rely on such professional guidance in the establishment of legal requirements.[19]

Because the *U.S.P.* and the *N.F.* establish the national standards for dosage forms, it is appropriate to devote some attention to their coverage. Dr. Lloyd C. Miller, Director of Revision, 1960–70, stated that the Pharmacopeia "offers a list of those drugs, and their accepted dosage forms, which are best known and of proven therapeutic value."[19] It also contains, according to Dr. Miller, information of general value to pharmacists and descriptions of desirable procedures to use in the preparation of certain dosage forms or in the conduct of official assays. The content of individual monographs is described as follows:

The U.S.P. monographs on drugs describe their physical properties, state their solubilities in the solvents common to pharmacy, provide minimum limits on their purity or potency, and state tests and assays for demonstrating compliance with these limits. Information on specific packaging and storage requirements is given which tells the story of the drug's stability.

A statement of the usual dosage is included, as is an indication of the pharmacologic or pharmaceutic category to which the drug belongs.

The *National Formulary* is quite similar to the *United States Pharmacopeia* except that the *National Formulary* has carried customarily more general information for the pharmacist and has included drugs and preparations which were unacceptable to the U.S.P. Committee. The standard for admission to the *National Formulary* has varied from the standard for admission to the *United States Pharmacopeia* primarily in the fact that "extent of use" was the major criterion for inclusion instead of "efficacy" as used by the Pharmacopoeia. This policy was changed with the *N.F. XII* and the criterion of efficacy has now been established for admission to either book of standards.

It should be noted that neither the *U.S.P.* nor the *N.F.* attempts to define in detail the procedures by which dosage forms are to be prepared, except where processes must be standardized in order to ensure uniformity of the product. "Secundum artem" decisions such as choice of equipment, order of mixing, solvent to be used, inert ingredients to be added and other related matters are left to the discretion of the individual pharmacist or manufacturer. It is at this point that the professional training and skill of the pharmacist are relied on, and expected to function, within the limits permitted by official assays. Needless to say, the quality of the ultimate product will be dependent on the reliability and the uniformity of procedures used.

It is important to note that this approach to the manufacture of official dosage forms suffers from two major disadvantages: (1) "Secundum artem" decisions made by the industrial pharmacist, which may indeed lead to an elegant pharmaceutical product, may also dramatically alter the in-vivo performance of that product (see below), and (2) by present official assays and tests it may not be possible, for the most part, to identify batches of the dosage form that will give unsatisfactory performance in vivo or in which there is unacceptable dose-to-dose variation in potency.

Dose-to-dose variation in potency is a quality control problem that has received considerable attention recently. The problem is particularly acute with very potent drugs administered in low doses, such as digoxin.[29] The very first step in the official assay procedure for digoxin tablets requires that 20 tablets be thoroughly ground and mixed in a mortar. If there were sub-potent and super-potent tablets in a given batch due to improper mixing during manufacturing, it is quite possible that a dangerous dose-to-dose variation in the individual tablets would be completely overlooked by the official assay method.

Many official assays are relatively old methods which were developed before some of the present-day sophisticated, sensitive analytical instruments were available. Now that such instrumentation is available, pharmaceutical scientists are actively developing assay methods for single dosage forms of even the lowest dose drugs. No doubt these methods will soon begin to appear in the official compendia, making official dosage forms more uniform and reliable than has previously been possible.

Besides the *United States Pharmacopeia* and the *National Formulary,* which exert major control over the quality and the purity of dosage forms used in the United States, there is a second type of authority which exerts an increasing influence on these products. This is the Food and Drug Administration acting through the authority of the Department of Health, Education and Welfare under powers granted by the Food, Drug and Cosmetic Act of 1938 and its further amendments. It is beyond the scope of this chapter to describe all the ways in which the FDA regulates the development, testing, manufacturing, quality control, marketing, and use of drug products in the United States. But certain of the FDA's activities are directly related to dosage forms; and it is worthwhile reviewing them.

Much of the impetus for improving control over dosage form performance, particularly the ability of the dosage form to release its active ingredient following administration, stems from the 1962 amendment to the drug law which requires, among other things, that drug products be both safe *and* *effective* for the condition(s) for which they are intended. (The previous law required only that drugs be safe.) It is easy to see how this new requirement for effectiveness adds a new dimension to the performance requirements for dosage forms if one considers, for example, an oral tablet of a potentially dangerous drug. If safety were the only consideration, it might be possible to formulate a tablet that would pass completely through a patient's gastrointestinal tract without dissolving. Thus, the tablet would meet the requirement for safety, because little if any drug would reach the patient's systemic circulation where it could do harm. It should be obvious that the tablet would also be ineffective. Such a tablet might even meet compendial standards for assay potency, since all compendial assays require that tablets first be ground in a mortar. The tablet might not meet the *U.S.P.* disintegration specification which requires that tablets disperse in artificial gastric or intestinal fluid into particles small enough to pass through a 10-mesh screen. But, if the tablet were prepared by compressing water-insoluble 20-mesh granules containing the active drug, it might be possible for the tablet to meet all compendial standards and yet be ineffective or show markedly reduced efficacy. Of course, no pharmaceutical formulator would attempt to do such a thing intentionally; but many have come close to achieving these results unintentionally.[8] (See Chapter 11 for a complete discussion of the preparation and evaluation of tablet formulations.)

Thus, the thrust of a significant part of the FDA's regulatory activities and of a large amount of clinical research presently being conducted by the pharmaceutical industry is directed toward proving that the dosage forms of drugs are performing in such a way that the drug is both safe *and* effective in clinical use. Since many widely used drug products have never been tested in this way, and new drug products are continuously appearing on the market, it is likely that these activities will continue at a high level for the foreseeable future.

Testing the performance of drug products in vivo is no simple matter,[7] but the science of biopharmaceutics has progressed to the point where a great number of drug products can be studied quantitatively. As a result, compendial revision committees are giving serious consideration to adopting standards for the in-vivo performance of a number of official dosage forms. As progress is made in biopharmaceutics and, perhaps more important, in developing sensitive quantitative analytical methods for drugs and metabolites in blood and body fluids, it is likely that standards will be adopted for the in-vivo performance of all official dosage forms. Thus, the official compendia are continuously moving toward the ultimate goal of the entire profession of pharmacy: to make the drug product the most reliable factor in the treatment of any patient.

REFERENCES

1. Berlinger, J.: A. Ph. A., *56*:901, 1908.
2. Breasted, J. H.: The Edwin Smith Surgical Papyrus (2 vols.). Univ. Chicago Press, 1930.
3. Charas, Moses: *Pharmacopoeia Regia Galenica,* 1684 (p. 203).
4. Chemist and Druggist, *106*:808, 1927.
5. Civil, Miguel: Ciba Journal, No. 12, pp. 1–7; Revue d'Assyriologie, vol. 54, no. 2, 1960, pp. 5–54.
6. Couch, J. F.: The early history of percolation. Am. J. Pharm., *91*:16, 1919.
7. Dittert, L. W., Cressman, W. A., Kaplan, S., Wagner, J. G., and Riegelman, S.: Guidelines for Biopharmaceutical Studies in Man. Pharm. Assoc., Washington, D. C., 1972.
8. Drug Information Bulletin *3,* January/June 1969. Drug Information Association, Cincinnati, Ohio, 1969.
9. Ebbel, B., The Papyrus Ebers. Copenhagen, Levin & Munksgaard, 1937.
10. Ellis, T. J.: Am. J. Pharm. *6*:274, 1835.
11. Gordon, B. L.: Medieval and Rennaisance Medicine. New York, Philosophical Library, 1959.
12. Greenblatt, R. B.: Search the Scriptures. Philadelphia, J. B. Lippincott, 1963.
13. Griffenhagen, G. B.: Tools of the Apothecary. Am. Pharm. A., 1957.
14. Kramer, S. N.: The Sumerians. Univ. Chicago Press, 1963.
15. Leake, Chauncey: Medical papyri. Ciba Symposium, *1*:311, 1940.
16. Matthews, L. G.: History of Pharmacy in Britain. Edinburgh, Livingston, 1962.
17. Medicine and Pharmacy, an Informal History. Schering Corporation, Bloomfield, N. J., 1955.
18. Meyerhof, M.: Pharmacology during the Golden Age of Arabian medicine. Ciba Symposia, *6*:1857, 1944.
19. Miller, L. C.: The U.S.P. in the practice of pharmacy. J. Am. Pharm. A., [Pract. Ed.], *18*:150, 1957.
20. Pharmaceutical Recipe Book. ed. 2. Am. Pharm. A., Washington, D. C., 1936.
21. Sigerist, H.: A History of Medicine. Vol. 1. New York, Oxford University Press, 1955.
22. Sonnedecker, Glenn: Kremers and Urdang's History of Pharmacy. Philadelphia, J. B. Lippincott, 1963.
23. Stedman's Medical Dictionary. ed. 21. Baltimore, Williams and Wilkins, 1966.
24. Stubb, S. G. Biaksland and Bleigh, E. G.: Sixty Centuries of Health and Physic. London, Sampson, Low, Marston, 1931.
25. Taylor, A. B.: Suppositories. Am. J. Pharm., *24*:211, 1852.
26. Thompson, R. C.: Assyrian Herbal. London, 1923.
27. ————: Assyrian medical texts. Proc. Roy. Soc. Med. [Sect. Hist. Med.], *17*:28, 1924.
28. Urdang, George: Pharmacopoeias as Witnesses of World History. J. Hist. Med., *1*:46, 1946.
29. Vitti, T. G., Banes, D., and Byers, T. E.: New Eng. J. Med., *285*:1433, 1971.
30. Wootton, A. C.: Chronicles of Pharmacy. London, Macmillan, 1910.

BIBLIOGRAPHY

Farber, E.: Great Chemists. vols. 1 and 2. New York, Interscience, 1961.
Lawall, C. H.: Four Thousand Years of Pharmacy. Philadelphia, J. B. Lippincott, 1927.
Schelenz, Hermann: Geschichte der Pharmazie. Berlin, Springer, 1904.
Sonnedecker, Glenn: *Kremers and Urdang's History of Pharmacy.* Philadelphia, J. B. Lippincott, 1963.

2

E. A. Brecht, Ph.D., *Professor of Pharmaceutics, Northeast Louisiana University*

Pharmaceutical Measurements

Pharmaceutical preparations, as the final forms used for medication, must be effective and safe. These requirements demand, qualitatively, that the identity of the ingredients be certain and, quantitatively, that the amounts be accurate.

The pharmacist uses in his work not only his knowledge of the profession and understanding of the principles, but also automatic procedures for the assuring and checking of the reliability of his products.

The student, while gaining the first requisite—knowledge—should be assiduous, both in the development of the understanding that enables the application of that knowledge to new procedures and in practicing and drilling himself in safety reflexes which he must acquire to prevent errors. The student's experience with accuracy is obtained most obviously in quantitative analysis and drug assay. The making of preparations should be equally valuable because the products can be assayed for accuracy by methods either official or extemporized.

The procedures of weighing and of measuring volume appear to be easy and uncomplicated, but experience proves that accuracy requires both understanding and care. It is a truism to say that a little carelessness makes a lot of mistake. This is serious when full medicinal action must be attained without toxic effect.

The work of Goldstein[1] as pharmaceutical chemist for the Maryland State Health Department was effective in showing the need for diligence to attain accuracy. About one hundred samples of each of a few prescriptions for several kinds of dosage forms were knowingly compounded by pharmacists to be assayed. The results showed a normal distribution of accuracy which was used as a basis for recommending tolerances for judging the acceptability of a product. The results also showed a few products with gross error almost always attributable not to lack of knowledge or equipment but to the lack of care. Recommendations for the improvement of techniques[2] and a series of five articles on weighing, measurement of volume, and calculation[3] were published. These provide a basis for some of the following information. The making of preparations in small quantities is comparable with the compounding of prescriptions.

QUALITATIVE ACCURACY

There must be constant vigilance in assuring the identity of ingredients. The safety reflex consists of reading each label carefully, not at a glance, and doing this three times: first, when the container is taken from the shelf; second, when it is used, and, third, after it has been used. The risk of taking a container from its usual location by habit rather than careful reading has caused some pharmacists to change the locations of potent ingredients or preparations periodically, but the inconvenience and the delay is hardly justified if the triple check is used rigorously. In the reading of either a formula or a label, the mind must be disciplined to avoid jumping to conclusions. It has happened that Opium Tincture has been touched, only because of failure to read three words: Opium Tincture, Camph. The former is 25 times as potent as the latter! Usually a second thought corrects the mistake, but this risk should be prevented by the application of the safety reflex.

Concern for qualitative accuracy goes beyond labeling. While mislabeling is rare, it does occur. There should be observation of the appearance such as color, shape and texture as well as the odor of every ingredient. Mistakes have been detected by pharmacists. Examples include packages labeled magnesium sulfate which contained boric acid (an extremely serious mistake), labeling on the carton different from the labeling on the bottle which it contained, tablets of different appearance in the same container, capsules of the wrong size, etc.

QUANTITATIVE ACCURACY

It is paradoxical that accuracy is required and that perfect accuracy is impossible. This does not apply to the *counting* of discrete objects such as pennies, tablets or bottles, for which perfect accuracy is possible. It applies to *measurement,* such as of weight or volume, for which each value could be determined more accurately by using a more refined measuring device. Therefore, accuracy is relative to purpose. An aspirin tablet of 300 mg. dose may contain from 285 mg. to 315 mg. of the drug. The official monograph states that the tablet must contain not less than 95 percent and not more than 105 percent of the labeled amount of $C_9H_8O_4$ (aspirin). This tolerance of 5 percent is reasonable when it is considered that the tablet may be taken by a woman weighing 120 pounds or a man weighing 200 pounds. This accuracy is easily attainable with reasonable care in manufacturing; a higher degree of accuracy increases the cost of production beyond the value of the slight improvement gained.

Significant Figures. The attainment of required accuracy is understood best through the concept of significant figures. Measurements are expressed numerically. The accuracy required of the measurement is specified by the number of digits which are certain, plus an additional digit which is certain within a value of plus or minus one, ± 1 (unless statistical evaluation indicates a different degree of uncertainty such as ± 3, etc.; it is assumed that the uncertainty is unity in the last digit unless specified otherwise). Zeros are not significant figures when they are used only to locate the decimal point. Three figure accuracy is found in a

number such as 15.4 which, in this case, means that its value is 15.35 or more, but less than 15.45. This shows that a fourth digit was rounded off, i.e., it was dropped if it had a value of less than 5 or 1 was added to the third digit if the value of the fourth digit was 5 or greater. Examples of four figure accuracy are 2,957, 29.57, and 0.02957. The accuracy of a number like 29,570 is uncertain; four figure accuracy can be specified by writing it in the form 2.957×10^4.

The concept of significant figures is not completely adequate for specifying accuracy. For the three figure numbers 101 and 999 a change of 1 in the last digit represents percentage changes of 1.0 percent, or 1 part in 100, and 0.1 percent or 1 part in 1,000 respectively. This is a tenfold difference of variation. It is well to include the consideration of percentage accuracy in using the concept of significant figures. Nevertheless, significant figures are useful in that they help to avoid unnecessarily tedious calculations, to specify the degree of accuracy, and to avoid long numbers which indicate false accuracy.

In calculations for addition and subtraction the answer can be no more accurate than the least accurate significant figure. The following addition shows the application of this statement:

The numbers	Method 1	Method 2
242.75	242.8	242.75
38.4	38.4	38.4
4.683	4.7	4.68
	285.9	285.83 = 285.8

The 4 in the second number is the limiting digit, not because it is the number with only 3 significant figures, but because its last digit in the first decimal place represents the lowest accuracy of the total. The addition is done by both methods, but Method 2 is better and shows the value, in practice, of retaining an extra digit during the calculation. The correct answer is 285.8.

In multiplication and division the answer is no more accurate than the least accurate measurement. For example, $11 \times 15.43 = 170$, and $11.00 \times 15.43 = 169.7$, not 169.73. It is recommended in a series of calculations for one final answer that one additional digit is retained in intermediate products and quotients to permit the final rounding off only in the last answer.

Official Guidance. For analytic accuracy the *U.S.P. XVIII*, p. 845, and the *N.F. XIII*, p. 902, state,

Where substances are to be "accurately weighed" in an assay or a test, the weighing is to be performed in such a manner as to limit the error to 0.1 percent or less. For example, a quantity of 50 mg. is to be weighed to the nearest 0.05 mg.; a quantity of 0.1 g. is to be weighed to the nearest 0.1 mg.; and a quantity of 10 g. is to be weighed to the nearest 10 mg.

Four significant figures are required to work within this required accuracy.

The *U.S.P.* and the *N.F.* (inside back covers) give a "Table of Metric Doses with Approximate Apothecary Equivalents" and authorization for interchanging final dosage forms labeled with either kind of unit. Maximum variations are found at 5.7 percent for 1,000 ml. as the equivalent of 1 quart, 2.9 percent for 1 g. as the equivalent of 15 grains, and 8.0 percent for 1 grain as the equivalent of 60 mg. It must be clearly understood that these tolerances apply only to finished dosage forms which are not subject to further change (to increase the error) and cannot be modified to gain greater accuracy, i.e., to change the weight of a finished tablet or volume of a sterile parenteral solution, etc. Both compendia emphasize that the approximate equivalents of the table are not applicable to any other use.

The *U.S.P.* (inside back cover and p. 1070) goes on to state, "To calculate quantities required in pharmaceutical formulas, use exact equivalents (see p. 1070). For prescription compounding, use the exact equivalents rounded to three significant figures." This statement is helpful but it does not really specify the accuracy appropriate to the making of preparations in small quantities, 1,000 g. or ml., or less. For these preparations six significant figures, for example 1 g. = 15.4324 grains, is unnecessarily and unrealistically exact; three significant figures, 15.4, while conforming to the Pharmacopeial recommendation for compounding, involves an error of 0.2 percent. Therefore, the practical equivalent for making preparations is 1 gram = 15.43

grains. The additional digit adds no great hardship in calculation, and it limits the error below 0.1 percent. The latter is important in a final result involving a series of calculations and manipulation because successive errors may be additive. The risk of additive error is limited by using the equivalent accurate to within 0.1 percent.

It is assumed that the reader of this text has a knowledge of the tables of measurement and pharmaceutical calculations. These were presented in the text of earlier editions of *American Pharmacy,* and may be found in the appendix. It is considered necessary only to emphasize a few points of information and list certain equivalents on an organized basis.

The simplicity of the metric system, and the ease of calculation based on decimal division of units have led to the wide adoption of this system throughout the world. The increasing use in the English speaking nations may be seen in the British Weights and Measures Act of 1963, which is an effort to secure the use of the metric system exclusively in that country. All of this prompts the question whether a second system of weights and measures, the U. S. Customary Measures, must be learned. Unfortunately, the answer for pharmacy students is that the second system must be learned because it is used to some extent, it will be used for some time to come, and a knowledge of it is needed to understand the literature of the past.

The units of measurement used in the *United States Pharmacopeia* and the *National Formulary* are:

Length

1 meter (m.) = 100 centimeters (cm.)
1 centimeter = 10 millimeters (mm.)
1 millimeter = 1,000 microns (μ)
1 micron = 1,000 millimicrons (mμ)

The International Bureau of Weights and Measures has proposed nm. as the abbreviation for nanometer (millimicron). *Nano* is the prefix meaning one billionth, 10^{-9}.

Weight

1 kilogram (kg.) = 1,000 grams (g.)
1 gram = 1,000 milligrams (mg.)
1 milligram = 1,000 micrograms (mcg.)
1 microgram = 1,000 nanograms (ng.)

There is no international convention, as yet, concerning the abbreviation for the microgram. While mcg. is used in pharmacy, μg is used in the literature of physics and physical chemistry, and γ is used in biochemical literature for a gamma, a microgram.

Volume
1 liter (l.) = 1,000 milliliters (ml.)
1 milliliter = 1,000 microliters (μl.)

The *U.S.P.* and the *N.F.* state that in these compendia one milliliter is used as the equivalent of one cubic centimeter (cc.). As a result of small error in the making of early standards, 1 liter = 1,000.028 cubic centimeters. *U.S.P. XIV, N.F. IX* and earlier editions of both used cc. as the standard unit of volume, specifying that it meant "the one thousandth part of the liter, or a milliliter." For all practical purposes the difference is insignificant.

The microliter is also called a lambda (λ) in scientific literature and equipment catalogs.

Practical Equivalents. It frequently is necessary to convert a weight or a measurement from units of one system to units of another. Such a calculation requires knowledge of an equivalent of the 2 units. Practical equivalents are used because the exact equivalents would require too many digits to be used conveniently and assume deceptive accuracy except when all equivalents have equal significance. The following equivalents are accurate to within 0.1 percent, except the one converting kilograms to pounds (which has a 0.2 percent error and is included on the basis of common usage).

Practical Equivalents
Length
1 inch (in.)   = 2.54 centimeters (cm.)
1 meter (m.) = 39.37 inches (in.)

Volume
1 milliliter (ml.) = 16.23 minims (♏)
1 fluidounce (f℥) = 29.57 milliliters (ml.)
1 pint (O.)   = 473 milliliters (ml.)

Weight
1 grain (gr.)   = 64.8 milligrams (mg.)
1 gram (g.)   = 15.43 grains (gr.)
1 ounce (oz.)   = 28.35 grams (g.)
1 ounce (℥)   = 31.1 (g.)
1 pound (lb.)   = 454 grams (g.)
1 kilogram (kg.) = 2.2 pounds (lb.)

Accurate Equivalents (legal definitions)
1 inch, U.S. and
British   = 25.4 millimeters, exactly
1 gallon, U.S.   = 3.785411784 liters
1 gallon, British
imperial   = 4.546087 liters
1 pound, U.S.
avoirdupois and
British imperial   = 453.59237 grams, exactly
1 grain   = 64.79891 milligrams, exactly

Household Measures. Although medicines are prepared in the pharmacy with professional accuracy, they are administered in the home with available measures, called household measures. For household purposes, the U.S.A. Standards Institute has established the American Standard Teaspoon with a volume of 4.93 ± 0.25 ml. The National Bureau of Standards recognizes this same volume (1⅔ fℨ) as corresponding more closely with the actual capacities of "measuring" spoons and silver teaspoons. Studies have shown that "teaspoons" may have capacities varying from 3 to 8 ml., but 5 ml. is the most realistic average.*

Household Measures
1 teaspoonful   =   5 ml. or 1⅓ fℨ
1 dessertspoonful =   10 ml. or 2⅔ fℨ
1 tablespoonful   =   15 ml. or 4 fℨ
1 wineglassful   =   60 ml. or 2 f℥
1 teacupful   = 120 ml. or 4 f℥
1 glassful   = 240 ml. or 8 f℥

The drop sometimes is included in the household measures. Since its volume is extremely variable, it ought to be avoided as a measure of potent medicines, because the size of a drop depends not only on the nature of the liquid but also on the size and the shape of the dropping surface. For the specifications of the international standard dropper, see page 35.

* Some references list a (medicinal) teaspoon equivalent to 4 ml. or 1 fℨ and a dessertspoon equivalent to 8 ml. or 2 fℨ. These volumes may be measured with special spoons or medicine glasses, but the availability of these measures is problematical. There are also plastic spoons made specifically for administering medicines which measure the standard teaspoonful of 5 ml. It is noteworthy that, in France (the source of the metric system), the Codex Medicamentarius Gallicus states the 5 ml. and the 10 ml. equivalents to be official.

WEIGHT

Weight is measured by means of a balance. Class A prescription balances[3] (Figs. 2-1 and 2-2) have a sensitivity of 2 mg. Sensitivity is the smallest weight that makes a perceptible change in the pointer which indicates equilibrium. What is perceptible to different operators varies greatly; the amounts may vary two or threefold. Sensibility reciprocal is a better measure of sensitivity. The sensibility reciprocal, introduced in *N.F. X* (1955), is the weight necessary to move the pointer of the balance one division on the index plate against which equilibrium is observed. Class A prescription balances were required by law to have a sensibility reciprocal of 13 mg. or less. The value is usually better, from 10 mg. down to 6 mg. The capacity of a prescription balance is 120 g. Larger amounts should not be weighed, owing to the danger of damaging the mechanism.

Sensibility reciprocal was replaced by sensitivity requirement (SR) in the NBS Handbook 44, ed. 3, 1965[4] with a less precise definition: the minimum change in the position of rest of the indicating element in response to the test-weight load. For a

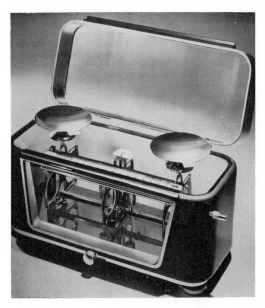

FIG. 2-1. Torsion prescription balance.

Class A prescription balance the SR shall be 0.1 grain (6 mg.). Unfortunately the new term was adopted in *N.F. XIII* but the definition was not changed. The *N.F. XIII Second Supplement* corrects the minimum amount to be weighed on a prescription balance to

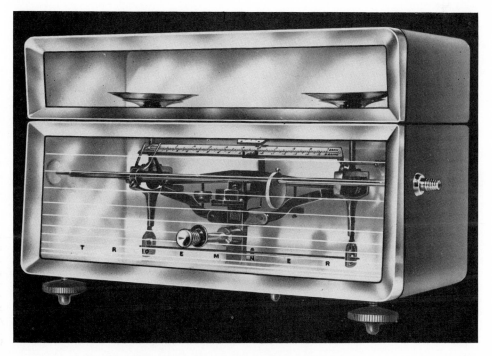

FIG. 2-2. Troemner prescription balance.

120 mg. (2 gr.) not 200 mg. (3 gr.). A 5.0 percent maximum tolerance is realized: 5 percent of 120 mg. is 6 mg.

Class B prescription balances must have a maximum maintenance sensibility reciprocal of 30 mg. and must be labeled "Class B—Not to be used in weighing loads of less than 648 mg. (10 grains)." The capacity is also 120 g. Since the Class B balance has no advantage, it is rarely seen and is no longer recognized in the N.B.S. Handbook 44.[4]

Amounts larger than 120 g. should be weighed in portions on a prescription balance or on a solution balance (Fig. 2-3) or its equivalent. It has a sensitivity of 1 g. (it does not have a pointer scale) and a capacity of 20 kg. (45 lb.).

Weights. Equally as important as the balance in the weighing process are the mass standards, the weights (Fig. 2-4). Any inaccuracy in either nullifies the accuracy of the other. Good weights commonly are made of polished brass. To increase resistance to corrosion, they may be lacquered or plated with nickel, chromium, gold or platinum. Weights of high accuracy also are made of stainless alloys. Metric weights of less than 1 g. are made of tantalum for 500 mg. to 50 mg. and aluminum for less than 50 mg. Apothecary weights of less than one half scruple are made of aluminum, a light metal, in order to increase the size of the weight. Good weights are purchased in covered blocks with a hole of appropriate size and shape for each weight. A forceps is kept with the weights to eliminate the need for handling them with the fingers. Coin weights of the apothecaries' system are illustrated because they were used widely in earlier times and are of historical interest. The use of coin weights is not recommended in the *National Formulary*; they can be handled conveniently only with the fingers, which quickly causes a loss in accuracy.

N.F. XIII specifies analytical weights for use with a prescription balance. The *Second Supplement* names National Bureau of Standards Class P or better but recognizes Class Q weights as acceptable. However, Class C, specified in earlier editions and less costly, are entirely satisfactory. They have a per-

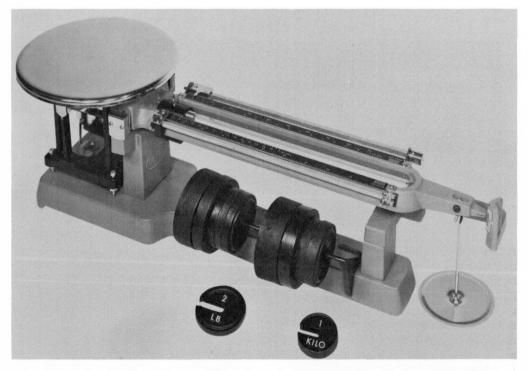

FIG. 2-3.   Solution balance. (From Ohaus Scale Corporation, Florham Park, N.J.)

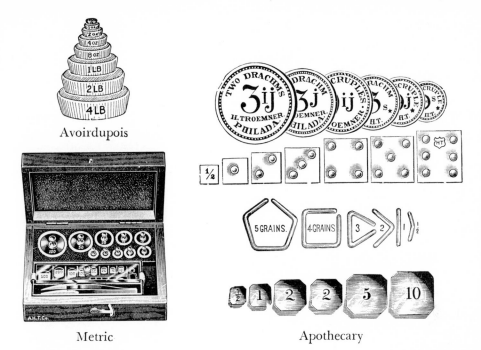

Avoirdupois

Metric   Apothecary

FIG. 2-4.   Weights: avoirdupois, metric and apothecary. (The apothecary weights shown are of historical interest only. Today, knob weights, similar to the metric set shown here, are the only type recommended for use.)

mitted tolerance 50 percent better than legally required for prescription weights.[4]

TECHNIQUE OF WEIGHING

In making a weighing, it is customary to place the weights on the right pan of the balance and the substance to be weighed on the left. All graduated beams are attached on this basis. Also, this position is more convenient for transferring powders from bottles to the pan. A left-handed operator will find it useful to learn to handle a spatula with the right hand.

When the weights on both pans are equal, a balance is said to be at equilibrium or in balance.

Balance may be determined by several methods. Down balance consists of adding the substance until the weights are overbalanced. Although this method is rapid, it is grossly inaccurate; if used at all, it is usually as a preliminary step in reaching true balance. Fixed balance is a more nearly accurate method, in which the pointer remains at the central position when the beam is made free to swing. Swinging balance is

most accurate and is indicated when the pointer swings an equal number of divisions to both sides of the central position.

Good technique in the weighing process is important to both accuracy and prolonged usefulness of the equipment. The following rules may serve as guides:

The balance should be located in a well-lighted place, as free as possible from vibration, dust, moisture and corrosive vapors.

The balance cover should be kept down except when the balance is in use.

The balance should be kept clean at all times. Any chemical spilled on the balance should be removed immediately with a soft brush or a clean, dry towel.

The pans should be protected from wear and corrosion; powder papers should be used routinely and tared watch glasses or stoppered bottles used for corrosive substances.

The knife-edges or steel bands should be protected from jarring and unnecessary wear; the pans should be supported at all times except when equilibrium is being tested. Weights and materials should never be added to or removed from the pans unless the pans are supported. The pan support is controlled by the knob at the front of the balance.

Weights should be protected from dust and corrosion by keeping them in covered boxes when they are not in use.

Weights should be handled only with forceps. Fingerprints not only increase their weight but also accelerate corrosion.

If the weights require cleaning, it should be done with a soft, clean towel. If this is not sufficient, a paste of precipitated calcium carbonate and glycerin may be used, to be followed by cleaning with a moistened towel and drying.

To avoid mistakes, weights are totaled 3 times: (1) as they are placed on the balance, (2) from the vacant positions in the weight box and (3) as they rest on the pan.

Sources of Error. The most common source of error in weighing is failure to adjust the scale to perfect balance before each weighting. This is particularly true when a new powder paper is placed on the pan. Tests of powder papers show that there may be as much as 60 mg. difference in the weights of 3½ by 4½ inch glassine papers taken from the same package. A very large error occurs when the counterbalancing paper is forgotten. Currents of air cause error; when greatest accuracy is needed, the final balance should be determined with the cover down. In this case, it is necessary to be sure that the papers are not touching the inside of the balance cover.

The Weighing of Small Amounts. The *National Formulary,* p. 1084, *Second Supplement,* states:

In order to avoid errors of 5 percent or more which might be due to the limit of accuracy of the Class A prescription balance, do not weigh less than 120 mg. (2 grains) of any material. If a smaller weight of dry material is required, mix a larger known weight of the ingredient with a known weight of dry diluent, and weigh an aliquot portion of the mixture for use.

This statement permits a maximum tolerance of 5 percent. The error can be reduced by careful technique and by increasing the amounts weighed to more than 120 mg.— the quantity that must be considered the minimum for each of the following: the active ingredient, the diluent, and the aliquot part of the mixture.

The mixture is also called a trituration, a mixture of powders of accurately known composition. The diluent is usually lactose, although an inorganic salt such as sodium chloride may be used when the organic sugar must be avoided, or talc may be used when the product does not need to be soluble. The diluent selected should be harmless and compatible. If the active ingredient is to be used in a solution, it may be better and quicker to use a suitable solvent such as water, alcohol or the vehicle to make a stock solution of known concentration and use the aliquot portion of it.

To obtain 15 mg. of atropine sulfate for a preparation, 20 times as much (300 mg.) may be weighed accurately and triturated thoroughly with 19×300 mg. of lactose (5.70 g.), to make 6.00 g. of triturate. One twentieth of the triturate (300 mg.) is weighed for use in the preparation. Check: 300 mg. $\times 1/20 = 15$ mg. of atropine sulfate. The remainder of triturate may be labeled "Atropine Sulfate Triturate in Lactose, 1 in 20." Atropine sulfate is very potent, so that a more dilute trituration should be more useful for other uses. The trituration might be 1 in 100. To make this, 300 mg. of atropine sulfate is triturated with 29.7 g. of lactose, and 1.50 g. of the 1 percent triturate is used to obtain 15 mg. of atropine sulfate for the preparation. If the lactose is objectionable, 300 mg. of atropine sulfate may be dissolved in water to make 100 ml. The calculation for the aliquot part is 100 ml. $\times$ 15 mg./300 mg. = 5 ml. of stock solution to be used. In general, triturations are more stable for future use due to their dryness. Stock solutions are subject to deterioration by the growth of organisms and some degree of chemical reaction.

In making a trituration, geometric dilution is used to assure thorough mixing with minimum effort. The active ingredient is placed in a clean, dry, smooth (glass preferred) mortar. An equal bulk (by estimation) of the weighed diluent is added. It is mixed quickly, and twice as much diluent, now equal to the amount in the mortar, is added and mixed. The amount of diluent is doubled for each addition. The final mixing must be vigorous and thorough to prevent any portion of the mixture from being more potent than any other part.

VOLUME

Volume is space. It is possible to describe a given amount of matter in terms of the quantity of space which it occupies, as well as by its weight. It is customary to measure amounts of liquids by volume and solids by weight. However, there are many exceptions to this generalization. The pharmacist buys many liquids by weight (glycerin, acids, oils). He dispenses them by volume.

An important factor in the accuracy of an instrument used for measuring volume is the surface area of the liquid in it (Fig. 2-5); the accuracy is increased as the surface area is decreased, because a perceptible difference in the height of the liquid represents a smaller volume. At the same time, as the surface is decreased, the convenience of transferring a liquid to and from the instrument is decreased. Therefore, there must be a compromise between accuracy and convenience.

Since it is seldom possible to pour all of a liquid from a vessel, a distinction must be made between receiving capacity (the true volume) and delivery capacity, the true volume plus an allowance for the liquid (water as a standard) which will adhere to the vessel. Unless specified otherwise, graduated vessels are calibrated to show delivery capacities. Volumetric flasks are an exception, usually being graduated to show receiving capacity. Some volumetric flasks and pipets have double calibrations, showing both receiving and delivery capacities.

Volumetric apparatus is usually calibrated at 20°. The change of volume due to fluctuations of room temperatures is so small that it can be ignored. (See *U.S.P. XVIII*, p. 844).

Conical graduates (Fig. 2-6) are used most frequently for measuring volumes in pharmacy. Many apparatus catalogs list them as pharmaceutical graduates. They possess several advantages. The wide mouth is convenient for filling and emptying and for cleaning and drying. A low center of gravity gives stability. Conical graduates usually are

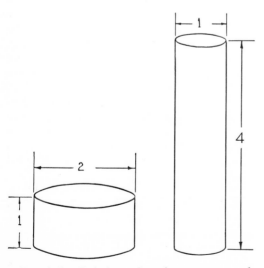

FIG. 2-5. Relation of surface area to volume. The volumes are equal. Therefore, a unit distance of height is four times more accurate on the taller cylinder.

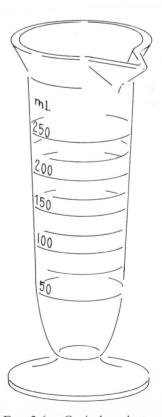

FIG. 2-6. Conical graduate.

graduated in both metric and apothecary units.

TECHNIQUE OF MEASURING LIQUIDS

Good technique in measuring liquids involves the following points (Fig. 2-7): the graduate is held at the bottom with the thumb and the forefinger and supported on the curved middle finger of the left hand. The bottle is grasped with the right hand so that the label of the bottle will be up while pouring: this prevents drippings from soiling the label. The stopper of the bottle is removed with the little finger of the left hand. The graduate is then raised level with the eyes to minimize the error in reading (error of parallax, Fig. 2-8). The liquid is poured into the graduate until the bottom of the meniscus exactly reaches the required mark, which should be level with the eyes.

Cylindrical graduates (graduated cylinders) (Fig. 2-9) can be used somewhat more accurately than conical graduates. The uniform diameter makes it possible to judge volumes between graduation markings more accurately. They usually are graduated only in metric units, but they are available with both metric and apothecary graduations.

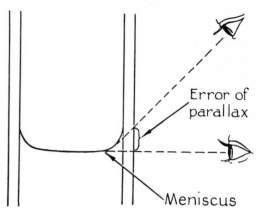

FIG. 2-8.   Error of parallax.

Important changes in the legal requirements for graduates were announced in the National Bureau of Standards Handbook 44 —Second Edition, effective July 1, 1956 for all new equipment and are in force in nearly all states. Previously acquired graduates and graduated cylinders were allowed to be used for their normal life, but they did not conform with one or more of the following specifications: (1) The smallest graduation may not be less than $\frac{1}{5}$ and not more than $\frac{1}{4}$ of the capacity of the graduate. (2) A graduate for a capacity of 4 fluid drams or less may not be conical (i.e., it must be cylindrical). (3) A graduate for a capacity

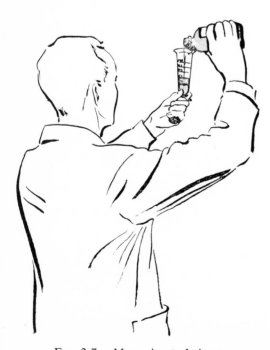

FIG. 2-7.   Measuring technique.

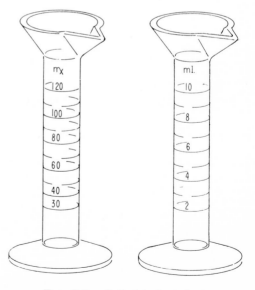

FIG. 2-9.   Cylindrical graduates.

of 4 fluid drams or less may not have a dual scale (both apothecaries' and metric graduations). These requirements apply to prescription work and enforce good pharmaceutical practice by elimination of attempts to measure small volumes in large graduates. These requirements became effective July 1, 1970 and rendered illegal further use of graduates in existence from times preceding 1956.[4] Graduates must be made of glass.

Pipets provide a means for greatest accuracy in measuring volume, by affording the smallest surface to the liquid. Ordinarily, a pipet is used to measure only one specific volume, e.g., a 25-ml. pipet. They are sometimes called transfer pipets. The graduated pipet may be used to measure various volumes within the capacity of the pipet. Especially useful to the pharmacist for measuring small volumes are a 10-ml. pipet graduated in tenth milliliters and a 1-ml. pipet graduated in hundredth milliliters (Fig. 2-10).

U.S.P. XVIII gives the international specifications for an official medicine dropper (Fig. 2-11). Such a dropper has a delivery tip with an outside diameter of 3 mm.; when held in a vertical position, it delivers drops of water that weigh between 45 mg. and 55 mg. This represents an effort to standardize the drop as a unit of volume. However, even with the same dropper, the volume of a drop will vary for different liquids, depending on the surface tension, the viscosity and the density of the liquid. A drop should not be used as a measure for medicine until its volume has been determined in each specific case.

There are several limitations to accuracy in the measuring of volumes. The 50 ml. buret used in drug assay has a graduated length of approximately 535 mm., an inside diameter of only 10.9 mm. and marked divisions of 0.1 ml. The instrument can be read, by estimating the tenth of a division, to 0.01 ml. ± 1 or 2. This is four significant figure accuracy in measuring volumes of more than 10 ml. Accuracy is enhanced by the numerous divisions etched in the glass, the uniform bore of the cylinder, and the small diameter of the column of liquid. The same advantages are found in graduated pipets recommended earlier in this chapter for measuring small volumes, i.e., less than 5 ml. In using graduated pipets it must be noted that the measured volume is delivered between two division marks on the pipet, not between a division mark and the tip.

It is estimated that the level of liquid in a pharmaceutical graduate can be judged with an accuracy of ± 1 mm.[3:IV] In a 120-ml. conical graduate, the errors resulting from this maximum deviation are 1.0 ml. at the 30 ml. level, 1.7 ml. at the 60 ml. level, and 1.9 ml. at the 120 ml. level. The error in a 100-ml. cylindrical graduate is 0.5 ml. at all levels. In the latter case, the error is 10 percent at the 5 ml. level but only 0.5 percent at the 100 ml. level. This is

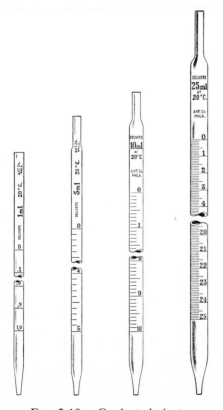

FIG. 2-10.   Graduated pipets.

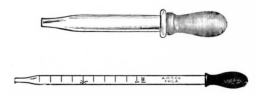

FIG. 2-11.   Medicine droppers.

the basis for the regulation of 1956 eliminating graduations, for prescription compounding, of marked divisions less than $\frac{1}{5}$ of the full volume. It also emphasizes that in using graduates, the smallest one that will measure the required amount should be selected, e.g., to measure 45 ml., a 50 or 60 ml. graduate, not 100 or 120 ml. graduate, should be used.

The same reference points out the importance of drainage time when liquids are viscous. The drainage of aqueous and alcoholic liquids was complete in $\frac{1}{2}$ minute, but when 25 ml. of glycerin was drained for the same time only 23.7 ml. was delivered from the graduate.

When small volumes (less than 5 ml.) must be measured and no suitable graduated pipet is available, either of the two following methods should be used: The aliquot part of a dilution, or the calibration of a medicine dropper. To measure 1.36 ml. of hydrochloric acid, 10 ml. of the acid may be diluted to 100 ml. and 13.6 ml. of the dilution used. The second method consists of using a medicine dropper, preferably held vertically to keep the drops smaller and give a more reproducible angle, and counting the drops to measure exactly as possible 3.0, 4.0 or 5.0 ml. As an example, 52 drops equals 3.0 ml. Then 1 ml. equals 17.3 drops and 1.36 ml. $\times$ 17.3 drops/ml. $= 23.5 = $ 24 drops. (A fraction of a drop cannot be measured reliably.) The half drop represents an error of 2 percent. Of the two methods the use of a dilution is usually better.

DENSITY AND SPECIFIC GRAVITY

Density is mass per unit volume. It is a recognition of the difference between a pound of lead and a pound of feathers. Every substance has its own characteristic density. Therefore, density can be a test of identity and a test of quality or concentration.

Density is useful also for determining the volume occupied by a specified weight of a substance and the reverse, the weight of a definite volume of a substance. Such calculations are necessary in pharmacy. The pharmacist buys some liquids by weight, such as glycerin and heavy acids, e.g., concentrated

sulfuric acid; he sells them by volume. Density must be used to relate weight and volume in calculating costs. Density may be used in other ways. For example, a reaction or preparation may require an accurate weight of a chemical such as H_2SO_4. The percentage strength of concentrated sulfuric acid is known, and the weight of the commercial product must be calculated to allow for its small but appreciable content of water. The acid is corrosive, and it is inconvenient to weigh the calculated amount. By the use of density the exact corresponding volume of the acid can be calculated and then measured easily.

The equation for density can be written and used in three forms:

$$\frac{W}{V} = D; \; VD = W; \; \frac{W}{D} = V$$

$$V \times D = W$$

$$W \div D = V$$

The expression of density *always* requires a unit of weight and a unit of volume. Since there are many of each, the number of possible combinations is very large.

The following are a few densities of water worth memorizing for general usefulness:

SOME DENSITIES OF WATER

AVOIRDUPOIS	METRIC
0.95 gr./♏	
0.95 ʒ/fʒ	1 g./ml.
0.95 ℥/f℥	1,000 g./l.
455 gr./f℥*	1 kg./l.
7280 gr./O.*	
1.04 lb./O.	
62.4 lb./cu. ft.	

* The metric unity relationship, at 4°C., is so convenient that it is used routinely. The densities marked with an asterisk are true at 25°, the official room temperature. This discrepancy is less than 0.4 percent and can be considered negligible. The density of water at 4° is 456.4 gr./f℥.

It is inconvenient that one substance can have so many different expressions for its density. It is convenient to have only one specific number for each of the thousands and thousands of known substances, and this is done by relating each substance to a standard.

Specific gravity is the density of a substance related to the density of a standard. It is also known as relative density. It can be stated in another way which is directly useful in determining its value: specific gravity is the weight of a substance divided by the weight of an equal volume of the standard.

$$\text{Sp. Gr.} = \frac{D_x}{D_s} \; or \; \frac{W_x}{W_s} \; (\text{of equal volumes})$$

In either case, the units cancel, and specific gravity is an abstract number independent of the units used in its determination. It simply states the ratio of its weight to that of the standard. Therefore, a substance has only one specific gravity.

Water is the standard for the specific gravities of solids and liquids. Water is a good choice because it is commonly available and easily purified. Air (a mixture) or hydrogen (the lightest gas) are used for the standards for gases.

Specific gravity *cannot* be used directly to convert weight to volume or vice versa. For example, it is wrong to calculate 10 ml. $\times$ 1.25 = 12.5 g. for the same reason that it is meaningless to calculate 3 apples $\times$ 2 = 6 oranges. The units don't check on each side of the equation. It is the unity relationship for the density of water in the metric system that is responsible for this erroneous conception. The conversion requires density. The equation above can be written in this useful form:

$$D_x = \text{Sp. Gr.} \times D_w$$

The density of the substance can be calculated from its specific gravity and the water density selected for its convenience in the problem. The calculation above becomes:

$$10 \text{ ml.} \times 1.25 \text{ g./ml.} = 12.5 \text{ g.}$$

The volume of a pound (avoirdupois) of glycerin, sp. gr. 1.25, can be calculated in two ways:

1. 1 lb. = 7,000 gr.
   7,000 gr. ÷ 1.25 = 5,600 gr., the weight of an equal volume of water.
   5,600 gr. ÷ 455 gr./f℥ = 12.3 f℥ or
   12 f℥ 144 ♏ or
   12 f℥ 2f℈ 24 ♏

2. 1 lb. = 7,000 gr.
   1.25 × 455 gr./f℥ = 569 gr./f℥, a density of glycerin
   7,000 gr. ÷ 569 gr./f℥ = 12.3 f℥, etc., above.

PERCENTAGE

Percentage means parts per hundred and, unless specified otherwise, means parts by weight, both of the solute and the solution. It is best to think of the percent sign as a modification of the decimal point: 0.5 = 50 percent, 0.02 = 2 percent, etc. The following equation is wrong:

$$\frac{5}{100} \times 100 = 5 \text{ percent}$$

The equation is best written:

$$\frac{5}{100} = 0.05 = 5 \text{ percent}$$

and the middle decimal can be omitted when there is accurate familiarity with the meaning of percentage. The equation can be written also in the form:

$$\frac{5}{100} \times 100\% = 5\%,$$

but it must be recognized that 100% = 1. Multiplying by unity does not change the equation; the "100%" is an unnecessary device for fixing the position of the decimal point.

The *U.S.P. XVIII*, p. 12, defines percent weight in volume as the number of g. in 100 ml. of solution, regardless of whether water or another liquid is the solvent. Preceding revisions specified that percent used in prescriptions without qualification means for solids in solids w/w, solids in liquids w/v, liquids in liquids v/v, and gases in liquids w/v. Preference for percentage weight in volume derives from the general custom of weighing solids and measuring liquids by volume and from the uniformity of solute content which is independent of the density of the solvent and the solution. Percentage volume in volume applies generally to liquid solutes and always to content of ethyl alcohol in a liquid.

INDIRECT MEASUREMENT

The active content is not always determined or specified directly in units of weight or volume. For example, Bacitracin, *U.S.P.* "has a potency of not less than 40 units of bacitracin activity per mg., except that when intended for parenteral use its potency is not less than 50 units per mg." Bacitracin, labeled 45 units per mg. is used to make 30 g. of bacitracin ointment, 500 units per g. The calculation of the amount of the bacitracin ingredient is as follows:

30 g. × 500 units/g. = 15,000 units
15,000 units ÷ 45 units/mg. = 333 mg. of Bacitracin, *U.S.P.*

CALCULATIONS

Calculations should be written and checked. It is helpful to write the units after each number as an added check, by their algebraic cancellation, on the correctness of multiplying *vs.* dividing and on the correctness of selecting the practical equivalent. Sometimes the decimal point is elusive. It needs to be checked with special attention to prevent a 0.5 percent solution from being 5 percent or a 1 percent ointment from being 10 percent.

In making percentage solutions the information is frequently used that a 1 percent solution contains 4.55 gr. per fluidounce. In making 3 fluidounces of a 5 percent solution, a substantial error is caused if an interruption causes forgetfulness to multiply the 4.55 gr. by the 3 and the 5. This method is useful in checking calculations made by another method.

MANIPULATION

Finally, careful and thoughtful manipulation is necessary after the calculation, the weighing and the measuring have been done correctly. Loss of material in transferring from a powder paper to a graduate, mortar or other container reduces the accuracy of the weighing. The spilling or splashing of a liquid or incomplete transfer from the measuring apparatus spoils the accuracy of the measurement. When a liquid must be filtered, last traces of the actual ingredients should be washed from the filter by using more of the solvent or vehicle to avoid loss. The final volume should be adjusted in a graduate because graduated prescription bottles are not sufficiently accurate for this purpose and are forbidden by law in some states.

The information and techniques presented in this chapter are important but should not appear formidable. Their understanding and practice are essential attributes of the qualified operator, for whom the satisfying confidence of his mastery will be its own reward.

REFERENCES

1. Goldstein, S. W.: Standard tolerances for pharmaceutical compounding; a basis for their establishment. 1. Ointments. 2. Liquid preparations. 3. Capsules. J. Am. Pharm. A. (Sci. Ed.), *38*:18–22, 1949; *38*:131–138, 1949; *39*:505–506, 1950; 4. Hand-made pills. Bull. Nat. Formulary Committee, *18*:125–130, 1950; 5. Divided powders. J. Am. Pharm. A. (Sci. Ed.), *39*:507–508, 1950.

2. ———: Improvement of prescription practices. J. Am. Pharm. A. (Pract. Ed.), *11*:605–609, 1950.

3. Goldstein, S. W., *et al.*: Professional equilibrium and compounding precision. 1. What is a prescription balance? 2. How to test your prescription balance. 3. How to weigh accurately. 4. How to measure accurately. 5. Careless arithmetic nullifies careful compounding. J. Am. Pharm. A. (Pract. Ed.), *12*:214–216; 293–295, 310; 362–364; 421–423; 485–487, 1951. (A reprint comprising all five parts is available from the American Pharmaceutical Association, 2215 Constitution Ave., N.W., Washington, D. C. 20037.

4. National Bureau of Standards Handbook 44, ed. 3. U.S. Department of Commerce, Superintendent of Documents, U.S. Government Printing Office, Washington, D. C. 20402, 1965 (with annual supplements; price $2.00).

3

Mitchell John Stoklosa, Sc.D., *Dean of Students
and Professor of Pharmacy, Massachusetts College of Pharmacy*

Solutions Containing Nonvolatile Materials

GENERAL CONSIDERATIONS

A solution may be defined as a one-phase system of two or more substances. For example, the addition of sucrose to water produces a single-phase system that is composed of two different chemical substances which are so intimately mixed with each other that a physically homogeneous system results. In other words, the dissolved substance is completely and permanently dissipated throughout the liquid, and a *true solution* results. Although such a system may be solid, liquid or gaseous in nature, the pharmacist deals most frequently with solutions in which the *solvent* is a liquid. The dissolved substance, or the *solute,* in this type of solution may be a liquid, a solid or a gas. When water is one of the components of the system, it is usually considered to be the solvent. But, in a system consisting of two liquids which are said to be miscible with each other, such as alcohol and water, the terms solute and solvent are interchangeable. The component of the system which is present in the larger amount usually is designated as the solvent. However, when a solid is dissolved in a liquid, the solid is considered as the solute and the liquid as the solvent regardless of the proportion of one to the other.

Solutions—more specifically, *true solutions*—make up one group of dispersions. In a *true solution,* such as that represented by sucrose dissolved in water, the particles of the solute dispersed in the solvent are so small that they consist of molecules or ions; hence, a true solution is a molecular dispersion. In a *suspension* of zinc oxide in water, the particles are larger than 0.1 micron and can be seen with the naked eye or with the aid of an ordinary microscope. In a *colloidal solution* or *dispersion,* such as silver protein in water or methylcellulose in water, the particles range in size from 0.1 micron to 1 millimicron and their presence may be detected by the use of an ultramicroscope.

TYPES OF SOLUTIONS

Solutions of Liquids in Liquids

When two liquids, such as *alcohol* and *water, glycerin* and *water,* or *acetone* and *water* are mixed, a homogeneous system is formed irrespective of the proportions in which the two are taken. Such pairs of liquids are said to be *miscible.* Other liquid pairs, such as *liquefied phenol* and *water* or *ether* and *water,* produce homogeneous systems only when mixed in certain ratios. These liquids are said to be *miscible in certain proportions.* Still other pairs of liquids, such as *mineral oil* and *water,* are practically insoluble in each other in any proportion and are, therefore, *immiscible.*

Solutions of Gases in Liquids

The solubility of different gases in liquids varies considerably. In general, the behavior of a gas in solution is described by Henry's Law which states that the solubility, by weight, of a gas is very nearly proportional to the pressure if the temperature remains constant, provided that the gas is only slightly soluble. The law applies less accurately to moderately soluble gases and not at all to very soluble gases. The great solubility of certain gases, such as ammonia and hydrogen chloride, must be due either to a chemical reaction between the gas and the solvent or to cohesive influences which the molecules exert on one another. Increased pressure in the latter case has little or no effect on their solubility.

39

The solubility of a gas is also influenced by temperature. As the temperature is raised the solubility of a gas in a liquid decreases. For example, carbon dioxide is twice as soluble at 0° as it is at 20° C. It is for this reason that gaseous solutions should be stored in a cool place, preferably in a refrigerator.

Containers holding gaseous solutions, such as strong ammonia solution, should always be cooled before they are opened in order to reduce the liberation and expansion of the gas.

In general, when a salt is added to a liquid containing a dissolved gas, a liberation of the gas occurs due to decreased solubility. This effect is referred to as a *salting-out* of the gas.

Solutions of Solids in Liquids

Most of the true solutions which are of pharmaceutical interest represent examples of solid-in-liquid solution. The preparation of such solutions involves some knowledge of solubility, factors affecting solubility and the use of solvents. Equally important is a clear understanding of the different methods which are used for expressing the strength, or concentration, of solutions.

SOLUBILITY

As a rule, not more than a certain amount of a solute will dissolve in a given quantity of solvent at a particular temperature. When an excess of a solid (*solute*) is shaken with a liquid (*solvent*) for a period of time, a maximum amount of it will be dissolved. The solvent is then saturated by the solute. The resulting solution is a *saturated solution* at a given temperature, and the extent to which the solute dissolves is called its *solubility*. Ordinarily, when a saturated solution is in contact with excess solute and the temperature is raised, more of the solute will dissolve. If such a solution is filtered and cooled to the original temperature, it often will retain the extra solute that it dissolved at the higher temperature. The resulting solution is called a *supersaturated solution*. Sodium thiosulfate and potassium acetate are examples of substances which form such solutions readily.

FACTORS AFFECTING SOLUBILITY

For a given solvent, the degree of solubility of a solute depends on temperature. Generally speaking, solids usually are more soluble in hot than in cold liquids. If, in the process of solution, an *endothermic reaction* takes place, increased temperature will cause more of the solute to go into solution. On the other hand, if a solute gives off heat during the process of solution (an *exothermic reaction*), its solubility is decreased with an increase in temperature. Certain compounds, such as methylcellulose and the calcium salts, are more soluble in cold than in hot water. For example, calcium hydroxide is soluble to the extent of 0.17 g. per 100 ml. of water at 15° but only to the extent of 0.14 g. at 25° C. And a solution of methylcellulose becomes cloudy when heated and yields a flaky precipitate which redissolves as the solution cools. When heat is neither absorbed nor given off in the process of solution, the solubility of a solute in a solvent is not affected significantly by variations in temperature. Sodium chloride, for instance, has almost the same solubility in water at 25° C. as it has in boiling water.

SOLUBILITY VS. RATE OF SOLUTION

A distinction should be made between *degree of solubility* and *rate of solution*. An increase in the rate of solution does not mean an increase in the amount of solute which a given solvent will dissolve. The rate of solution depends on (1) the particle size of the solute, (2) agitation and (3) temperature.

Since the mechanism of solution involves surface action, an increase in surface area will increase the rate of solution. It is for this reason that the particle size of a substance should be reduced before it is dissolved. Agitation increases the rate of solution by removing from the surface of the solute the more concentrated solution around it and bringing in the less concentrated solvent. Heating a liquid also causes solution to take place more rapidly by increasing the frequency with which solvent molecules collide with the surface of the dissolving material. With increased molecular motion, diffusion increases, and this hastens the removal of the material dissolved and tends to maintain a condition of unsaturation around the solid.

EFFECT OF MOLECULAR STRUCTURE ON SOLUBILITY

The solubility of solids in liquids varies within very wide limits. Solvents will dissolve certain substances quite readily and others only slightly or not at all. It is generally true that the more nearly solute and solvent are alike in molecular structure the greater is the solubility of one in the other. Moreover, the selectivity of solvent action is dependent on the ability of the solvent to overcome certain electronic forces which hold the atoms of the solute together and on its ability to act as the solute-solvent binding force.

A comparison of the molecular structure of water, carbon tetrachloride and ethyl alcohol illustrates the mechanism of solvent action of these liquids on solutes of different types.

The solubility of substances in water undoubtedly is linked to the dipole nature of the water molecules. Water is composed of covalent molecules which are described as polar structures with strong dipole characteristics (a negative and a positive region). Since the covalent bonds in the molecule are arranged asymmetrically, the molecule as a whole is polar. Molecules having dipoles show a tendency to join into groups of molecules and to associate with other polar substances. This attraction, in the case of the water molecules, is brought about by *hydrogen bonding,* which may be represented as:

$$\underset{H}{\overset{H}{|}}\;O \ldots \underset{H}{\overset{H}{|}}\;O \ldots$$

H—O ... H—O ... H—O ... H—O

where the hydrogen bond is established between the oxygen of one molecule of water and the hydrogen of another molecule of water.

When an electrovalent compound, such as sodium chloride, is placed in water, the water molecules have a strong tendency to orient themselves at the chloride and the sodium ions with sufficient energy to overcome the force which holds the ions in the crystal of sodium chloride. As a result, the water molecules attach themselves to the

ions and solvate them. Thus the polar molecules of the water form a stable union (a solution) with polar substances. In general, it may be stated that polar solvents, such as water, will dissolve salts and other electrolytes readily. However, they are poor solvents for nonpolar substances.

A polar liquid may also act as a solvent when it and the solute are capable of being complexed through hydrogen bond formation. For example, the water-solubility of alcohols having a low molecular weight may be explained on the basis of the ability of the alcohol molecules to couple or complex with the water molecules:

H—O ... H—O ... H—O ... H—O

However, as the molecular weight of the alcohol increases it becomes less polar and, consequently, less soluble in water.

The carbon tetrachloride molecule contains 4 covalent bonds. Since these bonds are distributed symmetrically, the molecule

$$\begin{array}{c} Cl \\ | \\ Cl{-}C{-}Cl \\ | \\ Cl \end{array}$$

Carbon tetrachloride molecule

is said to be nonpolar. Such a solvent will not solvate ions of a salt like sodium chloride. In this case, the molecules of carbon tetrachloride do not supply the attractive force (solvent force) which is required to overcome the force that holds the ions of the salt together. Consequently, the salt has little tendency to dissolve in a solvent of this type. Nonpolar liquids do not dissolve polar or ionic compounds to any appreciable extent, but they dissolve nonpolar or slightly polar substances.

The ethyl alcohol molecule has 5 essentially nonpolar carbon-hydrogen bonds and a carbon-carbon bond which is nonpolar.

$$\begin{array}{c} H \quad H \\ | \quad | \\ H{-}C{-}C{-}O{-}H \\ | \quad | \\ H \quad H \end{array}$$

Ethyl alcohol molecule

The carbon-oxygen bond and the hydrogen-oxygen bond are polar. The presence of distinct polar and nonpolar regions probably accounts for the fact that ethyl alcohol is a good solvent for some polar substances and for some nonpolar substances as well.

Although there are exceptions to any specific rules which might be formulated for the selection of solvents, the following generalizations should be of some value in predicting solubilities.

1. The more nearly solvents and solutes are alike structurally, the more rapidly solution takes place.

2. Polar liquids dissolve electrovalent compounds readily, but they are poor solvents for nonpolar substances. On the other hand, nonpolar liquids are required for nonpolar solutes.

3. Polar liquids should be miscible with other polar liquids. Conversely, nonpolar liquids dissolve only slightly in polar solvents, but they dissolve readily in solvents that are nonpolar.

4. Complex organic compounds which have polar and nonpolar groups in their molecules may dissolve in polar liquids, but their solubility in such solvents tends to decrease in proportion to the number of nonpolar groups.

5. Semipolar liquids, such as ethyl alcohol, possess some of the properties of both polar and nonpolar solvents.

EFFECT OF pH ON SOLUBILITY

Many of the organic substances which are used medicinally are either weak acids or weak bases, and their aqueous solubilities are dependent to a very substantial degree upon the pH of the solvent. These weak organic acids and weak organic bases dissociate only slightly, and their molecular or *undissociated* forms are only slightly soluble in water. But within certain ranges of pH they exist predominantly in ionic or *dissociated* forms which are very soluble in water and, consequently, their aqueous solubilities may be increased by adjusting the solvent to an appropriate pH.

The solubility in water of weak organic acids, such as the barbiturates and the sulfonamides, is increased as the pH is increased by the addition of a base. This increase in solubility is due to the formation of a water-soluble salt. For example, the solubility of phenobarbital (free acid) in water at 25° is about 1.25 g./1000 ml., and the pH of the solution is about 5.5. On the other hand, the solubility of phenobarbital sodium (salt) in water at 25° is about 1000 g./1000 ml., and the pH of the solution is about 9.3. If the pH of the phenobarbital solution is increased above 5.5 by the addition of a strong base, the solubility would increase. If the pH of the salt solution is lowered by the addition of a strong acid, phenobarbital (free acid) would precipitate.

Similarly, weak organic bases, which include many alkaloids and local anesthetics, are generally only slightly soluble in water; but, if the pH of the aqueous medium is lowered by the addition of an acid, the base is converted to a water-soluble salt. For example, the solubility of atropine (free base) in water at 25° is about 2.2 g./1000 ml., and the pH of the solution is over 10, whereas the solubility of atropine sulfate (salt) in water at 25° is about 2500 g./1000 ml., and the pH of the solution is about 5.4. However, if the pH of the aqueous solution of the salt is raised by the addition of a base, atropine (free base) would precipitate.

At a given pH, the degree of ionization of a weakly acidic or basic drug depends upon its pK_a value which is the negative logarithm of its dissociation constant. In the case of a weakly acidic drug, the total solubility of the drug in water is the sum of the concentrations of the *dissociated* (ionic) and *undissociated* (molecular) species; and it is related to pH according to the following equation:

$$pH = pK_a + \log \frac{S - S_0}{S_0}$$

where S = molar concentration of drug (dissociated + undissociated species) in the solution

and S_0 = molar solubility of the undissociated species

This equation is derived from the Henderson-Hasselbalch equation for weak acids, and it may be used to calculate the pH at which a weak acid will precipitate from a solution of its salt.

Example. At what pH will free phenobarbital precipitate from a 1 percent solution of phenobarbital sodium at 25° C.? The molar solubility of phenobarbital (free acid) is 0.005 and the pK_a value is 7.41. The molecular weight of phenobarbital sodium is 254.

The molar concentration of a 1 percent solution of phenobarbital sodium is

$$\frac{\text{g. per liter}}{\text{molecular weight}} = \frac{10}{254} = 0.039$$

$$pH = 7.41 + \log \frac{0.039 - 0.005}{0.005}$$

$$= 7.41 + \log 6.8$$

$$= 8.24$$

For substances containing a weak basic group, the equation is

$$pH = pK_w - pK_b + \log \frac{S_0}{S - S_0}$$

Example. At what pH will free cocaine begin to precipitate from a 1 percent solution of cocaine hydrochloride at 25° C.? The molar solubility of cocaine is 0.0056 and the pK_b value is 5.59. The molecular weight of cocaine hydrochloride is 340.

The molar concentration of a 1 percent solution of cocaine hydrochloride is

$$\frac{\text{g. per liter}}{\text{molecular weight}} = \frac{10}{340} = 0.029$$

$$pH = 14.0 - 5.59 + \log \frac{0.0056}{0.029 - 0.0056}$$

$$= 8.41 + \log 0.24$$

$$= 7.79$$

Effect of Other Substances on Solubility

The solubility of a substance is dependent upon the types and concentrations of other substances in solution. In general, the solubility of slightly soluble electrolytes is reduced by the addition of a second salt which contains a common ion. The extent of the reduction is governed by the law of mass action which states that *the product of the concentration of the ions of a slightly soluble salt, raised to a power equal to the number of ions in the formula has a constant value at a given temperature.* This value is called the *solubility product.* If, for instance, sodium chloride—which has an ion (Cl^-) in common with AgCl—is added to a saturated solution of silver chloride, some of the AgCl precipitates from the solution until the constant value (solubility product) is once again established. However, if a common ion forms a complex with a slightly soluble electrolyte, the solubility of the salt may be increased. Mercuric iodide, for instance, is practically insoluble in water, yet it is dissolved by solutions of soluble iodides. This effect is an example of complex-ion formation.

The water-solubility of nonelectrolytes may be either decreased or increased by the addition of electrolytes. When the solubility of a nonelectrolyte is decreased, the phenomenon is referred to as *salting-out*; if it is increased, the effect is described as *salting-in*.

It is interesting to note that iodine is very slightly soluble in water; but, when it is added to a concentrated solution of potassium iodide, it dissolves immediately. The increased solubility of the iodine probably occurs through the formation of the triiodide ion (I_3^-). Most volatile oils, such as peppermint, rose, and the citrus oils, are only very slightly soluble in water; but they may be solubilized by the use of certain nonionic surfactants.

Expression of Solubility

The solubility of a substance may be expressed in various ways, but, usually, it is designated as the number of ml. of a solvent required to dissolve 1 g. of the solute, or in the case of compounds that are ordinarily liquids at 25° C., to dissolve 1 ml. of the solute. For example, 1 g. of potassium iodide dissolves in 0.7 ml. of water and in 0.5 ml. of boiling water; and 1 ml. of paraldehyde dissolves in 10 ml. of water, and in 17 ml. of boiling water. Rate of solution is described by terms such as "slowly soluble," "quickly soluble" and "soluble with difficulty."

If the solubility of a substance has been determined accurately, it may be used as an index of purity for that substance. However, the statements on solubility in the *U.S.P.* and the *N.F.* are not intended as standards or tests for purity, but are provided primarily as information for those who use, prepare, and dispense drugs. The approximate solubilities of official substances are indicated by the use of the following descriptive terms:

Descriptive Term	Parts of Solvent Required for 1 Part of Solute
Very soluble	Less than 1
Freely soluble	From 1 to 10
Soluble	From 10 to 30
Sparingly soluble	From 30 to 100
Slightly soluble	From 100 to 1,000
Very slightly soluble	From 1,000 to 10,000
Practically insoluble; Insoluble	More than 10,000

SOLVENTS FOR PHARMACEUTICAL USE

It was pointed out earlier in the discussion that solubility is a property which is determined by the chemical nature and structure of both solute and solvent. Although structural similarity is significant and important in the selection of the proper solvent for a given solute, the choice of a suitable solvent for pharmaceutical use depends, to a large extent, on such factors as toxicity, volatility and stability. In the preparation of many solution dosage forms, a mixture of solvents is desirable to dissolve certain compounds.

Water has the widest range of usefulness of all the solvents employed in pharmaceutical dispensing and manufacturing. It is a good solvent for most inorganic salts and for many organic compounds. Its miscibility with other solvents, such as alcohol and glycerin, makes it a useful vehicle for many pharmaceutical preparations.

Alcohol is a good solvent for many organic substances, both natural and synthetic. It dissolves important plant constituents such as resins, volatile oils, alkaloids, glycosides and neutral principles. Next in usefulness to water, alcohol produces solutions which, in many instances, have a greater stability than their aqueous counterparts. Alcohol is often diluted with water in the manufacture of certain preparations. Such *hydroalcoholic* liquids are commonly used as solvents for

plant constituents because they effectively dissolve the active principles; yet, by their negative solvent action, they do not dissolve therapeutically inert plant materials like gums and starches.

Dehydrated Alcohol, or *absolute alcohol,* is practically free from water and, for this reason, it has a greater range of solvent power. Its chief use in pharmacy is in research and analytic work and in the preparation of synthetic organic medicinals.

Isopropyl Alcohol possesses solvent properties which are similar to those of ethyl alcohol. It is tax-free and finds its greatest use as an ingredient in rubbing alcohol compounds and as a solvent in cosmetic and dermatologic formulations.

Glycerin is miscible with both water and alcohol but not with chloroform, ether or fixed oils. It is an excellent solvent for tannins, phenol and boric acid. Because of its preservative qualities it is sometimes used as a stabilizer for solutions prepared with other solvents. When used as a solvent, glycerin must be heated in order to reduce its viscosity. If this is not done, considerable difficulty may be experienced in dissolving substances in it.

Propylene Glycol is miscible with water, acetone, alcohol and chloroform. It is soluble in ether and will dissolve many essential oils, but it is immiscible with fixed oils. It has a wide range of usefulness as a solvent and is frequently used as a replacement for glycerin in certain pharmaceutical and cosmetic preparations.

Polyethylene Glycol 400 is miscible with water, acetone, alcohol and other glycols. It dissolves many water-soluble organic compounds as well as certain water-insoluble substances such as acetylsalicylic acid, ethyl aminobenzoate and theophylline.

Ethyl Oxide, or *solvent ether,* is miscible with alcohol, benzene, chloroform, solvent hexane and both fixed and volatile oils. It dissolves in about 12 volumes of water. It is highly volatile and flammable, and its vapor may explode when mixed with air and ignited. It is a good solvent for oils, fats, resins and many alkaloids.

Chloroform is miscible with alcohol, ether, benzene, solvent hexane and both fixed and volatile oils. It dissolves in 210 volumes of water. It is not flammable, but its vapor is decomposed by naked flames, producing harmful gases. It is a solvent for many alkaloids.

Petroleum Benzin, or *solvent hexane,* is immiscible with water but is miscible with dehydrated alcohol and with ether, chloroform and most of the fixed and the volatile oils. It is highly flammable. One of its uses as a pharmaceutical solvent is for the removal of objectionable fats from certain drugs prior to the extraction of the active principles with alcohol or hydroalcoholic solvents.

Carbon Tetrachloride is only very slightly soluble in water but is miscible with the common organic solvents. It dissolves fats and oils and has the advantage of nonflammability, compared with petroleum benzin.

Acetone is miscible with water, alcohol, ether, chloroform and most of the volatile oils. Although it is flammable, its use as a solvent does not involve the danger of explosion that exists with ether.

METHODS OF PREPARING SOLUTIONS

The usual method for preparing solutions at the prescription counter requires the use of a mortar and pestle. The solute, which has been reduced previously to a fine powder by trituration in a mortar, is dissolved by pouring solvent on it and triturating it until solution takes place. In some instances, it may be desirable to dissolve the solute in a flask or bottle, or by heating the solute and solvent in a suitable vessel. Solutions of substances like pepsin and silver protein compounds may be prepared most efficiently by placing the solute on the surface of the solvent contained in a beaker or evaporating dish and allowing solution to take place by circulatory diffusion.

METHODS USED IN EXPRESSING CONCENTRATIONS OF SOLUTIONS

A number of methods are employed to express the relative amounts of the components of a solution in quantitative terms. These methods fall into two general categories: those employing physical units and those in which chemical units are used. The pharmacist employs physical units when he uses percentage as a convenient means of expressing concentrations of solutions. Percentage, as it applies to solutions, may have different meanings. Obviously, in a *true percentage solution,* the percentage refers to parts of solute, by weight, per 100 parts of solution, by weight. However, in pharmaceutical practice, the term percentage used without qualification refers to the number of g. (or ml. in the case of a liquid) of solute per 100 ml. of solution and is used regardless of whether water or another liquid is the solvent.

More recently, the pharmacist has encountered a different method for designating the concentration of solutions, one in which chemical units, rather than physical units, are employed. A *chemical unit,* the *milliequivalent,* is now used almost exclusively to express the concentration of electrolyte solutions, such as isotonic sodium chloride solution. This unit of measure is related to the total number of ionic charges in solution, and it takes note of the valence of the ions. In other words, it is a unit of measurement of the amount of *chemical activity* of the solute.

The meaning of the expressions and symbols used in the methods which have been discussed are summarized in Table 3-1.

OFFICIAL SOLUTIONS

The term "solution" as used by the *U.S.P.* and the *N.F.* has a more limited meaning than the general definition which was stated earlier. The official solutions are liquid preparations that contain one or more soluble chemical substances dissolved in liquid solvents and that do not, by reason of their ingredients (sucrose) or their method of preparation (injections) fall into another category of liquid dosage forms. The solute is usually nonvolatile.

The solvent most commonly used in preparing the official solutions is water. Other liquids, such as alcohol and glycerin, are specified in some of the monographs. The solutes vary widely as to their nature and include solids, liquids and gases. Differences in composition, method of preparation,

TABLE 3-1.   METHODS OF EXPRESSING THE CONCENTRATIONS OF SOLUTIONS

EXPRESSION	SYMBOL	DEFINITION
Percent weight in volume	% w/v	Percent weight in volume expresses the number of g. of a solute in 100 ml. of a solution.
Percent volume in volume	% v/v	Percent volume in volume expresses the number of ml. of a solute in 100 ml. of a solution.
Percent weight in weight	% w/w	Percent weight in weight expresses the number of g. of a solute in 100 g. of a solution.
Milliequivalent	mEq	A milliequivalent is a unit of measure which represents the amount, expressed in g. or mg., of a solute equal to 1/1,000 of its gram equivalent weight. In other words, a milliequivalent expresses the number of g. of solute contained in 1 ml. of a *normal solution.* It is a unit of measurement of the amount of chemical activity of an electrolyte.

strength, potency, mode of administration, use, and dosage contribute to the diverse nature of this class of liquid preparations.

USES

The official solutions are used for many and varied purposes. Some are intended to be used for the specific therapeutic effect, either internally or externally, of the ingredients which they contain; others are used as ingredients in the compounding of prescriptions or in the formulation of other official preparations; and still others serve as reagents in various processes, as solvents for certain substances and as coloring agents for pharmaceutical products.

PREPARATION AND CLASSIFICATION

The methods by which the official solutions are prepared are no less varied than the uses for which they are intended. Because the concentration of solutions varies widely, from 0.05 percent to 100 percent, weight-to-volume, and because nearly every solution is prepared by a special method, there is no general formula for the class, and no type processes can be given for the manufacture of the group as a whole. However, for the purpose of study, the following classification based on the type of procedure involved in the preparation of solutions seems to be practicable:

1. Solutions prepared by simple solution

2. Solutions prepared by chemical reaction

3. Solutions prepared by simple solution with sterilization
   A. Anticoagulant, irrigating, and physiologic solutions
   B. Ophthalmic solutions
   C. Ophthalmic solutions prepared from sterile ophthalmic powders

4. Solutions prepared by extraction

It is not intended to imply in the division given above that there is any fundamental difference in character between a simple solution and a chemical solution. Identical solutions of calcium hydroxide can be prepared by dissolving calcium hydroxide in water or by slaking lime (calcium oxide) with an excess of water in which it dissolves after first reacting to form calcium hydroxide. On the other hand, a solution made by chemical reaction is often more complex than a corresponding simple solution because it contains all the products of the reactions that have taken place during the method of preparation.

The official compendia direct the preparation of certain solutions by methods involving chemical reactions for three principal reasons:

1. The desired therapeutic substance may not be obtainable or readily usable in a form other than that of a solution (formaldehyde solution, hydrogen peroxide solution and others).

2. The pure solute may not dissolve readily from the solid state (aluminum subacetate solution).

3. The several products resulting from the chemical reaction may be desirable constituents of the preparation (magnesium citrate solution).

Some of the official solutions are prepared in sterile form for special uses. These include ophthalmic solutions, anticoagulant solutions for mixing with blood, irrigating solutions, and physiologic solutions that are intended to be used per se or as vehicles for other medicaments for application to delicate mucous membranes. Sterile solutions intended for parenteral administration are now classified as Injections.

OPHTHALMIC SOLUTIONS

Ophthalmic solutions, or *collyria,* are required by the *U.S.P.* and the *N.F.* to be sterile and, if packaged in multiple-dose containers, to contain a suitable substance or mixture of substances to prevent the growth of, or to destroy, microorganisms introduced accidentally when the containers are opened in use. These requirements are consistent with a ruling from the Food and Drug Administration in regard to liquid preparations for ophthalmic use.

Because of the very nature of their use, the *sterility* of ophthalmic solutions is one of the most important considerations in their preparation. Autoclaving in the final container is the preferred method of sterilizing ophthalmic solutions. However, since no specific procedure is directed in any instance (see monograph on Ophthalmic Solutions in both the *U.S.P.* and the *N.F.*), the methods of attaining sterility are determined by the character of a particular product. Sterilization methods and procedures are discussed in detail in Chapter 8.

Several *preservatives* have been suggested for use in ophthalmic solutions. These include: (1) phenylethyl alcohol in a concentration of 0.5 percent; (2) chlorobutanol in a concentration of 0.5 percent; (3) benzalkonium chloride in a concentration of 0.01 percent (1 in 10,000); and (4) phenylmercuric nitrate in 0.001 percent concentration (1 in 100,000). However, any preservative which is harmless yet effective in the concentration employed is acceptable. Ophthalmic solutions that are intended for surgical use must be sterile and must not contain any preservative. Such solutions should be packaged in single-use disposable containers.

Ideally, ophthalmic solutions should be *isotonic* with the lacrimal fluid. Although the eye can tolerate tonicity values above and below that corresponding to a 0.9 percent sodium chloride solution, an adjusted solution is less likely to produce discomfort or irritation to the eye. The amount of osmotic adjustment needed to make solutions which are isotonic with the lacrimal fluid varies with the amount and chemical nature of the active medicament. The methods which are used for adjusting the tonicity of ophthalmic solutions depend upon the *colligative* properties of solutions. In using any of the accepted methods, it is important to remember that the agent which is used to adjust the tonicity of solutions must be compatible with the active medicament.

The optimum pH for the stability and solubility of many drugs, notably the alkaloidal salts which are used in preparing ophthalmic solutions, may not be the same as the pH at which the optimum therapeutic response takes place. These drugs are most effective at pH levels that favor the undissociated free base because it is lipoid-soluble and can penetrate the cornea rapidly. The salt of the free base is water-soluble and does not penetrate the cornea easily. The lacrimal fluid has a pH of 7.4. Ideally, an ophthalmic solution should have the same pH as the lacrimal fluid. However, this is not usually possible because at this pH many drugs are not appreciably soluble in water, and most alkaloidal salts precipitate at this level. Therefore, a pH must be found which represents a compromise between optimum stability and maximum therapeutic effect, and this level must be held by means of *buffers.* The buffer system that is used should have the pH that is nearest to the physiologic pH of 7.4 and at which precipitation of the drug does not occur. The *U.S.P.* and *N.F.* give formulas for buffer vehicles which may be used for specific drugs.

Increased *viscosity* of ophthalmic solutions offers prolonged contact with the tissue, thus possibly enhancing the penetration and therapeutic effect of the drug. Thickening agents such as methylcellulose (1% if the viscosity is 25 cps, or 0.25% if 4,000 cps) may be added to ophthalmic solutions to increase the viscosity.

In the extemporaneous compounding of ophthalmic solutions, it is recommended that aseptic conditions be maintained throughout if contamination is to be avoided. All intermediate containers used in their preparation and the final container should be sterilized. If the dispensing container is a dropper-bottle unit, the accompanying dropper top may be stapled into a stiff paper envelope and autoclaved separately. The solvents used should be sterile distilled water or water for injection.

The *U.S.P.* recognizes two ophthalmic powders, Chloramphenicol and Echothiophate Iodide, and the *N.F.* includes Ophthalmic Chlortetracycline Hydrochloride, Ophthalmic Oxytetracycline Hydrochloride and Tetracycline Hydrochloride, which are intended for preparing solutions for use in the eye. Each of these preparations is official as a sterile, dry mixture with suitable buffers, preservatives and diluents. Prior to dispensing, sterile distilled water is added to the dry powder to make a solution of the desired concentration.

OTHER OFFICIAL SOLUTIONS

Two dry powders, Sodium Cloxacillin for Solution and Sodium Oxacillin for Solution, are included in the *U.S.P.*; and one dry powder, Potassium Phenethicillin for Oral Solution, is included in the *N.F.* From these powders, solutions suitable for oral administration may be prepared by the addition of water.

The *U.S.P.* recognizes two Tablets for Solution, Halazone and Potassium Permanganate, which are intended for the extemporaneous preparation of solutions.

One official solution, Epinephrine Solution, is prepared by extraction of the active principles from suitable animal tissues.

The official solutions prepared by these methods are summarized in Tables 3-2 through 3-9. The individual monographs of the *U.S.P.* and *N.F.* should be consulted for more detailed information concerning any specific solution. Former titles, common names or synonyms of certain official solutions are given in Table 3-10, and some unofficial solutions are summarized in Table 3-11.

TABLE 3-2. OFFICIAL SOLUTIONS PREPARED BY SIMPLE SOLUTION

OFFICIAL NAME	COMMERCIAL COUNTERPART(S)	STRENGTH OF OFFICIAL SOLUTION OR OF ITS COMMERCIAL COUNTERPART	CATEGORY OR USE(S)	COMMENTS
Amaranth Solution, U.S.P.		1% amaranth in purified water	Coloring agent	Imparts red color to clear liquid preparations.
Compound Amaranth Solution, N.F.		9% amaranth solution and 10% caramel in hydroalcoholic solution	Coloring agent	Imparts a reddish-brown color to clear liquid preparations.
Strong Ammonia Solution, N.F.		27-30% (w/w) ammonia in aqueous solution	Solvent; reagent; source of ammonia	Loses ammonia rapidly upon exposure to air. Store in tight containers preferably at a temperature not exceeding 25°C.
Antipyrine and Benzocaine Solution, N.F.	Auralgan	5.4% antipyrine and 1.4% benzocaine in dehydrated glycerin	Local anesthetic; otic decongestant	Administered by instilling into ear canal.
Benzalkonium Chloride Solution, U.S.P.	Zephiran Chloride Solution	1:750 aqueous solution; 17% buffered aqueous concentrate	Topical anti-infective; surface disinfectant; cationic detergent and germicide	Ordinary soaps which are anionic detergents may interfere with its germicidal action.
Benzethonium Chloride Solution, N.F.	Phemerol Chloride Solution	1:750 aqueous solution; 3% topical solution	Local anti-infective, surface-active germicide and antiseptic	Activity, like that of other quaternary ammonium compounds, is decreased by anionic detergents.
Calcium Cyclamate and Calcium Saccharin Solution, N.F.	Sucaryl Sweetening Solution	6% calcium cyclamate and 0.6% calcium saccharin in aqueous solution	Non-nutritive sweetener	Because of absence of sodium ion, it may be used by persons on low-sodium diets.
Dioctyl Sodium Sulfosuccinate Solution, N.F.	Colace; Doxinate	1% and 5% aqueous solution	Fecal matter softener	Usually administered in milk or orange juice to mask its bitter taste.
Diphenoxylate Hydrochloride and Atropine Sulfate Solution, N.F.	Lomotil Liquid	2.5 mg. diphenoxylate hydrochloride and 0.025 mg. atropine sulfate in each 5 ml.	Antidiarrheal (narcotic)	Atropine sulfate is added to minimize the addiction potential of diphenoxylate hydrochloride. Solution should not be administered with barbiturates.
Ephedrine Sulfate Solution, U.S.P.		3% ephedrine sulfate and 0.5% chlorobutanol in an isotonic solution	Adrenergic	For use on mucous membranes of the nose, it should be diluted with an equal volume of isotonic sodium chloride solution.
Ergocalciferol Solution, U.S.P.	Drisdol	250 mcg. (10,000 U.S.P. Vitamin D units) of ergocalciferol in each g.	Antirachitic	Clear liquid having the characteristics of the solvent used (edible vegetable oil, polysorbate 80, or propylene glycol).
Gentian Violet Solution, U.S.P.		1% gentian violet in hydroalcoholic (10% alcohol) solution	Topical local anti-infective	Used topically in undiluted form in infections caused by gram-positive bacteria or by certain parasitic fungi.

TABLE 3-2 *(Continued)*

Official Name	Commercial Counterpart(s)	Strength of Official Solution or of its Commercial Counterpart	Category or Use(s)	Comments
Haloperidol Solution, N.F.	Haldol	2 mg. haloperidol per ml.	Tranquilizer (major)	Used for control of moderate to severe psychomotor agitation, anxiety and tension.
Hexylcaine Hydrochloride Solution, N.F.	Cyclaine Hydrochloride Solution	5% isotonic solution	Local anesthetic	Concentrations of 1 to 5% used for topical application by spray, cotton applicator, or tampons to mucous membranes. As potent as equal concentrations of cocaine.
Iodine Solution, N.F.		2% iodine and 2.4% sodium iodide in aqueous solution	Local anti-infective	Used as a skin and surgical disinfectant.
Strong Iodine Solution, U.S.P.		5% iodine and 10% potassium iodide in an aqueous solution	Source of iodine	Commonly known as Lugol's Solution. Administered internally for systemic effect of iodine; the usual dose is 0.3 ml. diluted with water or milk, 3 times a day.
Naphazoline Hydrochloride Solution, N.F.	Privine Hydrochloride Solution	0.05 and 0.1% isotonic, buffered solution	Vasoconstrictor	Used to relieve congestion and swelling of nasal mucosa due to colds, hay fever and other allergic conditions.
Neomycin Sulfate Oral Solution, U.S.P.	Mycifradin Sulfate Oral Solution	125 mg. neomycin sulfate per 5 ml.	Antibacterial	Used in bacterial diarrheas. Also used preoperatively for intestinal antisepsis to "sterilize" the intestinal tract before abdominal surgery.
Nitrofurazone Solution, N.F.	Furacin Solution	0.2% (w/w) nitrofurazone in a mixture of polyethylene glycols	Local anti-infective	Used topically in the prophylaxis and treatment of mixed infections. Applied directly to the infected area or to bandage covering the area.
Nitromersol Solution, N.F.	Metaphen Solution	0.2% nitromersol	Local anti-infective	Dilutions should be prepared as needed since they tend to precipitate on standing.
Oxymetazoline Hydrochloride Solution, N.F.	Afrin	0.05% aqueous solution adjusted to suitable pH and tonicity	Vasoconstrictor; nasal decongestant	Used topically.
Paramethadione Solution, U.S.P.	Paradione Solution	30% paramethadione in dilute alcohol	Anticonvulsant	Solution should be diluted before administration. Indicated in the treatment of petit mal, myoclonic and akinetic epilepsy.

TABLE 3-2 (*Continued*)

OFFICIAL NAME	COMMERCIAL COUNTERPART(S)	STRENGTH OF OFFICIAL SOLUTION OR OF ITS COMMERCIAL COUNTERPART	CATEGORY OR USE(S)	COMMENTS
Phenylephrine Hydrochloride Solution, U.S.P.	Neo-Synephrine Hydrochloride Solution	0.125 to 10% isotonic solutions	Vasoconstrictor	Used topically to mucous membranes to relieve nasal congestion. An effective ophthalmic decongestant and mydriatic.
Potassium Iodide Solution, N.F.		Saturated solution of potassium iodide in purified water	Iodide supplement; expectorant	Each ml. of the solution contains 1 g. of potassium iodide. Should be well diluted with water or milk prior to administration.
Povidone-Iodine Solution, N.F.	Betadine Antiseptic Solution	5, 7.5, 10 and 30% solutions of povidone-iodine equivalent to 0.5, 0.75, 1 and 3% of available iodine	Local anti-infective	Used topically for the preoperative disinfection of the skin, and as a general microbicide.
Sodium Cyclamate and Sodium Saccharin Solution, N.F.	Sucaryl Sodium Sweetening Solution	6% sodium cyclamate and 0.6% sodium saccharin in aqueous solution	Non-nutritive sweetener	In sweetening power each 0.9 ml. (approximately 1/5 tsp.) is equivalent to about 2 tsp. of sugar.
Sodium Iodide I 125 Solution, U.S.P.		Available in such volumes as may be requested by the physician	Diagnostic aid (thyroid function determination)	Usual diagnostic dose, the equivalent of 50 to 100 microcuries of I 125.
Sodium Iodide I 131 Solution, U.S.P.		Available in such volumes as may be requested by the physician	Antineoplastic; diagnostic aid (thyroid function determination)	Usual diagnostic dose, the equivalent of 1 to 100 microcuries of I 131; the therapeutic dose, the equivalent of 1 to 200 microcuries of I 131.
Sodium Phosphate Solution, N.F.		75.5% sodium phosphate in a glycerin-water solution	Mild saline cathartic	Palatable dosage form of sodium phosphate.
Sodium Phosphate P32 Solution, U.S.P.	Phosphotope Solution	Available in such volumes as may be requested by the physician	Antineoplastic; antipolycythemic; diagnostic aid (tumor localization)	Usual diagnostic dose, the equivalent of 250 microcuries to 1 millicurie; the therapeutic dose, the equivalent of 1 to 12 millicuries of P32.
Sorbitol Solution, U.S.P.		70%, by weight, of total solids consisting essentially of sorbitol and a small amount of mannitol and other isomeric polyhydric alcohols	Flavored vehicle; humectant and sweetener	Used as an emollient and moisture-conditioning agent in various cosmetic and pharmaceutical formulations.
Tetrahydrozoline Hydrochloride Solution, N.F.	Tyzine Solution	0.05 and 0.1% solution adjusted to suitable tonicity	Vasoconstrictor; nasal decongestant	Applied topically by dropper or spray.
Thimerosal Solution, N.F.	Merthiolate Solution	0.1% thimerosal buffered with ethylenediamine and sodium borate	Local anti-infective	Used as an antiseptic or disinfectant for topical application to wounds and abrasions.

TABLE 3-2 (*Continued*)

OFFICIAL NAME	COMMERCIAL COUNTERPART(S)	STRENGTH OF OFFICIAL SOLUTION OR OF ITS COMMERCIAL COUNTERPART	CATEGORY OR USE(S)	COMMENTS
Thoridazine Hydrochloride Solution, U.S.P.	Mellaril Concentrate	3% thoridazine hydrochloride	Major tranquilizer	Must be diluted to appropriate strength with water or suitable juices prior to administration. Useful in a wide range of emotional and mental disturbances.
Tolnaftate Solution, U.S.P.	Tinactin	1% tolnaftate in a nonaqueous, homogeneous vehicle of polyethylene glycol 400	Antifungal	Used topically in the treatment of superficial fungous infections of the skin.
Tribromoethanol Solution, N.F.	Avertin with Amylene Hydrate	100% (w/v) tribromoethanol in amylene hydrate	Basal anesthetic	Must be diluted, just before use, with 40 times its volume of warm purified water.
Trimethadione Solution, U.S.P.	Tridione Solution	4% trimethadione in a flavored aqueous vehicle	Anticonvulsant	Useful in the petit mal type of epilepsy.
Tuaminoheptane Sulfate Solution, N.F.	Tuamine Sulfate Solution	1% tuaminoheptane sulfate in water adjusted to a suitable pH and tonicity	Adrenergic; nasal vasoconstrictor	Claimed to have the advantage of longer duration of action over solutions of ephedrine sulfate.
Xylometazoline Hydrochloride Solution, N.F.	Otrivin	0.05 and 0.1% xylometazoline hydrochloride in water adjusted to a suitable pH and tonicity	Adrenergic (vasoconstrictor)	Used topically for the relief of nasal congestion.

TABLE 3-3. OFFICIAL ORAL SOLUTIONS PREPARED FROM DRY POWDERS BY RECONSTITUTION

OFFICIAL NAME	COMMERCIAL COUNTERPART(S)	SIZES AVAILABLE	CATEGORY AND USE	COMMENTS
Potassium Phenethicillin for Oral Solution, N.F.	Chemipen; Darcil; Maxipen; Syncillin	Powder available in 60 ml. and 150 ml. containers and, when reconstituted, yields a solution containing 125 mg. (200,000 units) of phenethicillin as the potassium salt per 5 ml.	Antibacterial; used in the treatment of a variety of bacterial infections due to penicillin-susceptible organisms.	Reconstituted solution should be kept under refrigeration. May be kept for 2 weeks without significant loss of potency.
Sodium Cloxacillin for Solution, U.S.P.	Tegopen	Dry mixture available in 80 ml. and 150 ml. containers and, when reconstituted, yields a solution containing 125 mg. of cloxacillin as the sodium salt per 5 ml.	Antibacterial; used in the treatment of severe staphylococcal infections due to penicillinase-positive organisms.	Reconstituted solution should be stored under refrigeration. Unused portions should be discarded after 14 days.
Sodium Oxacillin for Solution, U.S.P.	Prostaphlin	Dry mixture available in 100 ml. containers and, when reconstituted, contains 250 mg. of sodium oxacillin per 5 ml.	Antibacterial; used in the treatment of infections known to be due to penicillinase-producing staphylococci which have been shown to be sensitive to it.	Reconstituted solution is stable for 1 week when stored under refrigeration.

TABLE 3-4.   OFFICIAL SOLUTIONS PREPARED BY CHEMICAL REACTION

OFFICIAL NAME	% STRENGTH	METHOD OF PREPARATION	CATEGORY OR USE	COMMENTS
Aluminum Acetate Solution, U.S.P.	5% neutral aluminum acetate, Al- $(C_2H_3O_2)_3$	Prepared by adding glacial acetic acid to aluminum subacetate solution and diluting with water.	Astringent; for topical application, it is usually diluted with 10 to 40 parts of water; an ingredient in dermatologic lotions, ointments and pastes.	Commonly known as Burow's Solution. Boric acid is used to retard or prevent the precipitation of the basic acetate. Dispense only when clear.
Aluminum Subacetate Solution, U.S.P.	8% basic aluminum acetate, Al (OH)- $(C_2H_3O_2)_2$	Prepared by reacting aluminum sulfate with acetic acid and precipitated calcium carbonate, removing the precipitate, and diluting with water.	Astringent; used topically, diluted with 20 to 40 parts of water, as a wash or wet dressing in eczematous conditions of the skin.	Stabilized by adding boric acid.
Saponated Cresol Solution, U.S.P.	50% cresol in an aqueous saponated solution	Prepared by the saponification of a mixture of cresol and vegetable oils or mixed fatty acids derived therefrom.	Disinfectant and deodorant; usually diluted with 50 to 100 parts of water.	Alcohol is used in its manufacture because of its catalytic effect on the saponification reaction.
Formaldehyde Solution, U.S.P.	Not less than 37%, by weight, of formaldehyde in water	Prepared by oxidation of methyl alcohol in the presence of catalysts. A small amount of unconverted methanol retards polymerization.	Disinfectant; for disinfection of inanimate objects, in full strength or as a 10% solution.	Commonly known as Formalin and Formol. An ingredient of embalming fluids.
Hydrogen Peroxide Solution, U.S.P.	3% hydrogen peroxide	Prepared by the decomposition of barium peroxide with phosphoric acid or diluted sulfuric acid; or by the hydrolysis of persulfuric acid.	Topical anti-infective; used for cleansing of wounds and suppurative areas.	Capable of liberating 10 times its volume of oxygen; hence, it is called "10 volume peroxide."
Magnesium Citrate Solution, N.F.	Each 100 ml. contains the equivalent of 1.55 to 1.9 g. of magnesium oxide	Prepared by reacting magnesium carbonate with citric acid, and sweetening, flavoring and carbonating the liquid.	Cathartic	The N.F. directs that the solution be packaged in bottles containing not less than 200 ml. Should be stored in a cool place, preferably in a refrigerator to prevent spoilage.
Sodium Hypochlorite Solution, N.F.	4 to 6% of sodium hypochlorite	Prepared by the electrolysis of a cold dilute solution of common salt.	Disinfectant; deodorant and bleaching agent	The N.F. cautions that the solution is not suitable for application to wounds.
Diluted Sodium Hypochlorite Solution, N.F.	0.45 to 0.50% of sodium hypochlorite	Prepared by diluting Sodium Hypochlorite Solution and adjusting its alkalinity.	Local anti-infective; used as a surgical disinfectant, undiluted or diluted with from 1 to 3 volumes of water.	Solution has a faintly alkaline reaction in order that it may best exert its therapeutic action.

TABLE 3-5.   OFFICIAL SOLUTIONS PREPARED BY SIMPLE SOLUTION WITH STERILIZATION
ANTICOAGULANT, IRRIGATING, AND PHYSIOLOGIC SOLUTIONS

OFFICIAL NAME	CONCENTRATION OF ACTIVE INGREDIENT(S)	SOLUTIONS AVAILABLE	CATEGORY AND USE(S)	COMMENTS
Aminoacetic Acid Sterile Solution, N.F.	Sterile solution of 1.5 and 15% aminoacetic acid in water for injection	1.5% in 1500, 2000, and 3000 ml.; 15% concentrate in 1000 ml.	Irrigating fluid in the transurethral resection of the prostate; a non-hemolyzing irrigant	Commercially available as Urogate Glycine Solution for Urologic Irrigation. The 15% concentrate requires dilution, aseptically, before use.
Anticoagulant Citrate Dextrose Solution, U.S.P.	Sterile solution of $$\begin{array}{cc} A & B \\ \hline \text{citric acid} & \\ 7.3\% & 4.4\% \\ \text{sodium citrate} & \\ 22.0\% & 13.2\% \\ \text{dextrose} & \\ 24.5\% & 14.7\% \end{array}$$ in water for injection	Solution A-37.5, 67.5, and 75 ml. Solution B-30, 60, 110, and 120 ml.	Anticoagulant for storage of whole blood	Solution must be labeled to indicate the number of ml. required per 100 ml. of whole blood. The U.S.P. states that 25 ml. of Solution A or 125 ml. of Solution B should be used for each 500 ml. of whole blood.
Anticoagulant Citrate Phosphate Dextrose Solution, U.S.P.	Sterile solution of 3.0% citric acid, 26.3% sodium citrate, 2.22% sodium biphosphate, and 25.5% dextrose in water for injection		Anticoagulant for storage of whole blood	Solution must be labeled to indicate the number of ml. required per 100 ml. of whole blood. The U.S.P. states that 70 ml. of the solution should be used for each 500 ml. of whole blood.
Anticoagulant Heparin Solution, U.S.P.	Sterile solution of 75,000 units of sodium heparin in sodium chloride injection	Containers holding 2025, 2125, and 2250 units	Anticoagulant for storage of whole blood	Solution must be labeled in terms of U.S.P. Heparin Units and to indicate the number of ml. required per 100 ml. of whole blood. The U.S.P. states that 30 ml. of the solution should be used for each 500 ml. of whole blood.
*Ringer's Solution, N.F.	Isotonic solution of 8.6% sodium chloride, 0.3% potassium chloride and 0.33% of calcium chloride in purified water		Irrigation solution; a physiologic salt solution which is used as a solvent for medicinal substances which are to be applied topically to delicate tissues.	Solution is not to be used for parenteral administration or in preparations to be used parenterally.

TABLE 3-5 (*Continued*)

Official Name	Concentration of Active Ingredient(s)	Solutions Available	Category and Use(s)	Comments
*Sodium Chloride Solution, U.S.P.	Solution of 0.9% sodium chloride in purified water.		Isotonic vehicle; used as a solvent for medications that are intended to be applied topically.	Designation "non-sterilized" or "not sterilized" must appear prominently on the label unless the solution has been rendered sterile. Not to be used for parenteral administration or for irrigation that may result in absorption of the solution into the blood.
Anticoagulant Sodium Citrate Solution, N.F.	Sterile Solution of 4% sodium citrate in water for injection		Anticoagulant for plasma and for blood fractionation	Prevents clotting of blood by combining with serum calcium ions to form nonionizing calcium citrate. Used in the proportion of 50 ml. to 500 ml. of normal plasma or blood.

* Although these solutions should be classified more properly with those made by simple solution without sterilization, they are included here because of their use.

TABLE 3-6.   OFFICIAL SOLUTIONS PREPARED BY SIMPLE SOLUTION WITH STERILIZATION
OPHTHALMIC SOLUTIONS

OFFICIAL NAME	COMMERCIAL COUNTER-PART(S)	CONCENTRATION(S) OF OFFICIAL SOLUTION OR ITS COMMERCIAL COUNTER-PART(S)	PRESERVATIVE, BUFFER AND TONICIC AGENTS	CATEGORY AND USE(S) COMMENTS
Antazoline Phosphate Ophthalmic Solution, N.F.	Antistine Ophthalmic Solution	0.5% sterile, aqueous solution of antazoline phosphate	Isotonic	Antihistamine; used for symptomatic relief of certain conditions of the eye resulting from allergies.
Atropine Sulfate Ophthalmic Solution, U.S.P.	Isopto Atropine; Murocoll Atropine	0.125, 0.25, 0.5, 1, 2, 3, and 4% of atropine sulfate in sterile, aqueous solution	Isotonic; may contain suitable stabilizers and antimicrobial agents.	Ophthalmic anticholinergic; produces mydriasis and cycloplegia; contraindicated in persons with glaucoma
Carbachol Ophthalmic Solution, U.S.P.	Carba-miotin	0.75, 1.5, 2.25, and 3% carbachol in a sterile, aqueous medium	Isotonic; may contain suitable preservatives and antimicrobial agents.	Ophthalmic cholinergic; used to produce effective miosis in the treatment of chronic congestive glaucoma.
Cyclopentolate Hydrochloride Ophthalmic Solution, U.S.P.	Cyclogyl	0.5, 1.0, and 2.0% cyclopentolate hydrochloride as a sterile, aqueous solution	Isotonic and buffered	Cycloplegic and mydriatic; suggested for routine office use to prepare the eye for refraction when fitting glasses; used in iritis and keratitis.
Demecarium Bromide Ophthalmic Solution, U.S.P.	Humorsol	0.125 and 0.25% demecarium bromide in sterile, aqueous solution	Contains a suitable antimicrobial agent.	Ophthalmic cholinergic; used topically in the treatment of chronic glaucoma.
Dexamethasone Sodium Phosphate Ophthalmic Solution, N.F.	Decadron Phosphate Ophthalmic Solution	0.1% dexamethasone sodium phosphate in sterile aqueous solution		Glucocorticoid; used in various forms of conjunctivitis, lid allergies and other inflammatory conditions of the eye.
Dyclonine Hydrochloride Solution, U.S.P.	Dyclone Solution	0.5 to 1.0% dyclonine hydrochloride in sterile, aqueous solution	May contain suitable stabilizers and antimicrobial agents.	Topical anesthetic; in minor surgical procedures, it produces anesthesia without mydriasis or miosis when instilled into the eye.
Epinephrine Bitartrate Ophthalmic Solution, U.S.P.	Adrena-trate; Epitrate; Mytrate	1 and 2% epinephrine bitartrate in sterile, aqueous solution	Contains a suitable antibacterial agent; may contain suitable preservatives.	Ophthalmic adrenergic; used topically for reducing intraocular pressure in certain cases of chronic simple glaucoma.
Homatropine Hydrobromide Ophthalmic Solution, U.S.P.		1, 2, and 5% homatropine hydrobromide in sterile, buffered, aqueous solution	May contain suitable antimicrobial agents.	Ophthalmic anticholinergic; used for its mydriatic effect and as a cycloplegic in eye examination; preferred to atropine because of the shorter mydriasis which it produces.

TABLE 3-6 *(Continued)*

OFFICIAL NAME	COMMERCIAL COUNTERPART(S)	CONCENTRATION(S) OF OFFICIAL SOLUTION OR ITS COMMERCIAL COUNTERPART(S)	PRESERVATIVE, BUFFER AND TONICIC AGENTS	CATEGORY AND USE(S) COMMENTS
Hydroxyamphetamine Hydrobromide Ophthalmic Solution, U.S.P.	Paredrine	1% hydroxyamphetamine hydrobromide in sterile, buffered, aqueous solution	Isotonic; it contains a suitable antimicrobial agent.	Ophthalmic adrenergic; used as an adjuvant to atropine or homatropine to induce a rapid cycloplegia for refraction.
Idoxuridine Ophthalmic Solution, U.S.P.	Dendrid; Herplex; Stoxil	0.1% idoxuridine in sterile, aqueous solution	May contain suitable buffers, stabilizers, and antimicrobial agents.	Ophthalmic antiviral; used in the treatment of herpes simplex; should not be mixed with other medications to insure stability. Store under refrigeration.
Isoflurophate Ophthalmic Solution, U.S.P.	Floropryl	0.1% isopropyl phosphorofluoridate in a sterile, vegetable oil solution		Powerful parasympathomimetic cholinergic; used primarily in the treatment of glaucoma. Must be labeled to indicate the expiration date which is not later than 2 years after the date of manufacture.
Neomycin Sulfate, Polymyxin B, and Gramicidin Ophthalmic Solution, N.F.	Neosporin Ophthalmic Solution	Each ml. contains 5000 units of polymyxin B sulfate, 2.5 mg. of neomycin sulfate, and 0.025 mg. of gramicidin in sterile, aqueous solution	Isotonic; contains thimerosal as a preservative.	Local anti-infective.
Phenylephrine Hydrochloride Ophthalmic Solution, U.S.P.	Neo-Synephrine Ophthalmic Solution	0.125, 2.5, and 10% phenylephrine hydrochloride in sterile, buffered, aqueous solution	Contains a suitable antimicrobial agent and may contain suitable antioxidants.	Adrenergic; used for its vasoconstrictor and mydriatic action.
Pilocarpine Hydrochloride Ophthalmic Solution, U.S.P.	Available commercially under various trade names	0.25, 0.5, 1, 2, 3, 4, 5, 6, 7, 8, and 10% pilocarpine hydrochloride in sterile, buffered, aqueous solution	May contain suitable antimicrobial agents and stabilizers, and suitable additives to increase its viscosity.	Ophthalmic cholinergic; used to control intraocular pressure in glaucoma.
Pilocarpine Nitrate Ophthalmic Solution, U.S.P.	Available commercially under various trade names	0.5, 1, 2, 3, 4, and 6% pilocarpine nitrate in sterile, buffered, aqueous solution	May contain suitable antimicrobial agents and stabilizers, and suitable additives to increase its viscosity.	Ophthalmic cholinergic; used in glaucoma.
Prednisolone Sodium Phosphate Ophthalmic Solution, U.S.P.	Hydeltrasol Solution	0.5% prednisolone sodium phosphate in sterile, buffered, aqueous solution		Adrenocortical steroid; used in inflammatory disorders of the eye, particularly in diseases of the anterior segment of the eye.

TABLE 3-6 (*Continued*)

OFFICIAL NAME	COMMERCIAL COUNTERPART(S)	CONCENTRATION(S) OF OFFICIAL SOLUTION OR ITS COMMERCIAL COUNTERPART(S)	PRESERVATIVE, BUFFER AND TONICIC AGENTS	CATEGORY AND USE(S) COMMENTS
Proparacaine Hydrochloride Ophthalmic Solution, U.S.P.	Ophthaine Solution	0.5% proparacaine hydrochloride in sterile, aqueous solution	Commercial product contains glycerin as a stabilizer, is buffered, and contains preservatives.	Rapid-acting local anesthetic for ophthalmic use; must be stored in refrigerator after the container is opened.
*Silver Nitrate Ophthalmic Solution, U.S.P.		1% silver nitrate in a water medium. Available in collapsible capsules containing about 0.3 ml.	May be buffered by the addition of sodium acetate.	Topical anti-infective; used primarily for the prevention of gonococcic infections of the eyes of newborn infants.
Sodium Fluorescein Ophthalmic Solution, U.S.P.		2% sodium fluorescein in sterile, buffered, aqueous solution	Contains a suitable antimicrobial agent, and may contain 3% sodium bicarbonate.	Corneal trauma indicator; used as a diagnostic aid for disclosing corneal injuries and ulcers.
Sodium Sulfacetamide Ophthalmic Solution, U.S.P.	Sodium Sulamyd	10 and 30% sodium sulfacetamide in sterile, aqueous solution	May contain suitable buffers, stabilizers, and antimicrobial agents.	Antibacterial; used topically in the eye for bacterial infections that are susceptible to sulfonamide therapy.
Tetrahydrozoline Hydrochloride Ophthalmic Solution, N.F.	Tyzine	0.05 and 0.1% tetrahydrozoline hydrochloride in sterile, aqueous solution		Adrenergic; possesses vasoconstrictor and decongestant properties when applied topically.
Tropicamide Ophthalmic Solution, U.S.P.	Mydriacyl	0.5 and 1% tropicamide in sterile, buffered aqueous solution	Contains a suitable antimicrobial agent, and may contain suitable substances to increase its viscosity.	Ophthalmic anticholinergic; used as a mydriatic and cycloplegic.
Zinc Sulfate Ophthalmic Solution, U.S.P.	Commercially available under various trade names	0.1 to 0.25% zinc sulfate in sterile, aqueous solution	Made isotonic by the addition of suitable salts.	Ophthalmic astringent; used for the treatment of conjunctivitis.

* Although this solution should be classified more properly with those made by simple solution without sterilization, it is included here because of its use.

TABLE 3-7.　OFFICIAL OPHTHALMIC SOLUTIONS PREPARED FROM STERILE OPHTHALMIC POWDERS

OFFICIAL NAME	COMMERCIAL COUNTERPART	SIZES AVAILABLE	CATEGORY AND USE(S)	COMMENTS
Chloramphenicol for Ophthalmic Solution, U.S.P.	Chloromycetin Ophthalmic	25 mg. chloramphenicol with boric acid-sodium borate buffer	Antibacterial; used topically in the treatment of bacterial conjunctivitis.	Solution is prepared by adding sterile distilled water to the powder in sufficient quantity to make a 0.16, 0.25, or 0.5% solution. It remains stable at room temperature for 10 days.
Ophthalmic Chlortetracycline Hydrochloride, N.F.	Aureomycin Ophthalmic Powder, Sterilized	25 mg. chlortetracycline hydrochloride with a suitable buffer	Antibacterial; used topically for the treatment of ocular viral and bacterial infections.	Powder is dissolved in 5 ml. of sterile distilled water; when stored under refrigeration, the solution remains stable for 2 days.
Echothiophate Iodide for Ophthalmic Solution, U.S.P.	Phospholine Iodide	1.5, 3, 6.25, 12.5, and 125 mg. echothiophate iodide with mannitol or other suitable diluent	Ophthalmic cholinergic; used topically to the conjunctiva for the control of intraocular tension in glaucoma.	Solutions of appropriate strength, 0.03, 0.06, 0.125, and 0.25% are freshly prepared by dissolving the powder in a sterile, buffered solvent.
Ophthalmic Oxytetracycline Hydrochloride, N.F.	Terramycin Hydrochloride Ophthalmic	25 mg. oxytetracycline hydrochloride with a suitable buffer and/or bacteriostatic agent	Antibacterial; used topically in the eye for the treatment of ocular infections caused by a wide range of pathogens.	Solution is prepared by dissolving the powder in 5 ml. of sterile distilled water; remains stable for 48 hours if stored in a refrigerator.
Tetracycline Hydrochloride for Ophthalmic Solution, N.F.	Achromycin Ophthalmic Powder, Sterilized	25 mg. tetracycline hydrochloride with one or more suitable buffers	Antibacterial; used topically by application to eyelid or conjunctiva.	Solution is prepared by dissolving the powder in 5 ml. of sterile distilled water; remains stable for 2 days if stored in a refrigerator.

TABLE 3-8.　OFFICIAL SOLUTION PREPARED BY EXTRACTION

OFFICIAL NAME	COMMERCIAL COUNTERPART	CONCENTRATION	CATEGORY AND USE	COMMENTS
Epinephrine Solution, U.S.P.	Adrenalin Chloride	1-1000 epinephrine in purified water prepared with the aid of hydrochloric acid; available in containers of 30 ml.	Vasoconstrictor; used to increase blood pressure, to prevent hemorrhage, and to prolong the action of local anesthetics.	U.S.P. notes that the solution should not be used if it becomes brown in color or if it contains a precipitate.

TABLE 3-9. OFFICIAL SOLUTIONS PREPARED FROM TABLETS

OFFICIAL NAME	STRENGTH OF TABLETS AVAILABLE	CATEGORY AND USE(S)	COMMENTS
Halazone Tablets for Solution, U.S.P.	4 mg. of halazone	Disinfectant; for the sterilization of drinking water, 1 or 2 tablets per liter may be employed.	The tablets should be labeled to indicate that they are not intended to be swallowed.
Potassium Permanganate Tablets for Solution, U.S.P.	60, 125, and 300 mg. of potassium permanganate	Topical anti-infective; applied topically to the skin and mucous membranes as a 0.004 to 1% solution or in a wet dressing.	Solution of the tablets has a deep violet-red color when concentrated and a pink color when highly diluted. Since potassium permanganate is incompatible with organic material such as might be present in tap water, only distilled water should be used in preparing solutions of it.

TABLE 3-10. FORMER TITLES, COMMON NAMES OR SYNONYMS OF SOME OFFICIAL SOLUTIONS

OFFICIAL TITLE	FORMER TITLE, COMMON NAME, OR SYNONYM
Aluminum Acetate Solution, U.S.P.	Burow's Solution
Strong Ammonia Solution, N.F.	Stronger Ammonia Water; Stronger Ammonium Hydroxide Solution
Anticoagulant Citrate Dextrose Solution, U.S.P.	A.C.D. Solution; Anticoagulant Acid Citrate Dextrose Solution
Calcium Cyclamate and Calcium Saccharin Solution, N.F.	Compound Calcium Cyclamate Solution
Calcium Hydroxide Solution, U.S.P.	Lime Water; Liquor Calcis
Carbol-Fuchsin Solution, N.F.	Castellani's Paint
Coal Tar Solution, U.S.P.	Liquor Carbonis Detergens; Liquor Picis Carbonis
Saponated Cresol Solution, N.F.	Compound Cresol Solution
Cyanocobalamin Co 57 Solution, U.S.P.	Radiocyanocobalamin Solution
Ergocalciferol Solution, U.S.P.	Calciferol Solution
Formaldehyde Solution, U.S.P.	Formalin
Gentian Violet Solution, U.S.P.	Methylrosaniline Chloride Solution
Hydrogen Peroxide Solution, U.S.P.	Hydrogen Dioxide Solution
Strong Iodine Solution, U.S.P.	Lugol's Solution; Compound Iodine Solution
Magnesium Citrate Solution, N.F.	Citrate of Magnesia
Potassium Iodide Solution, N.F.	Saturated Potassium Iodide Solution
Ringer's Solution, N.F.	Isotonic Solution of Three Chlorides
Sodium Chloride Solution, U.S.P.	Isotonic Sodium Chloride Solution; Normal Saline Solution
Sodium Cyclamate and Sodium Saccharin Solution, N.F.	Compound Sodium Cyclamate Solution
Diluted Sodium Hypochlorite Solution, N.F.	Modified Dakin's Solution
Sodium Iodide I 131 Solution, U.S.P.	Sodium Radio Iodide Solution
Sodium Phosphate P 32 Solution, U.S.P.	Sodium Radiophosphate Solution
Tribromoethanol Solution, N.F.	Bromethol

TABLE 3-11. UNOFFICIAL SOLUTIONS

TITLE	SYNONYM	DESCRIPTION	PREPARATION	USE
Diluted Ammonia Solution, U.S.P. XVI	Ammonia Water	Clear, colorless liquid, having a very pungent, characteristic odor	Prepared by diluting 308 ml. of strong ammonia solution to 1,000 ml. with purified water.	Possesses stimulant properties because of the ammonium ion which it contains. Its rubefacient properties make it useful as an ingredient in the formulation of stimulating liniments.
N.F. Antiseptic Solution, N.F. XII		Hydroalcoholic solution containing boric acid, thymol, chlorothymol, menthol, eucalyptol, methyl salicylate, and thyme oil	Prepared by dissolving the boric acid in water and the other ingredients in alcohol, mixing the two solutions, allowing to stand for 2 hours or more to ensure complete saturation, cooling to 10°C., and filtering at this temperature, using purified talc if necessary, to remove the excess of volatile principles.	Used as a mouthwash; when employed for this purpose, it should be used undiluted.
Boric Acid Solution, N.F. XII	"Saturated" Boric Acid Solution	An aqueous solution containing not less than 4.25 g. of boric acid in each 100 ml. Although commonly referred to as "Saturated Boric Acid Solution," it is actually undersaturated.	Prepared by dissolving 50 g. of boric acid in 350 ml. of hot distilled water, agitating to ensure complete solution, and immediately adding a sufficient quantity of cold distilled water to make 1000 ml.	Used as a wash and wet dressing for wounds, skin inflammations, and similar conditions. Also used as a cleansing wash for the eyes and as a vehicle in the preparation of collyria and eyedrops. For ophthalmic use, it may be diluted with an equal volume of water so as to produce a solution that is very nearly isotonic with tear fluid.
Ferric Chloride Solution, N.F. XI		A yellowish-orange liquid, having a faint odor of hydrochloric acid and an acid reaction	Prepared by the oxidation of ferrous chloride, using nitric acid, chlorine or hydrogen peroxide.	Hematinic and powerful astringent; sometimes employed as a styptic.
Ferric Subsulfate Solution, N.F. XI	Monsel's Solution	Dark, reddish-brown liquid, odorless or nearly so, with an acid, strongly astringent taste	Prepared by adding ferrous sulfate to a hot, diluted mixture of sulfuric and nitric acids and boiling the combined reactants until the chemical reaction is complete and the solution is free from nitrate ion.	Astringent; in undiluted form, it is used primarily as a styptic for external application by means of cotton swabs.
Sulfurated Lime Solution, N.F. XII	Vleminckx' Solution	Clear, orange liquid with a slight odor of hydrogen sulfide. It must be preserved in	Prepared by boiling a suspension of lime and sublimed sulfur in water.	Diluted with 9 volumes of water, it may be used as a scabicide. Sometimes prescribed

TABLE 3-11 (*Continued*)

TITLE	SYNONYM	DESCRIPTION	PREPARATION	USE
		completely-filled, tight containers, otherwise carbon dioxide will precipitate the calcium as the carbonate, and free sulfur will be liberated.		as an ingredient in dermatologic lotions and creams, particularly in combination with zinc sulfate with which it reacts to form polysulfides of zinc.
Merbromin Solution, N.F. XII		Clear, red liquid having a yellow-green fluorescence	Prepared by dissolving 2% of merbromin in purified water.	Nonirritating antiseptic for local application to minor wounds. When used for this purpose, its reliability is open to question, since merbromin, in aqueous solution, has been shown to have a low phenol coefficient. When combined with acids or acid salts, precipitation results.
Surgical Merbromin Solution, N.F. XII	Scott's Solution	Clear, red liquid with a yellow-green fluorescence	Prepared by dissolving 2% of merbromin in a solvent consisting of approximately 35% of purified water, 10% of acetone, and 55% of neutralized alcohol.	Skin disinfectant, particularly in preparing the skin for surgical operations. Merbromin has been shown to be more effective as a germicide in a vehicle consisting of acetone, alcohol, and water.
N.F. Mouthwash, N.F. XII	Alkaline Aromatic Solution	Clear, bright red liquid, with an aromatic odor and taste	A hydroalcoholic solution containing thymol, eucalyptol, methyl salicylate, and glycerin, alkalinized by sodium borate and potassium bicarbonate, and colored by amaranth solution.	Its uses are the same as those for N.F. Antiseptic Solution, N.F. XII. It possesses a mild alkalinity; and, when diluted with an equal volume of water, it is claimed to be almost isotonic with body fluids. For oral use, the solution should not be diluted; for use in the dental spray bottle, it should be diluted with 5 volumes of water.
Ammoniacal Silver Nitrate Solution, N.F. XII	Ammoniacal Silver Nitrate, Howe	Clear, colorless, almost odorless liquid	Prepared by adding strong ammonia solution to a solution of silver nitrate until all but the last trace of black precipitate is dissolved, and filtering the product.	Dental protective; used by dentists to deposit silver on exposed dentin and to fill up minute crevices in the teeth. For topical application, it is mixed with a reducing agent, such as formaldehyde (1 in 10) or eugenol, so as to deposit the metallic silver in the infected area in a state of fine subdivision.

TABLE 3-11 (*Continued*)

Title	Synonym	Description	Preparation	Use
Compound Sodium Borate Solution, N.F. XI	Dobell's Solution	Clear, colorless or yellowish liquid, with a phenol-like odor	Prepared by dissolving sodium borate and sodium bicarbonate in purified water, adding glycerin and liquefied phenol, allowing the liquid to react until effervescence ceases, and diluting to the required volume with purified water.	Nonirritating alkaline wash for mucous membranes. Used undiluted as a mouthwash and gargle.

BIBLIOGRAPHY

Goodman, L. S., and Gilman, A.: The Pharmacological Basis of Therapeutics. Ed. 4. New York, Macmillan, 1970.

Martin, E. W. (Ed.): Husa's Pharmaceutical Dispensing. Easton, Pa., Mack Publishing Co., 1966.

Martin, A. N.: Physical Pharmacy. Ed. 2. Philadelphia, Lea & Febiger, 1969.

Lewis, A. J. (Ed.): Modern Drug Encyclopedia and Therapeutic Index. Ed. 11. The Yorke Medical Group, New York, 1970.

Parrott, E. L.: Pharmaceutical Technology. Minneapolis, Burgess, 1970.

Remington's Pharmaceutical Sciences. Ed. 14 Easton, Pa., Mack Publishing Co., 1970.

Sprowls, J. B.: Prescription Pharmacy. Ed. 2. Philadelphia, J. B. Lippincott, 1970.

The United States Dispensatory and Physicians' Pharmacology. Ed. 26. Philadelphia, J. B. Lippincott, 1967.

4

Nicholas G. Lordi, Ph.D., *Professor of Pharmacy*
College of Pharmacy, Rutgers, The State University

Aqueous Solutions Containing Aromatic Principles: Waters, Syrups, and Juices

INTRODUCTION

The most efficient dosage forms are solutions—homogeneous mixtures of two or more components in liquid phases. The most important solvent for pharmaceutical solutions is water, the standards for which are found in the *U.S.P.* and specify 5 degrees of purity. These are entitled as follows:

Water
Purified Water
Water for Injection
Sterile Water for Injection
Bacteriostatic Water for Injection

Waters for pharmaceutical use also include a group of flavored and medicated preparations known as *aromatic waters.* These are aqueous solutions, usually saturated, of volatile substances characterized by very low water-solubilities. In aromatic waters, the medical practitioner possesses not only the solvent powers of water but also the enhancing aroma and flavor of natural plant essences or other volatile matter. In former revisions of the official compendia and in some modern foreign pharmacopeias, aromatic waters include solutions of many chemicals as well as essential oils used in flavoring and perfumery. The official aromatic waters are listed in Table 4-1, page 76.

Two important classes of aqueous pharmaceutical preparations which also generally contain aromatic principles are *syrups* and *juices.* Syrups may be defined broadly as sweet, viscous, aqueous liquids designed specifically for medicine to be administered orally. A juice is a liquid obtained by expression from the fresh part of a plant. The *U.S.P.* contains two monographs on juices

made from fresh fruits—Cherry and Raspberry Juices. Some of the foreign official compendia describe juices prepared from fresh leaves, succulent bulbs, etc. *The British Pharmaceutical Codex,* 1968, contains monographs for the juices of black currant and raspberry. In the past, juices frequently served as the base for syrups. Two such syrups are still retained in the *U.S.P.* Table 4-3 (p. 86) lists the official syrups.

Aromatic waters are examples of the simplest of formulated dosage forms, consisting only of the solvent water and the volatile solute. Juices, which may be extremely complex in composition, have characteristics which are not readily controlled by the pharmacist, since they are derived directly from natural sources. On the other hand, syrups are formulated preparations that often contain ingredients, so-called pharmaceutic necessities or adjuvants, which are added to improve the "elegance" of the product. Any pharmaceutical formulation is said to be "elegant" if it meets three standards of quality. It should be stable; it should be palatable, and it should be therapeutically effective.

Pharmaceutical preparations are stable if they show no loss in therapeutic activity and no undesirable chemical and physical changes over extended periods of time. Products should have shelf lives exceeding 2 to 3 years; otherwise, they should be dated. The shelf life may be defined as the time required for the drug level in a product stored at room temperature (nominally 25° C.) to degrade to 90 percent of its labeled potency. Consideration of the stability of a dosage form plays a most important role in formulation. Attention must be paid not only to the therapeutic ingredients but also to the other components of the formulation as well as the possible effects of environmental factors such as microbial contamination, light, atmospheric oxygen, humidity and temperature. In aqueous solutions, especially waters and syrups, growth of microorganisms, particularly molds, may be a problem. Chemical changes which may be observed include hydrolytic degradation and autoxidation. Physical changes which may be observed include precipitation and alteration in color, odor and viscosity. All lead to specification of storage requirements, designed to minimize deterioration of the preparation.

A pharmaceutical preparation is palatable if it is reasonably pleasant to the senses of the person who is to use the product. The problem of flavoring must be considered in the formulation of oral medication. At one time, medicine was viewed as something which should be distasteful (Chap. 1). Today, considerable effort is made to improve the palatability of medication. Emphasis is placed on the combined stimulation of the senses of taste and smell, as well as on "mouth feel" and the appearance of the product. The selection of flavors for pharmaceutical preparations is dictated by a number of factors—among them, the age group for which the medicine is intended, the color of the preparation, the taste to be masked by the preparation and the type of dosage form. Syrups and Aromatic Waters are designed to provide a base which will produce palatable medicinal products. It is important, especially in designing pediatric medication, that this effort should not be carried too far. The advantage of providing medication which is taken willingly by children must be weighed against the danger of making medication as attractive as candy.

A preparation may be perfectly stable and palatable and yet be therapeutically worthless. The therapeutic efficacy of dosage forms is determined by their ability to effect quick release of medicinal agents. Medicaments are physiologically available in syrups and aromatic waters, since these are aqueous solutions. However, if a product is unstable and/or unpalatable, it may also be therapeutically ineffective.

CLARIFICATION

Clarification is an operation which involves the removal of suspended matter from a fluid medium. Aromatic waters, juices, and syrups are designed to be clear liquids. The inadvertent introduction of foreign particles, the precipitation of undesirable materials during the course of manufacture and the presence of impurities in the raw materials used to manufacture the preparation result in requirements for clarification of the preparation as the last stage in its manufacture as well as in preceding steps.

The specific procedures and equipment which may be used to achieve clarification are dependent on a number of factors. These are:

The particle size of the suspended matter: The state of subdivision of the suspended particles may range from the coarse (discrete particles which may be seen by the eye) to the colloidal (particles which cannot be seen in the field of the ordinary microscope unless viewed by their reflected light).

The physical state of the suspended matter: The clarification of aromatic waters and syrups often involves the removal of finely divided insoluble liquids derived from the flavoring ingredients, whereas most clarification problems are concerned with the removal of finely divided solids.

The quantity of suspended matter: The liquid to be clarified may be a slurry, containing a high concentration of solids, or a colloidal dispersion in which the concentration of suspended matter is small.

The characteristics of the fluid medium: Viscosity, the temperature at which the fluid is to be clarified, the presence of volatile constituents in solution, etc., require special consideration.

The speed of the operation: This depends primarily on the quantity of liquid to be clarified.

The principal operations used in clarification are: (a) *settling,* (b) *filtration* and *colation,* and (c) *absorption* and *adsorption.*

SETTLING

The simplest method of clarification is to allow the liquid to stand in a suitable container until the suspended matter either has settled or has risen to the top of the liquid. The latter occurs when the density of the suspended matter is less than that of the fluid medium. The insoluble matter may be separated from the clear liquid phase by skimming, decantation or siphoning. When the suspended particles are large and settle rapidly, this procedure may be advantageous. Moreover, it also may be used to remove fine particles, especially those which tend to flocculate, if a long waiting-period is feasible. If the viscosity of the liquid is high, as is true of syrups, the waiting period may be excessive. In general, the method fails when the suspended matter is colloidal or when its density is approximately equal to that of the liquid phase.

Acceleration of the settling process can be accomplished by centrifugation. In this operation, the liquid is rotated in a special container at high speeds. The centrifugal forces developed in the rotating container drive the suspended particles to the bottom and the sides of the container. The effective force is proportional to the square of the speed of rotation and may be several thousand times the gravitational force involved in natural settling.

Centrifugal clarifiers which have capacities in excess of 20,000 liters per hour are available. Figure 4-1 shows a diagram of a clarifying bowl. Liquid is fed into the bowl at a rate determined by the character of the feed (e.g., viscosity, particle size and concentration of suspended matter) while rotating at high speed. The clear effluent is ejected from special ports. Continuous clarification of the liquid occurs until the holding spaces of the bowl are filled. Then the operation is stopped and the bowl is cleaned manually. Continuous clarifiers have also been designed which enable the sludge to be discharged automatically from the bowl at predetermined intervals.

FILTRATION AND COLATION

Theory. The process of removing solid particles from a fluid by passing the suspension through a porous, fibrous or granular substance is called filtration.[1,2] Colation or

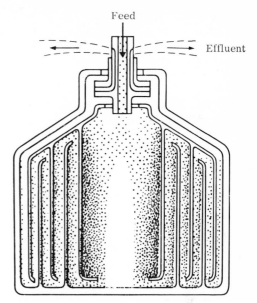

Fig. 4-1.   Clarifying bowl. (From Centrico, Inc.)

straining is crude filtration. The distinction between the two processes is based only on the degree of fineness of the straining or filtration media involved. A filter or strainer consists essentially of a medium which contains numerous pores which may vary considerably in size and shape and may be characterized by a high degree of tortuosity. These effects are achieved by intertwining fibers, layering granular materials or punching holes in suitable materials.

A filter (or strainer) functions primarily by impeding the passage of suspended particles with diameters greater than that of the pores, while allowing the liquid to pass. The retentiveness of filters varies over a wide range, depending on the average pore size. Ultrafilters are filters which are retentive to colloidal matter. Bacteria-, virus-, and pyrogen-retentive filters (see Chap. 14) as well as "microsieves" capable of separating molecules of differing sizes have been developed.

The theory of filtration involves consideration of the factors which influence the rate at which fluids can be passed through a porous medium. These factors are summarized in their simplest form in the following expression:

Rate of Filtration =

$$\frac{\text{(Filter Area) (Pressure Drop)}}{\text{(Liquid Viscosity) (Filter Resistance)}}$$

The rate of filtration, measured as the volume of liquid passed through the filter per unit time, will be reduced in proportion to the filter resistance and viscosity of the filtrate. It will be increased in proportion to the pressure drop across the filter and the filter area. The filter resistance is increased as the size of the pores is decreased and as the tortuosity of the channels through the filter is decreased.

In small-scale filtration the pressure drop is determined by the weight of the liquid above the filter. Usually, this is not great enough to effect filtration in reasonably short periods if highly retentive filters are employed or highly viscous liquids such as syrups are being filtered. Straining is the preferred operation as long as suspended particles are removed by the strainer, in order to take advantage of the higher speeds characteristic of colation. Suction filtration may be employed with properly designed equipment to increase the pressure drop by lowering the pressure beneath the filter, or pressure filtration (in which the pressure above the liquid is increased) may be used.

Another factor which has an important effect on the potential filtration rate is the blocking potential of the particles retained on or in the filter. Small particles which tend to be trapped in the pores can increase the efficiency of filtration, as measured by removal of insoluble matter, in addition to reducing the filtration rate. The caking of material on the filter also has the same effects. In many instances, if the initial filtrate is still cloudy, it should be recycled through the same filter to effect clarification. When high concentrations of solids are to be removed from the liquid, clogging of the filter by the resulting filter cake will drastically reduce the filtration rate and, therefore, the efficiency of the operation.

Filter Media. A filter medium used for clarification must be capable of delivering a clear filtrate at a suitable production rate. Consequently, it must withstand the mechanical stresses which may be imposed on it without rupturing or being compressed

significantly. Furthermore, no chemical or physical interactions with the components of the filtrate should occur. A large number of media are employed in filtration. These may be conveniently classified in the following categories:

Sheets of woven or felted material: These include wire screening; fabrics of cotton, wool, linen or synthetic materials such as nylon; felt or muslin; and filter paper. In pharmaceutical practice, as in the prescription laboratory, filter paper is the usual filter medium. This paper is a porous, unsized material which may be obtained in various degrees of retentiveness and purity. Wire sieves, muslin and surgical gauze are employed frequently as strainers.

Porous plates: These include perforated metal or rubber plates; natural porous materials, i.e., stone, procelain and other ceramics; and frittered or sintered glass. These are often used as supports for other filter media; they also can be obtained in forms which are highly retentive. Unlike other media, they frequently can be reused after cleaning instead of being discarded on completion of a single filtration.

Membrane filters: These are made by casting. One form, exemplified by the Millipore filters (see Chap. 14), is prepared from cellulose esters and is a thin porous membrane, the pores of which are essentially uniform channels through the membrane. In a typical Millipore filter the pore volume may occupy as much of 80 percent of the volume of the filter. This porosity characteristic permits very high liquid flow rates, with maximum retentiveness determined by the ratio of particle diameter to pore diameter. Since the sizes of the pores can be controlled with a high degree of precision, these membranes may be used in a wide variety of clarification operations.

Unwoven fibrous materials: These include cotton, asbestos fibers and paper pulp and are employed with woven or felted material or porous plates used as supports.

Granular or powdered materials, with suitable supports: These include sand, gravel, diatomaceous earth, charcoal, etc.

Filtration Equipment. This discussion will be restricted to pressure filtration—the clarification procedure most important to industry. Pressure filtration is carried out with plate-and-frame or leaf filters. Other special types of filtration apparatus used in the preparation of sterile solutions are described in Chapter 14.

Plate-and-frame filters, also known as filter presses, are available in a variety of shapes, sizes and designs and range in capacity from a few liters to many hundreds of liters per hour. Figure 4-2 is a diagram of a filter press. In designing a filter press, the aim is to secure maximum surface area of filter, with efficient use of space. This is accomplished by using many filters or plates (the diagram shows 4 plates) arranged in such a fashion that the liquid flows through them only once. A pump provides the energy needed to maintain flow and prevent backflow of the effluent through the filters. The filter pads usually employed consist of woven or felted material restrained on wire mesh or perforated plates.

Pressure filters may be included as components of liquid transfer systems. These so-called cartridge filters are placed in the pipeline carrying the liquid to be clarified. The leaf filter consists of vertical, narrow, hollow shells which are fitted with suitable filter media and suspended in a pressure vessel. Each leaf has an outlet which is tied into a common line.

ABSORPTION AND ADSORPTION

Filter media effect clarification through the operation of absorptive and adsorptive

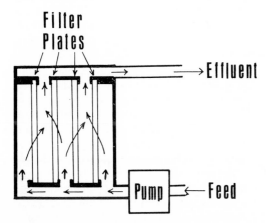

Fig. 4-2. Plate-and-frame filter press, flow diagram.

processes, in addition to their "sieve" action. In absorption, foreign particles are "soaked up" or trapped within the medium; in adsorption, foreign material adheres to the surface of the media. These processes are particularly important in the removal of finely divided solid and insoluble liquid material from solutions. Filter media which act by absorption have a high degree of porosity; filter media which act by adsorption present a large surface area to the liquid to be clarified. Frequently, agents other than the filtration medium itself, i.e., filter aids, are used to provide the absorptive and adsorptive functions.

Filter aids are finely divided materials or, in some instances, fibrous materials which deposit on the filter medium. They include talc, fuller's earth, boneblack, pumice stone, asbestos fibers, pulped filter paper and infusorial earth (Kieselguhr, or diatomaceous earth). Filter aids may be added directly to the liquid which is to be filtered or used in the form of a slurry in the solvent to precoat the filter.

Filtering aids used in the clarification of pharmaceutical solutions should be chemically inert, they should have a high adsorptive capacity, and they should be of such particle size that they can be readily filtered out of the solution. One must consider whether the filter aid dissolves in the liquid or reacts with it. Carbonates (e.g., magnesium and calcium) and other materials which dissolve to some extent in water and, thereby, alter the pH of the solution are not generally employed. They may be used as filter aids in the manufacture of preparations when an alkaline reaction is desired, e.g., Tolu Balsam Syrup, N.F. Filter interaction may take the form of adsorption. Consequently, due to adsorption by the filter or filter aid, active therapeutic agents or pharmaceutical adjuvants present in small concentrations can be depleted significantly from solution. For example, asbestos readily adsorbs coloring agents such as amaranth from aqueous solution.

Soluble materials which can be precipitated from solution may serve as filter aids. These function by trapping smaller particles within the precipitate, which then is removed readily by filtration or settling. Albumin, which is water-soluble and is coagulated by heating of the solution, is an example of a filter aid of this type.

As indicated in the foregoing discussion, selection of the proper filtration medium and filter aid is not arbitrary, but must be considered carefully.

WATER

STANDARDS FOR WATER

Water, U.S.P. Pharmaceutical manufacturers are permitted to use drinking water that conforms to the standards listed under Water, U.S.P., in the washing and the extraction of crude drugs, in the preparation of products for external use and in other preparations in which the difference between water and purified water is of no consequence. This is done because the huge amount of water employed in this phase of drug manufacturing would require enormous facilities for production and storage.

Water, U.S.P., is not suitable for general pharmaceutical use because of the considerable amount of dissolved solids present.[3] A 100-ml. portion of official water contains not more than 100 mg. of residue (0.1%) after evaporation to dryness on a steam bath and subsequent drying to constant weight in an oven at 105°, while an equal amount of purified water yields not more than 1 mg. of residue under the same conditions. These dissolved solids consist chiefly of the chlorides, the sulfates and the bicarbonates of sodium, potassium, calcium and magnesium. Practically the only difference between water and purified water lies in the amount of total dissolved solids. The development of precipitates and effervescence, which occurs when medicinals are prepared with water (in place of purified water), is the major objection to its use. Water is clear, colorless and practically tasteless and odorless, even near the boiling point. It meets the U.S. Public Health Service regulations for potable water with respect to bacteriologic purity. A pH range is given, but most tap water meets the requirements because it is neutral or just slightly alkaline. The deviaction from neutrality to slight acidity or alkalinity is due not only to the composition

of the dissolved solids, but also to dissolved carbon dioxide or ammonia.

Purified Water, U.S.P., is used in the preparation of all medication containing water except ampuls, injections, some official external preparations, such as liniments, and other specialized products. Water for Injection, U.S.P., must be used for aqueous solutions intended for injection.

With the exceptions of the amounts of dissolved solids and of oxidizable substances permitted, the standards for Purified Water, U.S.P., are similar to those for water. Purified Water, U.S.P., formerly official as Distilled Water, may be prepared by distillation or deionization. Freshly distilled water has a pH of about 5.6 and usually changes to about pH 6 on storage. Distilled water may be rendered carbon-dioxide-free by boiling after it is freshly prepared. Since purified water is obtained by distillation or deionization, it must be labeled to indicate the method of preparation.

Although deionization or demineralization procedures for the removal of dissolved salts from water have been used for more than 30 years, water purified in this manner was not given official recognition until the fourth and final supplement to *U.S.P. XIV*.

The deionization methods for the production of water of distilled-water quality, when compared with distillation, possess a number of advantages for the manufacturer, the laboratory worker and the prescriptionist. These include: (1) elimination of the use of heat, (2) simpler equipment, with less maintenance, (3) lower long-term costs and (4) ease of production and storage. However, demineralization units require special attention in order to ensure that they do not serve as sites for microorganism growth which could contaminate the effluent water.

The deionization methods in use today no doubt resulted from the well-known zeolite process of "softening" water of high mineral content.[3] The "exchangers" used are synthetic, polymeric resins of high molecular weight, which are insoluble in water and are characterized by an unusually high content of free amino, sulfonic acid or phenolic functions. These resins are mainly of 2 types: the cation, or acid, exchangers, which permit the replacement of the cations in solution with hydrogen ion, and the anion, or base, exchange resins, which permit the removal of anions.

The manner in which these resins function may be summed up, in simplified form, as follows:

1. *Acid, or Cation, Exchange Step:* In this step, the cation(s) of the salt(s) are replaced with hydrogen ions. The cations so replaced remain behind, "fixed" to the resin.

$$\text{H Resin} + M^+ + X^- \longrightarrow$$
$$\text{M Resin} + H^+ + X^-$$

where M^+ and X^- are the cation and the anion of a salt present in solution.

2. *Base, or Anion, Exchange Step:* The water is passed through a basic resin (usually a polyamine) and the anion remaining after step (1) is removed according to:

$$\text{Resin} - NH_2 + H^+ + X^- \longrightarrow$$
$$\text{Resin} - NH_2 \cdot HX$$

This anion exchange step also may be represented as:

$$\text{Resin} - NH_3OH + H^+ + X^- \longrightarrow$$
$$\text{Resin} - NH_3X + H_2O$$

Ion exchange as shown above effects removal of dissolved salts. In those instances in which the anion is a carbonate or a bicarbonate, the carbon dioxide formed usually remains dissolved and, most often, is present in amounts too small to alter the purity of the water. However, if large quantities of carbonates or bicarbonates give rise to substantial amounts of carbon dioxide, the gas may be removed by aeration.

Many types of ion-exchange resins are available. Simple units of the "mixed-bed" type, which may be installed easily in any prescription department or laboratory, make available a ready supply of purified water. Regeneration of the units is a simple procedure and does not require a great deal of time or material.

As an alternate to the permanent units, "cartridges" of mixed resins which fit into the top of a polyethylene bottle provide a simple means for readily converting tap water into purified water.

With the exception of preparations intended for parenteral administration for which Water for Injection is specifically intended, purified water prepared by deionization may be used in any formulation, preparation or prescription calling for distilled water.

Water for Injection, U.S.P. This is pyrogen-free water, purified by distillation, for the preparation of products for parenteral use. It is intended for use as a solvent only in solutions that are to be sterilized after preparation. If it is to be used as a solvent in parenteral solutions prepared under aseptic conditions (see Chap. 14), Water for Injection must be sterilized before use. It contains no added substance and meets the requirements of the tests for purified water. It must meet the requirements of the Pyrogen Test (for this test it must first be made isotonic by the addition of 900 mg. of pyrogen-free sodium chloride for each 100 ml).

Sterilization is the freeing of materials from all living organisms and their spores. This may be accomplished in various ways, but, in this case, the preferable method is *U.S.P. XIII* Process C., i.e., steam under pressure (heating in an autoclave). If an autoclave is not available, freshly distilled water may be sterilized by boiling the water for at least 60 minutes in a flask stoppered with a plug of purified nonabsorbent cotton covered with gauze, tinfoil or stout nonabsorbent paper; or the neck of the flask may be covered with cellophane and tightly fastened with cord. The water is allowed to cool without removing the stopper. If the cotton plug is used as a stopper, the top of the flask may be wrapped with paper in order to protect the mouth of the flask.

Pyrogens are fever-producing substances probably of bacterial origin. They probably consist of polysaccharide-bearing bacterial antigens. Distilled-water pyrogens are produced by specific bacteria which grow in water and are nonvolatile. Nevertheless, ordinary distillation will not assure removal of these pyrogenic substances. The manufacturer of pyrogen-free sterile water may employ any suitable method of preparation that will produce a product that conforms to the U.S.P. Sterility Test for Liquids, the Pyrogen Test, and the requirements of the tests prescribed in the official monograph of

Water for Injection. Everett[4] has described the factors to be considered in the design of water distillation equipment for production of high purity water.

The only satisfactory method for proving the absence of pyrogens in the final product is by conducting the pyrogen test (cf. Chap. 14).

Pyrogen- and bacterial-retentive filters are used widely. Models can be obtained with a steam-generating unit from which steam may pass through the filter to ensure complete sterilization of the circulatory passages as well as the filter disks themselves.

Water for injection prepared for immediate use must be distilled and sterilized within 24 hours and may be stored for not more than 24 hours in well-cleansed, tight containers at a temperature below or above that at which bacterial growth may take place. It can be stored for periods up to a month in special tanks containing ultraviolet lamps. Unused portions are to be discarded or resterilized, unless, following sterilization, the container is kept closed at all times and nothing enters except the filtered air needed for replacement as the water for injection is drawn off. When this freshly prepared water is stored and sterilized in hermetically sealed containers, it will remain in good condition indefinitely.

Sterile Water for Injection, U.S.P. Specifications are provided in this monograph for water for injection, sterilized and packaged in suitable single-dose containers, preferably of Type I glass, of not larger than 1,000-ml. size.

The preparation must meet the requirements of the Sterility Tests and the Pyrogen Test and the other tests under Purified Water. The following limits for total solids apply for Sterile Water for Injection in glass containers: up to and including 30-ml. size, 40 parts per million; from 30-ml. up to and including 100-ml. size, 30 parts per million; and for larger sizes 20 parts per million.

Bacteriostatic Water for Injection, U.S.P. This is sterile water for injection containing bacteriostatic agents. It may be packaged in single-dose containers of not larger than 5-ml. size and in multiple-dose containers of not larger than 30-ml. size, the label of which indicates the name and the proportion of added agent.

AROMATIC WATERS

Aromatic waters were known in antiquity; distilled waters were prepared in Egypt as early as the 4th century. Distilled rose water was an important article of export in Persia in the 8th and the 9th centuries. The introduction in Europe of distillation and of distilled aromatic waters has been attributed to the renowned Catalonian physician, Arnaldus de Villanova (1235–1312). Around 1500, the distilled waters were accorded much recognition in therapy. There developed a special trade of "water-brenners," and a number of books on the art of distillation appeared, of which those written by Hieronymous Brunschwygk (1430–1512) are best known. Until the end of the 18th century, the official pharmacopeias of many countries vied with each other in the number and the variety of their formulas for distilled waters.

Although the number of aromatic waters for which official standards are maintained presently is few, aromatic waters still provide a pleasantly flavored medium for the administration of water-soluble drugs when masking of undesirable tastes is not a problem and for the liquid phase of emulsions and suspensions (e.g., Cinnamon Water was a component of the vehicle in Chalk Mixture, N.F. XI). Aromatic waters are not therapeutically potent because of the very small proportion of active ingredient present in them. Aromatic waters prepared from essential oils, e.g., peppermint water, have been used as carminatives. Chloroform Water, N.F. XI, was used in expectorant preparations. Where doses are specified, they generally range between 5 and 15 ml.

Several aromatic waters are not used as vehicles for oral medication. These include Rose Water, Hamamelis Water, N.F. XI, and Camphor Water, N.F. XI. Rose Water is a perfume. Hamamelis Water, or Witch Hazel, is employed commonly as a rub and also is used as an astringent and perfume in aftershave lotions and other cosmetic products. Camphor water is frequently prescribed in eyedrops and eyewashes for its slight refreshing, stimulating effect.

PREPARATION

Most aromatic waters are prepared extemporaneously according to the simple procedures of the *U.S.P.* and the *N.F.* The *U.S.P.* prescribes 3 general methods: distillation, solution and alternate solution. The ultimate goal in preparing any pharmaceutical is to obtain a product that adheres to official standards. The compendiums permit deviation in detail from the official methods, provided that the final product meets official requirements. Formulas for concentrates of the aromatic principles, containing either alcohol or solubilizing agents, have been developed. To prepare an aromatic water, the concentrates are diluted with water. They provide an alternative to the official methods of preparation.

DISTILLATION

Most of the aromatic waters can be prepared by distillation. However, it is not practical or economically feasible to use this method in most cases, when an equally satisfactory product can be prepared as needed in the prescription laboratory at small cost and with little apparatus. Stronger Rose Water, N.F., Orange Flower Water, N.F., and Hamamelis Water, N.F. XI, are prepared directly from fresh plant material and, thus, cannot be prepared by any method other than distillation. The distillation method consists of placing the odoriferous portion of the plant or drug from which the aromatic water is to be prepared in a suitable still with sufficient purified water and then distilling most of the water, carefully avoiding the development of empyreumatic odors through charring or scorching of the substances. The excess oil is separated from the distillate. The aqueous phase, which may require further clarification, is the product.

Frequently, the labels of commercial witch hazel contain one or more X's, each X representing one distillation. For example, XXXX means that the water was a quadruple-distilled product, i.e., the distillate of the first distillation was returned to a fresh quantity of the drug and redistilled, the procedure, in this instance, being carried out 4 times. It is thought that the first distillation does not yield a saturated solution, thus necessitating subsequent distillations. The other waters prepared by distillation are treated in a similar fashion.

SOLUTION

The aromatic principles of most plants can be separated from the crude material by steam distillation. Consequently, they are available for use in the extemporaneous preparation of waters. Therefore, for most waters, the *U.S.P.* prescribes that the volatile substance be agitated with purified water for a period of 15 minutes. The mixture is then set aside for at least 12 hours, to ensure saturation, before it is filtered through wetted filter paper. A large excess of solute is used (2 mil. or 2 g., liquid or solid as the case may be, per liter) in order to obtain the maximal rate of solution. The filter paper must be wet to prevent the passage of excess oil into the filtrate and to eliminate absorption of the dissolved aromatics by the filter.

The disadvantage of this method is that, in spite of repeated filtration, it is difficult to obtain a brilliantly clear preparation, owing to the formation of extremely fine particles. This may be obviated by using boiling, purified water. Moreover, it is not necessary to make up to volume through the filter as the compendium directs, since a saturated solution is sought.

Chloroform Water, N.F. XI, is prepared by solution. No clarification problem exists in this case, since a slight excess of chloroform must remain in the bottle. A saturated solution is prepared and maintained by adding an excess of cholorform to a given quantity of purified water, shaking vigorously, and taking care that an excess of chloroform is always present. Since chloroform is heavier than water, the excess will remain at the bottom of the container. The high volatility of chloroform creates an equilibrium of loss and restoration of strength by evaporation. Naturally, when it is dispensed, the bottle should not be shaken, and only the supernatant liquid should be used.

ALTERNATE SOLUTION

The compendiums have recognized that clarification and the amount of time consumed present difficulties in the simple solution method. An alternative method is offered, in which the volatile material is mixed thoroughly with 15 g. of purified talc or with a sufficient quantity of purified siliceous earth or pulped filter paper. This mixture is agitated with a liter of purified water for 10 minutes, prior to filtration.

The talc or other inert material functions as both a filter aid and a distribution agent. In the latter capacity it serves to accelerate the rate of solution by adsorbing and facilitating the breaking up of the aromatic substance into fine particles, thus increasing the surface area exposed to solvent action. In the former capacity, it facilitates the clarification of the solution. The time-saving factor is an important advantage.

Unfortunately, the alternate method has not proved to be entirely satisfactory, owing to the problem of the purified talc or siliceous earth passing through the filter papers commonly used. Purified talc on the market is subdivided too finely, and it is difficult to obtain good purified siliceous earth free from soluble and finely divided extraneous matter. In order to remove finely divided material and possible soluble matter and, thus, produce a better filter aid for aromatic waters, these materials could be first treated with water in an elutriation process. The use of pulped filter paper does not solve the clarification problem. Several other substances have been recommended as substitutes. Calcium phosphate showed great promise at first; not only did it produce a clear water, but, also, the preparation possessed a more sparkling clarity. However, these waters developed a yellow tinge which was due to the slightly alkaline reaction of dissolved calcium phosphate with the dissolved volatile ingredients.

Many aromatic waters have been prepared from essential oils, e.g., Peppermint Water. Essential oils are complex mixtures of hydrocarbons, alcohols, ethers, aldehydes and ketones. The hydrocarbon fraction of many essential oils is made up of terpenes. These components of the oil are the least water-soluble and, consequently, constitute most of the insoluble matter removed in the clarification process. The other substances, unlike the hydrocarbon fraction, are the "aroma carriers." Terpeneless oils are commercially available. They are prepared by fractional distillation and/or extraction. They are concentrated products which, therefore, are stronger in aroma and more soluble; also, they may be more stable than the natural essential oil. Their use in the preparation of aromatic waters should result in less difficulties in clarification. However, the greater cost of the terpeneless oils makes it uneconomical to use them in the preparation of aromatic waters.

DILUTION

In an attempt to obviate the difficulties involved in the clarification of aromatic waters, formulas have been developed for concentrates which are designed to be diluted with an appropriate volume of water when needed.

The British Pharmaceutical Codex gives as an alternative to the three methods of making aromatic waters a procedure for preparing a concentrate. An alcoholic solution of the essential oil is mixed with water and talc. The mixture is agitated; after several hours it is filtered. The concentrate contains between 50 and 55 percent alcohol by volume. If prepared from essential oils, the concentrate, containing the dilute alcohol-soluble fraction of 2 ml. of oil in each 100 ml., is a solution of a terpeneless oil. One volume of concentrate is diluted with 39 volumes of water, producing an aromatic water which contains less than 1.5 percent of alcohol.

When "Rose Water" is called for, it may be prepared by diluting Stronger Rose Water with an equal volume of purified water. A large proportion of rose water in general use is not prepared from the official stronger rose water, but is made by diluting a specially prepared solution of 50 percent alcohol and rose oil or rose synthetic. Neither of these artificial substitutes compares in quality with the official products. Aqueous preparations that contain small amounts of alcohol are prone to alterations in flavor and aroma, as a consequence of oxidative degradation of the alcohol.

The introduction into commerce of nontoxic, nonionic surface-active agents, e.g., Polysorbate 80 U.S.P., (Tween® 80) has resulted in the exploitation of the principle of "solubilization" in the preparation of liquid dosage forms.[6] Solutions of these agents can dissolve significantly greater concentrations of normally water-insoluble materials. Because of their unbalanced structure (see Chap. 7), surface-active agents tend to associate in the bulk aqueous phase, forming aggregates of molecules known as micelles. In effect, the micelles function as a separate, microscopic phase into which nonpolar and semipolar compounds can distribute. Consequently, when mixed with a suitable quantity of a surfactant, essential oils can be made water-miscible.

One formula suggested for a peppermint oil concentrate was:[5]

Peppermint Oil	7.5 ml.
Tween 20	43 ml.
Purified Water qs	ad 100 ml.

To prepare an aromatic water, 1 ml. of the concentrate is diluted to 100 ml. with purified water. Such aromatic waters possess several objectionable characteristics.[7] The pH generally is lower than that of the official product, and they foam excessively on agitation. Also, they tend to develop a disagreeable taste more readily than official waters and are more easily subject to mold growth. Furthermore, in order to get the same aroma and flavor as in the official water, more oil must be dissolved than will saturate the aqueous phase, since most of the aromatic principles are dispersed into the miscellar phase. However, the concentrate is stable.

The use of solubilizing agents in the preparation of aromatic waters is an example of an undesirable application of solubilization to pharmaceutical formulation, in the sense that the agents which are used permit the solution of unwanted materials —e.g., the terpenes—which, ordinarily, are removed in the filtration step. In this instance, the simplification of the manufacture of the aromatic waters results in an inferior preparation.

STABILITY

Generally, instability in aromatic waters can be attributed to improper storage or failure to consider the properties of the preparations. Many waters support the growth of molds. This is particularly true of the distilled waters. For this reason, orange flower water frequently is prepared from orange flower oil, and a rose oil concentrate is used to prepare rose water. Witch hazel (Hamamelis Water, N.F. XI) is preserved by the addition of 15 percent of alcohol. However, as a rule, no preservatives are added to aromatic waters.

Excessive exposure to light and to changes in temperature cause aromatic waters to lose some of their desirable characteristics. Since the solutes are volatile materials, loss of aroma occurs on prolonged exposure to the atmosphere, particularly at elevated temperatures. Since aromatic waters are saturated solutions, lowering the temperature causes separation of the aromatic component, thus producing cloudiness. The aromatics may be salted out when the water is used as a vehicle for drugs which are electrolytes. The insoluble material may collect on the top of the liquid, imparting a burning taste to the first dose, Significant loss in flavor may be observed if aromatic waters are used in the external phase of dispersions, owing to adsorption of aromatic constituents by suspended matter.

Finally, instability in aromatic waters may occur because of the chemical nature of the solutes. Many of the aroma-bearing solutes, as well as the terpenes, are oxidizable compounds. Oxidative degradation, involving dissolved atmospheric oxygen, is likely. This autoxidation can be catalyzed by light and trace quantities of metal ions such as iron (III) and copper (II). Chloroform Water, N.F. XI, is stored in light-resistant bottles, since light catalyzes the oxidation of chloroform to the poisonous gas, phosgene. Bitter

TABLE 4-1.   AROMATIC WATERS OF THE *U.S.P.* AND THE *N.F.*

TITLE AND SYNONYMS	CATEGORY	DOSE
Cinnamon Water, N.F.	flavored vehicle	
Orange Flower Water, N.F.	flavored vehicle	
(Aqua Neroli)	perfume	
Stronger Rose Water, N.F.	perfume	
(Aqua Rosae Fortior)		
Peppermint Water, U.S.P. XVII	flavored vehicle	
(Aqua Menthae Piperitae)	carminative	15 ml.
Camphor Water, N.F. XI	vehicle	
Chloroform Water, N.F. XI	vehicle	
	expectorant, stomachic, antiemetic	15 ml.
Hamamelis Water, N. F. XI	astringent	
(Distilled Witch Hazel Extract)		
(Witch Hazel)		

Almond Water, N.F. VIII, deposits crystals of benzoic acid which result from the autoxidation of benzaldehyde.

In general, aromatic waters are not permanently stable preparations. Prolonged storage in sealed containers tends to make the water acquire the odor of stale air. Waters which were prepared aseptically with recently boiled, purified water and were filtered through bacterial retentive filters into sterilized resistant glass containers have remained in perfect condition for a year.

SYRUPS

Syrups are sweet, viscous aqueous liquids. Medicinally, they are divided into two groups: the *flavoring* syrups, which are used as vehicles, and the *medicated* syrups, which contain ingredients giving them therapeutic value. The syrup dosage form is used for antibiotics, antihistaminics, antitussives, sedatives and vitamins, as well as for other drugs. Products of this type are included in the official compendiums to provide legal standards for their medicinal content. In regard to the vehicles, there are no official formulas for their preparation and no detailed descriptions of the products are given in the compendiums.

Pharmaceutically, syrups are classified best according to their basic formulas: those which are concentrated solutions of a sugar and those which are formulated with artificial sweetening agents and viscosity builders.

Although there are many different sugars,

sucrose and dextrose have been the only ones used in the preparation of syrups. Sucrose is obtained from sugar cane, sugar beet or, less commonly, sugar maple. Before passage of the Food and Drug Act of 1906, the sucrose ordinarily available was often unsuitable for pharmaceutical use, owing to the addition of harmful whitening agents, such as ultramarine, or the use of bleaching chemicals. At that time, crystal sugar was preferred for pharmaceutical use. Honey was used as a base for thick liquid preparations known as Honey or Mels. Honey is the secretion deposited in the honeycomb of the bee and consists of a mixture of invert sugars. Oxymels (Sour or Acid Honeys), preparations containing acetic acid and honey, are still described in the British Pharmaceutical Codex. Liquid glucose, prepared by incompletely hydrolyzing starch, may also be used as a component of syrups. Sucrose is one of the purest of commercially available substances and is the preferred carbohydrate for syrups because of its purity, degree of sweetness, lack of color and ease of handling.

The development of liquid preparations which are intended as substitutes for syrups and contain no, or very little, available carbohydrates stems from an attempt to satisfy the need of persons who must exclude sugar from their diets. These "artificial" syrups have become the basis for a number of commercial formulations, since fewer problems may be associated with their long-term stability. From a historical viewpoint, syrups were first preparations based on natural products, such as honey, then concentrated sucrose solutions, the quality of which is controlled more easily, and, now, a general formula, perhaps more complex, which lacks carbohydrate and may or may not be advantageous in comparison with the sucrose-based syrup.

FORMULATION OF SUGAR-BASED SYRUPS

Stability of Aqueous Sucrose Solutions. In order to formulate a syrup properly, one must consider the properties of the basic vehicle, particularly its stability. Sucrose is subject to two degradative pathways in aqueous solution: fermentation and hydrolysis.

As a carbohydrate, sucrose in dilute aqueous solution provides a nutrient medium for the growth of microorganisms, particularly yeasts and molds. The consequences of this growth include turbidity, fermentation and changes in taste. The concentration of sucrose is an important factor in inhibiting mold growth. Nearly saturated solutions of sucrose, if stored properly, are self-preserving. In effect, such solutions contain no "free water"; thus, they behave as an anhydrous medium with respect to growth of microorganisms.

Preservatives may be specified in syrup formulations to prevent fermentation; however, most official syrups depend only on sufficient sucrose concentration for preservation. If the concentration of sucrose is significantly less than that of Syrup, U.S.P., that is, less than 85 percent (w/v) of sucrose, preservative should be added.[9] Some preservatives which are suitable for use in syrups are summarized in Table 4-2.[22] The benzoates, the parabens and sorbic acid are most effective in acid solutions; they are ineffective as preservatives in alkaline solutions. Mixtures of the parabens are frequently employed to take advantage of their potentiating effect.[21] A concentration of 1:4,500 of a mixture of equal parts of methylparaben and butylparaben has been recommended for syrups.

The amount of added preservative which is needed in those syrups containing reduced sugar concentrations may be estimated from

TABLE 4-2.   PRESERVATIVES FOR SYRUPS

PRESERVATIVE	CONCENTRATION USED (in percent)
Benzoic acid	0.1–0.2
Sodium benzoate	0.1–0.2
Butylparaben	0.02
Propylparaben	0.05
Methylparaben	0.1
Sorbic acid	0.1
Alcohol	15–20
Glycerin	45

a knowledge of the calculated "free water."[16] For example, 100 ml. of a 65 percent (w/v), sucrose solution is equivalent to 76.5 ml. of an 85 percent (w/v) syrup and 24.5 ml. of water; that is

$$65:x = 85:100$$

$$x = 76.5 \text{ ml}$$

The more free water, the more preservative required in the product. Calculations of this type show that the official syrups are adequately preserved. The fact that some syrups are still subject to deterioration due to mold growth can be explained on the basis of a difference in nutritive properties of other components in the syrup.

In some syrups alcohol is present in small amounts. It serves as a solvent for the alcohol-soluble ingredients. Although the concentration of alcohol is not sufficient to have a preservative effect, the alcohol concentrates in vapors above the syrup and thus prevents the growth of surface molds. In sealed containers, vaporization of water from the syrup and its subsequent condensation on the syrup result in the formation of a dilute solution of sucrose on the surface, and this can support mold growth.

Sucrose is a disaccharide and, consequently, can be hydrolyzed to give the monosaccharides dextrose (glucose) and levulose (fructose, fruit sugar), i.e.,

$$\underset{\text{Sucrose}}{C_{12}H_{22}O_{11}} + H_2O \longrightarrow \underset{\text{Dextrose}}{C_6H_{12}O_6} + \underset{\text{Levulose}}{C_6H_{12}O_6}$$

The hydrolytic reaction is specific-acid, i.e., hydrogen-ion catalyzed. This reaction is also called inversion. A solution of sucrose rotates polarized light to the right (dextrorotation), while the same solution, after hydrolysis, is levo-rotatory, since the levulose has a greater rotating power than the dextrose. The invert sugar formed on hydrolysis has several interesting properties: (1) Solutions of invert sugar are fermented more easily than are solutions of sugar. The first step in fermentation is inversion. (2) Invert sugar is sweeter than sucrose: if, in regard to sweetness, sucrose is rated 100, dextrose is rated 74 and levulose 173. (3) Finally, degradation of the levulose formed by inversion seems to be responsible for the brown discoloration which develops in some of the colorless syrups. This change is called *caramelization*. It takes place particularly in syrups containing strong acids.

Certain incompatibilities should be anticipated when syrups are mixed with other liquid preparations. If the preparations contain high concentrations of alcohol, sucrose will crystallize. Simple syrup can tolerate 10 percent alcohol without crystallization. When solutions containing pectins are mixed with sucrose syrups, gellation frequently is observed, since sucrose partially dehydrates the pectin. When syrups are diluted with aqueous solutions, the necessity for additional preservative should be considered.

Generally, syrups are stored at room temperature in tightly stoppered well-filled bottles. While refrigeration inhibits both mold growth and inversion and may be required for some syrups, it may cause crystallization of the sucrose. Large crystals which form are difficult to redissolve. The supernatant liquid may contain significantly lower concentrations of sucrose.

Syrup, U.S.P., contains 85 percent (w/v) of sucrose, corresponding to 64.74 percent by weight. Its specific gravity is 1.313. The latter parameter provides a ready means of standardizing the preparation. A saturated solution of sucrose is 67.9 percent (w/w) at 25° C.; the British Pharmacopoeia Syrup is 66.7 percent (w/w) sucrose. Simple syrup is a saturated solution at 4° C. Therefore, no crystallization should be observed in a properly prepared syrup, unless the temperature drops below 4° C. If the syrup is too concentrated, crystallization may be observed; if too dilute, simple syrup will readily support the growth of molds.

Syrup is made by dissolving sucrose in boiling water or, preferably, without heat by percolation with purified water (about 465 ml. total). Cotton is packed loosely in the neck of the percolator to remove mechanical impurities such as lint. The cotton is moistened after packing and before the sucrose is placed in the percolator so that the first, concentrated syrup will pass through satisfactorily. In making small quantities it is always necessary to pass the percolate through the percolator several times before all the sucrose is dissolved. This process has the advantage of requiring little attention and it is well suited to the manufacture of large quantities of syrup. Alternatively, the sucrose may be dissolved more rapidly in the proper amount of water by agitation in a graduated bottle. Syrup made without heat is practically colorless.

A so-called *hot process,* in which the syrup was heated to 100° C. to hasten solution of the sucrose, was described last in *U.S.P. XV.* An advantage gained by this method was some degree of sterilization from the heat. However, syrups prepared with heat have a pale amber color owing to caramelization. There is more inversion of the sucrose and, consequently, a reduction of the keeping quality of the product.

Other official syrups are prepared by the addition of ingredients to simple syrup or by the solution of sucrose in an aqueous solution of medicinal agents.

SYRUPS PREPARED BY SIMPLE ADMIXTURE

Several of the flavoring syrups are prepared most appropriately by mixing solutions of the flavoring ingredients with simple syrup.

Glycyrrhiza Syrup (Licorice Syrup), **U.S.P.,** is made by the addition of simple syrup to a blend of fennel oil and anise oil dissolved in fluidextract glycyrrhiza.

The same principles can readily be applied to the preparation of medicinal syrups. The medicament is dissolved in a small quantity of purified water which is diluted to volume with an appropriate flavoring syrup. The amount of drug used is such that a dose is obtained in 5 ml. (one teaspoonful) of syrup.

Hydrocodone Bitartrate Syrup, U.S.P., is prepared using cherry syrup. The official syrup contains 5 mg. of narcotic in each 5 ml.

Ipecac Syrup, U.S.P. Formerly, the compendium directed that this syrup be prepared by mixing ipecac fluidextract and glycerin and then adding enough syrup to make the required amount. The glycerin is added to inhibit precipitation of therapeutically inert extractives in the syrup. Since standards are no longer maintained for ipecac fluidextract, the compendium includes the directions for manufacture of the fluidextract (see Chap. 5) as part of the procedure for making the syrup. In this process the percolate obtained by exhausting powdered ipecac with a mixture of 3 volumes of alcohol and 1 volume of water is reduced in volume by evaporation at a temperature not exceeding 60° C. and subsequently mixed with a large volume of water. Precipitated resins are removed by filtration after a waiting period. The filtrate is again evaporated; hydrochloric acid and alcohol are added. The acid stabilizes the solution by converting the therapeutically active alkaloids emetine and cephaeline to their hydrochloride salts. The *U.S.P.* directs that the syrup be assayed for its alkaloidal content. Ipecac syrup is packaged in 1 fluidounce bottles, labeled for use in emergency treatment of poisoning. The fluidextract is not officially recognized in order to discourage its use and prevent its mistaken dispensing where the syrup is called for.

Syrups Prepared by Dissolution of Sucrose in Solutions of Ingredients

Most official syrups for which formulas are given are prepared by this method rather than by simple admixture. Several different techniques are employed to prepare the aqueous solution of medicaments and/or other ingredients.

Cherry and Raspberry Syrups, U.S.P., are made by dissolving sucrose in the appropriate juice. A small quantity of alcohol is added to inhibit the growth of surface molds. These syrups are acidic, owing to the acid content of the juices. They are clear red vehicles with very pleasant tastes.

Cherry Juice, U.S.P., is the liquid expressed from the fresh ripe fruit of the sour red cherry, *Prunus Cerasus* Linné (*Rosaceae*). It contains not less than 1.0 percent of malic acid. *Raspberry Juice, U.S.P.,* is the liquid expressed from the fresh ripe red raspberry, varieties of *Rubus idaeus* Linné or of *R. strigosus* Michaux (*Rosaceae*). It contains not less than 1.5 percent of acids calculated as citric acid.

The juices are manufactured by similar processes. The method of preparation will be described for Cherry Juice.

The cherries are stemmed but not pitted, washed with water, passed through a grinder to crush the kernels, and 0.1 percent of benzoic acid added to prevent fermentation. The kernels are crushed to add to the flavor of the juice. The mixture is allowed to stand at room temperature for several days to allow for the removal of pectin, a water-soluble product naturally present in fresh cherry juice. On standing, the pectin is hydrolyzed to pectic acid, which is insoluble in water. The hydrolysis is catalyzed by the enzyme pectase. (A small amount of methyl alcohol also results from the hydrolysis of pectin.) The absence of pectin is shown when a filtered portion of the juice gives a clear solution when mixed with one half its volume of alcohol. This solution should not become cloudy within 30 minutes if pectins are absent. The juice is then expressed and filtered. If the pectin is not removed from cherry juice, a syrup made from it is likely to gel.

Orange Syrup, U.S.P., is prepared by dissolving sucrose in an aromatic water containing citric acid. The water is made from sweet orange peel tincture, using talc as a distributing agent and filter aid. Heat must be avoided in dissolving the sucrose because the flavor of the finished product would be reduced by excessive volatilization of the aromatic constituents of the oil. Sweet orange peel tincture is preferred as the source of flavor rather than pure orange oil, since the latter tends to degrade, developing an objectionable odor. About 90 percent of orange oil is the terpene limonene which is susceptible to autoxidation, especially in the presence of moisture.

The products resulting from the oxidation are responsible for the changes in odor and flavor of natural orange-flavored preparations. The orange oil is significantly more stable in alcoholic solutions as exemplified by the tincture.

The *U.S.P.* cautions that Orange Syrup should not be used if it has a *terebinthine* odor or taste. This caution is also given in the monograph for **Citric Acid Syrup** (Lemon Syrup), **U.S.P.,** in which the flavor is derived from lemon oil, another source of limonene. Lemon syrup is prepared by mixing lemon tincture with simple syrup containing citric acid. The product has a faint opalescence which is caused by the precipitation of the terpenes contained in the tincture. The official syrup has been criticized for lack of definite flavor and for cloudiness and susceptibility to fermentation. Stoklosa[27] recommended that the syrup be prepared by the same technique used to manufacture Orange Syrup, i.e., sucrose is dissolved in an aromatic water prepared from the lemon tincture.

Tolu Balsam Syrup, N.F., also is prepared by a method in which an aromatic water is made with the aid of a distributing agent, and the sucrose is dissolved in the clear filtrate. Magnesium carbonate is used as the distributing agent for the tolu balsam tincture because its alkalinity aids in dissolving the resinous constituents of the tolu balsam. A small part of the sucrose is added to aid in the solution of the resins. The aqueous solution must be filtered until perfectly clear, since it is very difficult to remove a slight cloudiness after all the sucrose has been added. The remainder of the sucrose may be dissolved in the filtrate either by agitation with the aid of gentle heat, not over 50° C., or by percolation. The resulting product has a light yellow color which may vary in intensity from batch to batch, depending on the length of time during which the tincture, the distributing agent and the water are in contact. If, instead of magnesium carbonate, talc is used as a filtering aid, a colorless syrup will be obtained. Thurer et al.[30] have suggested that magnesium oxide is a more suitable distributing agent for the preparation of this syrup.

On aging, Tolu Balsam Syrup may develop an unpleasant odor resembling that of coal gas or benzene. This is caused by the growth of molds which reduce cinnamic acid (which is extracted from the balsam) to cinnamene.

Soluble tolu extracts, which have better keeping qualities than the tolu syrup, were commercially available for the extemporaneous preparation of unofficial tolu syrups. The British Pharmaceutical Codex (1968) gives a formula for Solution of Tolu (*Liquor Tolutanus*). Water and then talc are added to an alcoholic solution of tolu balsam. The mixture is heated, agitated and set aside for a day before being filtered. Sucrose is dissolved in the filtrate. The product contains 50 percent (w/v) of sucrose and 27 percent (v/v) of alcohol. One volume of this concentrate, when mixed with 7 volumes of simple syrup, yields a tolu syrup with good aromatic qualities.

Aromatic Eriodictyon Syrup, N.F. The technique of using reactive distributing agents to facilitate the water extraction of acidic constituents from crude drug extracts is applied in the preparation of this syrup also. In addition to magnesium carbonate, potassium hydroxide solution is used in the formulation in order to extract larger quantities of resinous materials from the fluidextract of eriodictyon than otherwise would be possible. The official Tolu Balsam and Eriodictyon Syrups are basic in reaction, a factor which must be considered as a possible source of incompatibility when using these syrups as vehicles. On the other hand, Tolu Syrups prepared from soluble tolu extracts are not basic.

Senna Syrup, N.F., is made by dissolving sucrose in a solution obtained by mixing senna fluidextract, in which coriander oil has first been dissolved, with purified water. The mixture is allowed to stand for 24 hours, with occasional agitation, to allow for solution of the active ingredients and precipitation of inert extractive before being filtered. The coriander oil imparts a pleasant flavor to the syrup and acts to reduce the griping action of the senna in the intestine. The active constituents are emodin and emodin glycosides.

Wild Cherry Syrup, U.S.P., and some other syrups are manufactured by dissolving sucrose in aqueous extracts of crude drugs made by percolation (see Chap. 5).

Wild Cherry Syrup, U.S.P., is prepared from the dried stem bark of *Prunus serotina* Ehrhart (*Rosaceae*). The extractive from 15 percent (w/v) crude drug is contained in this syrup.

The coarsely powdered wild cherry bark is percolated with water after 1 hour of maceration in the percolator. Sucrose is dissolved in the percolate by agitation without the aid of heat, as this syrup contains volatile constituents. Finally, glycerin, alcohol and sufficient water to make the required volume are added. The small amount of alcohol is used as a preservative; glycerin is added to prevent the formation of a sediment from the tannins dissolved by the menstruum. Formerly, glycerin was used in the menstruum, but this increased the extraction of tannins and resulted in a product which was too bitter. Since this syrup contains tannins, precipitation of insolube tannates may be observed when the syrup is used as a vehicle for alkaloidal salts.[25]

Wild cherry bark contains the glycoside of *d*-mandelonitrile and a thermolabile enzyme, emulsin, which catalyzes the hydrolysis of the glycoside.

$$C_{14}H_{17}O_6N + H_2O \xrightarrow{\text{emulsin}}$$
d-mandelonitrile
glycoside

$$C_6H_5CHO \quad + \quad HCN \quad + \quad C_6H_{12}O_6$$
benzaldehyde   hydrocyanic   glucose
acid

Benzaldehyde (synthetic oil of bitter almond) contributes to the odor and the flavor of this syrup. The amount of hydrocyanic acid is very small, but it may be sufficient to stimulate respiration slightly.

Compound White Pine Syrup, N.F. XI, is prepared from a percolate obtained by extracting a mixture of 6 botanic drugs: white pine, wild cherry, aralia, poplar bud, sanguinaria and sassafras. In addition to water the menstruum contains alcohol and glycerin to aid in extraction of the active constituents which are resinous for the most part. Amaranth solution is added to darken the color of the preparation. A small amount of chloroform is used, both as a preservative and for its local action in the throat.

Acacia Syrup, N.F., and **Cocoa Syrup, U.S.P.,** are characterized by a higher viscosity than that of simple syrup, owing to the presence of components which are colloidally dispersed or suspended in the syrup.

Acacia Syrup, N.F., is prepared by adding purified water to a mixture of the dry solid ingredients: sucrose, powdered or granualted acacia and sodium benzoate (0.1%). The solids are mixed first to avoid the lumping that would occur if the acacia were moistened separately. Solution is hastened by heating on a water bath. After the preparation is cooled, the scum which forms is skimmed from the surface of the syrup and vanilla tincture is added to impart a pleasant flavor. Even though sodium benzoate is added as a preservative, this syrup does not keep well at room temperature.

Cocoa Syrup (Chocolate Syrup), **U.S.P.,** is a suspension of cocoa powder in a vehicle containing liquid glucose, glycerin and sucrose. The liquid glucose prevents the cocoa powder from settling rapidly by adding viscosity to the syrup. Older formulas for Cocoa Syrup employed gelatin as a suspending agent. In the formula vanillin and sodium chloride function to accentuate and augment the chocolate flavor. Official cocoa may contain from 10 to 22 percent of nonvolatile, ether-soluble extractive which is chiefly cocoa butter, a fat. Breakfast cocoa contains about 20 percent of fat and gives a less satisfactory syrup than commercial cocoa (which contains near the lower limit of fat) because it tends to increase in viscosity owing to coalescence of the fat.[23]

Ephedrine Sulfate Syrup, U.S.P., is a good example of the complexity of flavoring often characteristic of liquid oral medication. The syrup contains 0.4 percent (w/v) of ephedrine sulfate dissolved in a vehicle flavored with lemon oil, orange oil, benzaldehyde and vanillin. It is given a tart taste with citric acid and is colored with amaranth solution and caramel. Alcohol is included in the formula to facilitate incorporation of the alcohol-soluble flavoring constituents. Sucrose is dissolved by agitation in water containing these ingredients.

Formerly, this syrup was prepared with cherry syrup as the vehicle, but the limited seasonal supply of the fresh fruit caused the adoption of this substitute formulation.

Syrups that contain active ingredients derived from natural products often required somewhat complicated techniques in their manufacture. When pure medicaments are used in the formula, complications in technique arise generally because of the complexity of the flavoring constituents which may be used rather than from difficulties involved in preparing solutions of the drugs.

Iron (II) salts frequently are administered in syrup form. Two preparations illustrate the problems involved in preparing "iron" syrups.

Ferrous Sulfate Syrup, N.F., contains 4 percent w/v $FeSO_4 \cdot 7H_2O$. The peppermint spirit, used as the source of flavor, has a persisting effect which masks the somewhat unpleasant ferruginous taste of the Fe^{++}. Care must be taken in preparing aqueous solutions of ferrous salts, since Fe^{++} is readily oxidized by dissolved oxygen to form Fe^{+++}, which precipitates as basic ferric salts, discoloring the solution. Ferrous sulfate is dissolved in purified water containing some sucrose which provides a reducing environment, thereby inhibiting the autoxidation. If all of the sucrose were added, the solution would be too viscous to allow perfect filtration. Citric acid is included in the formulation to prevent discoloration of the syrup, i.e., a change from a green to a reddish brown tint; it does this by preferentially chelating iron (III).

Ferrous Iodide Syrup, N.F. XI, contained 6.5 to 7.5 percent of (w/v) FeI_2. The ferrous iodide was prepared by the direct combination of iron, in the form of bright wire, and iodine. Either hypophosphorous acid or citric acid was added as a stabilizer. Citric acid functioned to chelate any Fe^{+++} which formed as a consequence of autoxidation, thereby preventing oxidation of the iodide by Fe^{+++}. Hypophosphorous acid is an antioxidant; it is also a strong acid which causes the syrup to caramelize after a few months storage. For this reason, citric acid was the preferred stabilizer in this syrup. Ferrous Iodide Syrup should be stored in well-filled, colorless glass containers exposed to light in order to take advantage of the reducing action of light. It was administered

in water through a drinking tube to avoid staining the teeth.

DEXTROSE-BASED SYRUPS

Dextrose may be used as a substitute for sucrose in syrups containing strong acids in order to eliminate the discoloration associated with caramelization. Formulas were adopted for *N.F. VII* (1942) in which dextrose was used in place of sucrose in Syrup of Hypophosphites and Compound Syrup of Hypophosphites. Hydriodic Acid Syrup, N.F. XII, was the only official syrup using dextrose. Ferrous Iodide Syrups containing dextrose have been formulated.[17] Dextrose-based syrups do not turn brown in acid solutions, but they are subject to other difficulties.

Dextrose forms a saturated solution in water at 70 percent (w/v), which is less viscous than simple syrup. Dextrose dissolves more slowly than sucrose and is less sweet. The saturated solution of dextrose readily supports the growth of microorganisms: consequently, it is more easily fermented. Preservatives are required to improve the keeping qualities of such syrups. Glycerin may be added in 30 to 45 percent (v/v) concentrations to act as a preservative, increase the viscosity and, also, give additional sweetness to the preparation.[14] However, syrups which contain glycerin and strong acid tend to develop a butyric odor on aging. Alternatively, other preservatives and artificial sweetening agents, e.g., saccharin sodium, could be used in place of the glycerin.

Hydriodic Acid Syrup, N.F. XII, is made by dissolving dextrose in a mixture of diluted hydriodic acid, containing 10 percent (w/v) of HI, and purified water. The syrup contains 1.3 to 1.5 percent (w/v) of HI and 45 percent (w/v) of dextrose. The *N.F. XI* syrup contained 45 percent (w/v) of sucrose; the unusually low concentration of sucrose served to reduce the amount of discoloration which otherwise would be observed. A syrup with the same viscosity as the *N.F. XI* product can be made by using 60 percent instead of 45 percent (w/v) of dextrose.[14] The acidity of the syrup is sufficient to prevent the growth of microorganisms.

The *N.F.* cautioned that this syrup should not be dispensed if it showed a red discoloration due to free iodine. The preparation should be stored in light-resistant containers, since the atmospheric oxidation of iodide ion to iodine is photocatalyzed. (The iron (II) in Ferrous Iodide Syrup prevents the formation of iodine.) This deterioration is inhibited by the hypophosphorous acid contained in the diluted hydriodic acid, because H_3PO_2 is oxidized more easily than is the iodide ion and will reduce iodine to iodide.

Hydriodic Acid Syrup should be administered well diluted with water through a drinking tube to protect the teeth. The acidity is sufficient to cause softening of the dentin.

APPLICATION OF SOLUBILIZATION TO SYRUP FORMULATION

Alternative formulations which are based on surfactants used as solubilizing agents have been proposed for Tolu Balsam, Aromatic Eriodictyon and Orange Syrups.[29] Ordinarily, these syrups require the use of distributing agents in their manufacture. Introduction of a solubilizing agent in the formulation enables considerable simplification in manufacturing procedure. For example, a Tolu Syrup could be prepared by combining simple syrup with Tween 20 (a nonionic surfactant), glycerin and tincture of tolu balsam. No clarification is required. Relatively large amounts of surfactant (*ca.* 30%) are needed for this purpose.

The problems arising from the use of solubilizing agents in liquid formulations have already been discussed with reference to Aromatic Waters. These include foaming, alteration in flavor (particularly the development of bitter aftertastes) and reduced stability with respect to mold growth. Syrups prepared with solubilizers may separate into two layers, one rich in surfactant and the other rich in water. These difficulties may be partially eliminated by proper selection of solubilizing agent for the formulation and the addition of other substances (e.g., antifoaming agents) to counteract some of the undesirable effects. However, the application of solubilization in syrup formulation should be precluded if the solubilizing agent functions largely to prevent the precipitation of undesirable constituents in the formulation, as is the case in these preparations.

FORMULATION OF "ARTIFICIAL" SYRUPS

Non-nutritive Syrups. Several formulas have been published for sugar-free vehicles which are intended as substitutes for syrups and are to be administered to persons who must regulate their sugar and/or caloric intake accurately.[28] For example, persons suffering from diabetes mellitus, which is characterized by hyperglycemia (higher than normal blood sugar levels), need such preparations. Some early formulas included glycerin in order to take advantage of its viscosity and sweetness. However, glycerin, as well as alcohol and propylene glycol (which is employed as a substitute for glycerin in oral liquid medication), are glycogenetic substances, i.e., they are materials which are converted into glucose in the body either directly or indirectly. Substances to be used as sugar substitutes should also be nonglycogenetic.[11]

Huyck and Maxwell have developed and tested formulas for non-nutritive syrups; the following general formula is an example of "Diabetic Simple Syrup":[18]

Sodium carboxymethylcellulose (medium viscosity grade)	1.5%
Sweetening Agent qs.	
Preservative qs.	
Purified Water qs.	

The carboxymethylcellulose, a derived gum, functions as a bodying agent (viscosity builder). Some investigators have proposed the use of natural gums such as acacia and tragacanth for this purpose.[35] However, syrups prepared from these gums are not colorless (tragacanth produces opalescent products) and tend to change their characteristics upon aging. Sodium alginate and methylcellulose also have been used as the base for sugar-free syrups. These substances are nonglycogenetic and produce clear, colorless products. Unlike methylcellulose, which is nonionic, the anionic alginate and carboxymethylcellulose may exhibit incompatibilities with cationic drugs. Strong dehydrating agents cause coagulation of aqueous dispersions of both natural and derived gums. Consequently, these syrups are incompatible with excessive amounts of alcohol and electrolytes. Evidence of incompatibilities may be either simple increases or decreases in viscosity or, in extreme cases, gelation or precipitation. Solutions of methylcellulose, unlike those of the other gums, gel when heated, since the methylcellulose is less soluble at elevated temperatures owing to dehydration of the polymer. Preservatives must be included in the formulation, since aqueous solutions of gums readily support growth of microorganisms.

Non-nutritive, synthetic sweetening agents are required in the formulation. Saccharin sodium, rated 300 to 550 times as sweet as sucrose, is one such agent. It may be used in concentrations of 0.1 to 0.2 percent, but it is characterized by a bitter aftertaste which detracts from the desirable properties of a syrup. Compound Sodium Cyclamate Solution was the recommended sweetener in these formulas. Sodium cyclamate is 30 to 40 times as sweet as sucrose and has significantly less aftertaste than saccharin. The preferred sweetening agent combined both of these substances to take advantage of the synergistic sweetening effect that saccharin has on sodium cyclamate, with minimum aftertaste.[31] However, the Food and Drug Administration has removed the cyclamates from the approved list of food and drug additives, owing to evidence of carcinogenic effects produced in rats. New synthetic sweeteners will no doubt be developed, which can be included in this type of formulation. Aspartylphenylalanine methyl ester is a potential new low-caloric sweetener reported to be about 160 times sweeter than sucrose in aqueous solution.[12]

The over-all taste of the diabetic simple syrup is described as being ". . . slick and demulcent, but not offending."[18] Non-nutritive formulas for syrups intended as substitutes for official sucrose-based syrups should not be expected to have the "mouth feel" characteristic of sucrose syrups.

Sorbitol-Based Syrups. Traditionally, syrups are concentrated sugar solutions. However, the commercial availability of sorbitol, a hexahydric alcohol ($C_6H_{14}O_6$) made by hydrogenation of glucose, has led to its use as a major component of proprietary syrup formulations. Crystalline sorbitol is a white, odorless and nonvolatile solid. It is used most in the form of a 70 percent (w/w) aqueous solution (Sorbitol Solution, U.S.P.), trademarked Sorbo.[12]

From both a physico-chemical and a physiologic standpoint Sorbitol Solution, in some respects, compares favorably with and, in other respects, is superior to simple syrup. Sorbitol Solution is not irritating to the membranes of the mouth and the throat. Unlike sucrose, it apparently does not contribute to the formation of dental caries. Studies have shown that sorbitol is metabolized and converted to glucose; however, it is not absorbed from the gastrointestinal tract as rapidly as sugars. No significant hyperglycemia has been found, and, consequently, it may be used as a component of non-nutritive vehicles.[34] On the other hand, the ingestion of excessive quantities of sorbitol may have a laxative effect.

Sorbitol solution is about 60 percent as sweet as sucrose and half as viscous as simple syrup. However, it has excellent "mouth feel" qualities and lacks the acrid characteristics of some polyols (e.g., propylene glycol). Improved flavor characteristics and reduced sweetness may result when sorbitol solution is included in sugar-based formulations (sometimes a desirable effect in medication intended for adults). It is compatible with other polyols and simple syrup; as much as 10 percent (v/v) of alcohol can be added before crystallization is observed. Sorbitol, in common with other polyols such as glycerin, is also added to sucrose-based syrups to reduce the tendency of concentrated sugar solutions to crystallize. A blend of 30 percent sorbitol solution with 70 percent Syrup U.S.P. shows very little tendency toward crystallization. Consequently, sorbitol inhibits the sticking or locking of bottle caps which occurs with high concentrations of sucrose.

Artificial syrup formulations based entirely on sorbitol may include saccharin sodium to intensify the mild sweetness of the sorbitol, which masks the aftertaste of the saccharin.[26] While Sorbitol Solution does not ordinarily support mold growth, preservatives should be used in solutions containing less than 60 percent (w/w) of sorbitol.[10] Sorbitol is chemically stable and practically inert with respect to drugs and other ingredients used in pharmaceutical preparations. Many drugs are more stable in sorbitol solutions than in sucrose syrups. Therefore, sorbitol-based syrups may have the extended shelf-lives required in proprietary products, a shelf-life not obtained readily in sucrose syrups.[8, 15]

APPLICATIONS OF SYRUPS

Syrups are intensely sweet vehicles which lack significant amounts of alcohol and can function to mask the taste of otherwise salty or bitter drugs. Their effectiveness as vehicles is due also to their high viscosity and "mouth feel" qualities. Syrups are often described as having "body" and "smoothness." For these reasons, they constitute the vehicles most widely used for pediatric medication.

An important advantage of syrups is their acceptability and wide variety of flavors. Besides traditional flavors such as orange, lemon and peppermint, more exotic flavors are employed more frequently. Flavored syrups of pleasing taste can be prepared from fresh fruits,[13] such as cranberries, peaches, etc., and from compounded imitation flavor concentrates such as maple, tutti-fruiti, grape, etc. Synthetic flavors are preferred in industrial formulation, although the corresponding natural flavors are generally superior. Wesley[32] has compiled information on the use of unofficial flavors which indicated that half the flavors employed and more than three quarters of the fruit flavors used were of the unofficial type. The flavors most frequently used in pharmaceuticals were cherry followed by orange, raspberry, chocolate and mint.[33] Cherry was preferred for antibiotics, cough preparations and sulfa-antibiotics; chocolate for sulfonamides; and orange for vitamins. Ladd and Lofgren[19] have documented the procedures involved in the formulation and selection of a flavored vehicle for dioctyl sodium sulfosuccinate.

The effectiveness of official syrups in masking the tastes of salty or bitter drugs has been the object of considerable study.[24]

Saline drugs (e.g., bromides, ammonium chloride, etc.) are masked most effectively by spicy (pungent) syrups such as ginger and cinnamon or by fruit syrups. The latter are characterized by a tart taste arising from the presence of weak acids in the syrup. Fruit syrups prepared from imitation flavors (e.g., cherry) are not effective in masking salty tastes unless weak acids are added.[20] For this reason citric acid is a component of Orange Syrup, U.S.P. The tartness of these syrups is required to mask the saline taste. Fruit syrups are effective in masking sour drugs also, because of their natural association.

On the other hand, fruit-flavored syrups are not effective masking agents for bitter drugs. Whether or not a weak acid is present in the syrup makes little difference. Preparations involving bitter drugs (e.g., amines and their derivatives) present a major taste problem in the design of vehicles. Since the threshold for eliciting a bitter taste is very low and the taste itself is persistent, this problem is difficult. When a bitter drug is administered in syrup form, the initial taste will be predominantly that of the vehicle, but a bitter aftertaste will characterize the product. Syrups which have proved most effective in masking bitter tastes are Compound Sarsaparilla, N.F. XI, Aromatic Eriodictyon and Cocoa Syrups. Eriodictyon Syrup is believed to be effective because its resinous constituents have a mild anesthetic effect on the taste receptors. Because of its alkalinity, this syrup may be incompatible with amine salts and cause their precipitation (which would go unnoticed in a dark syrup). The alkalinity of Eriodictyon Syrup may account for its effectiveness in reducing the bitter taste of alkaloids. Cocoa Syrup is the best vehicle for bitter drugs. To some extent this may be due to its popularity compared with that of other flavors. However, Cocoa Syrup is effective because of its high viscosity; in effect it coats the tongue and, thus, it tends to inhibit diffusion of the drug to the taste buds. Drugs which are present in low concentrations may be adsorbed significantly by the high concentration of suspended cocoa solids, thus accounting for the effectiveness of the syrup in masking taste. Like Cocoa Syrup, Acacia

TABLE 4-3.   SYRUPS OF THE *U.S.P.* AND *N.F.*

TITLE *Synonyms or Tradenames*	CATEGORY AND DOSE*

Syrup, U.S.P.
  Simple Syrup
  Sirup
	Vehicle

Cherry Syrup, U.S.P. Syrupus Cerasi	Flavored Vehicle
Chloral Hydrate Syrup, U.S.P.	Hypnotic
Chlorpheniramine Maleate Syrup, U.S.P. Chlor-Trimeton Maleate Syrup	Antihistaminic
Chlorpromazine Hydrochloride Syrup, U.S.P. Thorazine HCl Syrup	Tranquilizer
Citric Acid Syrup, U.S.P. (Imitation) Lemon Syrup	Flavored Vehicle

Cocoa Syrup, U.S.P.
  Cacao Syrup
  Chocolate Syrup
	Flavored Vehicle

Dimenhydrinate Syrup, U.S.P. Dramamine Liquid	Antinauseant
Ephedrine Sulfate Syrup, U.S.P.	Adrenergic
Glycyrrhiza Syrup, U.S.P. Licorice Syrup	Flavored Vehicle
Hydrocodone Bitartrate Syrup, U.S.P. Hycodan Bitartrate Syrup	Antitussive

Ipecac Syrup, U.S.P.	Emetic; Dose:
	  Adults 10-30 ml.
	  children 10-15 ml.
	
	Nauseant Expectorant
	  Dose: 1 ml.

Isoniazid Syrup, U.S.P.	Tuberculostatic

Orange Syrup, U.S.P.
  Syrupus Aurantii
  Orange Peel Syrup
	Flavored Vehicle

Piperazine Citrate Syrup, U.S.P. Phenergan HCl Syrup	Antiemetic
Pyridostigmine Bromide Syrup, U.S.P. Mestinon Bromide Syrup	Cholinergic
Raspberry Syrup, U.S.P. Syrupus Rubi Idaei	Flavored Vehicle
Wild Cherry Syrup, U.S.P. Syrupus Pruni Virginianae	Flavored Vehicle
Acacia Syrup, N.F.	Flavored Vehicle
Amantadine Hydrochloride Syrup, N.F. Symmetrel Syrup	Antiviral (Prophylactic)
Cyproheptadine Hydrochloride Syrup, N.F. Periactin Hydrochloride Syrup	Antihistaminic;
Dexchlorpheniramine Maleate Syrup, N.F.	Antihistaminic
Dextromethorphan Hydrobromide Syrup, N.F. Romilar Syrup	Antitussive
Dicyclomine Hydrochloride Syrup, N.F. Bentyl Hydrochloride Syrup	Anticholingeric
Dimethindene Maleate Syrup, N.F. Forhistal Maleate Syrup	Antihistaminic
Dioctyl Sodium Sulfosuccinate Syrup, N.F. Colace Syrup	Fecal matter softener

TABLE 4-3 (*Continued*)

TITLE *Synonyms or Tradenames*	CATEGORY AND DOSE*
Aromatic Eriodictyon Syrup, N.F. Syrupus Corrigens Aromatic Yerba Santa Syrup	Flavored Vehicle
Ferrous Sulfate Syrup, N.F.	Hematinic; Dose: 10 ml.
Glyceryl Guaiacolate Syrup, N.F. Glycotuss Syrup	Expectorant
Hydroxyzine Hydrochloride Syrup, N.F. Atarax Hydrochloride Syrup	Tranquilizer (minor)
Meperidine Hydrochloride Syrup, N.F. Demerol Hydrochloride Syrup	Analgesic (narcotic)
Methdilazine Hydrochloride Syrup, N.F. Tacaryl Hydrochloride Syrup	Antipruritic
Promazine Hydrochloride Syrup, N.F.	Tranquilizer (major)
Pseudoephedrine Hydrochloride Syrup, N.F. Sudafed Syrup	Adrenergic (decongestant)
Senna Syrup, N.F.	Cathartic; dose: 8 ml.
Tolu Balsam Syrup, N.F. Syrup of Tolu	Flavored Vehicle
Triamcinolone Diacetate Syrup, N.F. Aristocort Syrup	Glucocorticoid
Trimeprazine Tartrate Syrup, N.F. Temaril Syrup	Antipruritic
Bromides Syrup, N.F. XI	Central Depressant
Ferrous Iodide Syrup, N.F. XI	Tonic, Hematinic; Dose: 1 ml.
Hydriodic Acid Syrup, N.F. XII	Expectorant
Phenindamine Tartrate Syrup, N.F. XII Thephorin Syrup	Antihistaminic
Compound Sarsaparilla Syrup, N.F. XI	Flavored Vehicle
Compound White Pine Syrup, N.F. XI	Vehicle Antitussive

* Usual Doses are 5 ml. unless otherwise noted.

Syrup also has a "blanketing" effect but to a lesser extent.

The complicated flavor patterns that frequently are used in oral medication are developed in the attempt to mask the distastefulness of drugs, both the fore- and the aftertastes, effectively. This approach is most effective if the taste of the drug is made a component of the flavor.

Antitussive preparations (cough remedies) are a very important class of syrup products. Wild Cherry and Compound White Pine Syrups are used primarily as components of cough mixtures. The latter was classed as an antitussive. The cough-suppressant action of syrups is due partially to their soothing effect on the mucous membranes of mouth and throat. Studies have indicated that Sorbitol Solution has about the same antitussive effect as other commonly used syrup ingredients.[12]

Two other classes of pharmaceutical dosage forms illustrate the versatility of the syrup concept. Although syrups are usually classed as solutions, the syrup base serves as an effective vehicle for insoluble drugs. Certain suspension products (see Chap. 7), particularly those used for sulfonamides, employ syrup vehicles. Chocolate syrups have been particularly popular in this respect. Another type of dosage form consists of solids which, on addition of an appropriate quantity of water, reconstitute into a syrup. This type of product is designed for drugs such as antibiotics which deteriorate in aqueous solution but are stable in the solid state.

REFERENCES AND BIBLIOGRAPHY

CLARIFICATION

1. Burt, B. W.: Manuf. Chem., *32*:411, 1961.
2. Handbook of Filtration. ed. 1. Mt. Holly Springs, Pa., The Eaton-Dikeman Company, 1960.

STANDARDS FOR WATER

3. Discher, C. A.: Modern Inorganic Pharmaceutical Chemistry, pp. 129–159, New York, John Wiley, and Sons, 1964.
4. Everett, N. A.: Bull. Par. Drug Assoc., *15*(5):1, 1961.

AROMATIC WATERS

5. Monte Bovi, A. J.: J. Am. Pharm. A. (Pract. Ed.), *12*:565, 1951.
6. Mulley, B. J.: *In* Advances in Pharmaceutical Sciences. vol. 1. pp. 87–194. New York, Academic Press, 1964.
7. Steen, C. V., Marcus, A. D., and Benton, B. E.: J. Am. Pharm. A. (Pract. Ed.), *13*:180, 1952.

SYRUPS

8. Bandelin, F. J., and Tuschoff, J. V.: J. Am. Pharm. A. (Pract. Ed.), *15*:761, 1954.
9. Barr, M., and Tice, L. F.: J. Am. Pharm. A. (Sci. Ed.), *46*:219, 1957.
10. ———: J. Am. Pharm. A. (Sci. Ed.), *46*:221, 1957.
11. Bauer, G. W., and Wasson, L. A.: J. Am. Pharm. A. (Pract. Ed.), *10*:296, 1949.
12. Cloninger, M. R., and Baldwin, R. E.: Science, *170*:81, 1970.

13. Drommond, F. G., and DeKay, H. G.: J. Am. Pharm. A. (Pract. Ed.), *15*:232, 1954.
14. Ewing, C. O., and Graves, D. B.: Drug Standards, *19*:102, 1951.
15. Gerber, C. F., Hetzel, C. P., Klioze, O., and Leyden, A. F.: J. Am. Pharm. A. (Sci. Ed.), *46*:636, 1957.
16. Grote, I. W., and Walker, P.: J. Am. Pharm. A. (Sci. Ed.), *35*:182, 1946.
17. Husa, W. J., and Pedrero, E., Jr.: J. Am. Pharm. A. (Sci. Ed.), *39*:67, 1950.
18. Huyck, C. L., and Maxwell, J. L.: J. Am. Pharm. A. (Pract. Ed.), *19*:142, 1958.
19. Ladd, J. W., Jr., and Lofgren, F. V.: J. Am. Pharm. A. (Pract. Ed.), *20*:456, 1959.
20. Lankford, B. L., and Becker, C. H.: J. Am. Pharm. A. (Sci. Ed.), *40*:77, 1951.
21. Littlejohn, O. M., and Husa, W. J.: J. Am. Pharm. A. (Sci. Ed.), *44*:305, 1955.
22. Lord, C. F., Jr., and Husa, W. J.: J. Am. Pharm. A. (Sci. Ed.), *43*:438, 1954.
23. Narian, G., Ohmart, L. M., and Stoklosa, M. J.: J. Am. Pharm. A. (Pract. Ed.), *15*:97, 1954.
24. Pardum, W. A.: J. Am. Pharm. A. (Sci. Ed.), *32*:103, 1943.
25. Reed, C. C., Burrin, P. L., and Bibbins, F. E.: J. Am. Pharm. A. (Pract. Ed.), *1*:73, 1940.
26. Schumacher, G. E., and Berzin, A.: Am. J. Hosp. Pharm., *27*:762, 1970.
27. Stocklosa, J. M.: J. Am. Pharm. A. (Pract. Ed.), *9*:556, 1948.
28. Swafford, W. B.: Am. Profess. Pharmacist, *22*:880, 1956.
29. Swafford, W. B., and Nobles, W. L.: J. Am. Pharm. A. (Pract. Ed.), *16*:223, 1955.
30. Thurer, G., Stempel, E., and Fonda, L. D.: Drug Standards, *25*:42, 1957.
31. Vincent, H. C., Lynch, M. J., Pohley, F. M., Helgren, F. J., and Kirchmeyer, F. J.: J. Am. Pharm. A. (Sci. Ed.), *44*:442, 1955.
32. Wesley, F.: J. Am. Pharm. A. (Pract. Ed.), *20*:91, 1959.
33. ———: J. Am. Pharm. A. (Pract. Ed.), *18*:674, 1957.
34. Wick, A. N., Almen, M. C., and Joseph, L.: J. Am. Pharm. A. (Sci. Ed.), *40*:542, 1951.
35. Woo, M., and Huyck, C. L.: Bull. National Formulary Committee, *16*:140, 1948.

5

Thomas Dudley Rowe, PH.D., *Dean and Professor of Pharmacy*
University of Michigan College of Pharmacy
George Zografi, PH.D., *Professor of Pharmaceutics*
University of Wisconsin School of Pharmacy

Solutions Using Mixed Solvent Systems: Spirits, Elixirs, and Extracted Products

INTRODUCTION

The many advantages of water as a pharmaceutical solvent for the preparation of solution dosage forms have been discussed earlier in this text. When substances to be included in liquid dosage forms for oral administration are not water soluble or when they exhibit chemical instability in water, one must either prepare suspensions or utilize nonaqueous solvents alone or with a minimum amount of water. Although the technology associated with suspension formulation has progressed to a very advanced state, nonaqueous solution dosage forms may be preferred if one can solubilize the drugs in mixed solvent systems and still maintain their chemical stability. This chapter contains information concerned with the preparation of dosage forms containing solvents other than water. Since extracted products often fall in this category, they also are included.

SPIRITS

Spirits may be defined as solutions of volatile substances in alcohol. The volatile substances in the majority of cases are volatile oils. The amount of volatile material in spirits varies greatly, and no fixed percentage can be given. In past editions, the *N.F.* contained a monograph, "Spirits of Volatile Oils," which specified that 6.5 percent of volatile oil was to be used. This monograph is no longer official, presumably because the amount of oil indicated was considerably lower than that used in the majority of spirits and also because there was little demand for a general formula. In all cases, the volatile oil content of the official spirits is much greater than that of the corresponding aromatic waters.

Likewise, the alcohol content varies. The lowest percentage is in Aromatic Ammonia Spirit, N.F. XIII, with a permissible range of 62 to 68 percent. The highest is in Camphor Spirit, N.F. XIII, with 80 to 87 percent.

The term "essence" is often used in place of the word "spirit."

In preparing spirits, it must be kept in mind that the oils dissolved in alcohol are precipitated, causing turbidity when the solutions are mixed with water. In order to avoid this turbidity, water, except as specified in the formula, should be avoided. Graduates and other equipment used should be thoroughly dry. Filter paper should be moistened with alcohol.

HISTORY

Although it is known that spirits are an older class of preparations than elixirs, their historical background and development are not established clearly. The introduction of spirits into pharmacy and medicine was brought about by the development of distillation procedures. By these means, volatile oils first were separated from the other constituents of the crude drugs in which they are found.

Brandy and whisky are the first spirits of which there is historical record. The exact date of their discovery is uncertain. However, the distillation of wine was carried out by the early Egyptians.[5] Brandy and whisky differ in many respects from the usual spirits of today inasmuch as they are not prepared by dissolving a volatile substance in alcohol. The first reference in European pharmacy to a spirit made from wine was by Arnaldus of Villanova, in the 13th century. He distilled herbs such as rosemary and sage with it, and highly recommended the medicinal virtues of these preparations.

Alcoholic solutions of volatile oils are probably an outgrowth of the perfume industry. As more and more volatile oils became known, it was only natural that they should be mixed and made into fragrant blends. This industry developed during the 15th and the 16th centuries, and in 1725 J. Maria Farina of Cologne introduced eau de cologne.[5] The perfumed spirit of *N.F. VIII* is similar to one introduced by Farina.

By the beginning of the 19th century, many volatile oils were known and some of their chemistry had been worked out. However, the term "spirit" for alcoholic solutions of these oils came into common use only very gradually. The first *U.S.P.* classified many of the earlier spirits as tinctures, primarily because the liquids were prepared by extracting the volatile oils from the crude drugs by maceration or percolation with alcohol. Either volatile oils were not obtainable easily at that time, or else it was thought that extraction from the crude drug gave a more suitable product. Through *U.S.P. III,* many of the spirits were still classified as tinctures. There were some official spirits, but they consisted usually of both the crude drug extractive and a volatile oil. It was not until the 4th revision that the crude drugs were deleted as sources of volatile oils in the spirits. Prior to that time, some spirits were made from the crude drugs and some from the volatile oils.

The first *U.S.P.* (1820) had 3 spirits, all made by distillation after maceration. There is now 1 in *U.S.P. XVIII* and 3 in *N.F. XIII.* There were 4 spirits official in *N.F. XII.*

OFFICIAL SPIRITS

It is not possible to classify the official spirits (the total number of which is small) to any extent into therapeutic or pharmaceutical groupings. This situation exists because there is a different and separate medicinal action for nearly every one of the official spirits. Consequently, they are discussed for the most part individually rather than in groups.

Peppermint Spirit, N.F., is used as a carminative and flavor. Given orally in small doses, usually 1 ml., this spirit is an effective carminative, and it is used extensively for that purpose. Mixed with other drugs or preparations, it may be used also as a flavor.

Peppermint Spirit is more than a mere solution of the volatile oil in that a small amount of crude drug is used in its preparation, as follows: First the leaves are macerated in water to remove tannins, xanthophyll, and other principles soluble in water. The aqueous extract is discarded, and the leaves are expressed and then macerated in alcohol. The alcohol dissolves the chlorophyll so that the final product has a bright green color. To this alcoholic solution containing the chlorophyll, 10 percent of volatile oil is added. The leaves used do not impart any medicinal action to the preparation. This action comes from the volatile oil added to the alcohol.

Many of the commercial products of this spirit are colorless. Thus, they do not conform to the *N.F.* specification requiring green color, but they do have the same therapeutic value.

Compound Orange Spirit, U.S.P., is used almost entirely as a flavoring agent. It is a blend of several oils and is readily prepared by simple solution. It is an important ingredient of aromatic elixir.

Aromatic Ammonia Spirit, N.F., frequently referred to (improperly) as "ammonia," is one of the best-known spirits. It will be found in a handy location in practically every pharmacy. It acts as a carminative due to the volatile oils present, as an antacid, and as a mild reflex circulatory stimulant. The last-named effect is produced by the liberation of NH_3 from the ammonium carbonate which the spirit contains. This preparation occasionally is asked for by the dose and is used in cases of fainting. Because of the oils present, it makes a milky preparation when mixed with water. This precipitation does not affect its medicinal action and is behavior typical of all spirits which contain volatile oils.

In making Aromatic Ammonia Spirit, the *N.F.* specifies the use of translucent pieces of ammonium carbonate. This specification is included because of the peculiar chemical nature of this compound. The official ammonium carbonate is a mixture of ammonium bicarbonate and ammonium carbamate. Its chemical formula is $NH_4HCO_3 \cdot NH_4NH_2CO_2$. The bicarbonate portion is insoluble in alcohol while the carbamate portion is alcohol-soluble. On exposure to air, more of the insoluble bicarbonate is formed by the loss of CO_2 and NH_3. The entire compound eventually becomes opaque. The opaque form is composed primarily of the alcohol-insoluble bicarbonate and is unsuitable for use in this preparation.

Unless the original material is translucent, the conversion to the alcohol-soluble form is not complete, due to the presence of excess NH_4HOC_3 in the opaque form. Therefore, the use of this form would produce a spirit below the required strength.

Strong Ammonia Solution, *N.F.*, (10% NH_4OH) is used to dissolve the translucent amonium carbonate. It converts all of the official ammonium carbonate to $(NH_4)_2CO_3$, which readily is soluble in alcohol.

It takes several days to make this preparation. At the end of that time, it is usually colorless. On standing, it is likely to assume a pale amber color unless it is preserved according to *N.F.* directions. The color change is due to the oxidation of the oils. Apparently, the color change does not alter the medicinal action of the preparation.

Camphor Spirit, N.F., like aromatic ammonia spirit, is well known to the lay public. It is referred to as Tincture of Camphor and also as Camphor. This preparation is a simple solution of 10 percent camphor in alcohol. It rarely is used internally, but its external use is very common. Usually it is applied to "cold sores" and similar ailments.

ELIXIRS

Of the official liquid preparations for oral administration, elixirs probably are used the most widely. Their popularity is due to their pleasant flavor, their relative stability, and the ease with which most of them are prepared.

Elixirs originally were defined as sweetened hydroalcoholic solutions containing flavoring materials and, usually, medicinal substances. Their primary solvents were alcohol and water. This definition is now too limited. Originally, elixirs were distinguished from other classes of preparations by the presence of sugar and alcohol in the finished product. However, several of the official elixirs may not contain sugar or any other sweetening agent. Furthermore, some commercial elixirs do not contain alcohol; in some, sugar has been replaced by saccharin. Consequently, while the definition as presented covers many elixirs, it should be kept in mind that many commercial products and a few official ones do not meet those specifications. In the official elixirs, the alcohol content varies from 4 to 40 percent. Generally, there is just enough alcohol to keep volatile oils or the medicinal substances in solution.

Glycerin also is present in most elixirs. During World War II, the shortage of glycerin made it necessary to replace it with some other liquid. Propylene glycol was found to be satisfactory, and the Bulletin of the *N.F.* published the formulas in which propylene glycol could be used in place of glycerin.[2] In most cases today, glycerin has been reincorporated as part of the formulas; however, propylene glycol is still used in some of the official elixirs.

Although most elixirs can be prepared by simple procedures, their small-scale manufacture is often time-consuming and wasteful. These difficulties are encountered because of the need of filtering the liquids with talc. Under Aromatic Elixir, a more complete discussion of this problem is presented (p. 92).

Elixirs generally owe their pleasant flavor to the presence of sugar and the volatile flavoring agents. Their sugar content is lower than that of syrups.

HISTORY

Elixirs as we know them today are a comparatively new class of preparations. According to Lloyd,[11] the first published formular of an elixir containing sugar as a sweetening agent appeared in 1859. For centuries before that time, many substances were called elixirs, but the word was used to designate "the magical transformation powder, so much sought after, a pinch of which would convert a whole mass of base metal into gold."[11] Later, the word was used "to denote various preparations more or less alchemistic."[11] In the 18th century, the term was applied to liquid medicinal preparations. However, these preparations were more like our present-day tinctures and are not comparable with modern elixirs.

Lloyd probably is responsible for the accepted pharmaceutical concept of elixirs. His book of elixirs,[11] published in 1883, put them into a definite category and helped to end the confusion in regard to these liquids. This book contained 283 formulas of these preparations. According to the *History of the National Formulary,*[14] it was this book and the *New York and Brooklyn Formulary,* also published in 1883, which stimulated the American Pharmaceutical Association to consider the publication of a national formulary.

Although elixirs are still popular today, they reached the height of their demand during the latter part of the 19th century. The first *N.F.,* which contained a total of 435 preparations, included 86 elixirs. Today, there are 14 official elixirs in *N.F. XIII* of a total of more than 900 monographs included therein. *U.S.P. XVIII* recognizes 9 elixirs. This number is an increase of 2 over *U.S.P. XVII.* It is the first time in several revisions that the number of elixirs has increased rather than decreased. This change, which cannot yet be called a trend, does, however, reflect the progress in pharmaceutical technology and in therapeutics. As is well known, many new organic chemicals have been discovered in recent years. Some of these are insoluble in water or in low concentrations of hydroalcoholic solutions or are unstable in the latter. Yet the need for liquid dosage forms of these chemicals is well recognized. By using modern methods for producing stable solutions, it is now possible to produce liquid preparations of these drugs. Elixirs, because of their palatability, are often the dosage form of choice. Nearly all of the medicated elixirs now of-

ficial in both the *U.S.P.* and *N.F.* are solutions of these new organic medicinals. It seems likely that as new drugs are introduced in the future they too will be made available in elixirs. Thus, the popularity of this type of preparation, which has diminished during the past 20 years, is likely to increase in the future.

CLASSIFICATION OF ELIXIRS

Until *U.S.P. XVII* and *N.F. XII* were published, the number of official elixirs which contained no medication and were used primarily as palatable vehicles was about as large as that which contained medication. At that time, elixirs fell naturally into 2 classes—medicated and nonmedicated. In U.S.P. XVII and N.F. XII, there were 5 nonmedicated and 21 medicated elixirs. In the current revisions, there are only 3 nonmedicated and 23 medicated. While there are now still 2 types of elixirs, the nonmedicated ones play a much less important role. Medicated elixirs usually contain per 5 ml. (one teaspoonful) from 25 to 100 percent of the average single dose of the medicinal substance as listed in the U.S.P. or N.F.

NONMEDICATED ELIXIRS

The three nonmedicated elixirs which are presently official are: **Aromatic Elixir, U.S.P.; Iso-Alcoholic Elixir, N.F.;** and **Compound Benzaldehyde Elixir, N.F.**

While elixirs of the nonmedicated group are chiefly vehicles, it should be emphasized that classification as a medicated elixir does not preclude its use for solvent purposes. Thus, phenobarbital elixir has a decided therapeutic action, yet it frequently is prescribed as the vehicle for other drugs. The primary purpose of either type is to make it possible for medicines to be dispensed in a palatable form.

Aromatic Elixir, U.S.P. Of the elixirs in this group, Aromatic Elixir is by far the most widely used. By consulting the formula in the *U.S.P.,* it will be seen that Aromatic Elixir is a rather simple preparation. Yet it is a difficult elixir to make properly in small quantities. This difficulty arises because of the slowness with which it filters and the necessity for refiltration before the preparation becomes clear. Clearness is one requisite of all elixirs. On a small scale, it is not unusual for 10 to 20 percent of the entire volume to be lost during filtration, due to the number of times that the liquid is passed through the filter. The loss of liquid is costly, and a long time is required. Consequently, most pharmacists do not attempt to prepare their own aromatic elixir but buy it from manufacturing houses.

In past years considerable research was done to improve the method of making the preparation, but the results were not entirely satisfactory. Fantus,[4] Lee,[10] Smith[18] and their co-workers all suggested methods for making this solution. None of their suggestions was accepted by the *U.S.P.*, with the result that the preparation today is much the same as it was many years ago.

The slowness in filtration results from the syrup's being added before the preparation is filtered. This ingredient, plus the talc, makes it nearly impossible to get a good rate of filtration. It is necessary to use talc as a filtering agent to help absorb the excess oils present. Fantus et al.[4] suggested dissolving the sugar in the filtrate to increase the rate.

The cloudiness is due to the insolubility in water of the oils present in compound orange spirit, which is one of the basic ingredients of this elixir. Smith and Burlage[18] suggested the use of terpeneless oils (water-soluble) to avoid this difficulty. Both of these suggestions make it possible for the elixir to be made more rapidly.

Research in improvement of methods of manufacture of long established elixirs appears to be of minor concern today. With the *U.S.P.* and *N.F.* now trying to make these compendia more useful in pharmacy prescription practice, it is possible more interest will be shown in improving present small scale manufacturing methods. Unless this is accomplished, it seems that formulas such as that given for preparing aromatic elixir are of little small scale use except for College of Pharmacy laboratory experiments.

The sugar content of Aromatic Elixir is about 31 percent, or less than half that of syrup. The alcohol content is from 21 to 23 percent by volume. It should be noted that this elixir may be diluted with water without becoming turbid. Consequently, it can be used with aqueous preparations without producing a milky liquid.

Iso-Alcoholic Elixir, N.F., first appeared in *N.F. VI.* It is composed of 2 separate parts: low alcoholic elixir with an alcohol content of from 8 to 10 percent, and high alcoholic elixir with an alcohol content of from 73 to 78 percent. By mixing these 2 solutions according to the directions given in *N.F. XIII,* a final product may be obtained which has an alcohol content within the ranges given above.

There is need for this type of elixir. Doctors frequently prescribe aromatic elixir or some other liquid as a vehicle for drugs soluble only in high percentage alcohol. In such cases, the prescription must be dispensed as a shake mixture. If Iso-alcoholic Elixir were prescribed, the drug could be dispensed in solution by using the right proportion of the low and the high alcoholic elixirs. Unfortunately, this elixir has not become widely used. It is the type of preparation which pharmacists should call to the attention of physicians. It is easy to prepare, and both forms are stable. The product is similar in flavor and odor to aromatic elixir.

Compound Benzaldehyde Elixir, N.F., is prepared by simple solution and is used when a bitter-almond-like flavor is desired.

MEDICATED ELIXIRS

This group can be described best by further classifying them according to their therapeutic activity.

Antihistaminics. This is the largest group of elixirs having a definite therapeutic action. In all there are 6 elixirs in this classification. They are:

Chlorpheniramine Maleate Elixir, U.S.P.
Diphenhydramine Hydrochoride Elixir, U.S.P.
Tripelennamine Citrate Elixir, U.S.P.
Bromodiphenhydramine Hydrochloride Elixir, N.F.
Brompheniramine Maleate Elixir, N.F.
Carbinoxamine Maleate Elixir, N.F.

Diphenhydramine Hydrochloride was introduced originally under the trade name Benadryl, and Brompheniramine Maleate was marketed originally under the trade name Dimetane. Tripelennamine Citrate is the citrate form, rather than the hydrochloride of tripelennamine which, in the hydrochloride form, was introduced as Pyribenzamine.

Bromodiphenhydramine Hydrochloride is known commercially as Ambrodryl Hydrochloride, Carbinoxamine Maleate as Clistin, and Chlorpheniramine Maleate as Chlortrimeton Maleate and Teldrin. Thus, all official elixirs containing antihistaminics were first introduced as trade named preparations and are still best known by their trade names. There are on the market many other nonofficial elixirs containing other antihistaminics. Nearly all have extensive use. Those which are official in the *U.S.P.* and *N.F.* represent dosage forms of drugs whose therapeutic merit has been well established over a period of years.

Diphenhydramine was among the first antihistamines to be used medicinally. On the other hand, Brompheniramine is one of the more recently discovered antihistaminics. They represent 2 different chemical classes of antihistamines, but all have the same general therapeutic action.[1,3]

Diphenhydramine Hydrochloride Elixir was first official in *U.S.P. XV*. It was the first new elixir to appear in any *U.S.P.* since the 12th revision published in 1942. Brompheniramine Maleate Elixir was official for the first time in *U.S.P. XVII*. Bromodiphenhydramine Hyrochloride Elixir and Carbinoxamine Elixir are official for the first time in *N.F. XIII*.

Sedatives and Hypnotics. This is the second largest group of elixirs having a definite therapeutic action. In all, there are 6 elixirs in this classification, all of which contain some type of barbituate. In *U.S.P. XVII* and *N.F. VII* there were a total of 8 elixirs which contained sedatives and hypnotics. The current official elixirs are:

Phenobarbital Elixir, U.S.P.
Secobarbital Elixir, U.S.P.
Sodium Pentobarbital Elixir, U.S.P.
Aprobarbital Elixir, N.F.

Amobarbital Elixir, N.F.
Sodium Butabarbital Elixir, N.F.

Each of these preparations illustrates the primary function of an elixir—to present a drug in a palatable form. Since elixirs are true solutions, these preparations also accomplish another function of the dosage form—that is, they deliver the active drug to the blood stream rapidly and efficiently.

Phenobarbital is used for long-acting sedation; amobarbital and butabarbital for intermediate duration; and pentobarbital and secobarbital are commonly used short-acting barbiturates.[7,8,12] Each of these elixirs contains approximately 0.20 g. (⅓ gr.) of active ingredient per dose (5 ml.). When that amount of the drugs is taken, they act as mild sedatives. All five of the preparations often are used in combination with other drugs.

The method of dissolving the barbiturate differs in each case. In Phenobarbital Elixir, the active ingredient first is dissolved in alcohol before adding the other liquids. While phenobarbital dissolves readily in alcohol and will remain in solution when the alcohol content is lowered, it will dissolve with difficulty in the alcohol, water and glycerin mixture of the final product.

Actually, the amount of alcohol in the final product (12 to 15%) would not keep the phenobarbital in solution. The presence of the glycerin prevents the phenobarbital from precipitating. According to Krause and Cross,[9] "glycerin and glycerin water solutions are poor solvents for phenobarbital," but "the solubility of phenobarbital in alcohol is enhanced by the addition of glycerin." This point is illustrated further by one of their tables, which shows that 10 percent alcohol will dissolve 0.19 percent phenobarbital while 10 percent alcohol to which is added 40 percent glycerin will dissolve 0.5 percent phenobarbital.

A number of studies concerned with the prediction of drug solubility in mixed solvent systems have been reported.[6,13,15,19] In general, they involve an attempt to correlate the dielectric constant of these mixtures with the amount of drug solubilized. Although it is not yet of general practical value, this approach, if successful, eventually should allow one to predict the exact amount of each solvent in a formula required to solubilize a given amount of drug without the extensive number of "trials and errors" normally required.

In Amobarbital Elixir, methenamine is used to increase the solubility of the amobarbital. In Sodium Pentobarbital Elixir, the sodium salt, which is readily water-soluble, is used. This compound, after being dissolved, later is converted to pentobarbital by adding diluted hydrochloric acid. The conversion is necessary because sodium pentobarbital is not stable in solution but decomposes on standing. By starting out with the sodium salt, the solution is prepared more readily.

Sodium Butabarbital Elixir is a good example of this type of preparation in which neither sugar nor glycerin are used. Sodium saccharin is used as the sweetening agent and propylene glycol is used as a cosolvent.

The Durham-Humphrey law, a federal regulation, requires that preparations in which a barbiturate is one of the main ingredients must have a prescription, either oral or written, before they can be dispensed. This regulation applies to these 5 elixirs. These preparations are also subject to the provisions of the Federal Controlled Substances Act. Some state laws concerning the dispensing of barbiturate preparations are even more restrictive than the federal regulations. In such cases, the state regulations must be followed.

Before leaving this classification of elixirs, the absence of any inorganic bromide salts in elixirs should be noted. For many years, the sedative of choice was some form of inorganic bromide—sodium, potassium, or a mixture of these and others.[17] Until the advent of barbiturates and later, tranquilizers, the bromides were about the only as well as the best sedatives available. They had the disadvantage of having a strongly saline taste, even when masked in elixirs. Even so, they were widely used until rather recently. As late as *N.F. XII,* two elixirs containing bromides were recognized. None is official now. Thus, for the first time in modern therapy, no elixir containing an inorganic bromide is included in either of the official compendia. They have been replaced by better and more effective drugs.

Expectorants. Three elixirs included under this heading have extensive use. They are:

Terpin Hydrate Elixir, N.F.
Terpin Hydrate and Codeine Elixir, N.F.
Terpin Hydrate and Dextromethorphan Hydrobromide Elixir, N.F.

The latter two are made by dissolving the respective drugs in Terpin Hydrate Elixir.

These elixirs cannot be diluted with much water or the slightly water-soluble terpin hydrate will precipitate. In this inability to mix with water, they differ from most of the other elixirs, to which water may be added in any quantity.

These elixirs contain the highest percentage of alcohol (39 to 44%) of all elixirs in order to keep the terpin hydrate in solution. The terpin hydrate and codeine elixir contains approximately $\frac{9}{10}$ gr. of codeine per fluidounce and is, therefore, an exempt narcotic. The elixir containing dextromethorphan has been added in order to provide a standard formula for a non-narcotic expectorant elixir.

Because of the high percentage of alcohol and glycerin in these preparations, there are numerous nonofficial formulas in use. Most of these conform to the official preparations as far as the active constituents are concerned, but they are usually less viscous and less palatable.

They are probably the most efficacious cough remedies of all the official preparations.

Miscellaneous Medicated Elixirs. It is not feasible to place the other official elixirs into therapeutic groups because each one has its own medicinal activity. **Digoxin Elixir, U.S.P.,** is used as a cardiotonic. **Dextroamphetamine Sulfate Elixir, U.S.P.,** is used as a central stimulant. This preparation is official for the first time in *U.S.P. XVIII.* **Trihexyphenidyl Hydrochloride Elixir, U.S.P.,** is used as an anticholinergic. In addition to those *N.F. VIII* elixirs already discussed, the following elixirs are recognized: **Acetaminophen Elixir, N.F.,** which is used as an analgesic. This preparation is new in *N.F. XIII,* as is **Potassium Gluconate Elixir, N.F.,** which is used as an electrolyte replenisher. **Dexamethasone Elixir, N.F.,** contains a synthetic adrenocortical steroid and is used in the treatment of rheumatoid arthritis and other conditions for which corticosteroid therapy is indicated.

UNOFFICIAL ELIXIRS

There are on the market many elixirs not recognized by the *U.S.P.* or *N.F.* It would be impractical to include them in this chapter. Many of these are sold under trade-names, and may not be labeled as elixirs. Regardless of how named, the official and nonofficial elixirs, as indicated at the beginning of this section, probably have a more extensive use than any other liquid oral dosage form. Thus, they continue to be, as they have been, for more than 100 years, an important and widely accepted class of preparations.

EXTRACTED PRODUCTS

EXTRACTION PROCESSES

It was realized very early in history that plant and animal tissues contain chemical substances which provide relief and treatment for a variety of disease states. Reference to the extraction of medicinals from plants with water, wine, or vinegar can be found in the writings of ancient Egypt and Greece and in the Bible. The most significant period of development for pharmacy came in the 19th century when rapid advances were made in the technology associated with extraction. It was found that a solution of active principles in the form of tinctures, fluidextracts, decoctions, and infusions offered a number of advantages over the use of the crude drug itself. For example, by means of efficient extraction one could eliminate a variety of extraneous inert materials and obtain a more potent, more palatable, and more conveniently administered dosage form. It was during this time that the percolation and maceration techniques were made more efficient and inexpensive, as well as more suitable for large scale manufacturing. Needless to say, it was this activity which provided the basis for later significant contributions of the phar-

macist to the area of dosage form development.

It is rare today that the pharmacist in community or institutional practice is called upon to prepare an extracted product. However, such products are widely used and are prepared on a large scale by the pharmaceutical industry. Modern concepts and techniques of isolation and identification of chemical substances from natural sources allow one to obtain even the most complex therapeutic agents in a relatively high state of purity. In spite of this, some crude drugs, such as *Rauwolfia serpentina* and Veratrum, and some extracted products, such as belladonna tincture and ipecac syrup, are still in use. This is probably because of the traditionally proven utility of such products as well as the improved therapeutic effects due to mixtures of alkaloids in contrast to any one chemical principle in many cases.

As indicated above, the crude plant or animal tissue contains active principles of medicinal interest such as alkaloids, glycosides, tannins, resins, and oils. Associated with them are a variety of complex mixtures of proteins, lipids, and carbohydrates. In order to bring about efficient extraction of active principles with maximum selectivity, a variety of procedures and solvent systems can be used. Basically, the process of extraction requires that a solvent system penetrate into cellular material and dissolve the desired constituents with a minimum of undesired material. Consequently, a number of physical chemical processes must occur and the rate at which they occur will largely determine the suitability of a particular process. Since the rate of solvent penetration is enhanced by an increased amount of exposed surface area, comminution of the crude drug to reduce particle size is often desirable. Since crude drugs undergo a drying process in the initial steps of collection, storage, and shipment, it is possible that initial rates of solvent penetration may be slow. As we shall see later, pre-extractive soaking of the crude drug with solvent may be useful in such cases.

The process of liquid movement through the crude drug generally is diffusion controlled. To some extent the movement of liquid through the pores and capillaries found in natural systems is influenced by the surface tension of the liquid and its wetting properties. If air is entrapped in capillaries and is not easily removed, the high counter-pressures which develop may become a major deterrent to flow. Of considerable importance also is the rate at which active constituents are dissolved and tend to diffuse away from the site of dissolution. In the absence of agitation, a significant stagnant diffusion layer exists. This layer, which contains a saturated solution of principles, acts as a barrier to diffusion away from the site. Re-establishment of a steady and rapid diffusion is best accomplished by agitation and by replacement with fresh solvent.

Two major processes are officially recognized for the extraction of pharmaceuticals: maceration, and percolation.

Maceration. With maceration, the crude drug is generally placed into a solvent system, with or without the application of heat, and the mixture allowed to stand with occasional agitation for an extended period. After the appropriate time has elapsed, the system is filtered to remove undissolved material, and a sufficient quantity of solvent is added to the filtrate to bring the product to a desired volume. The solvent used is called the menstruum, and the undissolved portion is called the marc.

The process of maceration is well suited for the extraction of crude drugs containing little or no soft cellular tissue, such as benzoin. Apparently, the extended periods during which crude drug and solvent are in contact allow for sufficient solvent penetration. The usual procedure does not call for replacement of solvent. Consequently, it ordinarily is not possible to obtain complete exhaustion of active principles during one peroid of maceration. Continuous agitation is likewise generally omitted, making the procedure less efficient. One approach suggested to overcome this difficulty is to enclose the crude drug in a permeable membrane or sack, as in a tea bag. When this is suspended in the solvent, dissolved material falls away from the region near the crude drug because of its greater specific gravity, and fresh solvent takes its place. Special approaches used with various official products will be discussed later.

Percolation. The process of percolation is by far the most popular means of extraction in the United States for the preparation of tinctures, fluidextracts, and extracts. In general, the procedure involves packing the drug into a column, known as a percolator (see Fig. 5-1), slowing passing solvent through the column, and then collecting the extracted material dissolved in the solvent.

Percolation offers the opportunity to extract principles exhaustively with a minimum of solvent. This is important, because maximum yield is desired and because it is easier to bring a product to proper volume by adding solvent than by removing excess solvent. One variable which is useful in this regard is the shape and size of the percolator. For instance, in a long and narrow column, each particle of crude drug is exposed to nearly all of the solvent added to the column. If the rate of liquid movement under the influence of gravity or external

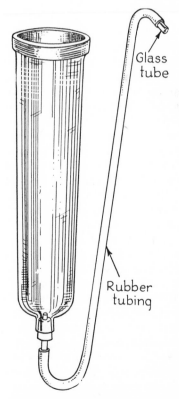

Fig. 5-1. Percolator with rubber-tube attachment for regulating flow of percolate.

pressure is controlled at the bottom of the column, one can make the rate slow enough to obtain very efficient extraction with a minimum volume of solvent.

On the other hand, consider a situation in which solvent movement is very slow because of the nature of the crude drug or the viscosity of the menstruum. Here, a wider and shorter column offers less distance for solvent travel and the hydrostatic pressure of the solvent is distributed over a greater surface area because of greater column cross-sectional area. Naturally, the amount of crude drug in the percolator determines the size of the percolator, as do the possible changes of the column because of cellular swelling. It should be stressed at this point that proper packing of the column of crude drug is important in order to maintain uniform movement of the menstruum. The control of flow rate at the orifice also can be used to ensure uniform and controlled solvent movement.

Often the problem of solvent penetration can be solved by allowing a period of maceration in the percolator. In this case, liquid is allowed to flow through the column, but outflow is stopped to allow the drug to soak in the solvent. The period of maceration varies with the nature of the crude drug. Usually the same solvent system is used for the maceration and the percolation steps, but there is no reason why different solvent systems cannot be used. For example, a crude drug containing alkaloids might be macerated with an acidified hydroalcoholic solvent in order to convert the basic alkaloids to their more soluble amine salts. This might then be followed by a normal hydroalcoholic solution for the percolation step. Selective removal of fats or tannins also may be carried out before the percolation step. Removal of fat might be particularly helpful in increasing the penetration of solvent system into plant or animal tissue.

As indicated earlier, the goal of percolation is to extract all of the active principles of a crude drug with a minimum of solvent. Exhaustive extraction can be monitored by the loss of color in the extracted solvent system, the loss of bitter taste characteristic of alkaloids, or the absence of principles as determined by spot tests with specific re-

agents. For most extractions of potent medication, the extract is quantitatively assayed so that the final adjustment of concentration may be made as exactly as possible. More details will be given, when of importance, as the various official extracted products are discussed.

Decoction, Digestion, and Infusion. Three other processes of extraction traditionally have been used, although no presently recognized product is made by these techniques. These are decoction, digestion, and infusion. **Decoction** involves placing plant material in water, bringing the water to a boil for about 15 minutes, and expressing and straining the remaining marc to obtain a maximum amount of water-soluble principles. At one time this was a widely used procedure for brewing tea and coffee. **Digestion** is actually maceration with continued heating during the maceration period. The temperature is usually maintained between 40 and 60°. **Infusion** involves first macerating the drug with cold water followed by the addition of boiling water in an amount equal to 90 percent of the desired volume. As can be seen, these processes are most applicable in obtaining water-soluble principles from plants, and this limitation is one reason for their general disuse today.

TINCTURES, FLUIDEXTRACTS, AND RESINS

The number of extracted products in use today is still quite significant, and no attempt will be made to discuss them all. The *U.S.P.* and *N.F.* recognize some of the more widely used products and set standards and procedures for their preparation. Three types of official dosage forms contain most of the extracted products being used. These are tinctures, fluidextracts, and extracts. The information that follows emphasizes those aspects of these dosage forms which are of general interest and are related to the preparation of these products. Reference should be made to the *U.S.P.* and *N.F.* for more specific information about the various preparations.

Tinctures are alcoholic or hydroalcoholic solutions of principles extracted from natural sources or of pure chemicals merely dissolved in these solvent systems. The amount of active ingredient in tinctures varies for different products; as a rule, however, tinctures of potent medication obtained by extraction are adjusted so that each ml. of tincture contains the potency equivalent of 0.1 g. of active crude drug constituents or 10 percent of activity. This is in contrast to fluidextracts, in which each ml. contains the equivalent of 1 g. of constituents or 100 percent of activity. Less potent drugs are prepared as tinctures with higher levels of potency equivalents, usually around 20 to 50 percent of activity.

Tinctures. A number of tinctures are prepared by maceration of crude drug as set forth in the official procedure known as **Process M.** This process is preferred for substances containing a high proportion of soluble constituents. In process M maceration takes place over a period of 3 days. Official tinctures prepared by maceration include: **Compound Benzoin Tincture, U.S.P.; Sweet Orange Peel Tincture, U.S.P.; Lemon Tincture, U.S.P.; Compound Cardamom Tincture, N.F.;** and **Tolu Balsam Tincture, N.F. Paregoric, U.S.P.,** formerly known as Camphorated Opium Tincture, also is prepared by maceration of the crude drug, opium. With the exception of Compound Benzoin Tincture, which is used as a topical protective, and Paregoric, which is used mainly to reduce peristaltic movement, all of the other tinctures given above are used as flavors. Making note of the solvent systems used we can see that two categories develop. Most of the products use alcohol as a menstruum; two products use Dilute Alcohol, *U.S.P.,* and a small amount of glycerin. The latter category includes Paregoric and Compound Cardamom Tincture. In both preparations the glycerin helps to prevent separation of tannins from the final product.

The *U.S.P.* and *N.F.* also recognize the process of percolation for extraction when preparing tinctures. This is known as **Process P.** The most widely used tincture, **Belladonna Tincture, U.S.P.,** is prepared by Process P using 10 g. of Belladonna Leaf for each 100 ml. of final product. This product is used widely as an anticholinergic agent because of atropine and other atropinelike

alkaloids extracted from the leaf. **Vanilla Tincture, N.F.,** which is used as a flavor, is prepared by first macerating the vanilla bean in water for 12 hours followed by 3 days of maceration with an additional equal volume of alcohol. The mixture is then added to a percolator which already contains a specified amount of sucrose. Percolation is then carried out with Diluted Alcohol. Thus, a combination of techniques is required to suitably extract the necessary principles from the vanilla bean.

The remaining official tinctures are prepared by simple solution of various chemicals. With the exception of Green Soap Tincture, N.F., all of these tinctures are used as disinfectants. They include: **Iodine Tincture, U.S.P.; Nitromersol Tincture, N.F.;** and **Thimerosal Tincture, N.F.** Iodine Tincture is prepared by dissolving 20 g. of iodine with 24 g. of sodium iodide in 1 liter of alcohol. Apparently the following reaction occurs:

$$I_2 + I^- \rightleftharpoons I_3^-,$$

and in this way the product is greatly stabilized against reaction between I_2 and ethyl alcohol. Since the I_3^- is quite water soluble, this product can be diluted with water to a considerable extent.

Green Soap Tincture, N.F., is prepared by dissolving Green Soap in alcohol and is used as a detergent solution, generally applied to the skin.

Fluidextracts. Fluidextracts are liquid preparations containing extracted principles from vegetable drugs prepared in such a way that each ml. contains the therapeutic constituents of 1 g. of the crude drug used to prepare the fluidextract. A number of processes involving percolation have been officially recognized. Percolation is preferred in all cases because of the exhaustive extraction required. The *N.F.* recognizes five processes labeled A, B, C, D, and E. The *U.S.P.,* which recognizes only two fluidextracts, does not recognize general processes; however for both *U.S.P.* fluidextracts the official procedure is the same as Process D in the *N.F.*

PROCESS A entails exhaustive percolation with an alcoholic or hydroalcoholic menstruum. In order to exhaustively extract a crude drug, more than 1,000 ml. of percolate per 1,000 g. of crude drug is often required. To facilitate any concentration of percolate that is necessary to bring the volume back to 1,000 ml., the first 850 ml. of percolate is set aside and the remaining percolate is collected separately. After complete extraction has taken place, the more dilute percolate is concentrated by slow evaporation and combined with the first percolate to give 1,000 ml.

PROCESS B involves the use of more than one menstruum for percolation. For example, in addition to alcohol or water-alcohol mixtures, glycerine or acid might be used to facilitate extraction. The procedure involves sequential use of the adjunct solvent, i.e., glycerine or acid, and the main solvent system, followed by the procedure outlined in Process A.

PROCESS C has been developed for use when the heating required for solvent concentration cannot be carried out. It is a fractional technique whereby the crude drug is divided into 3 portions. For example, 1,000 g. of crude drug is divided into 500-g., 300-g., and 200-g. portions, and each portion is percolated separately. From the first portion, 200 ml. of percolate is collected and set aside; then 5 300-ml. quantities are collected and numbered in order of collection. The second portion of drug (300 g.) is then percolated with the 5 300-ml. samples (from the first portion) in order of previous collection. In this case, the first 300 ml. of percolate is set aside, and 5 200-ml. quantities are collected and numbered. The process is then repeated with the third portion of drug and the 5 200-ml. quantities collected from the second portion. The first 500 ml. of percolate collected from the third portion is then pooled with the 200-ml. and 300-ml. portions collected from the first and second portions to give 1,000 ml. Thus, the crude drug is efficiently extracted with a minimum of solvent.

PROCESS D differs from Processes A and B only in that boiling water is used as the menstruum.

PROCESS E is a modification of Process C. The crude drug is packed into a column which has a length much greater than its width, or into a series of columns joined together. The column should be sufficiently long to allow complete extraction with 1,000 ml. of menstruum per 1,000 g. of crude drug. Percolation may be carried out by forcing the menstruum through with air pressure at one half the rate specified for other processes. One may apply air pressure from above with a closed cover on the percolator or one may pull the liquid through by means of suction applied at the bottom of the percolator.

Six *official fluidextracts* are recognized by the *U.S.P.* and *N.F.* Those prepared by Process A include: **Eriodictyon Fluidextract, N.F.,** used as a flavor; **Senna Fluidextract, N.F.,** used as cathartic; and **Belladonna Leaf Fluidextract, N.F.,** used as an anticholinergic agent (see Belladonna Tincture above). This last product may also be made by Process E. No official products are prepared by processes B or C. Three are prepared with boiling water, as in Process D. These include: **Glycyrrhiza Fluidextract, U.S.P.,** used as a flavor; and **Cascara Sagrada Fluidextract, N.F.,** and **Aromatic Cascara Sagrada Fluidextract, U.S.P.,** both use as cathartics. The latter product contains, in addition to the principles of Cascara Sagrada, pure glycyrrhiza extract, saccharin, anise oil, coriander oil, methyl salicylate, alcohol, and water.

At this point it is appropriate to include another extracted liquid preparation, **Ipecac Syrup, U.S.P.** Although categorized as a syrup, the product is prepared by percolation of powdered ipecac with 3 volumes of alcohol and 1 volume of water after 72 hours of maceration. After using enough menstruum to exhaustively extract the crude drug, the percolate is reduced in volume to a value equal to the weight of original crude drug. After filtering, the filtrate is further reduced in volume, and HCl and alcohol are added. Filtration, followed by more washing with HCl, alcohol, and water, leads to a solution ready to be brought back to a volume equal to the original crude drug weight. To this is added glycerin, and enough syrup to make the desired volume. Such a procedure of washing with acid, alcohol, and water ensures the complete extraction of alkaloids as their amine salts and the rejection of extraneous material. Ipecac Syrup is used widely as an antiemetic in case of poisoning.

Extracts. Although they are not liquid preparations, the official extracts are included in this chapter with their counterparts the fluidextracts. Extracts are concentrated preparations of animal or vegetable drugs which first have been extracted by procedures already discussed. They are potent preparations, usually 2 to 6 times as potent on a weight basis as the crude drug. In most cases, after percolation the volume is reduced by evaporation of solvent. Traditionally, three types of extracts have been prepared on the basis of consistency. These are: semi-liquid extracts with a syrupy consistency; pilular extracts with a plastic consistency; and powdered extracts, brought to complete dryness. For potent products, adjustment of potency is accomplished by the addition of inert diluents. Liquid glucose is often used for the pilular extracts; starch is added to powdered extracts.

Three plant extracts are officially recognized. These are: **Pure Glycyrrhiza Extract, U.S.P.; Cascara Sagrada Extract, N.F.;** and **Belladonna Extract, N.F.** Pure Glycyrrhiza Extract is prepared in the pilular state, whereas Cascara Sagrada Extract is made as the powdered extract. Both pilular and powdered forms of Belladonna Extract are officially recognized.

The *U.S.P.* recognizes one extract from an animal source, namely **Trichinella Extract, U.S.P.,** an aqueous extract of killed, washed, defatted, and powdered larvae of *Trichinella spiralis*. It consists of antigens of the larvae and is used as a dermal reactivity indicator.

Resins. The remaining group of extracted products that are officially recognized consists of resins. Natural resins are solid or semisolid exudations from plants or from insects that feed on plants. Chemically these exudations are the oxidized terpenes of the volatile oils of plants. Prepared resins are produced by exhaustively percolating a plant having a resin as the major ingredient. Percolation is usually carried out with alcohol as the menstruum. For example, **Podophyllum Resin, U.S.P.,** is obtained by percolation of the dried rhizome and roots of *Podophyllum peltatum*. Prepared as a dispersion in alcohol or in **Compound Benzoin Tincture, U.S.P.,** it is used as a topical caustic for the treatment of certain papillomas. **Rosin, N.F.,** is a solid resin which remains after the distillation of turpentine. It has many traditional uses; pharmaceutically it is widely used as an adhesive.

Oleoresins contain a mixture of volatile oils and resins. Turpentine, once official in the *N.F.*, is a good example. Now no oleoresins are officially recognized and their use in pharmacy is very limited.

REFERENCES

1. Beckman, Harry: Pharmacology: The Nature, Action and Use of Drugs. ed. 2. Philadelphia, W. B. Saunders, 1961.
2. Bull. National Formulary Comm., *11*:201, 1943.
3. DiPalma, J. R. (ed.): Drill's Pharmacology in Medicine. ed. 3. New York, McGraw-Hill, 1965.
4. Fantus, B., Dyniewicz, H. A., and Dyniewicz, J. M.: J. Am. Pharm., *22*:655, 1933.
5. Gildemeister, E., and Hoffman, F.: The Volatile Oils. ed. 2. vol. I. translated by Edward Kremers, New York, John Wiley and Sons, 1913.
6. Gorman, W. G., and Hall, G. D.: J. Pharm. Sci., *53*:1017, 1964.
7. Grollman, Arthur: Pharmacology and Therapeutics. ed. 7. Philadelphia, Lea and Febiger, 1970.
8. Krantz, J. C., and Carr, C. J.: The Pharmacologic Principles of Medical Practice. ed. 7. Baltimore, Williams and Wilkins, 1969.
9. Krause, G. M., and Cross, J. M.: J. Am. Ph. A., *40*:137, 1951.
10. Lee, C. O., and Close, M.: J. Am. Pharm. A., *23*:236, 1934.
11. Lloyd, J. U.: Elixirs. Cincinnati, Clarke, 1883.
12. Modell, W. (ed.): Drugs of Choice 1970-71. St. Louis, C. V. Mosby, 1970.
13. Moore, W. E.: J. Am. Pharm. A. (Sci. Ed.), *47*:855, 1958.
14. National Formulary, ed. 13. Washington, D. C., American Pharmaceutical Association, 1970.
15. Paruta, A., Sciarrone, B., and Lordi, N. G.: J. Pharm. Sci., *51*:704, 1962.
16. ———: J. Pharm. Sci., *53*:1349, 1964.
17. Salter, W. T.: A Textbook of Pharmacology. Philadelphia, W. B. Saunders, 1952.
18. Smith, W. J., and Burlage, H. M.: J. Am. Pharm. A., *25*:123, 1936.
19. Sorby, D. L., Bitter, R. G., and Webb, J. G.: J. Pharm. Sci., *52*:1149, 1963.

6

Hans Schott, Ph.D., *Professor of Physical and Colloid Chemistry,*
Temple University, School of Pharmacy
and
Alfred N. Martin, Ph.D., *Professor and Director, Drug Dynamics Institute,*
University of Texas, College of Pharmacy

Colloidal and Surface-Chemical Aspects of Dosage Forms

THE REALM OF COLLOIDAL PARTICLES AND INTERFACES

A system in the colloidal state is characterized by having one or more components with at least one dimension lying in the range between about 10 to 100 Å on the lower end and 1 μ on the upper end. There are 10^8 Å (Angstrom units) or 10^4 μ (microns) to the centimeter. Thus, the colloidally disperse phase can be a small three-dimensional solid particle or liquid droplet; a thread or rodlike particle or filament, like a muscle fiber or tobacco mosaic virus; a sheet or platelike particle, such as kaolin; a thin film, like a monolayer of denatured protein or a lamella encasing air in a soap bubble; or a biological membrane.

In view of their small size in at least one dimension, an appreciable fraction of the molecules or ions of a colloidal particle is located in the boundary region or interface between the particle, referred to as the disperse phase, and the medium surrounding it, called the continuous phase.[77] Owing to their location near an interface, these molecules are exposed to forces different from those to which the molecules in the core of the particle are exposed and are, therefore, more "energetic." This results in small liquid droplets having a higher vapor pressure than does a large bulk volume of the same liquid. Similarly, a solid subdivided into colloidal particles has a higher solubility in a given liquid than it does in the form of coarse pieces, a fact utilized to increase the rate of absorption of solid drugs. Coarsely powdered sulfur is poorly absorbed into the body when administered orally, but the same dose of *colloidal* sulfur is assimilated so completely and rapidly that it may cause toxic reactions and sometimes even death.

HISTORICAL ASPECTS

The applications of colloids in pharmacy preceded by a number of years the understanding of their underlying phenomena. Lotions, pastes, and soaps were widely used by the alchemists. It was only in 1861 that the Scotsman Thomas Graham, one of the early physical chemists, introduced the concept of *colloids,* a word from the Greek *kolla* meaning glue. He distinguished between "crystalloids" such as salts and sucrose, which had high rates of diffusion in water and dialyzed readily through membranes made of pig bladder or parchment paper, and "colloids" such as gelatin, starch, gums, tannins, Prussian blue (finely dispersed ferric ferrocyanide), and purple of Cassius (finely divided gold adsorbed on colloidal tin hydroxide). The colloids did not crystallize, diffused very slowly in water, and did not pass through dialysis membranes. Graham also coined the words *sol, gel, peptization,* and *syneresis.*[3,47] None of the colloids could be seen in the light microscope, but some could be detected by means of the Tyndall beam and the ultramicroscope (p. 123).

Colloid chemistry as a science in its own right began at the University of Leipzig with the work of Wolfgang Ostwald, who devoted his whole career to the study of the subject. In 1907 he became the first editor of the Kolloid-Zeitschrift. In 1906 he wrote a booklet entitled *The World of the Neglected Dimensions,*[44] in which he pointed out the difference between solutions of small mole-

103

TABLE 6-1.   CLASSIFICATION OF DISPERSE SYSTEMS BY PHYSICAL STATE

DISPERSE PHASE \ CONTINUOUS PHASE	SOLID	LIQUID	GAS
Solid	Glasses containing finely dispersed metals, e.g., ruby glass containing gold; alloys; pastes such as toothpaste	Sols, magmas, gels; suspensions such as Tetracycline Oral Suspension, U.S.P., Kaolin Mixture with Pectin, N.F.	Smokes, dust, solid aerosols, insufflations, e.g., isoproterenol sulfate, talc-based disinfectants
Liquid	Solid emulsions (rare); ointments such as Cold Cream, U.S.P., Hydrophilic Ointment, U.S.P.	Emulsions such as milk, mayonnaise, Sterile Phytonadione Emulsion, U.S.P.	Fog, mist, liquid aerosols; throat and nasal relief sprays, such as naphazoline hydrochloride solution
Gas	Solid foam, e.g., foamed plastics, sponges; pumice stone, meerschaums, xerogels	Foams; carbonated soft drinks	None

TABLE 6-2.   CLASSIFICATION OF DISPERSE SYSTEMS BY SIZE

CATEGORY	RANGE OF PARTICLE SIZE	CHARACTERISTICS	EXAMPLES
Molecular solutions of small molecules and ions	Below 10Å	At lower limit of resolution of electron microscope; high rates of diffusion; pass through filter paper, ultrafilter, and dialysis membranes; high osmotic pressure	NaCl, sucrose or alkaloidal salts in water; vitamin A acetate in cottonseed oil
Colloidal dispersions; solutions of macromolecules	Between 20 Å and 1 μ; 10^3 to 10^9 atoms per molecule or particle	Visible in electron microscope and often in ultramicroscope; invisible in ordinary microscope; low rates of diffusion; undergo Brownian motion; pass through filter paper, retained by ultrafilter and dialysis membranes; low osmotic pressure	Bentonite Magma, U.S.P.; Mild Silver Protein, N.F.; bacterial and virus suspensions; albumin and sodium carboxymethylcellulose in water; polystyrene in benzene; surfactant micelles
Coarse dispersions	Above 1 μ	Visible in ordinary microscope; retained by filter paper; no diffusion nor Brownian motion. Settle out or cream; negligible osmotic pressure	Most pharmaceutical suspensions and emulsions Erythrocytes in blood

cules and ions or molecularly dispersed systems, coarse dispersions which settle out readily, and colloidal dispersions which occupy an intermediate position. Thus, the colloidal state represents a general state of matter like the solid, liquid, and gaseous states.

The universality of the colloidal state was corroborated experimentally by von Weimarn,[78] who prepared an extraordinary variety of colloidal dispersions and gels in a score of liquids by proper adjustment of supersaturation, i.e., by regulating the rates of formation and growth of nuclei. Von Weimarn thus demonstrated that, contrary to Graham's hypothesis, there are no intrinsically colloidal substances, and that most substances can be prepared in the colloidal state of dispersion, including the "crystalloidal" substances. After all, during the processes of dissolution and precipitation, all systems pass through the colloidal size range, if only briefly. Von Weimarn prepared colloidal ice in liquid air, colloidal barium sulfate and sulfur in water, an aqueous barium sulfate gel, and colloidal dispersions of sugar and a gel of sodium chloride in organic liquids. On the other hand, some of Graham's "colloids," such as proteins, have been prepared as large, single crystals.

CLASSIFICATION OF DISPERSE SYSTEMS

Classifications based on three different criteria are discussed below.

Interaction Between Disperse Phase and Continuous Medium

This criterion is the basis for the most fundamental classification.

Lyophilic systems are characterized by a great affinity or attraction between the disperse phase and the dispersion medium, i.e., by extensive solvation.

Lyophobic systems are characterized by low affinity between the two. If the continuous phase is water, the disperse phases can be hydrophilic, i.e., attracted by water, or hydrophobic, i.e., water repelling. Hydrophobic phases are often lipophilic, oil attracting, or oleophilic. Hydrophilic materials include starch and methylcellulose, which have many hydroxyl groups; gums acacia and tragacanth, which have carboxyl groups as well; gelatin, which consists largely of amide groups; kaolin, whose surface is covered with hydroxyl and oxygen ions; and bentonite, whose surface is covered with oxygen ions. Owing to high concentrations of hydrophilic groups, these compounds swell and disperse spontaneously in water; most of them dissolve molecularly.

Hydrophobic materials include sulfur, silver chloride, magnesium stearate, steroids, polystyrene, activated charcoal, cottonseed oil, and paraffin. The last six compounds are lipophilic, i.e., they spontaneously disperse or dissolve in liquids of low polarity such as hydrocarbons. Dispersions of hydrophobic substances in water are intrinsically unstable and require surfactants or other stabilizing agents.

Association colloids form the third category of disperse systems according to this classification. These are surfactant molecules or ions which have hydrophilic and lipophilic moieties in a single molecule. This dual or *amphiphilic* nature causes them to form colloidal aggregates in solution.

Physical States of Disperse and Continuous Phases

The physical states of the disperse phase and of the continuous phase or matrix is the basis of the second classification (Table 6-1). The only combination that does not form colloidal systems is that of two or more gases. They form molecularly homogeneous mixtures. A *sol* is the colloidal dispersion of a solid in a fluid. *Aerosols* are dispersions in air, *hydrosols* in water, *organosols* in organic solvents.

Particle Size

The particle size of the disperse phase is the third criterion for classifying colloidal systems, as discussed at the beginning of the chapter. This classification is summarized in Table 6-2.

As the size of the particles decreases, the proportion of atoms or ions in their surface, and the interface with the continuous medium, increase. So does the specific surface area, A_{sp}, which is the number of square centimeters of surface area A per cubic centimeter of volume V or per gram of mass M of the dispersed substance. For a sphere of

TABLE 6-3. EFFECT OF A SUBDIVISION OF A SOLID CUBE ON THE SPECIFIC SURFACE AREA

NUMBER OF CUBES	L	A_{sp} cm.^{2}/cm.^{3} = cm.$^{-1}$
1	1 cm	6
10^3	1 mm.	60
10^6	0.1 mm.	600
10^9	0.01 mm.	6,000
10^{12}	1 μ	60,000
10^{15}	0.1 μ	600,000
10^{18}	0.01 μ	6,000,000
10^{21}	10 Å	60,000,000
10^{24}	1 Å	600,000,000

Shaded region corresponds to the colloidal state.

diameter D, the specific surface area, expressed as cm.^{2}/cm.^{3}, is

$$A_{sp} = \frac{A}{V} = \frac{\pi D^2}{\pi D^3/6} = \frac{6}{D} \qquad (1)$$

For a cube of edge length L,

$$A_{sp} = \frac{A}{V} = \frac{6L^2}{L^3} = \frac{6}{L} \qquad (2)$$

The increase in specific surface area for a cube of $V = 1$ cm.^{3} as it is subdivided into an increasing number of progressively smaller cubes is illustrated in Table 6-3.

Problem 1. Calculate the specific surface area, in m.^{2}/g., of serum albumin in aqueous solution, given that each molecule is a compact sphere of density $d = 1.34$ g./cm.^{3} and of diameter $D = 18\text{Å} = 18 \times 10^{-8}$ cm. The abbreviation m. is used for meter.

On a volume basis, from Equation 1,

$$A_{sp} = \frac{A}{V} = \frac{6}{D} = \frac{6}{18 \times 10^{-8}\text{ cm.}} =$$

$$3.33 \times 10^7 \text{ cm.}^2/\text{cm.}^3$$

On a weight basis, since mass $M = Vd$,

$$A_{sp} = \frac{A}{M} = \left(\frac{A}{V}\middle/d\right) = \left(\frac{3.33 \times 10^7 \text{cm.}^2}{\text{cm.}^3}\right)\left(\frac{\text{cm.}^3}{1.34\text{ g.}}\right) =$$

$$\frac{2.49 \times 10^7 \text{cm.}^2}{\text{g.}} = \left(\frac{2.49 \times 10^7 \text{cm.}^2}{\text{g.}}\right)\left(\frac{\text{m.}^2}{10^4 \text{cm.}^2}\right) =$$

$$2.49 \times 10^3 \text{ m.}^2/\text{g. or 2,500 m.}^2/\text{g.}$$

This area, the surface area of one gram of serum albumin in colloidal solution, equals 0.62 acre!

RHEOLOGY

Rheology is the science of deformation and flow. The systematic examination of the properties of liquids began only in the early 1910's, chiefly through the efforts of Bingham, Hatschek, and Reiner.[53] Rheology is important in physiology (flow of blood, stressing of muscles, deformation of bony structure), in many pharmaceutical manufacturing operations (stirring, mixing, extruding, filling, compressing), and in the application of pharmaceutical and cosmetic products (flow through a hypodermic needle, pouring from a bottle, spreading of an oint-

ment on the skin, squeezing a paste from a tube). The mechanical properties of packaging materials (strength and toughness of bottles and wrapping films, deformability of rubber stoppers and tubing) are also rheological properties.

Rheological Systems and Stresses. From the rheological viewpoint, solids are characterized by having constant volume and permanent shape, and are capable of supporting loads. Liquids have constant volumes at constant temperature and at all but very high pressures, variable shape, and support no loads. Gases have neither constant volume nor permanent shape.

Loads are expressed as stresses, τ, which have the dimensions of force F per area A, and the units of

$$\frac{\text{dyne}}{\text{cm.}^2} = \left(\frac{\text{g. cm.}}{\text{sec.}^2}\right)\frac{1}{\text{cm.}^2} = \frac{\text{g.}}{\text{cm. sec.}^2}$$

Stresses can produce tension, bending, torsion, compression, and shearing. These are different types of deformation or strain.

Mechanical Properties of Solids. Solids are elastic: They deform under stress, but once the stress is removed, they regain their original shape, and the strain returns to zero.

If a weight is hung from a piano wire, rubber band, or muscle, each will elongate from length L to $(L + \Delta L)$, where Δ designates increment. The deformation or strain, $\gamma = \Delta L/L$, is dimensionless because it is expressed as a fraction or percentage of the original length. Strain γ or elongation is proportional to the tensile stress, τ, according to Hooke's law:

$$\tau = E\gamma \qquad (3)$$

or

$$\frac{F}{A} = E\left(\frac{\Delta L}{L}\right) \qquad (4)$$

Here, A is the cross-sectional area of the muscle or wire which decreases during elongation in order to keep the volume constant. The proportionality constant E is called the *modulus of elasticity* or *Young's modulus.* It is a characteristic property of solids, representing their stiffness or hardness. The units are those of stress, namely, dyne/cm.^{2}

Representative values of E at room temperature are 2×10^{12} dyne/cm.^{2} for steel, 7×10^{11} for glass, 2×10^{11} for bone, 1.5×10^{11} for silk, 2×10^9 for polyethylene, 1×10^9 for tendon, 2×10^7 for vulcanized rubber, 6×10^6 for muscle, and 2×10^6 for a gelatin gel containing 20 percent solids.[24,53]

Typical stress-strain diagrams are presented in Figure 6-1. Initially, the curves are linear, indicating that Hooke's law is obeyed. The modulus of elasticity is the reciprocal slope of these straight-line portions, or the tangent of the angles θ. If the stretching process of polyethylene or steel is stopped before point Y, they will snap back to their original length and retrace the stress-strain curve. Point Y is the yield point or elastic limit, and the corresponding stress is the yield stress. If stressed beyond Y, the solids undergo permanent deformation from which they do not recover upon the removal of stress. This is called *creep* or *cold flow,* and represents liquidlike behavior. Point B is the breaking point; the corresponding strain is the elongation to break, and the corresponding stress, the tensile strength.

Glass has a high modulus but a very low elongation to break: it is hard and brittle. Plastics used in packaging, such as polyethylene and polyvinyl chloride, are rather soft and have relatively high elongations to break: they are tough and do not rupture easily. Toughness is defined as the energy required per unit volume of material to cause rupture. It is represented by the area between the stress-strain curve and the strain axis.

Flow of Liquids. The flow of liquids is produced by tangential forces or shear stresses. Liquids do not retain their shape; the smallest stresses, if applied for long enough times, produce infinite deformation: $E = 0$, therefore $\gamma = \tau/E = \infty$. What matters is the rate of deformation

$$\dot{\gamma} = \frac{d\gamma}{dt} \cong \frac{\Delta\gamma}{\Delta t} = \frac{\gamma_2 - \gamma_1}{t_2 - t_1} \qquad (5)$$

where d designates derivative and t time. The dimensions of $\dot{\gamma}$ are reciprocal time. Since the deformation is in shear, $\dot{\gamma}$ is called rate of shear.

If water and castor oil are poured from

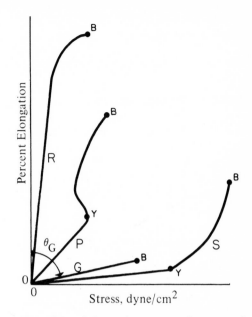

Fig. 6-1.   Schematic stress-strain curves for rubber (R), polyethylene (P), glass (G), and steel (S). Abscissa is true tensile stress, corrected for actual cross section. Y, yield point; B, break point.

bottles, water flows a thousand times faster, i.e., its rate of shear is a thousand times greater. The force is the same in both cases, namely, the pull of gravity, and so is the force per unit area or shear stress. Viscosity η is defined as the ratio of shear stress to rate of shear.

$$\eta = \frac{\tau}{\dot{\gamma}} \qquad (6)$$

Thus, the viscosity of castor oil is a thousand times greater than that of water. The unit of viscosity in the C.G.S. system,

$$\eta = \frac{F/A}{1/t} = \frac{\text{dyne/cm.}^2}{1/\text{sec.}} = \frac{\left(\frac{\text{g. cm.}}{\text{sec.}^2}\right)\text{sec.}}{\text{cm.}^2} = \frac{\text{g.}}{\text{cm. sec.}},$$

is called a *poise;* 0.01 poise is a *centipoise.* Air, water, olive oil, and castor oil have viscosities of 2×10^{-4}, 1×10^{-2}, 1, and 10 poise, respectively, at room temperature.

Isaac Newton, the English physicist, defined viscosity in 1687 as follows.[53] Consider

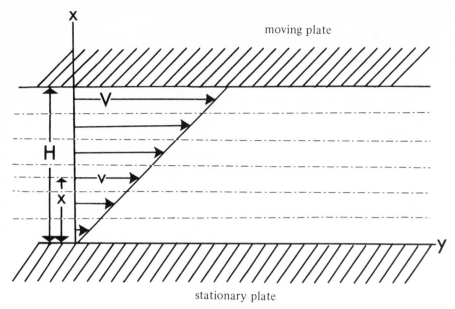

Fig. 6-2.   Velocity gradient in laminar flow between two parallel plates.

a liquid contained between two parallel plates separated by a distance, *H,* as shown in cross-section in Figure 6-2. The top plate moves while the bottom plate is stationary. Imagine the liquid to be divided arbitrarily into a large number of very thin, parallel layers indicated by the broken lines. The top plate moves in the *y*-direction with velocity *V*. The layer of liquid next to it adheres without slip and moves with the same velocity. The tangential or shear stress is transmitted to the adjacent layers by friction, with some loss in velocity from layer to layer. The layer next to the stationary plate adheres to it and is itself stationary. The velocities *v* of the individual layers, represented by the vectors or arrows in Figure 6-2, vary linearly with distance *x* in the direction perpendicularly to the lines of flow.

This velocity gradient

$$\dot\gamma = \frac{V}{H} = \frac{dv}{dx} \qquad (7)$$

has the units of

$$\frac{\left(\dfrac{cm.}{sec.}\right)}{cm.} = sec.^{-1}.$$

It is essentially identical with the rate of shear $\dot\gamma$ defined by Equation 5.[53]

In this context, viscosity is the proportionality constant between shear stress and velocity gradient. It is a measure of the efficiency with which liquids transmit shear stresses. If two parallel flat surfaces immersed in a liquid are one centimeter apart, the tangential force in dynes per square centimeter of area required to cause one plane to move relative to the other with the velocity of one centimeter per second is equal to the viscosity of the liquid in poise. These considerations refer to *laminar* or *streamlined flow,* where all layers of liquid flow parallel to each other in the *y*-direction, without turbulence or eddies.

When liquid flows through a cylindrical tube of small diameter or a capillary, the imaginary liquid layers are hollow concentric cylinders which telescope along the longitudinal axis of the tube in the direction of flow (Fig. 6-3). This is shown in cross-section in Figure 6-4, where the velocity distribution is seen to be parabolic. The velocity is zero at the wall of the tube, because the outermost layer of liquid adheres to it, and maximum in the center. Therefore, the radial velocity gradient

$$\dot\gamma = \frac{dv}{dr}$$

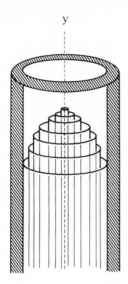

FIG. 6-3. Schematic representation of laminar liquid flow in a capillary.

is zero in the center and maximum at the wall.

Some typical shear rates are listed in Table 6-4.

Viscometry. The two most common types of viscometer are based on flow through a capillary tube and flow between two concentric cylinders. When a liquid flows through a capillary tube of length L and radius R under the influence of a pressure difference ΔP (neglecting the effect of gravity), the rate of flow is V cm.$^3/t$ sec. The maximum rate of shear, at the wall, is

$$\dot{\gamma} = \frac{4}{\pi R^3}\left(\frac{V}{t}\right) \qquad (8)$$

and the shear stress, also at the wall, is

$$\tau = \frac{R\Delta P}{2L} \qquad (9)$$

Combining the two by means of Equation 6 results in

$$\eta = \frac{\pi R^4 \Delta P}{8L}\left(\frac{t}{V}\right) \qquad (10)$$

This is called Poiseuille's law, after the French physician who discovered it while

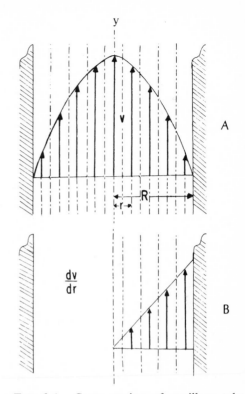

FIG. 6-4. Cross section of capillary tube, showing (A) velocity profile, and (B) velocity gradient in the radial direction.

TABLE 6-4. REPRESENTATIVE RATES OF SHEAR FOR VARIOUS PHARMACEUTICAL OPERATIONS

OPERATION	SHEAR RATE, sec.$^{-1}$
Pouring from a bottle	50
Spreading ointment on skin	400–900
Rubbing ointment on tile	500
Nasal spray from plastic squeeze bottle	2,000
Flow through hypodermic needle	10,000
Colloid mill processing	100,000

investigating the flow of blood in small blood vessels.

Problem 2. A dose of epinephrine increased the blood pressure by 20 percent and constricted the capillary blood vessels, reducing their radius by 10 percent. How will this affect the rate of flow of blood through these capillary vessels? Express the flow rate of blood after drug administration (subscript d) as percentage of the original flow rate (subscript o).

From Equation 10,

$$\left(\frac{V}{t}\right)_o = \frac{\pi R_o^4 \Delta P_o}{8L\eta} \quad \text{and} \quad \left(\frac{V}{t}\right)_d = \frac{\pi R_d^4 \Delta P_d}{8L\eta}$$

Dividing the first by the second equation and replacing ΔP_d by $1.2\Delta P_o$ (20% increase) and R_d by $0.9 R_o$ (10% decrease) results in

$$\frac{(V/t)_o}{(V/t)_d} = \frac{R_o^4 \Delta P_o}{R_d^4 \Delta P_d} = \frac{R_o^4 \Delta P_o}{(0.9 R_o)^4 1.2 \Delta P_o} =$$

$$\frac{1}{(0.9)^4 1.2} = \frac{1}{0.787}$$

$(V/t)_d = 0.787 \ (V/t)_o$. The flow rate after drug administration decreased to 78.7 percent of the original flow rate, a 21.3 percent drop. Since the flow rate varies as the fourth power of the radius, even a small change in the latter produces a large change in the former.

The most common instrument is the glass capillary Ostwald, Ubbelohde, or Cannon-Fenske viscometer, where the pressure difference is the hydrostatic head, $\Delta P = h \, d \, G$, of a liquid column of height h and density d; G is the acceleration of gravity. The liquid is drawn into the upper bulb of the instrument (Fig. 6-5). The time required for the liquid level to drop from the first to the second calibration mark as the liquid flows out through the capillary is measured with a stop watch. Unfortunately, the hydrostatic height h does not remain constant but rather decreases as the liquid flows into the lower reservoir. Using an average value h_{av} for the height of the liquid column, replacing ΔP by $h_{av} \, d \, G$ in Equation 10 and rearranging gives

$$\eta = \left[\frac{\pi R^4 h_{av} G}{8LV}\right] td = Ktd \qquad (11)$$

The quantities inside the bracket are either constants or characteristic dimensions of the viscometer. They are combined into a single constant K, which is determined experimentally by means of a liquid of known density and viscosity. Once K is known, the viscosity of any liquid of known density can be measured with the instrument using Equation 11. Alternatively, one can compare a reference liquid of known viscosity η_1, known density d_1 and measured efflux time t_1 directly with a liquid of unknown viscosity η_2, known

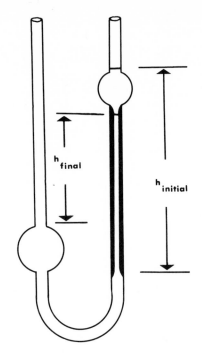

FIG. 6-5.   Glass capillary viscometer.

density d_2, and measured efflux time t_2. Combining the equations

$$\eta_1 = K \, t_1 d_1 \quad \text{and} \quad \eta_2 = K \, t_2 d_2$$

results in

$$\frac{\eta_1}{\eta_2} = \frac{t_1 d_1}{t_2 d_2} \qquad (12)$$

In designing viscometers, the closest that one can come to Newton's geometrical arrangement of shearing a liquid between two infinite parallel sheets is to form these sheets into two concentric cylinders. The inner cylinder or bob is solid; the outer cylinder or cup is closed at the bottom, and the liquid is contained between the two. These are called rotational or concentric-cylinder viscometers. In some, the cup is stationary and the bob is driven, for example, by a weight connected to its shaft via a pulley and gears or by a motor and a series of gears. In the former case, the rate of shear is measured as the speed of rotation of the bob (Stormer viscometer). In the latter case, the rate of shear is fixed at a selected value and the stress is measured by a torsion spring on the shaft of the bob (Haake and Drage viscometers) or by a strain gauge or spring on the cup (Merrill-Brookfield and Hercules Hi-Shear viscometers). In the MacMichael viscometer, the cup is rotated at one of several fixed speeds; and the stress on the bob is measured by the angle of twist of the torsion wire from which the bob is suspended. The viscous drag exerted by the liquid on the bottom of the bob (the end effect) can be compensated for by adding 10 percent to the bob height h in Equation 13. This correction is automatically included in the instrument constant K of Equation 14 (see below).

In all rotational instruments, the rate of rotation at equilibrium, ω (radians/sec.), is directly proportional to the rate of shear. It is constant, and the applied torque T (dyne cm.), which is directly proportional to the shear stress, is

$$T = 4\pi \left(\frac{R_c^2 \times R_b^2}{R_c^2 - R_b^2} \right) h\eta\omega \qquad (13)$$

R_c and R_b are the radii of the cup and bob, respectively[18,22,53,76]. In the case of the Stormer viscometer, for instance, $T =$ weight load in grams $\times$ acceleration of gravity $\times$ effective length of lever arm. Combining the characteristic dimensions of the cup and bob and the conversion factor of radians/sec. to r.p.m. $(60/2\pi)$ into an instrumental constant K results[76] in an equation of the type

$$\begin{aligned} \tau \text{ (torque, weight, scale divisions} \\ \text{or angle of deflection)} \\ = K\,\eta\,\dot{\gamma} \text{ (r.p.m. or radians/sec.)} \quad (14) \end{aligned}$$

for all rotational instruments. The instrument is calibrated, i.e., K is determined, with a liquid of known viscosity. Aqueous sucrose solutions, or oils supplied by the National Bureau of Standards, are often used as calibrating liquids.

Newtonian Liquids are liquids whose viscosity depends only on composition and temperature but not on shear stress, rate of shear, and time or duration of testing. Their flow or consistency curves are obtained by plotting rate of shear or r.p.m. versus shear stress, torque, scale divisions or angular deflection. The plots yield straight lines going through the origin as required by Equations 6 and 14. Viscosity is the reciprocal slope of the consistency curve, or tan θ in Figure 6-6. Curve B represents the more viscous liquid: the same stress produces a lower shear rate for B—or, stated otherwise, a given shear rate corresponds to a higher stress for B than for A. *Fluidity* is the reciprocal of viscosity; it is measured by the slope of the consistency curve.

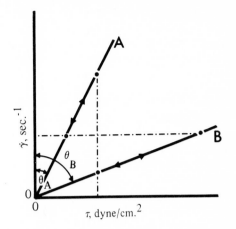

FIG. 6-6.   Consistency curves for two Newtonian liquids.

Effect of Temperature on Viscosity. The viscosity of liquids decreases exponentially with increasing temperature according to the expression

$$\eta = Ae^{\Delta E/RT} \qquad (15)$$

or

$$\log \eta = \log A + \Delta E/2.303\ RT \qquad (15a)$$

where ΔE, the apparent activation energy for viscous flow, is a measure of the magnitude of the temperature dependence of the viscosity; R is the gas constant (1.987 cal./mole degree Kelvin); and T is the absolute temperature. Some ΔE values are: 3,000 to 4,000 cal./mole for water, 1,700 for acetone, and 13,200 for castor oil.[53,76] This means that for a 10-degree temperature rise, say from 27° to 37° C., the viscosity of water decreases by 17 percent and that of castor oil by 51 percent.

The foregoing shows the necessity for close temperature control during viscosity measurements. The energy which causes liquids to flow, overcoming their viscous friction, is transformed into heat. In concentric-cylinder viscometers, where the same portion of liquid is sheared for long periods of time, the temperature often rises by several degrees unless cooling water is circulated through the instrument.

Pseudoplasticity. Many pharmaceutical preparations contain aggregates of particles or of molecules which are broken up by shear. Examples are solutions of polymers, such as methylcellulose or sodium carboxymethylcellulose and gums, such as tragacanth or acacia. They are all long-chain molecules which form random, entangled coils in solution. Other examples are sols of fine solid particles in liquids where the particles tend to aggregate, provided that these dispersions are dilute enough not to have yield values. Examples are carbon black and bentonite in water, and colloidal silicas in polar and nonpolar liquids.

The flexible, threadlike macromolecules in aqueous solution are constantly buffeted by the surrounding water molecules in thermal motion. This causes translation of chain segments as well as rotation around the carbon-carbon and carbon-oxygen bonds which make up the backbone of the macromolecular chains, resulting in constant segmental motion. Since this motion is random, the macromolecules tend to assume roughly spherical shapes and become entangled with one another (Figure 6-7a). The polymer chains are surrounded by a sheath of water of hydration; the hydrated coils are opened wide and permeated by solvent molecules.

Once the solution is made to flow in a shear field, the unidirectional laminar motion discussed above is superimposed on the random motion of the water molecules; and the randomly coiled, entangled macromolecules tend to disentangle themselves and align in the direction of flow, as shown in Figure 6-7b. The viscosity of the solution, which is determined largely by the concentration, chain length, flexibility, and solvation of the dissolved polymers, is reduced in three ways: (1) The polymer chains become elongated and thus offer less resistance to flow than the original, roughly spherical shapes. (2) Simultaneously, the amount of water trapped inside the coils decreases, and so does the size of the flow unit. (3) Finally, as the number of intermolecular entanglements decreases, the amount of work required to break remaining entanglements which are an obstacle to flow is reduced.[42] At each rate of shear there is an average equilibrium degree of disentanglement and alignment of the dissolved macromolecules, resulting from the balance between the shear-induced disentangling and aligning of chains, and the entwining and random coiling ten-

Fig. 6-7. Three randomly coiled polymer chains (A) at rest; (B) in a shear field.

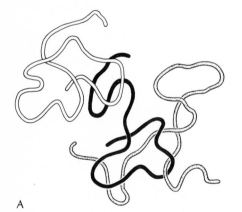

A

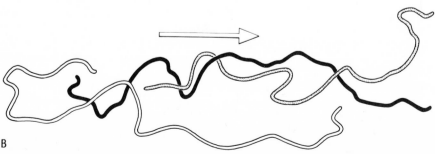

B

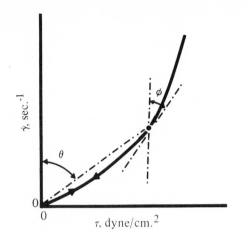

FIG. 6-8. Consistency curve of a pseudo-plastic or shear-thinning liquid.

There are two ways of describing the apparent viscosity of a pseudoplastic liquid, as shown in Figure 6-8. One method employs the reciprocal slope of the secant to the flow curve at the specified rate of shear, or the tangent of θ. This is equivalent to dividing the observed shear stress by the observed rate of shear. According to this definition, the apparent viscosity of the pseudoplastic liquid is the same as the viscosity of a Newtonian liquid whose consistency curve passes through the point of measurement.[5,22,76] The second method describes the apparent viscosity as the reciprocal slope of the tangent to the flow curve at the specified rate of shear, or the tangent of ϕ, or $d\tau/d\dot{\gamma}$.[18,50]

At extremely low shear rates, well below 1 sec.$^{-1}$, the alignment of polymer chains or of particle aggregates in the direction of flow, and the shear-induced disentanglement of chains or breaking up of aggregates are negligible. In this region, these systems exhibit Newtonian flow behavior, and their viscosity is designated as lower Newtonian or zero-shear viscosity, η_0. At extremely high shear rates, the particulate aggregates are completely broken up, and the polymer chains are wholly disentangled and well aligned in the direction of flow. Further increments in shear rate cannot reduce the viscosity any further when this, the upper Newtonian viscosity η_x is reached.[53,76] Dissolved macromolecules often undergo shear-induced rupture at these very high stresses. Schematic representations of the lower and upper Newtonian regions and the intervening pseudoplastic region are given in Figure 6-9.

Solutions of macromolecules have pronounced pseudoplastic behavior and ex-

dency caused by Brownian motion. The entwining is constant, while the disentanglement increases with shear. Thus, the viscosity of pseudoplastic or shear-thinning liquids decreases as the rate of shear increases; and the flow curve (Figure 6-8) is concave toward the shear rate axis. The opposite behavior, namely, an increase in viscosity with increasing shear, is called *dilatancy*. It is rarely observed.

In the case of dispersions of partly flocculated particles, increasing shear progressively breaks up the aggregates while Brownian motion tends to reconstitute them. Again, there is an average equilibrium size for the aggregates which decreases as the shear increases, because the aggregating forces remain constant while the breaking-up forces increase with increasing shear rates.

FIG. 6-9. Schematic representation of the three flow regions of a pseudoplastic liquid; (*left*) consistency curve, and (*right*) viscosity versus shear curve. 0A, lower Newtonian region; AB, pseudoplastic region; and BC, upper Newtonian region.

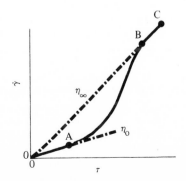

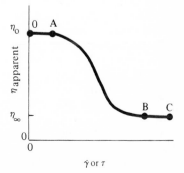

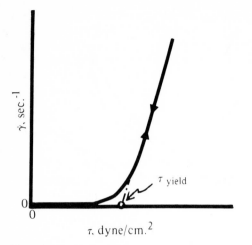

FIG. 6-10. Consistency curve of a plastic material.

tremely high viscosities when compared with solutions of their monomeric "building blocks" at comparable solids contents. If the polymer chains in Figure 6-7 were chopped into their monomeric units, the viscosity of the solutions would decrease enormously. For instance, a 2 percent aqueous solution of a typical U.S.P.-grade high-viscosity methylcellulose has a low-shear apparent viscosity of approximately 80 poise at 20° C. The molecular weight being about 300,000 and the degree of substitution 1.8 methoxy groups per anhydroglucose unit, there are on the average $300,000/187 = 1,600$ anhydroglucose repeat units per macromolecule. If the dissolved methylcellulose were quantitatively degraded to methyl-glucose, the viscosity of the solution would drop about eight thousand-fold. Even a 50 percent glucose solution has a viscosity of less than 0.1 poise, and is Newtonian.

The very high viscosity and the pronounced pseudoplasticity of macromolecular solutions, compared with the low viscosity and Newtonian behavior of solutions of the monomer units of the same weight-percent concentration, are due to the cooperative effect of many hundreds of monomer molecules joined into one giant molecule. All segments of this macromolecule move almost simultaneously when the solution flows. This phenomenon together with the highly asymmetrical shape of the linear macromolecules and with their tendency to become entangled with one another and to

immobilize large volumes of solvent within their randomly coiled chains results in the high viscosity. This is why natural and synthetic mucilages, gums and other polymers are efficient thickening agents for liquid pharmaceutical preparations.

Plasticity, Elasticity, and Yield Stress. If small stresses are applied to a paste or gel, it undergoes slight and reversible deformation but no flow. In retaining their shape, pastes and gels act like solids. As the stress is increased, a sudden onset of liquidlike flow occurs at a characteristic stress called the *yield stress*. Once the yield stress is exceeded, the material behaves like a liquid. Pastes, gels, ointments, creams, salves, butter and margarine, dough, mayonnaise, putties, and modeling clay exhibit yield stresses. Because of its plasticity, toothpaste does not sink into the toothbrush; ointments, clay slips and butter do not drip from the fingers, the spatula or the knife but hold their shape until sheared by a spreading pressure higher than their yield values.

As is seen in Figure 6-10, a plastic material sometimes flows at stresses slightly below its yield value, but in chunks ("plug flow") rather than in laminar flow where layer glides past layer. The yield stress is obtained by extrapolating the linear portion of the flow curve to the stress axis. The plastic viscosity η_{plast} is calculated as

$$\eta_{plast} = \frac{\tau - \tau_{yield}}{\dot{\gamma}} \qquad (16)$$

This is equivalent to moving the origin of the consistency plot to the yield stress and treating the system as a Newtonian liquid beyond that stress, i.e., taking its viscosity as the reciprocal slope of the linear portion. Some materials have a yield stress and show shear-thinning or pseudoplastic flow beyond the yield point, i.e., the flow curve above the yield stress is convex toward the stress axis.

The rheological distinction between *gels* and *pastes* or between elasticity and plasticity is not a sharp one. Both types have yield values. Gels possess a high degree of *elasticity:* they can undergo considerable reversible deformation, i.e., deformation from which they recover when released from stress, before they flow or suffer permanent deformation. Examples are gelatin or agar gels. Pastes, on the other hand, have little elasticity. They cannot recover their shape except from very small deformations; otherwise, they flow. Pastes have a doughlike consistency or moldability. This behavior is called *plasticity*.[3,40] Examples are Zinc Oxide Paste, U.S.P.; Aluminum Paste, U.S.P.; butter; and modeling clay.

The cause of plastic or elastic behavior is a continuous network of agglomerated small particles or of entangled polymer chains extending throughout the material to give it solidlike properties. The liquid is immobilized inside this network. Small stresses deform the network elastically, without rupturing aggregates or disentangling macromolecules. Gels are usually formed by the entanglement of macromolecules which are highly swollen or dissolved in the liquid. Pastes consist usually of aggregated solid particles and are more concentrated than gels. These differences in constitution cause gels to have much higher elastic limits than pastes, i.e., gels can undergo much greater elastic deformation below the yield value. However, their yield values need be no larger and are not infrequently smaller than those of pastes. Once the yield stress is exceeded, the continuous bridges or networks of agglomerated particles or entangled chains are broken in many places, and the pastes and gels begin to flow. If the stress is reduced below the yield stress, the networks are re-established by Brownian motion and flow ceases.

Thixotropy. The apparent viscosity of pseudoplastic and plastic systems depends on composition, temperature, and shear rate or shear stress. It does not depend on the previous history of shear treatment to which the material was subjected, i.e., duration and intensity of previous stirring inside or outside the viscometer. One can start measurements at any point or rate of shear on the flow curves of Figures 6-6, 6-8, 6-9, and 6-10 and increase or decrease the shear. The shear stress-shear rate points always fall on the same curve whether produced by increasing or decreasing the shear. This is the meaning of the arrows superimposed on these curves. In these systems, the re-establishment by Brownian motion of aggregates or entanglements broken by shear is very fast, and viscometers are too slow

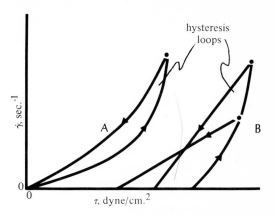

FIG. 6-11. Consistency curves for thixotropic systems: (A) without yield value, and (B) with yield value. Upturned arrows indicate direction of increasing stress, downward arrows indicate direction of decreasing stress.

to detect the parallel processes of structure build-up and regeneration of viscosity. There is a true equilibrium degree of entanglement for polymeric chains and of aggregation for colloidal particles corresponding to each rate of shear, which decreases only as the rate of shear increases.

While this applies to dilute and hence fluid polymer solutions and particulate dispersions where segments of the very thin polymer chains and small colloidal particles undergo rapid Brownian motion, it does not apply to viscous solutions and dispersions nor to suspensions of larger colloidal particles, whose Brownian motion is far too slow to afford almost instantaneous re-establishment of interparticle bonds. Continuous shearing at a constant rate of shear will gradually lower the apparent viscosity of the latter systems because the aggregation or structure-building process is slower than the breakdown process. Therefore, the size of the aggregates or the number of points of entanglement gradually decrease even while the shear rate is maintained constant. Such systems are said to be thixotropic, and the flow curves for increasing and decreasing shear stress do not coincide. Directly after being stirred at a high shear rate, the apparent viscosity of a thixotropic system at an intermediate shear rate is lower than if that intermediate shear rate had been reached starting from zero. More or less extensive periods at rest are required for Brownian motion to fully rebuild the structure of thixotropic systems so that they regain their high initial viscosity.

The two curves for increasing shear rate in Figure 6-11 correspond to higher apparent viscosities than those for decreasing shear. The area of the *hysteresis loop* between the ascending and the descending curves provides a measure of the amount of structure broken down. The smaller of the two loops in Figure 6-11B indicates that the shear stress was not raised to as high a value as in the full loop; therefore, less structure was destroyed.

Aqueous suspensions of bentonite and kaolin are typical of thixotropic systems. These clays consist of platelets with positively charged edges due to broken aluminum valences and negatively charged faces due to silicate cation exchange sites. Aggregation of the suspended clay particles occurs largely by electrostatic attraction between the edges of one platelet and the face of another. This builds up a house-of-cards structure which, if the suspensions are concentrated enough, extends throughout the entire suspension and produces a yield stress. Once the clay suspensions are stirred, the house-of-cards structure is partly destroyed. Because of the relatively large size of the clay platelets or the high viscosity of the suspensions, it is so slow in rebuilding that no yield stress is observed for periods at rest varying between minutes and hours, depending on the clay concentration and the duration and intensity of stirring.[75] Many pastes and gels exhibit thixotropy, i.e., they turn liquid under high shear but solidify and regain their yield values at rest.

Because there are many types of flow, a preparation must be studied over a range of shear rates to characterize its rheological behavior. Measurements are usually made first at increasing speeds and then at decreasing speeds to assess the extent of thixotropy. Measurements at a single shear rate do not differentiate between a Newtonian liquid, a non-Newtonian liquid, and a paste with a yield value.

Flow Relationships for Dispersions. The Einstein viscosity equation[3,5,23,30,36,42,50,53,76] is the simplest equation describing the flow of sols and suspensions. It is a limiting law which refers to Newtonian flow:

$$\eta_{12} = \eta_1 \left(1 + 2.5\phi\right) \qquad (17)$$

where η_{12} is the viscosity of the dispersion, η_1 that of the liquid medium or solvent, and ϕ is the volume fraction of the disperse phase. This equation is valid only for the following conditions: (a) The effects of gravity and inertia are negligible, and turbulence is excluded. (b) The particles are spherical. (c) The particles are large compared to the solvent molecules but small compared to the dimensions of the apparatus (radius of the capillary or gap between the concentric cylinders). (d) The particles are rigid. (e) There is no interaction between the particles, neither attraction nor repulsion. This excludes electrically charged particles, which make up the majority of dispersions encountered in practice. (f) The system is so dilute that the disturbance of the flow lines and deviation from laminar flow around one particle does not overlap with those around neighboring particles. If *a, b, c, e,* or *f* are not obeyed, the resistance to flow and η_{12} are higher than predicted by Equation 17. The increase in viscosity arising from the repulsion of particles of like charge is called *electroviscous effect.*[3] If *d* does not apply, as in the case of emulsions, η_{12} will be too small.

Solutions of globular proteins near the isoelectric point come close to following Einstein's equation if the hydration layer is included in their volume. Other examples are suspensions of glass beads, spherical spores or fungi, and polymer latices containing enough electrolyte to swamp the electroviscous effect (see below). Bentonite dispersions, which grossly violate conditions *b* and *e,* have viscosities 70 times greater than those calculated by Equation 17 at concentrations as low as $\phi = 10^{-4}$. An interesting feature of Einstein's viscosity equation is that η_{12} does not depend on particle size but only on the total volume of solvent replaced by the disperse phase.

Problem 3. A physiological saline solution has

a viscosity of 0.01 poise. Erythrocytes are suspended in it to the extent of 5 percent v/v. Assuming that the Einstein viscosity equation holds, calculate the viscosity of the suspension in poise and in centipoise.

$$\phi = \frac{5\% \text{ v/v}}{100\% \text{ v/v}} = 0.05. \quad \text{From Equation 17,}$$

$$\eta_{12} = 0.01 \text{ poise } [1 + (2.5)(0.05)] =$$

$$0.01125 \text{ poise} = 1.125 \text{ centipoise.}$$

Erythrocytes are disc shaped and concave on both sides rather than spherical, which increases the viscosity somewhat. The negative charge of the erythrocytes is swamped by the 0.15 M salt, so that the electroviscous effect is strongly reduced or possibly eliminated.[3]

The abnormal flow behavior of blood in small capillaries is called the tubular pinch or sigma effect.[11]

Two general equations describing a variety of types of non-Newtonian flow behavior in terms of structural parameters are given.[13, 20,21]

BROWNIAN MOTION, DIFFUSION, AND SEDIMENTATION

The molecules of liquids are in constant random motion, perpetually colliding with each other and changing direction. Colloidal particles suspended in liquids undergo continual bombardment by the surrrounding molecules. Being buffeted in a random fashion by the molecules of the liquid, the colloidal particles are engaged in a continuous, erratic motion called Brownian motion, after the Scottish botanist who first observed it with pollen grains suspended in water. The Brownian motion provides a magnified picture of the random motion of the molecules of the liquid themselves.

The mean displacement x of a colloidal particle during a period of time t was calculated by Einstein to be:

$$x = \sqrt{2\,\mathbf{D}\,t} \tag{18}$$

where $\mathbf{D}$ is the diffusion coefficient. Translational diffusion is the tendency of colloidal particles and of dissolved molecules to migrate from a region of high concentration to one of low concentration under the influence of Brownian motion. The diffusion coefficient of the colloidal particles is related to their friction factor $\mathbf{F}$ by Einstein's law of diffusion

$$\mathbf{D}\mathbf{F} = k\mathbf{T} = \frac{\mathbf{R}T}{\mathbf{N}} \tag{19}$$

where k is the Boltzmann constant (i.e., the gas constant $\mathbf{R}$ divided by Avogadro's number $\mathbf{N}$) and T is the absolute temperature. The resistance to diffusion, expressed by $\mathbf{F}$, is due to the viscosity of the liquid.

For spherical particles of radius R in a medium of viscosity η,

$$\mathbf{F} = 6\,\pi\eta R \tag{20}$$

This is *Stokes' law*, which is a limiting law derived with assumptions similar to those of Equation 17 and the added assumption that the particles move extremely slowly.[3,30,42,48, 72,77]

Combining Equations 19 and 20 results in an expression for the diffusion coefficient:

$$\mathbf{D} = \frac{\mathbf{R}T}{6\pi\eta R\mathbf{N}} \tag{21}$$

Combining Equations 18 and 21 gives the following expression for the mean displacement of colloidal particles by Brownian motion:

$$x = \sqrt{\frac{\mathbf{R}Tt}{3\pi\eta R\mathbf{N}}} \tag{22}$$

These considerations assume that the settling of particles under the influence of gravity is negligible.

For the globular protein, serum albumin, R is equal to 35 Å including the layer of hydration. According to Equation 21, in water at 20° C. or 293.2° K. where the viscosity is 0.010 poise:

$$\mathbf{D} = \left(\frac{8.314 \times 10^7 \text{ g. cm.}^2}{\text{mole } °\text{K. sec.}^2}\right)\frac{(293.2°\text{K.})}{6\pi}\left(\frac{\text{cm. sec.}}{0.010 \text{ g.}}\right)\frac{1}{(35 \times 10^{-8} \text{ cm.})}\left(\frac{\text{mole}}{6.023 \times 10^{23}}\right) = 6.13 \times 10^{-7}\frac{\text{cm.}^2}{\text{sec.}}$$

The mean displacement in a day or $24 \times 60 \times 60 = 86,400$ sec. is, according to Equation 18,

$$x = \sqrt{2(6.13 \times 10^{-7} \text{ cm.}^2/\text{sec.})(8.64 \times 10^4 \text{ sec.})}$$

$$= 0.326 \text{ cm.}$$

Perrin used Equation 22 to determine Avogadro's number, based on microscopic measurements of the Brownian displacement of fractionated mastic and gamboge suspensions in water and in aqueous glycerin.[48,72]

Brownian motion, convection currents, and vibration tend to keep particles uniformly distributed throughout dispersions. Gravity tends to cause particles to settle. If they are less dense than the liquid medium, the particles will rise. The driving force for sedimentation is the effective weight of the particle, i.e., the weight of the particle minus the weight of the liquid it displaces, or its volume V multiplied by the net density and by the acceleration of gravity G. The resisting force is the friction factor $\mathbf{F}$ multiplied by the velocity of sedimentation v. Constant velocity is reached rapidly. At that time, the two opposing forces become equal. If the particles are spherical and the conditions are such that Stokes' law is applicable,

$$\frac{4}{3}\pi R^3(d_P - d_L)G = 6\pi\eta Rv$$

where d_P and d_L represent the densities of the particle and of the liquid, respectively. If the particles are so large that settling under the influence of gravity is not disturbed by Brownian motion, the size of the particles can be determined by measuring the velocity of sedimentation v. The expression for the particle radius is

$$R = \sqrt{\frac{9\eta v}{2(d_p - d_L)G}} \qquad (23)$$

An equivalent radius is determined for non-spherical particles. Alternatively, by measuring the rate of sedimentation of spheres of known radius through a liquid, or the rate of rise of air bubbles, one can determine the viscosity η of the liquid medium.

Disperse particles near the lower end of the colloidal range are prevented by Brownian motion from settling. One can calculate a critical radius R_c for which the random displacement by Brownian motion just equals the downward displacement due to gravitational settling.[12] Particles with a smaller radius will not settle in the allotted time interval. Since the velocity of sedimentation equals the downward displacement h divided by time t, Equation 23 can be rewritten as

$$h = \frac{2(d_P - d_L)R^2Gt}{9\eta} \qquad (24)$$

The critical radius R_c is that radius for which the distance through which the particle settles in a given time interval equals the mean displacement x due to Brownian motion, i.e., for which h of Equation 24 equals x of Equation 22. Combining these two equations yields

$$R_c = \left[\frac{27\eta RT}{4\pi N(d_p - d_L)^2G^2t}\right]^{\frac{1}{6}} \qquad (25)$$

For a sulfur particle ($d_P = 2.0$ g./cm.^{3}) suspended in water at 20°C., the critical radius is 6.2×10^{-5} cm. or 0.62 μ for a one-second period. For a 100-second period, $R_c = 0.25 \mu$. In view of convection currents due to temperature fluctuations,[42] sulfur particles with radii below 0.62 μ are unlikely to settle out of aqueous suspensions. As d_P approaches d_L, the critical radius increases rapidly.

One publication[37] deals with the application of Equation 25 to the sedimentation of pharmaceutical suspensions. While Equation 25 as written in that paper placed t erroneously in the numerator, a tabulation correctly lists increasing values of R_c for shorter time intervals.

METHODS FOR DETERMINING THE WEIGHT OF PARTICLES AND OF MACROMOLECULES

If the particles in a colloidal dispersion or the molecules in a polymer solution were all of the same size (monodisperse systems), all methods for determining their weight would give the same results. This is the case of many native proteins. Simple organic molecules, like most synthetic drugs, are monodisperse, i.e., all molecules of a given compound contain the same number of C, H, O, N, etc. atoms and, hence, have the same molecular weight. During polymerization reactions, not all polymer chains begin to form at the same time nor do they all grow to the same size. Some macromolecules will have longer chains than others. In colloidal dispersions, it is rare for all particles to have the same size. This applies to dispersions made by comminution techniques as well as by precipitation techniques. Therefore, polymers and other colloidally dispersed particles are usually polydisperse, i.e., they have a range of particle sizes or molecular weights. Different methods for determining the average weight of polydisperse particles or macromolecules give different values depending on whether, in effect, they count the number of particles or assess their weight or size. The former averages are called number-average weights. Among the latter kind, weight-average weights are the most important averages.

Molecular or Particle Weight Averages

Colligative properties, like osmotic pressure and lowering of the vapor pressure or of the freezing point of solutions or dispersions, measure the *number-average size or weight* $\overline{M}_n$, which is computed by adding the number N of molecules or particles, each multiplied by its molecular weight or particle weight M, and dividing the sum by the total number of molecules or particles. The mathematical expression for this computation is:

$$\overline{M}_n = \frac{\sum\limits_{i=1}^{\infty} N_i M_i}{\sum\limits_{i=1}^{\infty} N_i} \qquad (26)$$

where the subscript i refers to one of the many sizes of particles or molecules, and Σ represents the summation over all sizes pres-

ent. If a polymeric material or colloidal dispersion contains 1,000 species of different molecular or particle weights, i assumes all values from 1 through 1000, and

$$\Sigma N_i M_i = N_1 M_1 + N_2 M_2 + N_3 M_3 + \cdots \cdots + N_{1,000} M_{1,000}.$$

M_n is the total weight divided by the total number of molecules. The number of moles or moles/liter can be used instead of the number of molecules or particles. Small and large particles contribute equally to $\overline{M}_n$.

Each particle or molecule contributes to the *weight-average size or weight* $\overline{M}_w$ in proportion to its weight w, so that larger particles or molecules affect $\overline{M}_w$ more than smaller ones. The expression for $\overline{M}_w$ is:

$$\overline{M}_w = \frac{\sum\limits_{i=1}^{\infty} w_i M_i}{\sum\limits_{i=1}^{\infty} w_i} \qquad (27)$$

The number of grams or grams/liter w_i of material with a particle or molecular weight M_i is multiplied by that particle or molecular weight. The sum of these products is divided by the total weight of the material in grams or grams/liter. Since $w_i = N_i M_i / N$, where N_i is the number of particles or molecules and N is Avogadro's number, Equation 27 can be rewritten as follows:

$$\overline{M}_w = \frac{\sum\limits_i N_i M_i M_i / N}{\sum\limits_i N_i M_i / N} = \frac{\sum\limits_i N_i M_i^2}{\sum\limits_i N_i M_i} \qquad (28)$$

The average particle or molecular weight obtained by light scattering is the weight-average value. Ultracentrifugation gives an average even more strongly dependent on the particle weight. In the format of Equation 28, that average contains M_i^3 instead of M_i^2 in the numerator, and M_i^2 instead of M_i in the denominator.[4,9,38,42,74] For monodisperse systems, $\overline{M}_n = \overline{M}_w$. For polydisperse systems, $\overline{M}_w$ is always greater than $\overline{M}_n$, and the magnitude of the ratio $\overline{M}_w / \overline{M}_n$ is a measure of the degree of polydispersity or the width of the molecular or particle weight distribution.

Problem 4. The following three monodisperse globular proteins were available as 5 percent w/v solutions: Lysozyme (M = 15,000), serum albumin (M = 65,000), and urease (M = 480,000). Calculate the number- and weight-average molecular weights of a mixture made by combining equal volumes of the three solutions.

The mixture contains equal weights of the three proteins. The weight-average molecular weight is readily calculated by Equation 27. Assuming that the weight of each protein equals one gram,

$$\overline{M}_w =$$
$$\frac{(1 \times 15,000) + (1 \times 65,000) + (1 \times 480,000)}{1 + 1 + 1}$$
$$= 186,670$$

In order to calculate $\overline{M}_n$, it becomes necessary to know the number of moles of each protein. For convenience, the weight of 100,000 grams is selected for each of the three proteins. Then, for lysozyme,

$$N = \frac{100,000 \text{ g.}\left(\frac{\text{mole}}{15,000 \text{ g.}}\right)}{} = 6.667 \text{ moles.}$$

For albumin, N = 100,000/65,000 = 1.538 moles, and for urease, N = 100,000/480,000 = 0.208 moles. From Equation 26,

$$\overline{M}_n = \frac{(6.667)(15,000) + (1.538)(65,000) + (0.208)(480,000)}{6.667 + 1.538 + 0.208} =$$

$$\frac{300,000}{8.413} = 35,660. \ \overline{M}_w \text{ is over five times larger than } \overline{M}_n.$$

the hydrostatic pressure of the liquid column in that capillary, which opposes the osmotic pressure Π, becomes equal to it in magnitude; that is: $hdG = -\Pi$, where h is the difference in height between the menisci in the two capillaries, d is the density of the solution, and G the acceleration of gravity.

The following are some of the experimental precautions and pitfalls in osmometry. Small solution volumes result in appreciable reductions in concentration on the solution side due to influx of solvent. With large solution volumes, on the other hand, the osmometer acts like a thermometer; the capillary level changes with temperature. Rigorous temperature control is therefore essential. Another problem is the extended period of time, from 7 to 50 hours, required to attain equilibrium. During this long time interval, low molecular weight fractions of dissolved polymers may diffuse into the A compartment. If the membrane were completely impermeable even to the smallest solute molecules, the rate of passage of the

Osmotic Pressure Measurements [4,9,38,42,74]

Osmometers like the one shown (Fig. 6-12) consist of two compartments A and B, each equipped with a vertical open end capillary glass tube. The compartments are separated by a semipermeable membrane, i.e., a membrane freely permeated by the solvent but with pores too small to permit the passage of dissolved macromolecules. Membranes are made of cellulose and its derivatives, e.g., cellophane, cellulose acetate or collodion, or of polyvinyl alcohol, polyvinyl butyral, polychlorotrifluoroethylene, or rubber. If compartment B is filled with a polymer solution and A with the pure solvent, solvent will diffuse through the membrane from A into B to equalize the concentration. The solute cannot diffuse in the opposite direction. Therefore, the liquid level in the capillary tube of compartment B rises until

solvent through the membrane would be so slow that equilibration would require excessively long time intervals. The loss in Π during the measurement due to diffusion of solute can be corrected by extrapolating h as a function of time back to zero time after steady state has been reached. Another method for preventing this error is to overfill compartment B so that the meniscus in its capillary is somewhat too high, or just at the estimated equilibrium level. If $h d G$ exceeds Π, reverse osmosis or flow of solvent from compartment B to A takes place. Plotting the h values for direct and reverse osmosis as a function of time produces two curves which converge to an equilibrium height corresponding to zero osmotic flow. Extrapolation of the two curves leads to that equilibrium value of h after less than 20 minutes observation.[4]

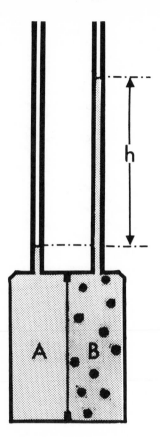

Fig. 6-12. Schematic drawing of a membrane osmometer.

of buffer salts, which diffuse through the membrane, to both compartments further reduces the error in osmotic pressure due to the few ionized groups of the protein molecules. Donnan equilibria in polyelectrolyte solutions require special treatment.[42,74]

In order to apply to most polymer solutions, the van't Hoff equation, $\Pi = cRT/\overline{M}_{n,2}$, for ideal solutions must be modified by the introduction of a correction term. This term contains a coefficient B, which in turn is related to the so-called *second virial coefficient* A_2 through the relationship $B = RTA_2$. Virial coefficients express deviations from ideal behavior. For solutions, B and A_2 are a measure of the intermolecular attraction between solvent and solute molecules, i.e., solvation. Positive values indicate that this attraction is greater than the attraction between solvent molecules and the attraction between solute molecules. Negative values indicate that the solute-solute attraction is greater than the solute-solvent attraction, which eventually leads to precipitation. Zero values connote equality between the three types of interaction. This occurs at the so-called θ temperature or Flory point, at which the solution behaves ideally.

The modified van't Hoff equation is

$$\frac{\Pi}{c} = \frac{RT}{\overline{M}_{n,2}} + Bc \qquad (29)$$

The solute concentration c is expressed in g./cm.[3]. Ideal behavior for values of B different from zero occurs at infinite dilution ($c \rightarrow 0$) where Equation 29 reduces to the van't Hoff equation. Typical plots of reduced osmotic pressure, Π/c, versus c are shown in Figure 6-13. According to Equation 29, the extrapolated intercept on the vertical axis is inversely proportional to the number-average molecular weight. The slope is equal to the coefficient B; the values of B and A_2 are a measure of the interaction between solvent and dissolved polymer. Lines 1 through 4 in Figure 6-13 represent different fractions of a single polymeric material in the same solvent, and at the same temperature. Thus, the four straight lines have the same slope. According to their intercepts, the molecular weights increase from 1 to 4. Lines 4 through 7 represent solutions of a single polymer

Late model osmometers have a horizontal rather than a vertical capillary tube connected with the solution compartment. Gradually increasing hydrostatic pressure is applied through that capillary until there is no net flow of solvent across the membrane. At that point, the applied pressure equals $-\Pi$. Flow of solvent is detected by the movement of an air bubble inside the capillary. Osmotic pressure measurements with such an instrument take only minutes.

The osmotic pressure of proteins must be measured at their isoelectric point. The countercations required to neutralize the carboxylate ions at higher pH values and the counteranions required to neutralize ionized basic groups such as amino, imidazole or guanidino at lower pH values gives excessively high osmotic pressure values. The addition

sample in four different solvents at the same temperature. The solvent of line 4 is the best. Line 6 corresponds to an ideal solution, with $B = A_2 = 0$, and line 7 corresponds to the poorest solvent. If the slope were more negative than that of line 7, phase separation would occur.

In practice, osmotic pressure measurements to determine particle or molecular weights are limited to lyophilic systems such as solutions of macromolecules and surfactant micelles. Lyophobic colloidal dispersions also exert an osmotic pressure. The semipermeable membrane is bombarded equally on both sides by solvent molecules in thermal motion, which produces no pressure difference and hence no osmotic pressure. However, disperse particles in Brownian motion impinge on the semipermeable membrane from one side only, thereby producing an osmotic pressure.[42]

Osmotic pressure measurements of lyophobic sols have not met with success. Aqueous hydrophobic dispersions, which are of prime pharmaceutical importance, are stabilized by electric charges on the particle surface. For electroneutrality, a large number of counterions are associated with each particle. Since each counterion produces the same osmotic pressure increment as the particle itself, the particle weight derived from osmotic pressure measurements would be far too small. These charge effects can be overcome by adding an excess of electrolyte to the aqueous dispersion, or by working in a liquid of low dielectric constant where there is no dissociation. In these cases, however, since each particle contributes only one kT unit to the energy of the system regardless of its size, the osmotic pressure of most colloidal dispersions will be too low to be measured accurately.

Light Scattering [4,9,38,42,74]

When light passes through a gaseous, liquid or solid single-phase or multiphase medium, it is either transmitted or absorbed or reflected or scattered. Light is an electromagnetic radiation. It causes electrons of molecules which it meets to vibrate in unison with it. These oscillating electrons act as weak secondary emitters, sending out radiation of the same frequency as the incident light in

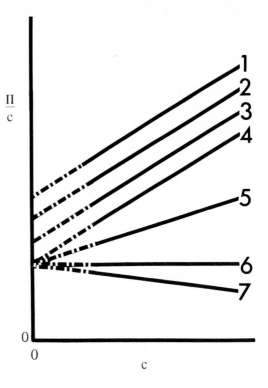

FIG. 6-13. Plots of reduced osmotic pressure versus concentration for polymer solutions.

all directions. This process is light scattering. In crystals, there is complete destructive interference between light scattered by individual ions or molecules because they are arranged in a regular lattice. In gases and pure liquids, thermal motion produces temporary fluctuations in density on a molecular scale. At any given moment, different portions with equal volumes contain different numbers of molecules, so that there is an excess scattering of light from one volume element which is not completely cancelled by the light scattered from another volume element through interference. When a solute is dissolved in a liquid, additional light is scattered because of nonhomogeneities resulting from fluctuations in the concentration of the solute.

Turbidity, τ, defined by the following equivalent equations

$$\frac{I}{I_o} = e^{-\tau L} \text{ and } \tau = \frac{2.303}{L} \log \frac{I_o}{I} \quad (30)$$

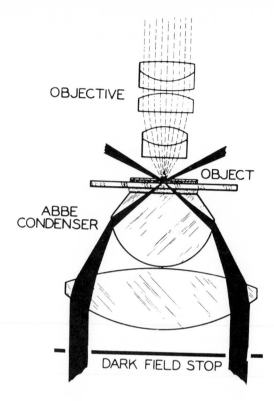

OBJECTIVE

OBJECT

ABBE
CONDENSER

DARK FIELD STOP

FIG. 6-14.   Dark-field illuminator made by equipping Abbe condenser with central stop. (Courtesy of Bausch & Lomb)

is a measure of the ability of a medium to scatter light. I and I_o are the intensities of the transmitted and incident light beams, respectively, and L is the length of the optical path or of the photometer cell containing the solution. The difference between I_o and I constitutes the intensity of the scattered light, provided that no light is absorbed or reflected. For this reason, light scattering cannot be used to measure the weight of opaque and of metallic or electrically conducting particles. Fluorescent and colored materials also present difficulties. Except for very turbid solutions or dispersions, I is nearly the same as I_o. Therefore, the intensity of the scattered light is measured directly rather than as the difference $I_o - I$. Instead of measuring the intensity of light scattered in all directions, it is usually possible to measure the scattered intensity at a single angle or at three angles, and from this to calculate

the total amount of light scattered in all directions and hence the turbidity.

From light-scattering measurements, one can obtain the weight-average molecular weight of macromolecules and of colloidal particles through the appropriate mathematical treatment. The angular distribution of the intensity of the scattered light and its depolarization provide information on the size as well as on the shape of these small particles.[4,9,38,74]

Related Optical Phenomena

Many colloidal dispersions, particularly lyophobic ones, exhibit pronounced turbidity. A narrow and intense beam of light passing through air or through a sol can be seen laterally, especially against a dark background, because of the light scattered in all directions by the particles of airborne dust or of colloids dispersed in a liquid. This is called the Tyndall effect, and constitutes the basis of the dark-field or ultramicroscope.[30,42,72] The best ordinary light microscopes equipped with immersion objectives have a limit of resolution of about half the wavelength of visible light or 3,000 Å. This restricts their usefulness to the upper limit of the colloidal range.

In the dark-field or ultramicroscope, a hollow cone of illuminating light comes to an apex which is located in the sample of colloidal suspension. This effect can be obtained either with a special cardioid (heart-shaped) condenser, or by placing a central stop on a regular Abbe condenser (Fig. 6-14). The central stop can be a disc of black paper covering all of the base of the condenser except for an annulus cut out of the paper, which allows only a hollow cylinder of light to pass. The condenser converges that cylinder into a hollow cone, focusing it on the sample. After passing through the liquid sample, the cone of light diverges and passes outside of the objective of the microscope. Since no light enters the objective, the field of the microscope appears dark. The presence of colloidal particles in the sample is revealed by the light which they scatter in all directions, some of which enters the objective. A small particle thus appears as a single bright blur against a dark background. The observer sees the particle only indirectly by its Tyndall effect. Even particles much smaller than the wavelength of light can be detected in the ultramicroscope. For instance, colloidal gold particles are observable down to 50-Å diameters, because they are very strong scatterers and reflectors. Lyophilic colloidal particles, such as dissolved proteins and synthetic polymers, as a rule do not scatter enough light to be perceptible, because the difference between their refractive indices and that of the solvent is small. For two particles to be individually "visible" in the ultramicroscope, they must be separated by a distance greater than the limit of resolution of the microscope. Ultramicroscopes do not have greater resolving powers than ordinary bright-field microscopes.

Very intense illumination is required in the dark-field microscope because only a small portion of the light beam is permitted to pass through the sample, and only a minute fraction is scattered by the colloidal particles into the objective. Of course, the intensity of the light passing through the sample is relatively high because the hollow conical beam is made to converge on the sample.

The dark-field microscope makes it possible to observe Brownian motion. Flat particles such as bentonite platelets scatter more light when their faces are perpendicular to the objective than when viewed edge-on. In the course of its Brownian motion, such a particle will twinkle in the dark field as the light scattered by the face is replaced by the much weaker light scattered by the thin edge whenever it flips. Since large particles scatter more light than smaller ones, they appear brighter. This makes it possible to follow the progress of flocculation in the dark-field microscope. By counting the number of particles and knowing their weight or volume concentration, it is possible to estimate their average particle size.

For coarse particles which are opaque or light-absorbing, the particle size can be estimated by optical extinction measurements. The optical density or turbidity of their suspensions depends on the projected area of the particles which, at constant concentra-

tion, increases as the particle size decreases. Unfortunately, the specific extinction coefficient is a function of particle size. Details of these measurements are given in a recent publication.[14]

Viscosity Relationships [30,42,74]

The Einstein viscosity equation (Equation 17) is the basis for the definition of the following four viscosity terms:

$$\frac{\eta_{12}}{\eta_1} = \text{relative viscosity}$$

$$\frac{\eta_{12} - \eta_1}{\eta_1} = \frac{\eta_{12}}{\eta_1} - 1 = \text{specific viscosity},$$

where η_1 is the viscosity of the solvent and η_{12} that of the solution.

According to Equation 17, the *specific viscosity* equals 2.5 ϕ. The *reduced viscosity* is defined as specific viscosity/ϕ or

$$\frac{\eta_{12} - \eta_1}{\eta_1 \phi}.$$

According to Equation 17, it is 2.5 for all disperse systems obeying Einstein's viscosity equation. That is a limiting law, however, and even most systems satisfying the conditions listed for the applicability of Equation 17 obey it only at high dilution. The *intrinsic viscosity* [η], also designated as limiting viscosity number, refers to infinite dilution:

$$[\eta] = (\text{reduced viscosity})_{\phi \to 0} = $$

$$\left(\frac{\text{specific viscosity}}{\phi}\right)_{\phi \to 0} = \left(\frac{\eta_{12} - \eta_1}{\eta_1 \phi}\right)_{\phi \to 0} \quad (31)$$

Ideally, it should be 2.5. Experimental [η] values for globular proteins at their isoelectric point in moderately concentrated salt solutions are 3.3 to 4.0 cm.^{3}/g., in comparatively good agreement with the theory. The difference between 2.5 and 3 or 4 is due to the layer of bound water hydrating the protein and/or to deviation from spherical shape. The hydration layer moves with the protein molecule and therefore affects its solution viscosity. Both asymmetry and solvation increase the intrinsic viscosity, but it is very difficult to separate the relative contributions of the two factors to such increases.

Polymer Molecular Weights from Solution Viscosity [4,9,38,42,74]

Staudinger, one of the pioneers of polymer chemistry, as well as Mark and Houwink, established the following relationship between intrinsic viscosity and molecular weight of dissolved polymers:

$$[\eta] = KM^a \qquad (32)$$

where K and a are constants which depend on the nature of polymer and solvent, on the temperature, and on the degree of branching. For randomly coiled polymer chains, $a \cong 0.5$. The reason that the intrinsic viscosity increases with the polymer molecular weight contrary to the Einstein equation is that the size of the coil increases not in proportion to the chain length but faster. The average distance between the two ends of the coiled polymer molecule and its radius of gyration increase with the square root of chain length or of molecular weight. The hydrodynamic volume of the random coil increases as the third power of the end-to-end distance or radius of gyration and hence with the $3/2 = 1.5$ power of the molecular weight M. Thus, the hydrodynamic volume increases faster than the dry molecular weight by a factor of $M^{1.5}/M = M^{0.5}$. The solvent molecules which solvate a dissolved polymer molecule and some of the solvent molecules mechanically trapped inside its randomly coiled chain move together with the chain, i.e., they are part of its hydrodynamic volume. Therefore, the values of the intrinsic viscosity of polymer solutions are large, often running into the hundreds of cubic centimeters per gram.

Once the values of K and a have been established for a particular polymer-solvent system at a given temperature by measuring $[\eta]$ for a sample of that polymer having a known molecular weight, Equation 32 can be used routinely for determining the molecular weights of other samples of the same polymer in the same solvent at the specified temperature. Viscosimetric techniques have been described earlier. Measurements are usually carried out in or close to the lower Newtonian region. Solution viscosimetry is the easiest and fastest method for determining polymer molecular weights. The molecular-weight average obtained from the intrinsic viscosity lies between the number-average and the weight-average values, being closer to the latter.

The molecular weight or intrinsic viscosity of polymer samples determine their effectiveness in thickening suspensions and emulsions and, thus, control the rates of settling or creaming as discussed in Chapter Seven.

Ultracentrifugation [3,38,42,74,]

In most sols of colloidal particles and macromolecules, Brownian motion prevents settling of the disperse phase under the effect of gravity (p. 118). Specially designed high-speed centrifuges called ultracentrifuges are capable of producing 60,000 or more revolutions per minute and accelerations equal to 250,000 times that of earth gravity or more. According to Equation 25, increasing G by a factor of a quarter of a million reduces the critical radius for settling by a factor of 144. The critical radius of a sulfur particle for a 100-second period would be 17 Å, which corresponds to the lower limit of the colloidal range. Colloidal sulfur particles thus settle out in the gravitational field of the ultracentrifuge, and their size can be determined by an equation similar to Equation 23 from their rate of sedimentation.

The particle size or molecular weight measured by the rate of sedimentation in the ultracentrifuge does not include the water of hydration of the particle. The average molecular weight determined by sedimentation velocity is a higher order average than the number-average molecular weight determined by osmotic pressure. Since protein solutions are essentially monodisperse, both methods should give the same average molecular weight (see p. 119). The molecular weight of lactoglobulin determined by osmotic pressure and sedimentation velocity is 35,000. For serum albumin, osmotic pressure gives a value of 69,000 while sedimentation velocity gives a value of 66,000.[74]

ADSORPTION[1,2,29]

*Ad*sorption is the accumulation of a substance at a surface or interface, whereas *ab*sorption is the accumulation and distribution of a substance throughout a phase. Drugs are *absorbed* by a tissue, organ or blood when they permeate its entire bulk or volume. They are *adsorbed* by a membrane, enzyme or cell wall when they are attached to its surface.

This section deals with adsorption at solid-liquid interfaces and, to a lesser extent, at solid-gas interfaces. (Adsorption at liquid-air and liquid-liquid interfaces is discussed in the following section.)

A solid immersed in a solution containing several dissolved substances may selectively remove one or the other solute or even the solvent by adsorbing it on its surface. The solid substrate is called the *adsorbent,* the substance being adsorbed, the *sorbate.* Drugs generally inhibit the metabolic activity of an enzyme because the drug molecules are adsorbed at the specific receptor sites of the much larger enzyme molecule, blocking these sites and impeding the adsorption and subsequent transformation of metabolic intermediates. In this case, the enzyme is the adsorbent. Enzymes and toxoids adsorbed from aqueous solution by gels of alumina or calcium phosphate are the sorbates. The antibacterial activity of quaternary ammonium halides is a result of their adsorption by the walls and membranes of bacteria.

If the adsorption process is limited to the surface of the solid adsorbent, is it possible to achieve the uptake of substantial amounts of sorbate? This depends on the specific surface area of the solid. It must be remembered that finely dispersed colloids have considerable specific surface areas (see Problem 1). Coarse grains of commercial adsorbents have very large internal surfaces, i.e., they are not solid throughout but porous, full of cavities, pores, cracks, and crevices.

Activated Charcoal, U.S.P., is an example. It is manufactured in two steps, the first being the pyrolysis (heating with exclusion of air) of such organic materials as wood, bone, sugar or coconut shells. The residue is largely carbon, with voids where the other atoms were. The second step is the activation process. It consists of heating the carbonaceous residue with air or steam. This removes some of the carbon via the reactions

$$2\,C + O_2 \rightarrow 2\,CO \text{ and } C + H_2O \rightarrow CO + H_2$$

from the interior as well as from the surface of the grains, and substantially increases their porosity and adsorptive power. Activated charcoals have specific surface areas of 100 to 500 m.^{2}/g. and can adsorb 10, 20, or even 100 percent or more of their weight in sorbate. Other solids with large adsorptive capacities include silica and alumina gels and clays like kaolin and bentonite.

Ions or atoms in the surface of a solid are not surrounded by the full complement of nearest neighbors; some of their valences are left unsatisfied (see discussion on liquid surfaces and Fig. 6-19). These unbalanced forces endow surfaces with special activity and bring about phenomena such as adsorption, catalysis, and adhesion. If the sorbate is attracted and bound to the solid surface through relatively weak secondary valences or van der Waals forces, the interaction is called *physical adsorption.* This type of adsorption is reversible (see below) and is characterized by relatively low heats of adsorption. If the sorbate interacts with the adsorbent by primary valence forces, i.e., if the two combine through a chemical reaction, the process is termed *chemisorption.* The heats of adsorption are much higher where chemisorption is involved, and the process is usually irreversible.

Physical adsorption is largely nonspecific. Activated charcoal physically adsorbs most organic solutes from aqueous solution. The solutes adsorbed include simple organic compounds like acetic acid, drugs, and more complex substances such as toxins and viruses. Chemisorption is much more specific; several examples are given below. Clays like bentonite and attapulgite have cation-exchange sites which consist of acidic silanol groups, of strength similar to silicic acid, built into their crystalline layer lattice. The protons of the acid silanol groups can be exchanged for other cations; the clays occur frequently in the sodium form. They chemisorb quaternary ammonium compounds like benzalkonium chloride and cetylpyridinium chloride by the following ion-exchange reaction:

The antibacterial agent, in this case cetylpyridinium chloride, is bound to the inorganic substrate by the electrovalence or ionic bond between the positive nitrogen and the negative silanolate group, forming essentially cetylpyridinium silicate. The ring and hydrocarbon chain of the organic compound are physically adsorbed on the silica surface, which removes them from the bulk of the water.[26] Cetylpyridinium chloride and benzalkonium chloride lose their antibacterial activity through chemisorption. Because of their incompatibility with cation-exchanging materials, quaternary ammonium compounds in particular and basic drugs in general should not be formulated together with clays like bentonite, kaolin or talc. Inactivation through chemisorption would occur otherwise.[8]

Bentonite, in its calcium form, chemisorbs sodium dodecyl sulfate via calcium bridges:[61]

$$-\underset{|}{\overset{|}{Si}}-O^-\,Ca^{++}\,(OH)^- + Na^+\,{}^-O_3SO-(CH_2)_{11}-CH_3 \longrightarrow$$

$$-\underset{|}{\overset{|}{Si}}-O^-\,Ca^{++}\,{}^-O_3SO-(CH_2)_{11}-CH_3 + NaOH$$

Again, electrovalences are involved, plus the physical adsorption of the dodecyl chain on the silicate surface so that it does not stick out into the water.

Toxins are proteins secreted by pathogenic organisms. In the stomach, toxins are positively charged as the hydrochloric acid transforms their amino, imidazole, and guanidino groups into the respective hydrochlorides while the carboxyl groups are undissociated. Attapulgite, kaolin and other clays probably adsorb these toxins by cation exchange with their basic groups similar to

the reaction shown for bentonite and cetylpyridinium chloride.[6] Physical adsorption of the remaining protein molecule onto the silicate surface takes place at the same time through hydrogen bonds and other strong dipole-dipole interactions; the protein molecule is at least partly denatured. This probably explains the specific action of Kaolin, N.F. and other clays against toxins like those produced by the bacteria Shigella and Salmonella, which cause dysentery and gastroenteritis.

By a similar cation exchange process, clays adsorb alkaloids which, at the low pH values of 1.2 to 1.7 prevailing in the stomach, are transformed into the hydrochloride salts. Activated charcoal is effective in removing free alkaloids by physical adsorption. Therefore, clays and activated charcoal have been used as antidotes for alkaloid poisoning.

Other gastrointestinal disturbances may also be alleviated by activated charcoal through adsorption. For instance, it adsorbs gases from the gastrointestinal tract. In industry, activated charcoal is frequently used for decolorizing, i.e., for removing colored impurities from solutions by adsorption.

Adsorption Isotherms

The quantitative relationship between the solution concentration of the sorbate and its uptake by the adsorbent is described by the so-called adsorption isotherms. As the word implies, adsorption isotherms characterize the adsorption process at a given temperature. The amount of sorbate taken up by

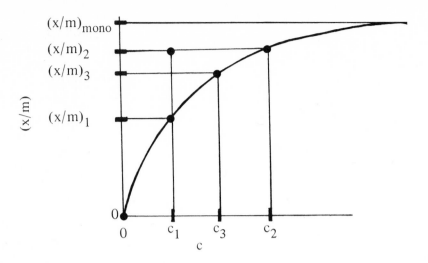

FIG. 6-15.   A typical adsorption isotherm.

the adsorbent, x, is expressed in grams or milligrams, or in moles or millimoles. This is referred to a quantity m of adsorbent, which is expressed either in grams, or in square centimeters or square meters. The dependent variable is thus x/m, viz., the amount of sorbate x adsorbed per unit weight or unit area m of adsorbent. The independent variable is the equilibrium concentration c of solute. This is the concentration of residual solute, or of solute remaining in solution after an equilibrium amount, x, has been removed by adsorption onto the solid. The extent of adsorption of the solute x/m increases as its equilibrium concentration c increases. When $c = 0$, $x/m = 0$, so that the adsorption isotherm goes through the origin (Fig. 6-15). Isotherms representing chemisorption processes usually have a steep initial rise, indicating that the adsorbent removes the solute almost completely from solution, i.e., that x/m increases much faster than c.

The isotherm of Figure 6-15 is typical of a physical adsorption process like the uptake of acetic acid by activated charcoal. If a mixture of aqueous acetic acid and charcoal comes to equilibrium at the point $[(x/m)_1, c_1]$, addition of glacial acetic acid increases the uptake to $(x/m)_2$ and the equilibrium concentration to c_2. If water is now added to the system until the concentration of acetic acid in solution drops to c_1

while the uptake is still at $(x/m)_2$, the system is not at equilibrium because the point $[(x/m)_2, c_1]$ is not on the isotherm. Desorption or release of adsorbed acetic acid from the charcoal proceeds until the concentration in water increases to c_3 and the amount adsorbed decreases to $(x/m)_3$ The equilibrium point $[(x/m)_3, c_3]$ falls again on the adsorption isotherm.

Reversible adsorption means that the isotherm describes both the adsorption and desorption processes, although hysteresis is sometimes observed. The adsorption equilibrium in physical adsorption is dynamic. There is a continual exchange between sorbate molecules adsorbed on the adsorbent and those dissolved in the liquid. On the average, for each sorbate molecule leaving the solid surface, another one becomes attached to it; the values of (x/m) and c remain unchanged.

The adsorption of gases and vapors on solids can be described by isotherms similar to those characterizing adsorption from solution. The gas pressure p or the relative vapor pressure p/p_0 replaces the concentration c in these and all subsequent considerations; p_0 is the saturation vapor pressure of the pure liquid at the temperature of the adsorption process, so that $100\ p/p_0$ represents the relative humidity in the case of water vapor.

Adsorption isotherms have many shapes;

TABLE 6-5. PHYSICAL ADSORPTION OF
ACETIC ACID BY ACTIVATED
CHARCOAL, U.S.P., AT 25°C.

ACID CONCENTRATION, NORMALITY		UPTAKE x/m
Initial	Equilibrium, c	g. acid/g. charcoal
0.500	0.325	0.103
0.250	0.127	0.0742
0.100	0.0268	0.0410
0.050	0.0079	0.0253
0	0*	0

* No leachable acid material in the charcoal.

many equations exist to describe them. Among the most widely used equations are the Freundlich and the Langmuir adsorption isotherms. A third isotherm, the so-called Brunauer-Emmett-Teller (B.E.T.) equation applicable to the adsorption of gases and vapors on solids, is discussed in Chapter Seven.

Freundlich Isotherm. The German chemist·H. Freundlich, one of the founders of colloid chemistry, observed that plots of x/m versus c on a double logarithmic scale were often linear. The relation between these two variables therefore follows the equation below in its two equivalent forms:

$$x/m = Kc^{\frac{1}{n}} \text{ and } \log (x/m) = \log K + \frac{1}{n} \log c \tag{33}$$

K and n are constants, n being usually greater than 1.

Problem 5. Five-gram portions of activated charcoal were equilibrated with 50-cm.^{3} volumes of acetic acid solutions of different strength. The equilibrium concentrations of acetic acid were determined by titrating aliquots of the filtrates with 0.1 N KOH against phenolphthalein (why was the charcoal filtered off prior to taking aliquots for titration?). The values of x/m were calculated from the decrease in concentration of acetic acid on treatment with charcoal. The data are given in Table 6-5. (a) Is the Freundlich adsorption isotherm obeyed? The four points on the double logarithmic plot of Figure 6-16 fall on a straight line, indicating that the process follows the Freundlich isotherm. (b) Determine the values for the constants K and n. Being a straight line, the plot of Figure 6-20 can be represented by the general equation of a straight line, $y = a + bx$. In the case of the logarithmic form of Equation 33, the dependent variable is $y = \log (x/m)$ and the independent variable is $x = \log c$. Note that x represents both the amount of acetic acid adsorbed and the independent variable. The extrapolated intercept of the straight line on the vertical axis, $a = \log K$, is the value for y or $\log (x/m)$ when x or $\log c$ is equal to zero:
$\log K = -0.812 = \bar{1}.188$ and $K = 0.154$. The slope $b = 1/n$ is obtained as

$$\frac{\log (x/m)_2 - \log (x/m)_1}{\log c_2 - \log c_1} =$$

$$\frac{-1.178 - (-1.544)}{-1.0 - (-2.0)} = \frac{0.366}{1} = 0.366$$

and $n = 1/0.366 = 2.73$

"Power-law" relationships between two variables as represented by Equation 33 are common. Log-log plots are often linear because, by taking the logarithms, the ordinate and abscissa scales are greatly compressed compared to the linear plots. The advantage of power laws including the Freundlich isotherm is that a linear relationship is easily handled—it can be described by two constants only, K and n. There are two disadvantages. First, the dimensions or units of K depend on the value of n. Second, the equation does not take into account that x/m cannot increase indefinitely with c. Sooner or later, the adsorbent becomes saturated with sorbate, and the adsorption isotherm levels off as shown in Figure 6-15. Evidently, the Freundlich isotherm is obeyed only at moderate concentrations, up to c_2 in Figure 6-15.

Langmuir Isotherm. I. Langmuir, the Nobel-prize winning surface chemist who worked in the research laboratories of the General Electric Company, derived an equation to characterize the complete adsorption isotherm having the shape given in Figure 6-15. He made two assumptions—first, that neighboring adsorbed molecules do not attract or repel each other laterally; second, that the adsorbent becomes saturated with sorbate when it is covered with a close-packed monolayer of adsorbed molecules, i.e., with a layer of sorbate one molecule thick in which these molecules are spaced as closely as possible. This saturation limit is designated as $(x/m)_{mono}$. The Langmuir adsorption isotherm is

$$(x/m) = \frac{(x/m)_{mono}\, bc}{1 + bc} \tag{34}$$

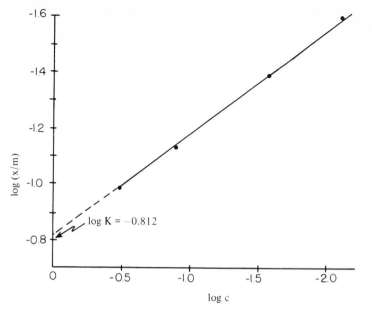

FIG. 6-16. Double logarithmic plot of the adsorption of acetic acid on charcoal according to the Freundlich isotherm.

where *b* is a constant related to the heat of adsorption. The ratio $\dfrac{(x/m)}{(x/m)_{mono}}$ represents the degree of coverage of the adsorbent by the sorbate as a fraction of saturation coverage. At high concentrations, $1 + bc \cong bc$, and Equation 34 becomes $(x/m) = (x/m)_{mono}$; the adsorbent has become saturated. Of course, not all adsorption processes stop when the adsorbent is covered by a close-packed monolayer of sorbate. When there is multilayer adsorption (sorbate accumulating on the adsorbent in a layer several molecules deep), the Langmuir isotherm does not apply. To test whether a set of experimental data follows the Langmuir adsorption isotherm, Equation 34 is best changed to a linear form. It is first inverted, and then multiplied through by *c*:

$$\frac{c}{(x/m)} = \frac{1}{(x/m)_{mono}b} + \frac{c}{(x/m)_{mono}} \quad (35)$$

This is the equation of a straight line, where the dependent variable is $y = \dfrac{c}{(x/m)}$ and the independent variable is $x = c$. The intercept on the vertical axis, for $c = 0$, is $a = \dfrac{1}{(x/m)_{mono}b}$. The slope is $b = \dfrac{1}{(x/m)_{mono}}$.

(Note that the letter *b* is used in two different ways—first, as the slope or coefficient of *x* in the general equation of a straight line, $y = a + bx$; second, as one of the two

TABLE 6-6.   ADSORPTION OF STRYCHNINE
ON CLAYS AT 24°C.*

c g. strychnine/liter	x/m mg. strychnine/g. clay	
	kaolin	attapulgite
0.05	3.65	43.4
0.1	5.40	52.4
0.2	7.08	58.6
0.4	8.39	62.2
0.6	8.94	63.5

Constants in Langmuir Adsorption Isotherm

	kaolin	attapulgite
b, liter/g.	11.0	38.0
$(x/m)_{mono}$, mg./g.	10.3	66.2

* Calculated from data of Ref. 17.

constants in the Langmuir adsorption isotherm.)

An example of adsorption which fits the Langmuir isotherm is that of several alkaloids by clays. The data for the adsorption of strychnine by kaolin and attapulgite, calculated from Reference 17, are listed in Table 6-6 and plotted in Figures 6-17 and

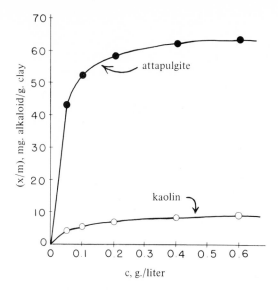

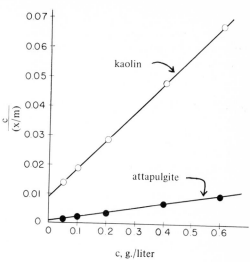

Fig. 6-17. Adsorption isotherms of strychnine on kaolin and on attapulgite at 24°C. Key: solid circles, attapulgite; open circles, kaolin.

Fig. 6-18. Adsorption isotherms of strychnine on kaolin and on attapulgite at 24°C., plotted according to the linear form of the Langmuir isotherm. Key: solid circles, attapulgite; open circles, kaolin.

6-18. The shapes of the two isotherms of Figure 6-17 show that attapulgite is a much more efficient adsorbing agent for strychnine than is kaolin. At a given equilibrium or residual concentration of strychnine, the former has a much higher uptake than the latter. At a given x/m value, kaolin is in equilibrium with a much larger residual strychnine concentration than attapulgite. The greater adsorptive power of attapulgite for the alkaloid can probably be ascribed to the fact that its cation exchange capacity is 3 to 6 times greater than that of kaolin. Of the two clays, kaolin has the smaller particle size[17] and presumably the larger specific surface area. The steep initial slope of the adsorption isotherm for attapulgite in Figure 6-17 is indicative of chemisorption, presumably by a cation exchange mechanism, since strychnine has one basic nitrogen.

To evaluate the two constants of the Langmuir adsorption isotherm, the data are plotted according to Equation 35 in Figure 6-18. Straight lines show that the Langmuir equation is followed. For kaolin, the intercept on the vertical axis in Figure 6-18 is $\dfrac{1}{(x/m)_{mono}b} = 0.00883$ and the slope is $\dfrac{1}{(x/m)_{mono}} = 0.0971$. The corresponding values for attapulgite are 0.0004 and 0.0151, respectively. The values of the two constants calculated from these data are listed in Table 6-6.

The slope of the linear plot for kaolin in Figure 6-18 is greater than for attapulgite, again indicating that the latter has a greater $(x/m)_{mono}$ value than the former. In the case of pure chemisorption via cation exchange, the magnitude of $(x/m)_{mono}$ is directly proportional to the cation exchange capacity of the adsorbent. For physical adsorption, it is directly proportional to its specific surface area. In fact, the specific surface area of a solid can be determined from the amount of sorbate adsorbed at saturation, i.e., from the $(x/m)_{mono}$ value, provided that the cross-sectional area per sorbate molecule in a close-packed monolayer is known. This is discussed in Chapter 7.

Adsorption is an exothermic process, i.e., it liberates heat. Therefore, adsorptions are more extensive at lower temperatures. An adsorption isotherm like the one in Figure 6-15, but determined at a lower temperature, would have a similar shape but would be shifted towards higher ordinates. The vertical distance between the isotherms determined at different temperatures is a measure of the heat of adsorption.

Several official dosage forms consist of drugs or biologics adsorbed on flocculent inorganic precipitates with high surface areas. Suspensions of these solids with the adsorbed drugs are administered by intramuscular injection. Gradual desorption and release of the adsorbed substances in the body makes their effect more lasting. Among such drugs are Sterile Corticotropin Zinc Hydroxide Suspension, U.S.P. Biologics adsorbed on aluminum hydroxide or aluminum phosphate include diphtheria toxoid, tetanus toxoid, pertussis vaccine, and their combinations. They are listed as Adsorbed Diphtheria (and/or Tetanus) Toxoid, U.S.P., and Adsorbed Pertussis Vaccine, U.S.P.

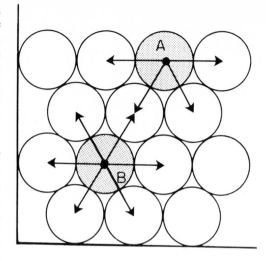

FIG. 6-19.   Unbalanced forces of attraction at a liquid surface.

PHENOMENA AT LIQUID INTERFACES AND SURFACE ACTIVITY

Surface and Interfacial Tensions [1, 2]

Molecules located in surfaces and interfaces are not surrounded by the full complement of nearest neighbors. This situation results in unsatisfied forces of intermolecular attraction, and endows these surfaces and interfaces with special energy. In the two-dimensional schematic drawing of Figure 6-19 representing spherical molecules of a liquid in a beaker, molecule B in the bulk of the liquid is symmetrically surrounded by six nearest neighbors which attract it by van der Waals forces represented by arrows. The attractive forces exerted on B are balanced, i.e., they are equal in all directions. By contrast, there are (in two dimensions) only four molecules adjacent to molecule A in the surface, two lateral and two beneath A. Therefore, molecule A is subjected to asymmetrically distributed intermolecular forces of attraction resulting in a net downward or inward force for lack of molecules

above it. The concentration of vaporized molecules of the liquid and of oxygen and nitrogen molecules in the air space above the liquid surface is almost 1,000 times smaller than the concentration of molecules in the liquid; it is negligible by comparison.

Molecules in the surface are thus subjected to a pull directed toward the interior of the liquid. Evidently, not all surface molecules can leave the surface for the interior, but as many as possible do. This causes liquid surfaces, which are mobile, to contract spontaneously in order to expose the smallest possible area. The geometric shape which has the smallest surface area for a given volume is the sphere, which explains why drops of liquid aerosols, nasal spray mists, and rain, as well as gas bubbles in effervescent liquids are spherical.

The tendency of liquid surfaces to contract in order to minimize their surface areas implies that work is required to enlarge the surfaces. This work is expended in pulling molecules from the bulk liquid, where they are symmetrically attracted from all sides, to the surface, where they are subjected to unbalanced force fields. Free energy is the general term for the net work supplied to or obtained from a given process. In the case of the expansion or contraction of liquid surfaces, it is called *surface free energy*.

The surface free energy γ of a liquid is defined as the work W required to increase its surface area A by 1 cm.^{2}:

$$W = \gamma \Delta A \qquad (36)$$

where ΔA is the increase in area or the difference between the final and the initial area. Its units are erg/cm.^{2}. The proportionality factor γ is also called *surface tension*. In that case, it is defined as the force acting at right angles to any line of 1 cm. length in the liquid surface, and its units are dyne/cm. The surface tensions and surface free energies of liquids are numerically equal: Water at 20°C. has a surface tension of 73 dyne/cm. and a surface free energy of 73 erg/cm.^{2}. The two are also dimensionally equivalent, since

$$\frac{\text{erg}}{\text{cm.}^2} = \frac{\text{dyne cm.}}{\text{cm.}^2} = \frac{\text{dyne}}{\text{cm.}}.$$

Problem 6. Isoproterenol hydrochloride solution is dispensed as an aerosol from a container pressurized with liquefied propellant for oral inhalation.

(a) Calculate the energy required to disperse a single dose, namely, 0.2 cm.^{3} of a 0.25 percent solution in 35 percent alcohol, into a mist of droplets having an average diameter $D = 1$ micron $= 10^{-4}$ cm. The surface tension of the solution is 30 dyne/cm.

The energy or work required is

$$W = \gamma \Delta A = \gamma (A_{\text{final}} - A_{\text{initial}}) \cong \gamma A_{\text{final}}.$$

The final surface area, namely, the surface area of the aerosol droplets, is so much greater than the initial surface area of the solution in the can of aerosol that the latter can be neglected.

The number of droplets equals the total volume of solution of the single dose, which is 0.2 cm.^{3}, divided by the volume of one droplet which is

$$\frac{\pi}{6} D^3, \quad \text{or} \quad (0.2 \text{ cm.}^3) \left(\frac{6}{\pi D^3} \right).$$

The total surface area is equal to the surface area of one droplet, which is πD^2, multiplied by the number of droplets, or

$$\frac{(\pi D^2)(0.2 \text{ cm.}^3)}{\pi D^3} \left(\frac{6}{\pi D^3} \right) = \frac{(0.2 \text{ cm.}^3)\, 6}{D} =$$

$$\frac{1.2 \text{ cm.}^3}{10^{-4} \text{ cm.}} = 1.2 \times 10^4 \text{ cm.}^2.$$

$$W = \gamma A_{\text{final}} = \left(\frac{30 \text{ dyne}}{\text{cm.}} \right)(1.2 \times 10^4 \text{ cm.}^2) =$$

$$3.6 \times 10^5 \text{ dyne cm.} = 3.6 \times 10^5 \text{ erg.}$$

(b) What supplies this energy? The answer is that it is the work of expansion of the liquefied propellant on vaporizing, namely,

$$\left(P_{\substack{\text{propellant} \\ \text{vapor}}} \times V_{\substack{\text{propellant} \\ \text{vapor}}} \right) -$$

$$\left(P_{\substack{\text{propellant} \\ \text{liquid}}} \times V_{\substack{\text{propellant} \\ \text{liquid}}} \right),$$

where P represents pressure and V, volume.

Analogous considerations apply to the interface between two immiscible liquids. An imbalance of intermolecular forces of attraction is imposed on both kinds of molecules in the interface similar to the imbalance at liquid-air interfaces, but of lower magnitude. The values of the interfacial tensions between pairs of immiscible liquids usually lie between the values of the two corresponding surface tensions. Representative data are listed in Table 6-7. Among the interfacial tensions against water, three are lower than the surface tensions of the two corresponding liquids, namely, those of ethyl ether, oleic acid, and octanol. Ether has a relatively high miscibility with water. The interfacial tension value listed is between water saturated with ether and ether saturated with water. It is to be expected that

TABLE 6-7. SURFACE TENSIONS OF VARIOUS LIQUIDS AND INTERFACIAL TENSIONS AGAINST WATER AT 20°C.

LIQUID	SURFACE TENSION (dyne/cm.)	INTERFACIAL TENSION AGAINST WATER (dyne/cm.)
water	72	—
mercury	480	415
glycerine	63	—
oleic acid	32	16
benzene	29	35
chloroform	27	33
carbon tetrachloride	27	45
n-octanol	27	8.5
n-octane	22	51
ethanol	22	—
ethyl ether	17	11

the presence of water molecules in ether and of ether molecules in water reduces the imbalance of intermolecular attractive forces at the ether-water interface. Oleic acid and octanol have hydrophilic groups which, at

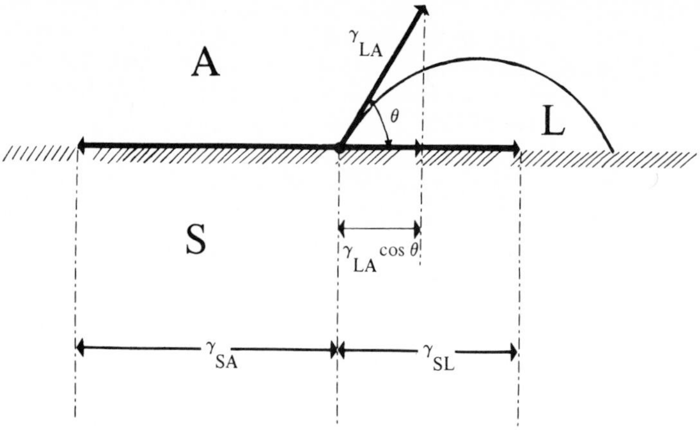

FIG. 6-20. Interfacial forces acting on a liquid drop placed on a horizontal solid surface.

the interface with water, are oriented toward the water phase. This makes the transition from the organic layer, which is primarily hydrocarbon and thus of low polarity, to the very polar water layer more gradual, reducing the imbalance of intermolecular forces at the interface and thus decreasing the interfacial tension.

Wetting Relationships [1, 2]

A solid is wetted by a liquid when the liquid spreads out on the solid surface and displaces the air. The solid-air interface is replaced by a solid-liquid interface. This process is important in the preparation of suspensions of powders in liquids, in the disintegration of tablets, in the spreading of lotions and topical formulations on skin, and in the displacement of air bubbles clinging to the inside of bottles filled with liquids.

Solids have a surface tension and a surface free energy, just as liquids do, but a solid cannot minimize its surface area by assuming a spherical shape unless it is heated above its melting point. The wetting of solids is studied by placing a drop of a liquid, small enough to neglect the effect of gravity, on a smooth horizontal solid surface. The three competing interfacial tensions are considered along the circular baseline of the drop, where the three phases meet. Subscripts S, L, and A indicate solid substrate, liquid drop, and air, respectively. As shown in Figure 6-20, the surface tension of the solid or rather, its interfacial tension against air γ_{SA}, is opposed by the solid-liquid interfacial tension γ_{SL}, and by the horizontal

component of the surface tension of the liquid γ_{LA}, namely, $\gamma_{LA} \cos \theta$. Here, θ is the angle which the vector or arrow representing γ_{LA} makes with the solid surface. The surface tension of the liquid (or better, its interfacial tension against air) acts along the tangent to the surface of the drop, because surface tension forces always act at right angles to lines in the surface. In order to add the three forces vectorially, that is, directionally, they must be in a common plane. The most convenient plane is that of the solid surface, in which γ_{SA} and γ_{SL} are acting. The projected length or magnitude of the γ_{LA} vector in that plane is $\gamma_{LA} \cos \theta$.

The Young-Dupré equation follows from Figure 6-20 when there is equilibrium:

$$\gamma_{SA} = \gamma_{SL} + \gamma_{LA} \cos \theta \qquad (37)$$

The *contact angle* θ, defined by the plane of the solid surface and the tangent to the liquid-air interface at the line where it meets the solid surface, can vary from $0°$ ($\cos \theta = 1$) through $90°$ ($\cos \theta = 0$) to almost $180°$ ($\cos \theta$ nearly equals -1). The value of θ depends on how much of γ_{LA} is needed in addition to γ_{SL} to balance γ_{SA}. If the contact angle is zero, $\gamma_{SA} - \gamma_{SL} \geqslant \gamma_{LA}$; the liquid drop spreads out on the solid surface as far as possible and wets it completely. A liquid spreads on a solid when its molecules are adsorbed by the solid more strongly than the gas or air molecules, with enough energy left over to overcome its own surface tension. Otherwise, the liquid remains on the solid as a distinct drop.

Critical Surface Tension

A measure of how well liquids wet a given solid surface is provided by the magnitude of the contact angles which the liquid drops make on that surface. Small angles and cosines close to unity indicate good wetting. The ability of liquids to wet solid surfaces increases as their surface tensions decrease. Zisman and collaborators at the U.S. Naval Research Laboratory[81] found a linear relationship between the cosines of the contact angles formed on a smooth solid surface by different liquids and the surface tension of these liquids:

$$\cos \theta = a - b\gamma_{LA} \qquad (38)$$

Typical plots, as shown in Figure 6-21, consist of straight lines ascending with decreasing surface tension until $\cos \theta$ reaches unity and $\theta = 0°$. Since a cosine cannot be greater than one, nor a contact angle smaller than zero, the plots then become horizontal. The surface tension at that point is called the *critical surface tension* for spreading, γ_c. Liquids with surface tensions equal to and smaller than the critical surface tension of a solid spread out completely on its surface.

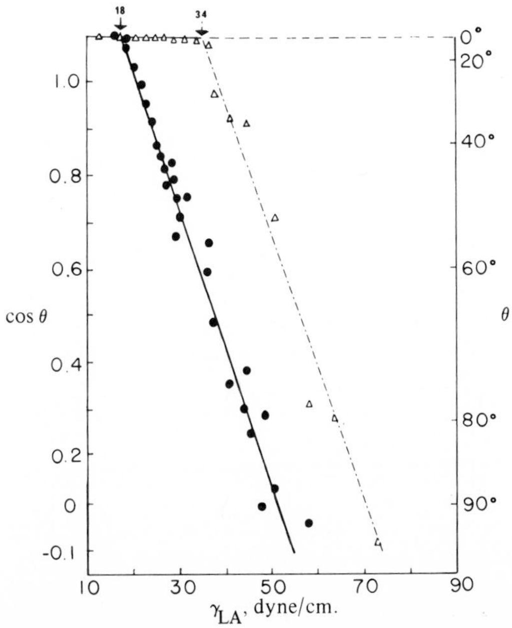

Liquids with surface tensions greater than γ_c remain as drops making finite contact angles. Since $\cos \theta = 1$ when $\gamma_{LA} = \gamma_c$, Equation 38 becomes

$$\cos \theta = 1 + b (\gamma_c - \gamma_{LA}) \qquad (39)$$

where b is a constant.

The critical surface tension is a characteristic property of the solid. It is thought to be close to its surface tension in vacuum. As is seen from Table 6-8, the critical surface tension depends on the polarity of the solid. For solid hydrocarbons, the values are low (25 to 33 dyne/cm). The presence of a chlorine atom in polyvinyl chloride, which introduces a permanent dipole, raises γ_c to 39 dyne/cm. The polar amide groups of 66-Nylon and hydroxyl groups of cellulose increase γ_c further. Inorganic compounds with ionic surfaces have high critical surface tension values, but small amounts of adsorbed water, which are difficult to remove from the surfaces, lower them significantly.

The foregoing considerations apply to smooth and clean surfaces. The effect of roughness and of impurities on contact angles is discussed in connection with the wettability of human skin. Its observed critical surface tension was in the 22 to 30 dyne/cm. range. This value is low for as polar a surface as keratin, if it were uniform, clean, and free of wrinkles.[63]

Fig. 6-21. Contact angles and their cosines versus the surface tensions of the corresponding liquids on polyethylene and polytetrafluoroethylene.

TABLE 6-8. CONTACT ANGLES OF WATER
ON LOW-ENERGY SURFACES AT 20° OR 25°,
AND CRITICAL SURFACE TENSIONS

SOLID	CONTACT ANGLE OF WATER (degrees)	CRITICAL SURFACE TENSION (dyne/cm.)
paraffin	111	25
sulfur*	90	30
polytetrafluoroethylene (Teflon)	107	17
polyethylene	92	31
polystyrene	90	33
polyvinyl chloride	86	39
polyhexamethylene adipamide (66-Nylon)	70	46
cellulose	38	45

* Rhombic.

Sulfur and organic, hydrophobic powders
have low-energy surfaces, on which water
makes large contact angles (see Table 6-8).
Poor wetting is the reason why these powders are so difficult to disperse in water.
Consider Equation 37 in the form

$$\cos \theta = \frac{\gamma_{SA} - \gamma_{SL}}{\gamma_{LA}}$$

For good wetting, liquids should have high
$\cos \theta$ values, close to 1, in order to make
low contact angles, close to zero. Barring
surface modifications, it is not possible to
change γ_{SA} without changing the solid. In
the case of water, the addition of surfactants
reduces γ_{SL}, which makes the numerator
larger, and also reduces the denominator
γ_{LA} (see next section). Both changes increase $\cos \theta$ and reduce θ, thereby facilitating the wetting and dispersal of the powders
in water. For the same reason, improved
wetting to speed up the disintegration of
tablets can be achieved by incorporating
small amounts of surfactants.

Another technique for wetting out hydrophobic powders, such as sulfur, with water
in order to prepare aqueous dispersions is
to mix them with a little alcohol first. Since
the surface tension of alcohol (Table 6-7)
is below the critical surface tension of sulfur (Table 6-8), alcohol makes a zero contact angle with sulfur surfaces and wets the
particles completely, i.e., it displaces all the
air, transforming the sulfur-air interface

into a sulfur-alcohol interface. When water
is added to the mixture, it dissolves the alcohol, producing the desired sulfur-water
interface.

Water wets surfaces of plastics poorly, as
shown by the high contact angles in Table
6-8. This is why plastic bottles filled with
aqueous media often have air bubbles clinging to the inside walls. The presence of
alcohol or of small amounts of surfactants
lowers the contact angle of the aqueous medium and improves its ability to wet the
plastic surface, thereby removing the air
bubbles. Air bubbles do not cling to glass
bottles filled with aqueous media because
glass, being an inorganic ionic compound,
has a higher critical surface tension than the
plastic materials of low polarity. Glass is
therefore well wetted by water despite the
high surface tension of the liquid.

Gibbs Adsorption Equation [1, 2, 3, 39]

The concentration of solutes in the surface layer of solutions is not always the same
as in the bulk of the solutions. There are
a number of substances, designated as surface active, that accumulate in the surface
layer and thereby lower the surface tension
of the solution, often to a fraction of the
surface tension of the pure solvent. The reduction in surface tension is understandable:
surface tension resists the expansion of the
surface. Molecules which tend to concentrate in the surface lower the resistance
against such expansion. Compounds concentrating in the surface layer are said to be
positively adsorbed at the surface. Negative
adsorption also occurs. For example, in the
case of electrolytes and sugars in aqueous
solution, where the forces of intermolecular
attraction between solute and solvent molecules exceed the solvent-solvent attractive
forces, the solute molecules tend to migrate
away from the surface region to the interior
of the liquid where they are totally surrounded by solvent molecules. This increases
the surface tension of the solution above
that of the solvent, but rarely by more than
a few percent.

J. Willard Gibbs, a Yale University professor of mathematical physics in the latter
part of the 19th century, pioneered in many
areas of physical chemistry. He derived an

equation to describe the situation of the previous paragraph:

$$\Gamma = - \left(\frac{c}{RT} \right) \left(\frac{d\gamma}{dc} \right) = \tag{40}$$

$$- \left(\frac{1}{2.303\ RT} \right) \left(\frac{d\gamma}{d\log c} \right)$$

Γ is the surface excess concentration of the solute. Since it refers to the surface, its units are moles/cm.^{2}; c is the bulk concentration in moles/cm.^{3}, and γ is the surface tension of the solution in dynes/cm. **R** and *T* are the gas constant and the absolute temperature, respectively. Because of the minus sign, the surface excess Γ increases as the rate of change of the surface tension with concentration, $d\gamma/dc$ or $d\gamma/d \log c$, decreases. This agrees with the earlier statement that surface-active or positively adsorbed solutes, for which Γ is positive, reduce the surface tension of the solution. Negatively adsorbed solutes, i.e., those having negative Γ values or a surface deficiency, increase the surface tension. The concentration of solutes in the surface layer, and Γ, can be obtained by analyzing collapsed foams or by using radioactive tracers.

Problem 7. For aqueous phenol solutions at 20°C, the slope of a plot of surface tension γ versus the logarithm of the phenol concentration is —19 erg/cm.^{2} at a concentration of 0.05 molar ($c = 5 \times 10^{-5}$ mole/cm.^{3}).

(a) Calculate the amount of phenol adsorbed in the surface of the solution above the amount that an equal volume in the bulk of the solution would contain.

$$\Gamma = - \left(\frac{1}{2.303\ RT} \right) \left(\frac{d\gamma}{d\log c} \right) =$$

$$- \frac{1}{2.303} \left(\frac{\text{mole °K}}{8.314 \times 10^7\ \text{erg}} \right) (293°K) \left(\frac{-19\ \text{erg}}{\text{cm.}^2} \right) =$$

$$3.39 \times 10^{-10}\ \text{mole/cm.}^2$$

(b) Calculate the area per excess molecule of phenol in the surface layer.
1 cm.^{2} or $(10^8\ \text{Å})^2 = 10^{16}\ \text{Å}^2$ contains 3.39×10^{-10} mole, or

$$\frac{(3.39 \times 10^{-10}\ \text{mole}) \left(\dfrac{6.023 \times 10^{23}\ \text{molecules}}{\text{mole}} \right)}{} =$$

$$2.042 \times 10^{14}\ \text{molecules.}$$

$$\text{Area} = \frac{1 \times 10^{16}\ \text{Å}^2}{2.042 \times 10^{14}\ \text{molecules}} = 49\ \frac{\text{Å}^2}{\text{molecule}}$$

There is a dynamic equilibrium between molecules of a surface-active solute in the bulk of the solution and in the surface layer, i.e., there is a continual exchange between the two. On the average, just as many solute molecules leave the surface region for the interior of the liquid in a given time interval as become adsorbed in the surface, so that Γ remains constant. The Gibbs adsorption equation is applicable not only to liquid-air interfaces but also to liquid-liquid and solid-liquid interfaces. Adsorption of surface-active substances in interfaces usually does not deplete their bulk concentrations markedly because the interfaces represent small volumes compared to the bulk of the solutions.

Relationships between Structure, Surface Activity and Pharmacological Activity [1, 2, 10, 29]

Surface activity is described by the Gibbs equation in terms of the surface excess Γ and the surface-tension lowering $d\gamma/dc$. The surface activity of a homologous series of compounds dissolved in water increases strongly and regularly with their chain length. *Traube's rule* states that in dilute aqueous solutions of compounds belonging to any one homologous series, the molar concentrations required to produce equal lowering of the surface tension of water decreases threefold for each additional CH_2 group in the hydrocarbon chain of the solute. For instance, the molar concentrations of normal primary alcohols required to reduce the surface tension of water at 20°C. from 73 to 50 dyne/cm. are 2.03 for ethanol, 0.60 for propanol, 0.18 for butanol, 0.06 for pentanol, and 0.02 for hexanol.

Traube's rule also applies to interfacial tensions at oil (e.g., benzene)-water interfaces. Although solid-liquid interfacial tensions cannot be measured directly, regular increases in the uptake of solutes by adsorbents are commonly found on ascending a homologous series. The adsorption of normal fatty acids from aqueous solution by activated charcoal is an example. The x/m values corresponding to the equilibrium concentration of 0.01 millimole acid/liter are 1.0, 1.8, 2.7, 3.3, and 3.6 millimoles acid/g. charcoal for acetic, propionic, butyric, valeric, and caproic acids, respectively. The amount adsorbed at the solid-liquid interface, x/m, is identical with the surface excess Γ; both can be expressed as mole/cm.^{2}, and Γ is directly proportional to the interfacial tension lowering $d\gamma/dc$.

This is reminiscent of the *Meyer-Overton theory* of narcosis, which states that the anesthetic activity of a series of compounds increases as the oil-water partition coefficients increase. The partition or distribution coefficient of a compound between oil and water is the ratio of its equilibrium concentration in "oil," meaning a liquid of low polarity, such as octanol, and its equilibrium concentration in water when these two immiscible liquids are in contact, permitting the compound to migrate from one phase to the other until the equilibrium distribution is attained.

Regular increases in both anesthetic activity and oil-water distribution coefficients are frequently observed within homologous series and within series of otherwise related compounds: plots of the logarithms of the minimum effective narcotic concentration versus the logarithms of the oil-water partition coefficient are often linear. Comparable correlations within a series of similar or homologous compounds are also found between other pharmacological effects, such as bactericidal activity, and the oil-water partition coefficient.

Surface activity (the accumulation in interfaces and the lowering of interfacial tensions as characterized by the Gibbs adsorption equation) is related to the oil-water partition coefficient. Both depend on the balance between the hydrophilic and lipophilic properties of a compound. This balance shifts gradually in favor of lipophilicity (or hydrophobicity) on ascending a homologous series, thereby increasing simultaneously the surface activity in water, i.e., the tendency to accumulate at water-air and oil-water interfaces, and the oil-water partition coefficient. Pharmacological effectiveness depends not only on the specific activity of a drug embodied in specific functional groups but also on its ability to be absorbed from the blood stream by a given tissue or microorganism. The *Ferguson principle* states that compounds present in a given biological system at the same fraction of their saturation concentration have the same pharmacological activity.

The absorption of a series of related drugs having the same functional groups by a lipoidal tissue such as the central nervous system is improved as their surface activity and their oil-water partition coefficients increase. Such increases can be brought about by going to higher members in a homologous series. The limitation is the water (or plasma) solubility, which decreases rapidly with increasing lipophilicity. Greater surface activity in a homologous series of compounds means that, for a given bulk concentration in water or plasma, there is a higher concentration of the compound in the water-air, oil-water, and cell membrane-plasma interface as the hydrocarbon chain length increases. This, in turn, leads to higher absorption by the tissue or microorganism of the more surface-active drug. For instance, the bacteriostatic activity of quarternary ammonium compounds has been correlated with their surface activity, i.e., with their ability to reduce the surface tension of water, which follows Traube's rule. The pharmacological activity of general and local anesthetics increases within a series of similar compounds with increases in their surface activity as well as with their oil-water partition coefficients, because the two are related. A well-presented, detailed account of this topic is given by Buechi.[10]

SURFACTANTS[65,66 68]

Surfactants, also called surface-active agents and association colloids, are compounds which, while soluble in a given liquid, tend to accumulate or be positively adsorbed at its interfaces with air, another liquid, or a solid.

Functional Classification

According to their intended use, surfactants can be divided into the following main categories. One surfactant sometimes can be used in several categories.

Wetting agents promote the wetting of solid surfaces by liquids, as discussed in the preceding section.

Detergents aid in personal cleanliness, washing of fabrics, and cleaning of hard surfaces.

Emulsifying agents promote the formation

of emulsions and stabilize them once they are formed, as discussed in Chapter 7.

Demulsifying agents break emulsions, such as water emulsified in petroleum.

Solubilizing agents promote the solubility in water of water-insoluble compounds.

Dispersing, suspending, deflocculating or peptizing agents deflocculate solids suspended in liquids and stabilize their dispersions.

Foaming agents promote the formation of foams and stabilize them, e.g., in toothpastes and in fire-extinguishing compositions.

Antifoaming agents destroy foams and reduce frothing, e.g., in aerobic fermentations, steam boilers, and papermaking machines.

Structural Classification

A single surfactant molecule contains one or more hydrophobic portions and one or more hydrophilic groups. The hydrophobic or oleophilic portions usually consist of hydrocarbons—paraffinic, unsaturated, alicyclic, aromatic, or combinations of these—although some surfactants contain fluorocarbons. Hydrophilic groups include ionic groups as well as organic functional groups with strong dipole moments, preferably capable of hydrogen bonding, such as hydroxyl, ether, carbonyl, carboxyl, sulfoxide, etc. The subsequent discussion in this chapter deals primarily with water-soluble surfactants. Oil-soluble surfactants are discussed in Chap. 7.

If the surfactant molecule contains ions, it is classified as ionic, otherwise the surfactant is said to be nonionic. *Anionic surfactants* contain the surface-active moiety including the hydrophobic portion in the anion or negative ion. Their cation is commonly an alkali metal ion, ammonium, or an organic monofunctional base. This simple, nonsurface-active ion, whose presence is necessary to establish electroneutrality, is called the counterion. *Cationic surfactants* contain the surface-active part of the molecule in the positive ion or cation. Their counterion or negative ion is commonly a simple inorganic ion such as chloride or sulfate. When the surfactant molecule as a whole forms a zwitterion, i.e., when it has both positively and negatively charged groups attached to the hydrocarbon portion by covalent bonds, the surfactant is said to be *ampholytic*.

Given the large number of hydrophilic and hydrophobic groups and the many different ways in which they can be combined, it is not surprising that there are millions of surface-active structures and thousands of commercially available surfactants. A few surfactants in each category of pharmaceutical, cosmetic, or biochemical importance are discussed below.

Anionic Surfactants. Soaps are the oldest surfactants. They are the metal salts of long-chain fatty acids, $CH_3(CH_2)_nCOO^-M^+$. Acids such as lauric (n = 10), myristic (n = 12), palmitic (n = 14), stearic (n = 16), oleic (n = 16, monounsaturated), and ricinoleic (n = 16, monounsaturated, with one hydroxyl group) and their mixtures are the major fatty acid ingredients of soap stock. Sodium, potassium, and triethanolamine are the most important cations. Sodium Stearate, N.F., consists of a mixture of sodium stearate and palmitate. Green Soap, N.F., is a potassium soap with a high enough oleic acid content and sufficient glycerine and water to leave it soft.

Among the alkyl sulfates, sodium dodecyl sulfate or Sodium Lauryl Sulfate, U.S.P., is used in toothpaste and ointments; triethanolamine dodecyl sulfate, $CH_3(CH_2)_{11}$-$OSO_3^-{}^+NH(CH_2CH_2OH)_3$, is used in shampoos and other cosmetic preparations. Sodium dodecylbenzene sulfonate

$$CH_3(CH_2)_{11}\!-\!\!\bigcirc\!\!-\!SO_3^-\,Na^+$$

is a detergent and has germicidal properties. Sodium dialkylsulfosuccinates are good wetting agents. Sodium bis(2-ethylhexyl)-sulfosuccinate, Dioctyl Sodium Sulfosuccinate, U.S.P.,

$$Na^+\,{}^-O_3S\!-\!CH\!-\!COO\!-\!CH_2\!-\!\underset{\underset{\displaystyle C_2H_5}{|}}{CH}\!-\!(CH_2)_3\!-\!CH_3$$
$$\underset{\underset{\displaystyle C_2H_5}{|}}{\overset{|}{CH_2}}\!-\!COO\!-\!CH_2\!-\!CH\!-\!(CH_2)_3\!-\!CH_3\text{,}$$

manufactured by American Cyanamid Company under the tradename Aerosol OT, is soluble in water as well as in oils. It is used internally as a fecal softener. Ichthammol,

N.F., is obtained by the destructive distillation of bituminous shales, followed by sulfonation of the resultant hydrocarbons and neutralization with ammonia to form ammonium ichthosulfonate. The product is used as a local antibacterial agent. The bile salts sodium glycocholate

and sodium taurocholate

emulsify triglycerides in the intestine and solubilize monoglycerides—essential steps in fat metabolism.

Cationic Surfactants.[27] These are chiefly quaternary ammonium compounds. They have bacteriostatic activity probably because they combine with the carboxyl groups in the cell walls and membranes of microorganisms by cation exchange, causing lysis. Among the most popular antiseptics in this category are cetylpyridinium chloride (formula on p. 127), benzalkonium chloride,

and, in Great Britain, cetyltrimethylammonium bromide,

$$CH_3(CH_2)_{15}N^+ (CH_3)_3Br^-.$$

Ampholytic Surfactants. These are the least common. An example is dodecyl-β-alanine, $CH_3(CH_2)_{11}N^+H_2$—CH_2—CH_2—COO^-.

Nonionic Surfactants.[56, 58] These are for the most part addition products of ethylene oxide. Any active hydrogen, such as the one

in an aliphatic or a phenolic hydroxyl, thiol, carboxyl, or amino group, can produce a ring-opening reaction, usually with the aid of an alkaline catalyst:

$$R{-}OH + H_2C{-}CH_2 \rightarrow R{-}O{-}CH_2{-}CH_2{-}OH$$
$$\underset{O}{\diagdown\diagup}$$

The reaction product has a terminal hydroxyl group and can add many more molecules of ethylene oxide. A typical surfactant is $CH_3(CH_2)_{11}O(CH_2CH_2O)_8H$. The addition of ethylene oxide, like many polymerization reactions, is a random process—some molecules grow faster than others. The number of ethylene oxide molecules incorporated into the surfactant molecule, shown as 8, is an average value; the extremes may be as low as 2 or 3 and as high as 20 or more.

The hydrophilic moiety in polyoxyethylated surfactants is the polyethylene glycol portion. Each ether oxygen binds 2 water molecules through hydrogen bonds, which in turn associate with additional water molecules. Hydration of ether linkages is not as efficient in achieving water solubility of the surfactant as the introduction of ionic groups. For the dodecyl moiety, the presence of a single sulfate or ammonium ion, as in $C_{12}H_{25}$-$OSO_3^-Na^+$ and $C_{12}H_{25}N^+H_3Cl^-$, brings about excellent water solubility. By comparison, about n $= 5$ ethylene oxide groups are required to make $C_{12}H_{25}O(CH_2CH_2O)_nH$ water-soluble at room temperature.

The hydration of ether linkages is exothermic, i.e., it evolves heat. Therefore, the extent of hydration decreases with increasing temperature, and the polyoxyethylated surfactants become less soluble. When heating such surfactant solutions, they become turbid at a characteristic temperature called the *cloud point,* owing to precipitation. The solution becomes clear again when cooled below the cloud point, as the surfactant molecules become rehydrated and redissolved. Cloud points are largely independent of the concentration of a surfactant but depend on its composition. For a given hydrocarbon moiety, the cloud point increases as the number of ethylene oxide units per molecule increases. At constant ethylene oxide content, cloud points decrease as the chain length of the hydrocarbon moiety increases.[62] Dispersions or emulsions stabilized with polyoxyethylated nonionic surfactants may be destroyed when heated above the cloud point of the surfactant, a problem to be kept in mind when sterilizing by heat. Polyoxyl 40 Stearate, U.S.P., consists of a mixture of the monostearate and distearate esters of polyethylene glycol with an average size of 40 ethylene oxide units.

Other nonionic surfactants have sucrose as their hydrophilic moiety—for example, the mono- and diesters of palmitic or oleic acids. Of pharmaceutical importance are surfactants based on sorbitan. Electrolytic reduction of glucose produces the hexahydroxy alcohol sorbitol, which on dehydration forms a mixture of five- and six-membered rings called sorbitan:

Esterification of the primary hydroxyl group with lauric, palmitic, stearic or oleic acid forms sorbitan monolaurate, monopalmitate, monostearate or monooleate, water-insoluble surfactants called Span* 20, 40, 60 or 80, respectively. Addition of about 20 ethylene oxide molecules produces the water-soluble surfactants called polysorbate or Tween* 20, 40, 60 or 80. The formula for the derivative of the six-membered ring is

where $x + y + z = 20$. Polysorbate 80, sorbitan monooleate with 20 ethylene oxide molecules, is listed in the U.S.P.

Other Surface-active Compounds. The only requisite for a water-soluble substance to be surface active is that it contain enough hydrophobic groups to cause it to accumulate at interfaces. Many organic compounds are thus surface active, even though they are not used as surfactants. The following classes of drugs are cationic surfactants: Phenothia-

zines—e.g., Chlorpromazine Hydrochloride, U.S.P.; Fluphenazine Hydrochloride, N.F.; Acetophenazine Maleate, N.F.; and Promazine Hydrochloride, N.F.[59] Many alkaloids, such as the hydrochloride and nitrate of pilocarpine, the hydrochlorides and sulfates of morphine and of codeine,[49] all listed in the *U.S.P.* or *N.F.*, as well as many local anesthetics—e.g., the hydrochlorides of cinchocaine or dibucaine, lidocaine, and procaine (Novocaine), all of the *U.S.P.*—are also cationic surfactants.[25] Besides the antibacterials already listed among the quaternary ammonium salts under cationic surfactants are salts of the acridines, which are cationic, and phenols, which are nonionic except in alkaline media, where they become anionic. Many water-soluble dyes are surface active. For instance, Orange II

is anionic, Methylene Blue, U.S.P., is cationic, and Congo Red,

is ampholytic.

Oriented Adsorption at Interfaces[1, 2, 3, 29]

The Gibbs adsorption equation describes quantitatively the extent of the accumulation of surfactants in interfaces. How surface-active molecules orient themselves in interfaces is illustrated in Figure 6-22. A surfactant molecule is depicted schematically as a cylinder representing the hydrocarbon portion with a sphere representing the polar group attached at one end.

* Span and Tween are trademarks of ICI America, Inc.

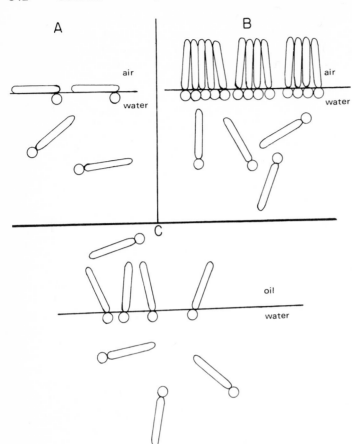

FIG. 6-22. Orientation of surfactant molecules adsorbed in water-air and oil-water interfaces: A, water-air interface, low coverage; B, water-air interface, higher coverage; C, oil-water interface.

In reality, the hydrocarbon chains are seldom straight, because rotation around carbon-carbon bonds bends, coils, and twists them.

Surface-active substances contain a hydrophilic and a hydrophobic or oleophilic portion. It is to be expected that in a monolayer adsorbed at an *oil-water interface,* surface-active molecules will be oriented so that the hydrophobic portion is inside the oil phase and the hydrophilic portion inside the water phase (Fig. 6-22C). This is in keeping with the maxim that like dissolves like and explains why surface-active substances tend to accumulate in the oil-water interface. This is the only region of a two-phase oil-water system where their hydrophilic polar groups and their hydrophobic and lipophilic hydrocarbon portions both find the proper environment simultaneously.

Hydrocarbon molecules by themselves have very low solubilities in water because they contain no polar groups with which to attract water molecules. For this reason, and because they interfere with the attraction between water molecules, hydrocarbon molecules are pushed out of the water. In the molecules of surface-active compounds, however, the hydrocarbon chains have hydrophilic portions attached to them which tend to dissolve in water and become hydrated. The *water-air interface* is the only location in an aqueous solution where both tendencies can be satisfied. The hydrocarbon chains of surface-active molecules adsorbed in water-air interfaces are pushed out of the water and rest on the surface, while the polar groups are inside the water. Perhaps the polar groups pull the hydrocarbon chains partly into the water. At low surfactant concentrations, the hydrocarbon chains of surfactant molecules adsorbed in the interface lie more or less flat on the water surface (Fig. 6-22A). At higher concentrations, they stand upright because this permits more surfactant molecules to pack into the interfacial mono-layer. The hydrocarbon chains protruding above the water surface are in lateral contact and attract each other by weak London or dispersion forces. The orientation of surfactant molecules in a close-packed mono-layer in the water-air interface is such that the hydrocarbon chains are perpendicular to the water surface (Fig. 6-22B). This is deduced from the fact that the cross-sectional area per molecule in several homologous series of normal paraffin derivatives, calculated as in Problem 7-b, is between 20.5 and 22 Å² regardless of the length of the paraffin chain. If the orientation were that of Figure 6-22A, the area per molecule occupied in the water-air interface would increase as one ascends the homologous series. Furthermore, the crosssection of a normal paraffin chain is 20.5 to 22 Å².

As an increasing number of surfactant molecules becomes adsorbed in the water-air interface, they tend to cover the water progressively with a layer of hydrocarbon chains. Thus, the water-air interface is gradually transformed into an oil-air interface. Since the γ_{LA} values of hydrocarbons are much lower than that of water (see Table 6-7), this process results in a decrease in the surface tension of water.

How does one predict whether a given compound is water soluble and yet surface active? A large hydrophobic portion is required for significant surface activity (see Traube's rule). If it is too large, however, it may reduce the water solubility to practically zero by overwhelming the hydrophilicity of the polar group. The presence of polar and hydrophilic groups in the surfactant molecules is also essential. If their hydrophilicity outweighs the hydrophobicity of the hydrocarbon portions by too much, the compounds will have little or no surface activity because the hydrophilic groups drag the entire molecule, hydrocarbon portion included, into the bulk of the water. Surface activity without loss of water solubility requires a proper and rather delicate balance between the hydrophilicity of the polar groups and the hydrophobicity of the hydro-

carbon portion of the surfactant molecule.

For nonionic surfactants, there is a convenient system used to predict the surface activity and water solubility. It is called the *H.L.B. system* and is outlined in Chapter 7. Ionic groups confer considerably more water solubility than merely polar hydrophilic groups like hydroxyls or ether links, and thereby reduce the surface activity considerably more. Phenol

is surface active (cf. Problem 7) because it contains a small hydrocarbon portion which, moreover, is rather polarizable, and one relatively weak hydrophilic group. Sodium benzene sulfonate,

on the other hand, has negligible surface activity. The hydrophilicity of the sulfonate ion by far outweighs the hydrophobicity of the benzene ring. A dodecyl group is required in addition to the benzene ring to bring the two opposite characteristics more into balance and to achieve significant surface activity:

is a surfactant. Two sulfonate groups on the alkylated benzene ring would shift the balance towards too great a hydrophilicity. On the other hand,

is practically insoluble in water because the weaker hydrophilicity of the hydroxyl group is completely outweighed by the hydrophobicity of the large hydrocarbon portion. Butyl alcohol and butyric acid are surface active, sodium butyrate is not. To balance the hydrophilicity of the carboxylate ion requires a $C_{11}H_{22}$ group as found in sodium laurate or larger. Lauryl alcohol and lauric acid, on the other hand, have already lost their solubility in water because the hydroxyl and undissociated carboxyl groups are much less hydrophilic than the carboxylate ion.

Surfactants physically adsorbed at *solid-water interfaces* are usually oriented with their hydrocarbon chains in contact with the solid surface and the polar groups directed toward the water, particularly if the solid substrate is activated charcoal or an organic solid of low polarity. The situation depicted in Figure 6-22A and 6-22B applies with the solid replacing air, except that the surfactant molecules are pushed by the solid into the water rather than by the water into the air as shown. Surfactants chemisorbed by a reaction between their ionic groups and the solid substrate have the opposite orientation. When glass or clay surfaces adsorb cationic surfactants by cation exchange and anionic surfactants by calcium bridges as shown on page 127, the ionic groups of the surfactant molecules are in contact with the solid surfaces, leaving the hydrocarbon chains directed outward, toward the aqueous phase. This effectively covers the formerly hydrophilic silicate surfaces with a monolayer of hydrocarbon chains and renders them hydrophobic. Aqueous dispersions of clays (bentonite, attapulgite, kaolin) treated with cationic surfactants coagulate as the clay surfaces become hydrophobic (see p. 127). Water spreads on clean glass surfaces, making a zero contact angle. After treating the glass with cationic surfactants and rinsing off the excess, the contact angle of water is almost as high as on solid hydrocarbons.

Surface Activity of Water-Soluble Polymers

The ability of water-soluble macromolecules to concentrate at oil-water and solid-water interfaces is important to their effectiveness in stabilizing emulsions and aqueous suspensions. The same structural features which contribute to the surface activity of small molecules are important to that of macromolecules. High concentrations of hydrophilic groups along the macromolecular chain reduce or eliminate surface activity.

Polyvinyl alcohol

$$\left(\!\!\begin{array}{c} CH_2\!\!-\!\!CH \\ | \\ OH \end{array}\!\!\right)_n$$

is produced by hydrolysis of polyvinyl acetate

$$\left(\!\!\begin{array}{c} CH_2\!\!-\!\!CH \\ | \\ O \\ | \\ O\!\!=\!\!C\!\!-\!\!CH_3 \end{array}\!\!\right)_n$$

Polyvinyl acetate is not soluble in water, but progressive hydrolysis, which replaces the ester groups with the more polar hydroxyls, renders it increasingly more soluble. The surface activity of the water-soluble polymers, measured by the surface excess Γ and the lowering of the surface tension $d\gamma/dc$, decreases simultaneously. Pure polyvinyl alcohol has little surface activity. Water-soluble proteins are also surface active owing to the hydrophilic amide links on the backbone and the hydrocarbon groups in the side chains of these macromolecules.

The presence of ionic groups reduces the surface activity strongly. Methylcellulose, a derivative of cellulose in which on the average from 1 to 2 hydroxyls per glucose repeat unit have been transformed into the much less polar methoxyl groups, has considerable surface activity. Sodium carboxymethylcellulose, which is cellulose containing 0.6 to 0.9

$$Na^{+} \; {}^{-}OOC\!\!-\!\!CH_2\!\!-\!\!O\!\!-\!\!\overset{|}{\underset{|}{C}}\!\!- \text{ groups per glu-}$$

cose unit, has none.

Incompatibilities Involving Surfactants

Ionic surfactants have anionic or cationic groups capable of reacting with compounds possessing ions of the opposite charge. These reactions may bind the surface-active ions, sometimes with precipitation. The compounds which react with the surface-active ions are also changed, and this may be harmful from the physiological or pharmacological point of view.

Among the soaps or salts of long-chain normal fatty acids, only those of most alkali metals and ammonium are water soluble.

Soaps of calcium and other di- and trivalent metals are hydrophobic and have extremely low solubilities in water, but they are frequently soluble in oils. They are formed by metathesis reactions with soluble alkali metal soaps:

$$2 Na^+ \ ^-OOC—C_{15}H_{31} + Ca^{++}Cl_2^= \ \rightleftharpoons$$
$$Ca^{++}(^-OOC—C_{15}H_{31})_2 + 2 Na^+Cl^-$$

Since the calcium soap precipitates quantitatively, the equilibrium is displaced completely toward its formation. Other anionic surfactants such as alkyl sulfates and alkylbenzene sulfonates have varying resistance to precipitation by water hardness (calcium and magnesium salts naturally present in waters) and by heavy metal ions. The tolerance of all anionic surfactants toward polyvalent metal ions which may be present in the same formulations needs watching.

Many insoluble inorganic salts, such as barium sulfate, chemisorb anionic surfactants via heavy metal bridges similar to the calcium bridge shown on page 127. This chemisorption depletes the concentration of the dissolved surfactant and alters the surface characteristics of the dispersed solid. Coagulation often occurs (see p. 158). The incompability of surface-active quaternary ammonium compounds with bentonite, kaolin, talc, and other solids having cation exchange capacity is also described on p. 127.

The reaction between anionic and cationic surfactants produces hydrophobic, sticky, oil-soluble, 1:1 precipitates. A typical reaction is the formation of cetyltrimethylammonium dodecyl sulfate:

$$C_{16}H_{33}—N^+Br^- + Na^+ \ ^-O_3SO—C_{12}H_{25} \rightleftharpoons$$
$$\underset{(CH_3)_3}{|}$$
$$C_{16}H_{33}—N^+ \ ^-O_3SO—C_{12}H_{25} + Na^+Br^-$$
$$\underset{(CH_3)_3}{|}$$

The reaction goes to completion because of the nearly quantitative precipitation of the product. Because the ionic groups in the precipitate are surrounded by hydrocarbon chains, they do not come into contact with water and cannot dissociate. This type of reaction is called complex coacervation; the insoluble product is called a *coacervate*.[31] Pyrvinium Pamoate, U.S.P., is another complex coacervate. The insoluble product is formed by metathesis between the water-soluble cationic surfactant pyrvinium methyl sulfate and the water-soluble anionic surfactant disodium 4,4'-methylenebis(3-hydroxyl-2-naphthoate). Benzathine Penicillin G, U.S.P., and Procaine Penicillin G, U.S.P., are also complex coacervates. Their water solubility is much lower than that of Potassium Penicillin G, U.S.P., because of the replacement of the small potassium cation by the large organic cations.

Precipitation may also occur when cationic drugs (alkaloidal salts, local anesthetics, most sympathomimetic, cholinomimetic, adrenergic blocking, and antimuscarinic agents and skeletal muscle relaxants, antihistamines, and many tranquilizing and antidepressant agents) react with anionic surfactants. Even in the absence of precipitation, the drugs may lose potency or availability because of combination with these surfactants. Drugs with carboxylic, sulfonic or phosphoric acid groups like salicylic and *p*-aminobenzoic acids interact likewise with cationic surfactants.

Cationic surfactants form complex coacervates with water-soluble polymers containing negatively charged groups, i.e., negatively charged polyelectrolytes or polyanions. Among those containing carboxylic acid groups are the natural gums (acacia, tragacanth, agar, carrageenin), pectate, alginate, sodium carboxymethylcellulose, and Carbopol* and other copolymers of acrylic acid. Polymers containing phosphoric acid groups include ribonucleic acids (RNA) and deoxyribonucleic acids (DNA). If P represents the chain of one of the carboxylated polymers,

$$P—COO^- Na^+ + C_{16}H_{33}—N^+Br^- \rightarrow$$
$$\underset{(CH_3)_3}{|}$$
$$P—COO^- \ ^+N—C_{16}H_{33} + Na^+Br^-.$$
$$\underset{(CH_3)_3}{|}$$

The cetyltrimethylammonium carboxylate groups hardly dissociate. Because polyelectrolytes owe their water solubility mainly to

---

* B. F. Goodrich Chemical Co. trademark.

the presence of dissociating groups and also because the reaction with quaternary compounds having one long alkyl chain builds a large number of these hydrophobic hydrocarbon chains into the macromolecule, precipitation occurs. The resulting coacervates usually consist of gels swollen with water of hydration.

Interaction of Ionic Surfactants with Proteins. Proteins consist of polypeptide chains, or condensed α-amino acids, with the repeat unit

$$\left(-NH-CH-\underset{\underset{O}{\parallel}}{C}-\right)$$
$$\underset{R}{\mid}$$

Among the substituent groups R are hydrogen, alkyl, phenyl, and hydroxyl. Some amino acids contain carboxyls in the side chain R; others contain basic groups such as amino, guanidino or imidazole. In alkaline media, the carboxyl groups dissociate to carboxylate ions while the basic groups are largely uncharged. The protein molecules are negatively charged and react with cationic surfactants. For a glutamic acid residue, the reaction is

$$\left(-NH-CH-\underset{\underset{O}{\parallel}}{C}-\right)$$
$$\underset{\underset{\underset{COO^- Na^+}{\mid}}{\underset{CH_2}{\mid}}}{\underset{CH_2}{\mid}} + Br^- \, {}^+N-C_{16}H_{33}$$
$$\underset{(CH_3)_3}{\mid} \longrightarrow$$

$$\left(-NH-CH-\underset{\underset{O}{\parallel}}{C}-\right)$$
$$\underset{\underset{\underset{COO^- \, {}^+N-C_{16}H_{33}}{\mid}}{\underset{CH_2}{\mid}}}{\underset{CH_2}{\mid}} + Na^+Br^-$$
$$\underset{(CH_3)_3}{\mid}$$

In acid media, the carboxyl groups are undissociated but the basic groups are in the protonated form, conferring a positive charge to the protein molecules. The latter now can chemisorb anionic surfactants. For a lysine residue, the reaction is

$$\left(-NH-CH-\underset{\underset{O}{\parallel}}{C}-\right)$$
$$\underset{\underset{H_3N^+Cl^-}{\mid}}{\underset{(CH_2)_4}{\mid}} + Na^+ \, {}^-O_3SO-C_{12}H_{25} \longrightarrow$$

$$\left(-NH-CH-\underset{\underset{O}{\parallel}}{C}-\right)$$
$$\underset{\underset{H_3N^+ \, {}^-O_3SO-C_{12}H_{25}}{\mid}}{\underset{(CH_2)_4}{\mid}} + Na^+Cl^-$$

In both alkaline and acid media, the surface-active ions are bound to the protein. The long chains of many protein molecules, in solution as well as in the solid state, are regularly coiled into a helical conformation. Two types of secondary valence forces hold the helices together: The $\diagdown{N}H$ and $\diagup{C}=O$ groups of the amide links in the backbone of the polypeptide chain form hydrogen bonds across successive turns of the helix. Hydrocarbon groups in the side chains fill the interior of the helix and are bound together by dispersion forces. This second type is called hydrophobic bonding. The hydrocarbon chains of chemisorbed surfactants interact with the hydrocarbon groups of the proteins and weaken their hydrophobic bonding to the point where the helices unfold, assuming the shape of random coils. Protein molecules undergoing this transformation are said to be denatured.

Because ionic surfactants are chemisorbed by proteins and because they promote protein denaturation, preparations designed to be taken internally are usually formulated with nonionic rather than ionic surfactants. The interaction between nonionic surfactants and proteins is weak and readily reversed. Nonionic surfactants in general have few incompatibilities with drugs and are preferred over ionic surfactants even in formulations for external use, except where the germicidal properties of cationic and anionic surfactants are important. Nonionic surfactants do, however, form relatively weak complexes with phenols, including esters of *p*-hydroxybenzoic acid, and with acids like benzoic and salicylic via hydrogen bonds. This reduces the antibacterial activity of these compounds somewhat.[69]

Micelle Formation [2, 3, 31, 39, 65, 66, 68]

As the bulk concentration of surfactants in aqueous solution is increased, their surface excess, Γ, also increases. When the surfactant molecules adsorbed as a monolayer in the water-air interface have become so closely packed that additional molecules cannot be accommodated with ease, they begin to agglomerate in the bulk of the solution, forming aggregates called micelles. At a given concentration, temperature, and salt content, all micelles of a given surfactant usually contain the same number of molecules, i.e., they are usually monodisperse. For different surfactants in dilute aqueous solutions, this number ranges approximately from 25 to 100. The diameters of micelles are approximately between 30 and 80 Å. Because of their ability to form aggregates of colloidal size, surfactants are also called *association colloids.*

Micelles are not permanent aggregates. They form and disperse continually, so that each surfactant molecule finds itself randomly alternating between the single and the aggregate state. The lowest concentration at which micelles first appear is called the *critical concentration* for micelle formation, abbreviated *CMC.* On increasing the surfactant concentration, practically all molecules added in excess of the CMC aggregate into micelles; the number or concentration of micelles increases proportionally with the total surfactant concentration. On dilution, the reverse process takes place; the number of micelles decreases until none is left when the concentration drops below the CMC.

Micelles formed in dilute aqueous solutions are approximately spherical (Fig. 6-23 A and E). The polar groups of the surfactants are in the periphery. The hydrocarbon chains are oriented toward the center, forming the core of the micelle. They are randomly coiled, just as in a liquid. This arrangement accomplishes the following: The polar groups are in contact with water, where they are hydrated and, if ionic, dissociated. The hydrocarbon portions are out of contact with water and do not interfere with the intermolecular attraction between water molecules. Some additional energy is gained from the intermolecular attraction between the hydrocarbon chains by dispersion forces. These "hydrophobic bonds" between methylene groups are weak, but they are far from negligible owing to the large number of methylene groups in a micelle.

Aggregation of surface-active molecules can also take place in solvents of low polarity or oils. These micelles are turned inside out or inverted compared to the micelles in aqueous media. The polar heads of the surfactant molecules face inward to form the core of the micelle while the hydrocarbon chains are oriented outward and associated with the molecules of the continuous hydrocarbon phase (Fig. 6-23B).

In more concentrated aqueous solutions of surfactants, micelles change from spheroidal either to cylindrical or to lamellar shapes (Fig. 6-23C and D). The polar groups make up the outer surface of the cylinders or lamellas which are in contact with the surrounding water; the hydrocarbon moieties fill the interior. At still higher concentrations, usually above 25 percent surfactant, many such cylindrical micelles often tend to line up parallel to each other in hexagonal packing, i.e., each cylinder is surrounded by 6 equidistant cylinders arranged on the points of a hexagon. Likewise, the laminar or lamellar micelles are often parallel and equidistant from each other, i.e., the layers of water between adjacent double lamellas are equally thick. Such solutions are liquid but quite viscous. Furthermore, they have different refractive indices parallel and perpendicular to the micellar cylinders or lamellas, i.e., they are birefringent and exhibit optical double refraction. This is a property

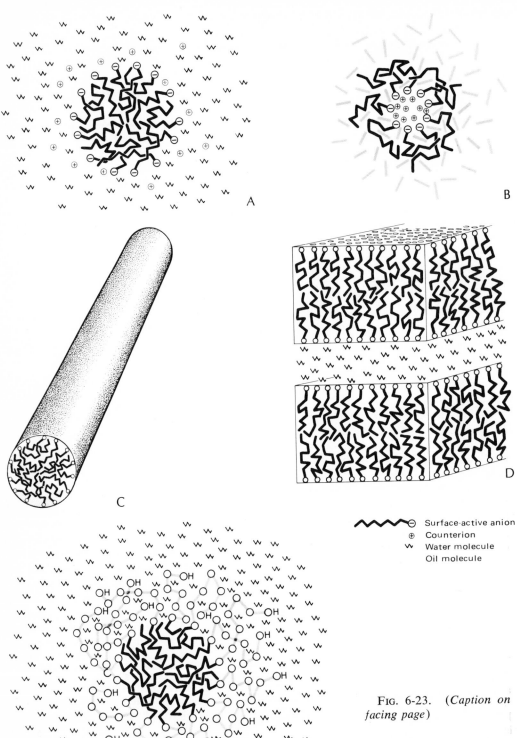

Surface-active anion
⊕ Counterion
w Water molecule
Oil molecule

Fig. 6-23.   (*Caption on facing page*)

characteristic of crystalline solids, and such structured liquids are said to be in the *liquid crystalline* or *mesomorphic* state. In simple liquid solutions, the cylindrical or laminar micelles are randomly arranged and move with respect to each other in Brownian motion, so that the liquid has the same optical properties in all directions, i.e., it is isotropic. Cell membranes and cell protoplasm may have structures like those of liquid crystals.

Critical Micelle Concentrations and Micellar Sizes.[3, 31, 39, 65, 66, 68] Many properties of surfactant solutions undergo abrupt changes at the CMC (Fig. 6-24). Surface and interfacial tensions level off to nearly constant values, owing to crowding of surfactant molecules adsorbed at surfaces and interfaces. The osmotic pressure (and all other colligative properties, lowering of the vapor pressure and of the freezing point, for example), rises much more slowly with increasing surfactant concentration above than it does below the CMC, because it depends on the number of dissolved particles. One single or nonaggregated nonionic surfactant molecule contributes just as much to the osmotic pressure as a micelle of 50 aggregated molecules. For ionic surfactants, the equivalent conductivity drops sharply above the CMC. Equivalent conductivity is the electric conductivity of the solution divided by the normality of the solute. The counterions of aggregated surfactant molecules are kinetically part of the micelle even when a D.C. voltage is applied to the solution. Only the counterions of nonassociated surfactant molecules can carry current.

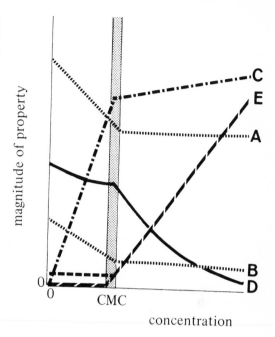

FIG. 6-24. Solution properties of surfactants as a function of concentration. Key to properties: A, surface tension; B, interfacial tension; C, osmotic pressure; D, equivalent conductivity; E, solubility of compounds with low or zero solubility in water.

Furthermore, the counterions associated with micelles reduce the micellar velocity of migration in the electric field because of their tendency to migrate to the opposite pole. Other solution properties changing more or less abruptly at the CMC are intrinsic viscosity and turbidity, which increase (see pp. 124 and 122), diffusion coefficient, which decreases (cf. p. 117), and the rates of change of refractive index, density, dielectric constant, and sound velocity with surfactant concentration.

All of these properties and others have been used to determine the CMC. Typical values are listed in Table 6-9. For nonionic surfactants, the CMC decreases and the micellar size increases with increasing temperature, i.e., in the direction of the cloud point and phase separation. The CMC values of ionic surfactants are generally higher

FIG. 6-23. (*On facing page*) Schematic drawings representing several types of micelles of anionic and nonionic surfactants: A, spherical micelle of anionic surfactant; B, inverted micelle in oil of anionic surfactant; C, cylindrical micelle of anionic surfactant; D, laminar micelle of anionic surfactant; E, spherical micelle of nonionic polyoxyethylated surfactant. See illustration for key.

TABLE 6-9.   TYPICAL VALUES OF CRITICAL MICELLE CONCENTRATIONS, AGGREGATION
NUMBERS, AND MICELLAR MOLECULAR WEIGHTS AT ROOM TEMPERATURE

SURFACTANT	CMC*	AGGREGATION NUMBER†	MICELLAR MOLECULAR WEIGHT
Sodium dodecyl sulfate	0.232	125	36,000
Dodecyltrimethylammonium bromide	0.463	99	30,500
$CH_3(CH_2)_{17}O(CH_2CH_2O)_{18}H$	0.0134	105	111,000
Polysorbate 20‡	0.0044	—	—

* Critical micelle concentration as percent weight-in-volume.
† Number of surfactant molecules per micelle.
‡ Formula on p. 141.

than those of nonionic surfactants. As is seen in Fig. 6-23A, the negatively charged groups in the micelle of an anionic surfactant are in close proximity. To overcome the resulting repulsion requires electric work. This defers the drive of ionic surfactants toward micelle formation to higher concentrations in comparison to nonionic surfactants, which have no electric repulsion to overcome in order to aggregate. The addition of salts to solutions of ionic surfactants reduces the electric repulsion between the charged groups in the periphery of the micelles because counterions from the added salt are drawn toward that region. Lower CMC values result.

The size or molecular weight of micelles is determined by the methods used for dissolved macromolecules. The same equations apply, except that the concentration c in Equation 29 is replaced by $(c - CMC)$. Subtracting the critical micelle concentration or concentration of single surfactant molecules from the total concentration c leaves the concentration of surfactant aggregated into micelles, which is the appropriate concentration term for determining micellar molecular weights. Typical values are given in Table 6-9.

Micellar Solubilization [16,19,35,41,43,67,68, 69, 73, 80]

As is shown in Figure 6-23, the interior of micelles A, C, D, and E is filled with disordered hydrocarbon chains. These micellar cores consist of regions having all of the characteristics of a liquid of low polarity like decane. The cores of the spherical micelles A and E are essentially oil droplets, while those of micelles C and D are cylinders and

layers of oil. Being pools of oil, these interior portions of micelles can dissolve molecules of water-insoluble, oil-soluble compounds, bringing them into solution in an over-all aqueous medium. This phenomenon is called micellar solubilization.

How do the molecules of water-insoluble compounds get into the interior of micelles —how are they able to traverse regions of water and penetrate the outer layer of hydrated polar groups which surrounds the hydrocarbon core? The answer is, they cannot! Surfactant molecules accumulate in the interfaces between water and solid masses or liquid layers of water-insoluble, oleophilic compounds. Their hydrocarbon chains penetrate the outermost layer of such solid or liquid masses and intermingle with the water-insoluble molecules. The latter thus become associated with and bound to the hydrocarbon portions of the adsorbed surfactant molecules. Micelles actually form around the molecules of the water-insoluble compound which are pre-associated with adsorbed surfactant molecules.

Being hydrophobic and oleophilic, the solubilized molecules are located primarily inside the hydrocarbon core of the micelles. However, even water-insoluble drugs usually contain hydroxyl, carbonyl, amino or amine hydrochloride, carboxyl or carboxylate, and other polar groups. Upon solubilization, these are located in the periphery of the micelles, among the polar groups of the surfactant, where they become hydrated. The nonpolar portions of the solubilized drug molecules are immersed in the hydrocarbon core.

Micelles of nonionic surfactants consist of an outer shell containing their polyethylene glycol moieties mixed with water and an inner core formed by their hydrocarbon moieties (Fig. 6-23E). Some compounds like phenols and benzoic acid form complexes with polyethylene glycols by hydrogen bonding and/or are more soluble in liquids of intermediate polarity like ethanol or ethyl ether than in liquids of low polarity like aliphatic hydrocarbons. These compounds locate in the aqueous polyethylene glycol outer shell of nonionic micelles on solubilization.[54] Micellar solubilization is nonspecific: any drug which is appreciably soluble in oils and lipids can be solubilized.

The inverted micelles formed by an oil-soluble surfactant like sodium dioctyl sulfosuccinate dissolved in a hydrocarbon solvent, as shown in Figure 6-23B, can solubilize water. The solubilized water is located in the center of the micelle, out of contact with the solvent, where it hydrates the $-SO_3^-$ and Na^+ ions of the surfactant. It may contain dissolved salts.

Micellar solubilization evidently depends on the existence of micelles; it does not take place below the CMC. This affords another means of determining the CMC. When the amount of a water-insoluble compound solubilized by aqueous surfactant solutions is plotted against the surfactant concentration, as in curve E of Figure 6-24, dissolution begins at the CMC. Above the CMC, the amount solubilized is directly proportional to the surfactant concentration because virtually all surfactant added to the solution in excess of the CMC exists in micellar form, and as the number of micelles increases, so does the extent of solubilization. Water-insoluble, oil-soluble dyes are frequently used to determine CMC values because their concentration is readily obtained by spectrophotometric measurements. Plots of optical density versus surfactant concentration are linear and intersect the horizontal axis at the CMC.[60] If the substance to be solubilized has a limited solubility in pure water, the plot of its concentration versus the surfactant concentration starts out as the broken horizontal line of Curve E in Figure 6-24.

Just as a compound soluble in oil or water has a solubility limit dependent only on temperature, so does a compound solubilized in aqueous surfactant solutions have a limit of solubilization, which is constant for a given surfactant provided that the temperature and the surfactant concentration are constant. For instance, the solubilization limit of Clove Oil, U.S.P., is 0.25 in polysorbate 20, 0.24 in polysorbate 40, 0.24 in polysorbate 60, and 0.19 in polysorbate 80. The corresponding values for Anise Oil, U.S.P., which has less polar components, are 0.11, 0.11, 0.11, and 0.089, respectively. The units are gram of oil per gram of surfactant associated in micelles, and the temperature is 20°C.[69] The solubilization limit for Progesterone, N.F., at 20°C. is 0.262, 0.150, and 0.009 g./g. micellar surfactant for sodium dodecyl sulfate, tetradecyltrimethylammonium bromide, and polysorbate 20, respectively.[69]

Compounds that are extensively solubilized increase the size of micelles in two ways. The micelles swell because their core volume is augmented by the volume of the solubilizate. Moreover, the number of surfactant molecules per micelle increases. Solubilization frequently lowers the CMC of surfactants somewhat.

Micellar solubilization produces dosage forms of considerable pharmaceutical importance. Oil-soluble, water-insoluble drugs administered orally or parenterally are frequently better absorbed from aqueous surfactant vehicles than from solutions in oils. Even though the surfactant solutions may be diluted below the CMC in the body and the solubilized drugs are precipitated, their particle size will be so small that adsorption is fast and complete. Percutaneous absorption is also considerably more efficient for drugs solubilized in surfactant solutions than for the same drugs dissolved in oils.[69]

The oldest official pharmaceutical preparation involving solubilization is Saponated Cresol Solution, N.F., which consists of cresol solubilized in soap solution. In addition to phenolic disinfectants, preservatives like hydroxybenzoic acid and its esters and other germicides like iodine are formulated in aqueous media as solubilizates. Essential oils are extensively solubilized by micellar surfactant solutions, as are alkaloidal drugs, glycosides, the fat-soluble Vitamins A, D, E, and K, many hormonal steroids, analgesics, sedatives and hypnotics like barbituric acid derivatives, sulfonamides, antibiotics like chloramphenicol, tyrothricin, and griseofulvin; anticoagulants based on biscoumarin; and many others. Octoxynol, N.F., an adduct of *p*-(1,1,3,3-tetramethylbutyl)phenol with an average of 10 ethylene oxide groups, is used to solubilize the versatile local antibacterial agent Nitrofurazone, N.F. Hexachlorophene Liquid Soap, U.S.P., a clear liquid, contains the anti-infective agent solubilized in a 10 to 13 percent aqueous solution of a potassium soap at the level of 0.25 percent.

Micellar Solubilization Versus Emulsification. While micellar solubilization bears a superficial resemblance to emulsification, the two processes are fundamentally quite different. They have two points in common: both require surfactants, and both can produce oil-in-water and water-in-oil dispersions. In the latter systems, oil is the continuous phase and water is solubilized in the core of inverted micelles as shown in Figure 6-23B. The differences are many. While solubilization occurs only if the surfactant concentration exceeds the CMC, emulsions are often prepared at lower surfactant concentrations. Solubilization requires a large excess of surfactant over the weight of the solubilizate, usually 4- to 20-fold or 400 to 2,000 percent. Emulsions are stabilized by an amount of surfactant in the vicinity of 5 percent of the weight of the disperse phase.

Solubilizates are much more finely dispersed than emulsions. Micelles measure about 30 to 100 Å in diameter, which is so small compared with the 4,000- to 6,600-Å range for the wavelength of visible light that surfactant solutions containing solubilized substances are perfectly clear to the naked eye. Their turbidity can only be detected with a light-scattering photometer. Because emulsion droplets range from 1,000 to 200,000 Å in diameter, emulsions are milky and opaque. Their droplets can be seen individually in a light microscope, in contrast to micelles. Micelles in a given system with or without solubilizates are monodisperse, while a wide range of droplet sizes is present in most emulsions.

A surfactant solution containing micellar solubilizates constitutes a single phase, whereas emulsions consist of two phases. The vapor pressure of solubilized liquids is lower than the vapor pressure of the pure liquids, just as is observed in solutions. The emulsification of one liquid in another does not lower the vapor pressure of either one. Micellar solubilization is a spontaneous process producing stable systems. Emulsification requires work, which can be calculated by Equation 36 and is commonly supplied by colloid mills or homogenizers described in Chapter 7. Emulsions are inherently unstable, even though they may have very long shelf lives. The order of addition of the ingredients can have a profound effect on the stability of emulsions, but none on the stability of micellar solubilizates. Micellar solubilzation has an upper limit or saturation point, whereas there is no fixed upper limit for the amount of disperse phase which can be emulsified.

LYOPHOBIC COLLOIDAL SYSTEMS[3,30,42]

Lyophobic or solvent-hating dispersions are intrinsically unstable. Once prepared, they must be stabilized by additives such as surfactants or protective colloids (see below). Examples of hydrophobic colloidal dispersions are those of gold, e.g., Gold Au 198 Injection, U.S.P., of silver, e.g., Mild Silver Protein, N.F., of sulfur, and of many organic water-insoluble compounds including medicaments, as well as latexes of natural and synthetic polymers. Emulsions, and suspensions of solid drugs which are too coarse to be classified as colloids, are treated in Chapter 7. There is no sharp dividing line between the two. The forces of interaction between colloidal particles described below are also operative between coarse particles.

Lyophobic dispersions have low relative viscosities even at high concentrations because of low solvation and of low attraction between the particles compared to the repulsion. High net interparticle attraction would lead to coagulation. Low solvation usually results in large differences in refractive index between the liquid medium and the disperse phase, which produces marked light scattering and strong Tyndall beams (pp.

123, 124). Lyophilic systems have the opposite behavior. Lyophobic sols form distinct granules on coagulation whereas lyophilic sols form gels. At high concentrations, lyophobic systems turn into pastes.

Preparation of Lyophobic Dispersions
3, 30, 42, 72

As discussed on pages 104–105, all elements and compounds—gaseous, liquid, or solid, organic or inorganic—can be prepared in the colloidal state. Emulsions and aerosols are discussed in Chapters 7 and 12, respectively. Sols or dispersions of solids in liquids are prepared by dispersion and condensation methods. Among the equipment used in dispersion or comminution are mills such as hammer, ball, jet, roller, and colloid mills described in Chapter 10. Ultrasonic vibrations and electric arcs inside liquids, which cause evaporation of the electrode material followed by condensation, are also employed. Condensation methods can be physical, such as the precipitation of sulfur by adding its solution in alcohol to water; or chemical, such as the reactions in aqueous solution between hydrogen sulfide and sulfur dioxide, between a strong acid and sodium thiosulfate, or between a strong acid and calcium polysulfide, all of which form elemental colloidal sulfur. The reduction of salts of gold, silver, copper, platinum, mercury, and tellurium produces sols of these metals. Precipitation reactions between barium chloride and sodium sulfate or between silver nitrate and potassium chloride can be carried out under conditions producing sols of barium sulfate or silver chloride.

Precipitation by physical or chemical means occurs in two stages: (a) nucleation, or the formation of submicroscopic nuclei or seeds, and (b) particle growth by deposition of precipitating material onto these nuclei. Two conditions can produce colloidal precipitates, namely, concentrated systems with high supersaturation, and dilute systems with low supersaturation. In dilute systems, there are few nuclei but so little total material precipitating that no nucleus can grow very large. In concentrated systems, many nuclei are formed so quickly that the amount of precipitating material per nucleus still is small. In systems of intermediate concentrations and moderate supersaturation, the number of nuclei is small compared to the amount of material precipitating from solution, so that most nuclei can grow into coarse particles.[2,42,77,78]

Colloidal particles are unstable compared to coarse particles of the same material because they have much larger surface areas and hence higher total surface free energies. On standing, colloidal particles recrystallize spontaneously into large particles to minimize the total surface free energy of the system. For instance, in quantitative analysis, barium sulfate precipitates are digested in hot water for several hours before filtering in order to let all particles grow to sizes large enough to ensure retention by the filter. Since the solubility of the salt is greater at higher temperatures, the recrystallization proceeds faster in hot mixtures. Surfactants adsorbed at the solid-liquid interface often inhibit or retard this recrystallization.

Stability of Lyophobic Dispersions [30, 42]

Particle Attraction. Molecules of solid, liquid, and gaseous compounds attract one another by secondary valences or van der Waals forces, which are operative over very short distances only. The resulting attractive energy declines with the sixth power of the distance between the molecules. The total attractive energy between two colloidal particles is essentially the sum of the energies of attraction of each atom or ion in one particle for each atom or ion in the other. This energy falls off only with the second or third power of the interparticle distance (curve A in Fig. 6-25). The attraction between colloidal particles reaches much farther than the attraction between isolated molecules. By convention, energies of attraction have negative values and energies of repulsion positive values. When particles suspended in a liquid or in air come within close range, the interparticle attraction causes them to stick together, coagulating the dispersion into coarse flocs or grains.

Electrostatic charges in the surface of the particles cause them to repel one another and tend to prevent coagulation. This repulsive energy varies exponentially with the interparticle distance (curve B in Figure 6-25).

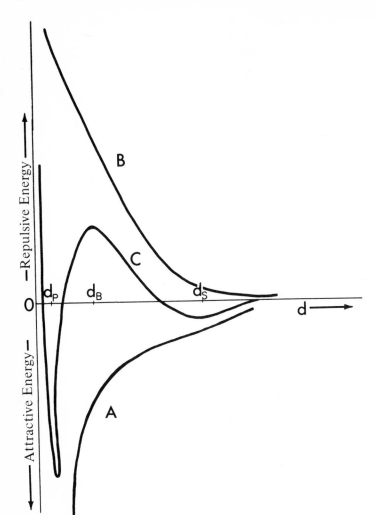

FIG. 6-25. Energy of attraction (curve A), energy of electrostatic repulsion (curve B), and net energy of interaction (curve C) between two particles as a function of the interparticle distance d.

Origin of Electric Charges. If silver chloride is formed by the metathetical reaction

$$AgNO_3 + NaCl \rightarrow AgCl + NaNO_3$$

the precipitated particles contain just as many Ag^+ ions as Cl^- ions except in the surface. If the reaction was carried out with an excess of silver nitrate, the outermost layer of the solid contains more Ag^+ than Cl^- ions; this confers a positive charge to the particles. An excess of sodium chloride produces surfaces richer in Cl^- than Ag^+ ions, and hence negatively charged particles. The first case is represented schematically in the upper half of Figure 6-26. The positively charged surface attracts the negative nitrate ions from the solution but repels the positive sodium ions. The excess concentration of nitrate counterions surrounding the particle surface is large enough to establish electroneutrality. The combination of the positively charged surface and the atmosphere of nitrate counterions surrounding it is called the *electric double layer*. The thermal motion of the water molecules tends to mix the solution surrounding the particle with the bulk solution, dispersing the excess nitrate ions. Therefore, the outer half of the double layer is diffuse.

The electric potentials associated with the double layer are plotted on the vertical axis in the lower half of Figure 6-26. The horizontal axis, representing the distance from the particle surface, is the same for the upper and lower halves of Figure 6-26. The excess of nitrate counterions in the immediate vicinity of the positive surface reduces the effectiveness of the positive surface charges to attract additional nitrate ions and to repel additional sodium ions farther away from the particle surface. This "screening effect" of the nitrate ions is cumulative, becoming more pronounced as the distance from the surface increases, i.e., on moving from the vicinity of the surface toward the bulk of the solution. It causes the potential to fall off with increasing distance from the surface. The concentration of the nitrate ions gradually decreases and that of the sodium ions gradually increases on moving away from the surface until they become identical and equal to their bulk concentration. At that point, the diffuse outer part of the double layer terminates and the potential is reduced to zero.

The potential is maximum directly at the particle surface and gradually drops off across the double layer, owing to the screening effect of the nitrate counterions, rapidly at first and more gradually farther out; it is zero in the bulk of the solution. The potential ψ_0 directly at the surface is the thermodynamic potential which is obtained by measurements made with reversible electrodes. For colloidal particles, it cannot be measured directly.

Determination of Zeta Potential by Electrophoresis. The so-called zeta potential can be determined directly by means of electrophoretic measurements. Colloidal particles migrate towards the oppositely charged electrode when an electric field is applied to their dispersions. The velocity of migration (v) depends (a) on the density of the surface charges or on the potential of the surface, (b) on the thickness of the double layer and the dielectric constant within, and (c) on the viscosity of the medium, but (d) not on the particle size. It is measured with a dark-field microscope by clocking the number of seconds required for particles to traverse a given number of divisions of the eyepiece micrometer. The electric field is generated by immersing two inert electrodes in the dispersion and applying an external potential across them. The force driving the particles is the potential gradient, or the

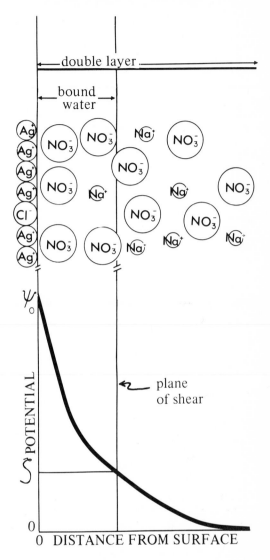

FIG. 6-26. Electric double layer at the surface of a silver chloride particle (upper part) and the corresponding potentials (lower part). The distance from the particle surface, plotted on the horizontal axis, refers to both the upper and lower part of the figure.

D.C. voltage E divided by the distance L between the electrodes in centimeters. The zeta potential, ζ, for approximately spherical, nonconducting particles is calculated by the Smoluchowski equation,

$$\zeta = \left(\frac{4\pi\eta}{\epsilon}\right) v \left(\frac{L}{E}\right) = 13v \left(\frac{L}{E}\right) \quad (41)$$

where η is the viscosity and ϵ the dielectric constant of the dispersion medium. The constant, 13, applies to water at 25° C. when ζ is expressed in millivolts and v in microns/sec.

When the silver chloride particle of Figure 6-26 migrates toward the negative pole, some of the nitrate ions very close to its surface are dragged along rather than migrating towards the positive pole because they are strongly attracted by the highly charged positive surface. Even though silver chloride has been described as hydrophobic, a thin shell of water of hydration is bound to the particle and moves along with it. The boundary between the bound and free water is designated the plane of shear (Figure 6-26). Ions trapped within the hydration layer for the most part move along with the particle in the electric field. The zeta potential is the potential measured at the plane of shear. It is considerably smaller than the potential ψ_0 at the particle surface because the counterions trapped in the hydration layer screen or neutralize a large fraction of the charge of the surface.

Further Sources of Electric Surface Charges. The charges of ionic solid particles originate from the excess of positive or negative ions in their surface. Bismuth subnitrate or subcarbonate particles usually have an excess of BiO^+ ions in their surface in neutral and acid media and are therefore positively charged. They move toward the negative pole in an electrophoresis cell. Aluminum hydroxide particles produced by treating aluminum chloride with ammonia or sodium carbonate are positively charged in neutral or slightly acid media owing to the presence in the particle surface of such species as

$$P\!-\!O\!-\!Al^+Cl^- \text{ and } P\!-\!O\!-\!Al^{++}2Cl^-,$$
$$\mid$$
$$OH$$

where P represents the particle. In strongly acid media, the particles dissolve with the formation of Al^{+++} ions. In basic media, the particles have negative surface charges because of $P\!-\!N\!-\!Al(OH)_3{}^-Na^+$ groups. In strongly basic media, they dissolve with the formation of sodium aluminate, $[Al(OH)_4]^-Na^+$. At pH 8, the surface consists exclusively of uncharged $P\!-\!O\!-\!Al(OH)_2$ groups. This is the *isoelectric point,* or point of zero charge, of aluminum hydroxide, at which its zeta potential is zero, i.e., its particles move neither to the positive nor to the negative pole in an electrophoresis cell but remain stationary.

Proteins have negative charges above their isoelectric points owing to the presence of carboxylate groups and of few or no groups containing protonated basic nitrogen. They have positive charges at lower pH values owing to the presence of protonated ammonium or guanidinium groups with few or no carboxylate ions with which to form zwitterions. The carboxyl groups are in the undissociated —COOH form. Particles of insoluble organic medicaments are negatively charged if they contain sulfonate or carboxylate groups and positively charged if they contain amine hydrochloride or other basic ionic groups. Bacteria are negatively charged at the physiologic pH of 7.4 because of carboxylate groups in their cell wall. They move to the positive pole in an electrophoresis cell.[64] Another source of surface charges is the adsorption of foreign ions from solution, such as those of ionic surfactants, or the Ca^{++} and Mg^{++} ions which constitute water hardness. Since aqueous solutions always contain ions, at least hydroxyl and hydrogen ions, it is exceedingly rare for a hydrosol to have zero charge.

Net Interaction Between Two Colloidal Particles. When two identical colloidal particles, like those of silver chloride depicted in Figure 6-26, approach each other, impelled by Brownian motion, convection currents, stirring or gravitational settling, they are subject to two opposing energies, electrostatic repulsion and van der Waals attraction. The resultant or net interaction energy often varies with the interparticle distance (curve C of Fig. 6-25). The repulsive energy (curve B) is an exponential function of the distance; the attractive energy (curve A) decreases as an inverse power of the distance. Consequently, attraction predominates at small and large distances, whereas repulsion may predominate at intermediate distances.

As the two particles approach, i.e., as the distance d between them decreases, the net energy of interaction represented by curve C passes through a minimum at a distance d_S. The net energy at d_S is negative; therefore, the minimum corresponds to a net attraction between the two particles. If the minimum is sufficiently deep, and hence the attraction is sufficiently large, the two particles remain attached to each other while separated by the comparatively large distance d_S. Coarse particles or small particles that are large in one or two dimensions (rods or plates) usually have pronounced minima at large distances of separation, and *flocculate* or aggregate. Because the minimum at d_S is relatively shallow, these aggregates are held together by relatively weak energies and can usually be broken up, *deflocculated* or *peptized* by stirring. The minimum at d_S is therefore called the *secondary minimum*. It is usually responsible for the caking of sediments of coarse dispersions, as discussed in Chapter 7. For particles smaller than about 200 Å, the secondary minimum either does not exist or is too shallow to cause flocculation.

Charged particles surrounded by their electrical double layers are electrically neutral; there is no net electrostatic interaction at large distances of separation. Electrostatic repulsion sets in when the particles are so close to one another that their double layers begin to interpenetrate. As two identical, small colloidal particles on a collision course approach to within distances smaller than d_S, the electrostatic repulsion becomes increasingly more important, as shown by the steep rise in curve C. In the case of two positively charged silver chloride particles, the two diffuse outer layers of nitrate counterions begin to overlap and repel each other. If the two particles possess high enough velocities or kinetic energies to continue their approach, pushing the intervening nitrate ions and water molecules out of the way, the positive charges of their two surfaces cause even higher repulsion; the inter-

action curve C approaches the maximum at d_B. If this energy barrier, the magnitude of which is related to the zeta potential, is sufficiently high, electrostatic repulsion deflects the two particles from their course and they move off in different directions. Otherwise, as they continue to approach each other, attraction begins to predominate over repulsion as curve C descends, passes through zero and then goes into the deep "primary" energy minimum at d_P. This corresponds to a very strong attraction between the particles at small distances. They touch and stick together so strongly that it becomes difficult to separate them again. As more and more particles of a sol become attached to other particles in the primary minimum, *coagulation* sets in.

Further reduction in the distance between the two particles could take place only through interpenetration of the two solid masses, which is practically impossible to achieve. This is the meaning of the steep rise in the interaction curve C at distances smaller than d_P. The difference between flocculation and coagulation is that flocculated particles adhere through weaker attraction energies and at larger interparticle distances than coagulated particles, and that flocculation can usually be reversed.

In order to stabilize a dispersion, the barrier or maximum in curve C should be high, i.e., the particles should have large zeta potentials, and the distance d_B should be large, i.e., the diffuse outer part of the electric double layer should extend far into the solution, to distances where the van der Waals attraction beween the particles is low. The zeta potential of particles with weak surface charges can be increased by the adsorption of ionic surfactants of the same sign as that of the surface. If the charge density of the particle surface is high, such surface-active ions are not adsorbed because electrostatic repulsion outweighs their tendency to adsorb at interfaces.

Coagulation of Hydrophobic Dispersions. Salts added to hydrophobic dispersions compress the double layer, reducing the absolute value of the zeta potential of the particles and hence the height of the repulsive barrier of curve C in Figure 6-25. This effect in-

TABLE 6-10. MINIMUM COAGULATION
CONCENTRATIONS* FOR A NEGATIVELY
CHARGED GOLD SOL

ELECTROLYTE	MCC*
monovalent cations	
NaCl	24
1/2 Na_2SO_4	24
KNO_3	25
1/2 K_2SO_4	23
mean	24
morphine hydrochloride	0.54
$C_{12}H_{25}NH_3Cl$	0.10
bivalent cations	
$CaCl_2$	0.41
$BaCl_2$	0.35
$MgSO_4$	0.30
mean	0.38
trivalent cations	
1/2 $Al_2(SO_4)_3$	0.06
$Ce(NO_3)_3$	0.03
1/2 $Cr_2(SO_4)_3$	0.04
mean	0.0325

* Lowest concentration capable of coagulating the sol, in millimoles/liter.

creases with increasing salt concentration and leads to coagulation. The effectiveness of salts in coagulating hydrophobic dispersions increases strongly with the valence of the counterion. The lowest salt concentrations capable of coagulating a negatively charged gold sol are far lower for salts with trivalent cations than for salts with divalent cations, which in turn cause coagulation at far lower concentrations than salt of monovalent cations, as is seen in Table 6-10. The negatively charged particle surface attracts Al^{+++} ions far more strongly than Ca^{++} ions, with the monovalent alkali metal cations being attracted the least. Electrostatic attraction between opposite charges always increases rapidly with increasing magnitude of either charge. The valence of the anions does not affect the minimum coagulation concentration of the negatively charged sol significantly.

The theory which deals quantitatively with the stability of lyophobic dispersions outlined in this section and embodied in Figure 6-25 was developed simultaneously by Derjaguin and Landau in Russia and by Verwey and Overbeek in the Netherlands in the mid 1940's. One of the predictions of this D-L-V-O theory is that the minimum concentrations of added salts required to coagulate hydrophobic sols vary as the inverse sixth power of the valence of the counterions. The minimum coagulation concentrations of salts with mono-, di-, and trivalent counterions for a given sol should be in the ratio of $\frac{1}{1^6}:\frac{1}{2^6}:\frac{1}{3^6}$, or 100:1.56:0.138. The average minimum coagulation concentrations for the negatively charged gold sol listed in Table 6-10 are in the ratio of 24:0.38:0.325, or 100:1.56:0.130 for salts with mono-, di-, and trivalent cations, in excellent agreement with the D-L-V-O theory and thereby confirming it.

The dependence of the minimum salt concentration required for coagulation on the valence of the counterion is sometimes called the Schulze-Hardy rule after the two investigators who emphasized it, based on experimental observations made at the turn of the century and earlier.

Aqueous disperions of hydrophobic solids can be flocculated or coagulated by the addition of alcohol and other water-miscible solvents. Lowering of the dielectric constant of the medium reduces the zeta potential according to Equation 41 and weakens the mechanism of stabilization by electrostatic repulsion. The minimum coagulation concentrations of salts for hydrosols are considerably reduced if alcohol (or acetone or dioxane) is also added.

Specific Effects in Coagulation. The exceptions in Table 6-10 to the Schulze-Hardy rule are morphine hydrochloride and dodecylamine hydrochloride, which have minimum coagulation concentrations typical of salts with divalent cations, even though their cations are monovalent. These two salts are cationic surfactants. Not only are their cations attracted, like other cations, by the negatively charged particle surface through electrostatic forces, but they have, in addition, a pronounced tendency to be positively adsorbed at solid-water interfaces in general. The solid attracts the organic portion of these molecules by van der Waals forces. Additional energy is gained because their removal from water increases the attraction among the water molecules. The dual attraction between the particle surface and the cationic surfactant enables the latter to coagulate the sol at much lower concentrations than other salts with monovalent cations. Traube's rule applies: the minimum coagulation concentration for a homologous series of surfactants decreases on ascending the series, paralleling the increases in surface activity and in van der Waals attraction of the surface for the hydrophobic moieties.

Another exception to the Schulze-Hardy rule is that the positively charged silver chloride sol (Fig. 6-26) is coagulated by the monovalent chloride, bromide, and iodide anions at concentrations equal to or lower than the minimum coagulation concentration of trivalent anions. This is because halide ions do not merely enter the double layer, nor are they merely physically adsorbed at the particle surface; rather they are incorporated by chemisorption into the silver chloride particle itself and become part of its surface. Thus, they change the ψ_0 potential at the particle surface rather than merely the zeta potential at the plane of shear. They are therefore called *potential-determining ions,* and their effect is highly specific. For a negatively charged silver chloride sol prepared with excess sodium chloride, Ag^+ is the potential-determining ion; lead and mercurous ions, whose halides also have low solubilities, are also potential-determining ions. Among the potential-determining ions for aluminum hydroxide sols are Al^{+++}, $[Al(OH)_4]^-$, Fe^{+++}, Mn^{++}, and OH^-, because they are incorporated into the particle proper, and H^+.

Charge Reversal. On adding increasing amounts of sodium chloride to a colloidal dispersion of positively charged silver chloride schematically represented in Figure 6-26, the ψ_0 and zeta potentials decrease because the charge density of the particle surface, produced by an excess of Ag^+ ions in the surface is reduced as more Cl^- ions enter the surface. This produces instability of the dispersion and eventually causes coagulation. As the concentration of added sodium chloride in solution is elevated further, an in-

creasing number of chloride ions enter the particle surfaces. The positive potentials are gradually reduced and go through zero when the concentrations of Ag^+ and Cl^- ions in the surfaces are equal. As the surfaces acquire a growing excess of chloride ions over silver ions, the potentials become increasingly negative: the charge of the particles has been reversed from positive to negative, and the counterions which originally were nitrate anions are now sodium cations. Due to a high negative zeta potential, the sol is again stabilized.

Ionic surfactants with charges opposite in sign to the charge of the particle surface can also reverse the charge. A first surfactant layer is adsorbed at the surface with its ionic head groups directed toward the charged surface (see pp. 127 and 158). Because of the added van der Waals attraction of the particle for the hydrocarbon moiety of the surfactant counterions, they displace the non-surface-active counterions from close proximity to the particle surface. This lowers the surface charge and the zeta potential of the particles and also covers the particles partly with hydrocarbon chains, reducing their hydration. Both factors lead to coagulation. At higher concentrations of dissolved surfactant, a second layer of surfactant molecules is adsorbed at the surface but with the opposite orientation. The hydrocarbon chains are directed toward the particle surface and bound by van der Waals forces to the hydrocarbon chains of the first layer of adsorbed surfactant ions; the ionic headgroups are oriented toward the aqueous phase. The charge of the particle is thereby reversed, i.e., it has acquired the same sign as that of the ionic surfactant.

Charge reversal can also be caused by polyvalent counterions—e.g., the positively charged bismuth subnitrate suspension and its charge reversal by the trivalent orthophosphate anion, which is depicted in Figure 7-14.

The foregoing considerations were discussed in terms of colloidal particles; however, they apply equally to coarse suspensions, such as the many aqueous suspensions of organic, hydrophobic drugs used as dosage forms. Coarse particles settle out of their dispersions rather than remaining in suspension through Brownian motion as do colloidal particles. The underlying factors which determine the state of aggregation of their sediments, the sedimentation volume, and the caking described in Chapter 7 are fully explained by the D-L-V-O theory.

Stabilization of Hydrophobic Dispersions by Nonionic Surfactants.[46] The previous sections describe the stabilization of aqueous dispersions by ionic surfactants of like charge and their flocculation or coagulation by salts or by ionic surfactants of opposite charge. Nonionic surfactants stabilize both positively and negatively charged dispersions. The hydrocarbon moieties of the nonionic surfactant molecules are physically adsorbed on the solid surface of the particles, as far from contact with water as possible. The polyethylene glycol moieties are immersed in the aqueous phase, much as in the nonionic micelle of Figure 6-23E. They are surrounded by water of hydration because each ether oxygen binds two water molecules through hydrogen bonds. Additional water is mechanically trapped inside the entangled coils of these randomly coiled polyoxyethylene chains. This extensive hydration layer, associated with the polyoxyethylene moieties of the adsorbed surfactant molecules, renders the formerly hydrophobic particle surfaces hydrophilic.

When two particles converge because of Brownian motion or while settling out, they cannot approach each other close enough to come within effective range of the van der Waals attractive forces. The polyoxyethylene portions of the adsorbed nonionic surfactant molecules extending into the water and the deep layer of hydration associated with them surround each particle, forming a steric barrier which prevents them from approaching within distances of the order of d_P of Figure 6-25. Coagulation is thereby prevented. The hydrophilic character conferred to the surfaces of hydrophobic particles by adsorbed nonionic surfactants considerably increases the resistance of their dispersions to coagulation by salts. Salting-out concentrations of the order of several molar are required for flocculation, rather than the low concentrations listed in Table 6-10.

Stabilization of Hydrophobic Dispersions by Water-Soluble Polymers. Dissolved macromolecules stabilize dispersions in several ways. A general mechanism of stabilization, effective with all soluble polymers, results from the considerable increases in the viscosity of the suspending medium caused even by small amounts of dissolved polymers (see pp. 113, 114). This slows down the Brownian motion of the colloidal particles. According to Equation 22, the square of the displacement per unit time is inversely proportional to the viscosity of the medium. A reduction in Brownian motion results in fewer interparticle collisions in a given time interval and hence slows down coagulation, since coagulation takes place only when particles collide inelastically.

The second mechanism of stabilization depends on the polymer being adsorbed from solution onto the solid-water interface. The structural features that promote the surface activity of polymers are discussed on page 144. Concerning the substrate, hydrophobic materials like organic drugs which have high interfacial free energies in water adsorb polymers more extensively than hydrophilic materials like cellulose or aluminum hydroxide. When a polymer chain is adsorbed as a monolayer in a solid-water interface, some segments are actually in contact with and lie flat against the solid substrate. Other segments extend into the water in the form of loops and coils. Since the polymer is water-soluble, all segments are hydrated. The hydration sheath surrounding the macromolecular chain is displaced at the areas of contact between polymer and solid surface.[55,71] The adsorbed polymer chains, portions of which extend into the aqueous phase, and the water of hydration associated with them form steric barriers around the particles which prevent them from approaching one another close enough for van der Waals attraction to become significant. If the adsorbed polymer has charged groups, its stabilizing action is enhanced by adding electrostatic repulsion to the steric protection. As with nonionic surfactants, the adsorption of hydrophilic polymers confers hydrophilicity to the surfaces of dispersed hydrophobic particles, and markedly increases the salt concentrations required to produce coagulation.

Polymers that stabilize aqueous disper-

TABLE 6-11. PROTECTIVE NUMBERS*

POLYMER	GOLD NUMBER	SILVER NUMBER	PRUSSIAN BLUE NUMBER	SULFUR NUMBER	Fe_2O_3† NUMBER
Gelatin	0.002–0.01	0.007	0.01	0.000025	—
Sodium caseinate	0.01	—	—	—	1
Egg albumin	0.02–0.5	0.3	5	—	—
Gum arabic	0.1–0.25	0.25	1	0.005	3
Gum tragacanth	2	—	—	0.005	5
Dextrin	1–7	20	50	0.025	—
Soluble starch	5–25	—	—	0.1	4

* Milligrams of water-soluble macromolecule per 10 cm.³ From Ref. 32.
† Graham sol.

sions are called *protective colloids.* Among them are the following[32]: proteins, such as albumin, and their degradation products like gelatin and sodium caseinate; polysaccharides including gums and mucilages such as acacia or gum arabic, tragacanth, agar, chondrus (carrageen), pectin, and sodium alginate; soluble cellulose derivatives like methylcellulose and hydroxyethylcellulose; soluble starch and its hydrolysis product dextrin; and synthetic polymers such as polyethylene glycol, polyvinylpyrrolidone, polyacrylamide, and sodium polyacrylate.

An example of protective colloid action is provided by the local anti-infective, Mild Silver Protein, N.F. It consists of 19 to 23 percent silver, mostly as colloidal metallic silver and/or silver oxide, which gives it the dark brown color. The balance consists of water-soluble protein. The concentration of silver ions is low, otherwise they would form a precipitate with the protein. Nonstabilized colloidal dispersions of silver or silver oxide, once dried, cannot be redispersed in water whereas Mild Silver Protein, consisting of solid granules, disperses readily in water. Each colloidal silver or silver oxide particle is surrounded by a multilayer of adsorbed protein. On adding water, some of the protein dissolves while a monolayer remains adsorbed on each particle, rendering its surface hydrophilic and protecting it from adhesion to other particles. Gold Au 198 Injection, U.S.P., is colloidal radioactive gold stabilized with gelatin.

In order to compare the protective action of water-soluble macromolecules quantitatively, Zsigmondy[32] defined a *gold number* as the minimum weight of dry polymer, in milligrams, which must be added to 10 cm.³

of a red gold sol to prevent its flocculation to a blue sol by the addition of 1 cm.³ of 10 percent sodium chloride solution. Other such "protective numbers" include the silver, carbon, Fe_2O_3, As_2S_3, Prussian blue (ferric ferrocyanide), and sulfur number. As is seen in Table 6-11, the protective action of a given water-soluble macromolecule, and even its qualitative ranking, varies from substrate to substrate. Protective numbers also depend strongly on the mode of preparation, concentration and pH of the dispersion, and on the salt used for the coagulation experiments.

Even some of the best protective colloids cause flocculation of hydrophobic dispersions when used at low concentrations. For instance, gelatin is an excellent protective agent for negatively charged gold sols, having a gold number of about 0.005 mg./10 cm.³ or 0.5 mg./liter. However, it flocculates these sols, in the absence of sodium chloride, at concentrations of 0.00005 to 0.0005 mg./liter in acid media. This is an example of charge inversion of the gold sol from negative to positive by adsorption of excess positively charged gelatin; flocculation occurs when the particles have near zero charge. When the experiments were conducted above the isoelectric point of gelatin, no flocculation was observed at any concentration.[52] The flocculation produced by very low concentrations of the cationic gelatin is an example of *sensitization.*

Several water-soluble macromolecules that serve as protective colloids for hydrophobic dispersions at higher concentrations sensitize them at lower concentrations without reducing their charge. For instance, polyacrylamide is an effective protective colloid, yet it is used as a flocculant in water treatment at the parts per million level. This is thought to be caused by a bridging mechanism. Good protective colloids are extensively adsorbed by hydrophobic particles. At low concentration, there is not enough polymer available to completely cover each particle with an adsorbed monolayer. Therefore, single polymer molecules are adsorbed on two or more particles. They bridge the gap between the particles and cement them together, thereby promoting flocculation. When enough polymer is added to surround each particle completely with adsorbed macromolecules, the situation is reversed inasmuch as there are several polymer molecules adsorbed on a single particle. Peptization and stabilization result.

LYOPHILIC COLLOIDAL SYSTEMS[31,74]

Lyophilicity is the tendency of particles, surfaces or functional groups to become extensively wetted, solvated, swollen, or dissolved by solvents. Mucilages and gelatin, clays and glass, Colloidal Silicon Dioxide, N.F., cellulose and starch, hydroxyl and carbonyl groups, and many ions are *hydrophilic* or water-loving. Petrolatum, margarine, cholesterol, essential oils, polystyrene, heavy metal soaps, vitamins A, D, E, and K, hundreds of oil-soluble drugs, groups like ethyl, phenyl, and trichloromethyl are *oleophilic,* or *lipophilic,* i.e., they have affinity toward solvents of low polarity. Lyophilic materials usually disperse spontaneously in the appropriate solvent as completely as is possible without breaking primary valence bonds. Highly crystalline polymers constitute occasional exceptions. The resultant dispersions are intrinsically stable.

Molecularly dissolved lyophilic materials are in the colloidal range only if they consist of macromolecules. In aqueous sucrose solutions, the size of the individual solute molecules is only about 9 Å and their molecular weight is 342. The molecules of methylcellulose discussed on page 114, on the other hand, weigh 900 times more and their size is about 10 times larger than sucrose molecules, so that their aqueous solutions are colloidal dispersions.

Dissolution of lyophilic polymers can be reduced to mere swelling of the material by *cross-linking,* a process whereby different chains or molecules are linked together by primary valence bonds. For instance, sodium polystyrene sulfonate is a water-soluble polyelectrolyte. In order to use it as a cation exchange resin (Sodium Polystyrene Sulfonate, U.S.P.), a water-insoluble form is produced by copolymerizing styrene with a few percent of divinylbenzene to give the following structure, after sulfonation and neutralization:

Chain v—x is tied to chain y—z and to other chains farther along through phenylene groups, building up a three-dimensional network. Without the cross-links, chains v—x and y—z would dissolve in water and separate. Being cross-linked, the polymer grains swell in water until the phenylene cross-ties are strained. Each grain is a single molecule, where each atom is linked to every other atom by primary valence bonds. The grains cannot dissolve without breaking many primary valence bonds, and these are strong enough to resist rupture and prevent dissolution.

Cholestyramine Resin, U.S.P., has the same backbone of cross-linked polystyrene chains but contains quaternary ammonium chloride groups instead of sodium sulfonate groups. It is an anion exchange resin, i.e., it can exchange the chloride ion for hydroxide, sulfate, alkylsulfonate, and other anions. When ingested, cholestyramine binds bile acid anions such as cholate and glycocholate, increasing their fecal excretion.

Another example of a cross-linked polymer is Polycarbophil, N.F., which is polyacrylic acid cross-linked with divinyl glycol. Owing to the weakly acidic carboxyl groups which dissociate into carboxylate ions in the alkaline intestines but not in the acid stomach, swelling by osmotic forces occurs mainly in the intestines. The ether cross-links prevent dissolution of the inert polymer. Through imbibition of water caused by its sodium and carboxylate ions, the polymer removes free fecal water in the intestinal tract and decreases the fluidity of the stool in diarrheal disorders.

Aqueous dispersions of hydrophilic materials and dispersions in oil of lipophilic materials are viscous even at low concentrations of the disperse phase, in part because of solvation and in part because of the attraction among the disperse particles. Interparticle attraction causes thickening of the dispersion medium, for example, in the entanglement of dissolved macromolecules and the house-of-cards aggregates of platelike clay particles with negatively charged faces and positively charged edges (pp. 112 to 114, and 116).

Gels or Jellies [3,31]

For lyophilic polymeric systems like those discussed below, the terms "gel" and "jelly" are equivalent. If the interparticle attraction in a lyophilic dispersion results in the formation of a continuous network or scaffold of the dispersed solid phase throughout the entire liquid, the dispersion solidifies or sets to a gel or jelly (p. 115). Two properties are necessary for a disperse phase to form a gel: the particles must be extensively solvated and they must be able to adhere to one another at the points of contact.[34,79] A gel consists of two continuous phases mixed together and interpenetrating—the solid matrix and the immobilized liquid. Some systems set to gels at surprisingly low concentrations of the disperse phase. As little as 2 or 3 percent by volume of sodium bentonite or pectic acid gel can immobilize 97 to 98 percent of water.

The following are among the techniques available to bring about gelation or the setting of gels and their liquefaction to sols.

Interparticle Attraction. In the case of particulate colloids (as opposed to molecularly dissolved macromolecules), high surface-to-volume ratios combined with some kind of strong attraction between the particles can produce a flocculated, continuous mesh or brush-heap structure throughout the liquid and cause gelation at low concentrations of the dispersed solid. For instance, bentonite dispersed in water has a specific surface area of several hundred square meters per gram. Attraction between the negatively charged faces and the positively charged edges of the bentonite platelets produces a house-of-cards structure and causes even dilute bentonite magmas to gel while standing at rest (p. 116). Shear breaks some of the interparticle contacts and liquefies the gel to a sol. This phenomenon is called thixotropy (p. 115).

Colloidal Silicon Dioxide, N.F., (Aerosil*) consists of roughly spherical particles with diameters ranging from 100 to 400 Å and specific surface areas of about 190 m.^{2}/g. This silica is prepared by pyrolysis of silicon tetrachloride in the presence of hydrogen and air or water vapor. It is used as a thickening agent for a wide variety of liquids. Liquids of low polarity, unable to form hydrogen bonds with the colloidal silica, are gelled at concentrations as low as 3 to 5 percent. Stable gels are formed at somewhat higher concentrations. Apparently, a continuous network or skeleton of flocculated silica spheres, held together by hydrogen bonds among surface silanol groups in the areas of contact between spheres, forms throughout the liquid. Because of the very small particle size or the high surface-to-volume ratio of the silica spheres, flocculation builds up 3-dimensional networks throughout the bulk of the liquid medium at such low concentrations.

In hydrogen-bonding liquids such as propanol, silica can be dispersed in concentrations as high as 30 percent without conferring yield values to the mixture. Each silica particle is surrounded by a shell of propanol molecules which solvate it through hydrogen bonds plus van der Waals forces. This prevents the silica particles from approaching

* Trademark, DEGUSSA (Germany).

one another closely enough to adhere, avoiding flocculation and gel formation. The addition of 10 percent or less of an alcohol to hydrocarbons is enough to prevent gel formation by colloidal silica. The alcohol molecules are selectively adsorbed by the silica particles.[28]

Phase Separation of Polymers. In the case of molecularly dissolved polymers, reducing the solubility limit of the disperse phase below its concentration in the sol by varying the temperature causes it to precipitate and produces gelation. The network of polymer chains solidifies because precipitated macromolecules adhere to one another at their points of contact. Segments of the precipitated macromolecules may even crystallize. Changing the temperature in the opposite direction may cause the gels to "melt" to sols. Renewed solvation of the polymer chains surrounds each macromolecule again with a solvent layer, detaching the chains from one another and dissolving the crystallized regions.

Plastibase* (referred to in Chap. 8) consists of 5 percent polyethylene, $-(CH_2-CH_2)_n$, and 95 percent mineral oil. Above 90°C., which is close to its melting point, polyethylene is soluble in the oil and the preparation is liquid. Below 90°C., the polymer precipitates and the solution sets to a gel because the precipitated and entangled chains form extensive networks throughout the oil, and even associate into small crystalline regions.

Aqueous gelatin solutions gel on cooling and melt on heating. The transition temperature is in the 35 to 50°C. range. Other polymers, such as methylcellulose and polyethylene glycol, are more soluble in cold than in hot water. Heating their solutions reduces the hydration of the macromolecules (cf. p. 140) and causes the separation of a gel phase consisting of entangled chains which immobilize the water in their interstices. The temperature at which this phase separation occurs is analogous to the cloud point of nonionic surfactants.

Polymer Precipitation by Nonsolvent Liquids. Another means of promoting the precipitation of dissolved macromolecules and the formation of gels is the addition to their solutions of a liquid which is miscible with the solvent but is a nonsolvent or precipitant for the solute. An example is ethanol which, when added to aqueous solutions of polyelectrolytes, lowers the dielectric constant of the medium and reduces the degree of dissociation of the ionic groups and, hence, the solubility of the polymer, causing gelation. Aqueous solutions of nonionic polymers are gelled by the addition of ethanol through precipitation via dehydration. Dilution with water reverses the gelation in both cases.

Salting Out of Dissolved Polymers. Aqueous polymer solutions and other dispersions of hydrophilic materials can in effect be rendered more concentrated if some of their water is tied up through the addition of dry salts of high water solubility which are extensively hydrated. If the solubility limit of the polymer in the water remaining attached to it is exceeded, it precipitates, and gelation occurs if enough polymer is present to form an extensive network structure. This process is called *salting out;* it requires high salt concentrations, usually several molar. Proteins are frequently salted out by adding enough ammonium sulfate to their solutions to produce salt concentrations of up to 3 M or 40 percent w/v.

The ability of salts to salt out hydrophilic materials dispersed or dissolved in water increases with the amount of water of hydration their ions are capable of binding. The *lyotropic* or *Hofmeister series* arranges ions in the order of increasing hydration and increasing effectiveness in salting out or precipitating hydrophilic colloids. The series is

$$Ba^{++} < Ca^{++} < Mg^{++} <$$
$$NH_4^+ < K^+ < Na^+ < Li^+$$

for the cations, and

$$SCN^- < I^- < Br^- < ClO_3^- < NO_3^- <$$
$$Cl^- < acetate < CO_4^= < tartrate < citrate$$

for the anions.[34] The salting-out process is reversible. Salt removal by dialysis or dilution with water redisperses the precipitated material and liquefies any gels which had been formed by the addition of salt.

Chemical Reactions Forming Precipitates. Chemical reactions like the precipitation of

---

* Trademark, E. R. Squibb & Sons.

flocculent or gelatinous aluminum hydroxide, aluminum phosphate, and silicic acid produce gels at sufficiently high concentrations. For instance, silica gel results when concentrated solutions of sodium silicate are acidified with hydrochloric acid. The orthosilicic acid formed initially polymerizes on standing by the elimination of water between silanol groups to form *oxo* bridges:

This condensation reaction gradually builds up a 3-dimensional silica network. The sol formed initially thickens to a soft jelly which, in turn, becomes increasingly more rigid as it loses water by evaporation and by exudation or syneresis (see below). The polymerization process can be reversed only in the early stages. Once the soft, transparent jelly has set to a rigid, opaque gel, its viscoelasticity can be reduced only by adding alkalis which tend to depolymerize the gel of condensed silicic acid back to monomeric alkali silicates.

Complex coacervation involving one or more water-soluble polymers (p. 145) often leads to gelation. The reaction between two polyelectrolytes of opposite charges, such as the negatively charged gum acacia and gelatin below its isoelectric point, where it is positively charged, produces gels. This involves the metathesis between the sodium carboxylate groups of the former and the amine hydrochloride and guanidinium chloride groups of the latter, eliminating sodium chloride and forming alkylammonium or guanidinium carboxylate cross-links between polysaccharide and polypeptide chains. Complex coacervation is the basis of the microencapsulation process of the National Cash Register Company.

The formation of alkaline earth or heavy metal salts of carboxylated polyelectrolytes such as cupric carboxymethylcellulose, calcium polyacrylate, or zinc or aluminum polyarabate causes precipitation. Gels may be formed at high polymer concentrations. The reaction involved is metathesis between the sodium salts of the polyelectrolytes and soluble salts of the heavy metal cations with inorganic anions (cf. pp. 168–169).

Syneresis. The edifice of particles in contact with each other or the mesh of entangled polymer chains which confer the solid structure to gels sometimes tightens further on standing because of crystallization of additional segments of adjacent polymer chains or in flocculent precipitates, or because the chemical reaction which produced the gel proceeds further. Aluminum hydroxide and silicic acid gels gradually eliminate water of constitution by further condensation of hydroxyl or *ol* groups to *oxo* bridges as shown above. These processes cause the gel structure to shrink and to exude some of the trapped liquid, a phenomenon called syneresis.[34] If the gel contains dissolved drugs, the amount remaining in the gel decreases in proportion to the fraction of the liquid phase containing the drug which is squeezed out.

OFFICIAL LYOPHILIC PREPARATIONS

Cellulose and Cellulose Derivatives

Many hydrophilic vehicles are based on cellulose derivatives. The raw material is obtained by purifying cotton linters or wood pulp. Cellulose consists of β-glucose residues joined by 1,4-glucosidic linkages, i.e., the 1-carbon atom of one glucopyranose ring is connected with the 4-carbon atom of the next ring by an ether linkage which is part of an acetal group. Polysaccharides or polymers based on sugars have the cyclic structures; hexoses are in the pyranose form and pentoses are in the furanose form. Acetals are resistant to alkalis but they are subject to hydrolysis in the presence of acids. In the cellulose structure below, the carbon atoms in the rings are numbered but omitted. The prefix *beta* indicates that the 1,4-ether linkage and the 6-carbon atom bearing the primary hydroxyl are on the same side of the 6-membered ring, either above or below it.

Glucose and its dimer cellobiose, which is the building block of cellulose, are extensively soluble in water whereas cellulose is insoluble. In cellulose, the long chain molecules are lined up more or less parallel to each other. Adjacent chains are held together by hydrogen bonds between their hydroxyl and ether groups. The chains are evenly spaced and in good register in crystalline regions called *crystallites,* and less well ordered in interspersed domains called disordered or *"amorphous" regions* where the density is somewhat lower. Water does not dissolve cellulose because the attraction among the water molecules themselves plus the attraction between adjacent cellulose chains is greater than the attraction between the water molecules and the cellulose chains. Thiocyanate and iodide ions reduce the attraction among the water molecules; consequently, concentrated thiocyanate and iodide solutions dissolve cellulose.

When cellulose is treated with aqueous solutions of mineral acids, they penetrate first the "amorphous" regions, where they hydrolyze the acetal groups linking the glucopyranose rings and break up the chains into water-soluble fragments. Diffusion into the crystalline regions is much slower. If the acid is washed out before it penetrates and hydrolyzes the crystallites to any great extent, the isolated crystallites are left intact and can be separated from one another by mechanical treatment. Individual crystallites are rod-shaped particles measuring on the average 3,000 Å in length and 200 Å in width.[7] This selective hydrolysis produces a novel material, Microcrystalline Cellulose, N.F.* It forms thixotropic dispersions in water at low concentrations and stable gels at somewhat higher concentrations, which can be used as vehicles and dispersants. In tablets, it serves as a binder and, since it swells in water, as a disintegrant as well.[51]

Cellulose derivatives are often prepared by pretreating cellulose with concentrated sodium hydroxide solutions which swell even the crystalline regions. Reagents added afterward penetrate the entire mass of cellulose.[45] *Alkali cellulose* is produced by

pressing out most of the lye and shredding the softened mass into crumbs. Subsequent chain scission by controlled air oxidation reduces the molecular weight of the alkali cellulose. This makes it possible to produce derivatives of different chain lengths which, according to Equation 34, have different solution viscosities. The extent of the substitution reactions of the cellulosic hydroxyls is expressed as *degree of substitution, D.S.,* viz., the number of substituted hydroxyls per glucose residue. Each glucopyranose residue in a cellulose molecule (except for the terminal ones) has three hydroxyls, of which the primary hydroxyl on the 6-carbon is the most reactive. The highest value for the D.S. is three, as in cellulose triacetate. All others are averages, and fractional values are the rule. In a cellulose derivative with a D.S. = 0.4, some glucose residues have no substituents while others have one or even two.

Treatment of alkali cellulose with methyl chloride introduces methoxy groups and produces **Methylcellulose, U.S.P.** The hydrochloric acid formed is neutralized by the caustic soda of the alkali cellulose. Commercial pharmaceutical grades have D.S. values between 1.6 and 2.0. The polymer is more soluble in cold than in hot water; reversible precipitation or gelation occurs when solutions are heated above 40° to 68°, the temperature of gelation depending on the D.S., molecular weight, and concentration. Being nonionic, methylcellulose is compatible with acids, alkalis, and salts. High salt concentrations decrease its hydration and salt it out, gelling its solutions or lowering the gelation temperature. Unlike many polyelectrolytes, its aqueous solutions can tolerate high concentrations of alcohol.

To dissolve methylcellulose in water, the powder is first dispersed in about one quarter of the total amount of water heated above 80°. Hot water wets the powder better and prevents the formation of gelatinous lumps encasing dry polymer which occurs often when a dry polymer is mixed with a good solvent; once formed, these lumps are difficult to disperse. The remainder of the water is added cold, sometimes with ice, while stirring.

Methylcellulose is used to thicken aqueous media. Because of its surface activity (see

---

* Manufactured by FMC Corp. under the trade-name Avicel.

p. 144), methylcellulose is extensively adsorbed at solid-water and oil-water interfaces. This makes it a good protective colloid, effective in dispersing and stabilizing aqueous suspensions. Aqueous methylcellulose gels are used as a greaseless ointment base. Methylcellulose is sometimes added to lotions, cataplasms, and burn medications to produce tough and flexible films which adhere to the skin when the product dries yet can be washed off readily. Methylcellulose as well as other gums and mucilages discussed below are demulcents, i.e., they protect abraded skin and mucous membranes from chemical and mechanical irritants. They are also bulk cathartics.

Aqueous solutions of these water-soluble polymers are viscous and sticky, and form strong films on drying. Moreover, the polymers are adsorbed from solution by suspended solids. These properties make them suitable binders for tablets, forming granules by causing powder particles to adhere to each other. When the tablets are ingested, the polymers swell and then dissolve, speeding up the disintegration of the tablets.

Treatment of methylcellulose with propylene oxide produces **Hydroxypropyl Methylcellulose, N.F.,** as some of the non-methoxylated hydroxyl groups are converted into $-OC_3H_6OH$ or hydroxypropoxy groups; 84 to 93 percent of the substituted hydroxyl groups are in the methoxy form, the rest in the hydroxypropoxy form. This treatment increases the temperature of gelation and improves the resistance to salting out of methylcellulose.

Treatment of alkali cellulose with sodium monochloroacetate produces **Sodium Carboxymethylcellulose, U.S.P.** The official limits for the D.S. are between 0.4 and 1.0. Sodium carboxymethylcellulose or cellulose gum is used as a thickening agent, protective colloid or suspending agent, and as a nongreasy ointment base. It is a bulk laxative and, as such, the active ingredient of Sodium Carboxymethylcellulose Tablets, N.F.

Treatment of alkali cellulose with ethyl chloride produces **Ethylcellulose, N.F.** The official products have D.S. values between 2.2 and 2.6. They are insoluble in water and propylene glycol but soluble in the common organic solvents. They find use as tablet binders, particularly for moisture-sensitive materials. Ethylcellulose absorbs less moisture from air than most of the water-soluble polymers, and its films have lower water vapor transmission rates.

Other official water-insoluble cellulose derivatives include pyroxylin and cellulose acetate phthalate. They are oleophilic rather than hydrophilic colloids. **Pyroxylin, U.S.P.,** is cellulose nitrate with a D.S. = 2. Dissolved in a mixture of 75 percent v/v of ether and 25 percent v/v of alcohol, it forms Collodion, U.S.P. Topically applied collodion leaves a protective film of nitrocellulose on drying. Camphor and castor oil are sometimes added to plasticize the film, i.e., to make it more flexible. This product is designated as **Flexible Collodion, U.S.P.** Collodions serve as vehicles for topical medicaments. For instance, the keratolytic salicylic acid is incorporated into flexible collodion. The product, Salicylic Acid Collodion, U.S.P., leaves a flexible plastic film containing salicylic acid on the portion of the skin to be desquamated.

Cellulose Acetate Phthalate, U.S.P., is a mixed ester of acetic and phthalic acids soluble in acetone or dioxane but insoluble in water. It is used as an enteric coating material for tablets because it remains intact until hydrolyzed by esterases of the intestine.

Starch, U.S.P., contains 10 to 20 percent of amylose, a linear polymer soluble in hot water, and 80 to 90 percent of amylopectin, a branched polymer which strongly swells but is insoluble in hot water. Both consist of glucose residues joined by α-1,4-glucosidic linkages, which are on the opposite side of the rings from the 6-carbon atoms. The branches of the amylopectin molecule are connected to the main chain by 1,6-glucosidic linkages. Starch is used in tablets as a diluent and disintegrant, and is the chief ingredient of dusting powder. *Dextrins,* obtained by hydrolytic degradation of starch, are more soluble in water. Dextriferron Injection, N.F., is a ferric hydroxide sol stabilized with partially hydrolyzed dextrin as a protective colloid. A similar product, Iron Dextran Injection, N.F., is a ferric hydroxide sol stabilized with partially hydrolyzed dextran. *Dextrans* are complex polysaccharides based on glucose, which are synthesized by some microorganisms from sucrose. They are used as plasma expanders after their molecular weight has been reduced to below 100,000 by controlled acid or enzymatic hydrolysis.

Polyelectrolytic Polysaccharides [40, 70]

Gums are dried plant exudates secreted when the bark is cut; *mucilages* are normal components of bark, roots, leaves, and seeds. In pharmacy, the term *mucilage* usually designates the viscous aqueous solutions of polymers. Gums find wide pharmaceutical application as thickening agents and as protective colloids to stabilize suspensions and emulsions. **Acacia, U.S.P.,** or gum arabic, is the dried gummy exudate of acacia trees. It consists mainly of the calcium salt of polyarabic acid but also contains some magnesium and potassium ions. On complete hydrolysis, it yields the hexoses arabinose, galactose, rhamnose, and glucuronic acid. The latter is glucose in which the 6-carbon atom was oxidized from a primary hydroxyl group to a carboxyl group. These sugar molecules, joined by glucosidic linkages, are the building blocks of polyarabic acid. The polymer has a molecular weight of about 240,000, indicating that a single molecule consists of about 1,400 hexose repeat units. The macromolecule is branched rather than linear. **Tragacanth, U.S.P.,** the dried gummy exudate from the genus Astragalus, is an even more complex gum. It is a mixture containing 30 to 40 percent of the water-soluble constituent tragacanthin, and 60 to 70 percent of a gel fraction called bassorin, which swells but is insoluble in water. Bassorin is a neutral polysaccharide comprising mainly arabinose and galactose units. Tragacanthin is a linear polymer consisting of galacturonic acid, the hexose fucose, and the pentose xylose. Some of the carboxyl groups of galacturonic acid are in the form of the methyl ester.

Related polysaccharides of simpler structure are pectin and sodium alginate. **Pectin, N.F.,** is a linear polymer of alpha 1,4-polygalacturonic acid, with many of the carboxyl groups in the form of the methyl ester. Pectin is widespread in nature. Commercially, it is obtained from the rind of citrus fruit or from apple pomace. Its use as a suspending and thickening agent is exemplified in Kaolin Mixture with Pectin, N.F., in which it acts as a demulcent as well.

Sodium Alginate, N.F., extracted from kelp, is the sodium salt of alginic or β-1,4-polymannuronic acid. In addition to their pharmaceutical applications, pectin and sodium alginate are widely used in foodstuffs—e.g., pectin as a gelling agent for jellies, and sodium alginate to thicken ice cream and to give it a smooth and uniform texture.

Agar, U.S.P., is also extracted from seaweed. It is a polysaccharide containing mostly galactose units. A few hydroxyl groups are esterified with sulfuric acid as monoesters. The second proton of the acid is replaced mainly by calcium ions. Cross-linking by the latter is probably responsible for the fact that agar is soluble in hot water but gels reversibly on cooling. Agar is used in bulk cathartics.

Sodium Heparin, U.S.P., is an anticoagulant of mammalian origin, being found in lung, liver, spleen, and blood. The active ingredient, heparin, is classified as a mucopolysaccharide, indicating that uronic acids and aminosugars are its chief components. Heparin is a polymer of glucuronic acid and glucosamine. The amino groups in the glucosamine residues, which replace the hydroxyls on the number 2 carbon atoms of glucose, are combined with sulfuric acid to form the monoamide, $-\overset{|}{\underset{|}{C}}-NH-SO_2-OH$, and most repeat units have one hydroxyl group in the form of the monoester of sulfuric acid, $-\overset{|}{\underset{|}{C}}-O-SO_2-OH$. The strongly acid heparin is usually dispensed in the sodium or potassium form. Its molecular weight is about 20,000.

Incompatibilities of Gums and Mucilages. The gums and mucilages discussed above, as well as sodium carboxymethylcellulose and Carbopol, a copolymer of acrylic acid, have carboxylate groups, i.e., they are anionic polyelectrolytes. Some of their reactions may lead to gel formation (p. 165). They have the following incompatibilities:

1. Mineral acids transform the salts into the carboxylic acid forms which are only slightly dissociated and usually precipitate. Therefore, gums should not be used in preparations with pH values below 3.

2. In the presence of heavy metal ions,

the soluble sodium, potassium or ammonium polycarboxylates undergo metathesis to the insoluble heavy metal carboxylates, causing precipitation. Alkaline earth ions may cause gelation instead of precipitation. The polyvalent metal ions form salt bridges which cross-link or tie polymer chains together. Schematically, if R_1 and R_2 represent different macromolecular chains,

$$R_1 - COO^-Na^+ + R_2 - COO^-Na^+ +$$

$$Pb(NO_3)_2 \rightarrow R_1 - COO^-Pb^{++}\ ^-OOC - R_2$$

$$+ 2\,NaNO_3$$

Precipitation of the lead polycarboxylate drives the metathetical equilibrium reaction to completion. Another example is the interaction between BiO^+ ions in solution and tragacanth[33,57] or sodium carboxymethylcellulose[33] in bismuth subnitrate suspensions thickened with those two carboxylic polyelectrolytes.

3. Cationic surfactants, and drugs listed on page 141 which behave as such, form complex coacervates with polycarboxylated polymers that are insoluble, as described on pages 145 to 146.

4. Complex coacervation also occurs with positively charged polymers, such as proteins below their isoelectric point, as discussed on page 165.

5. Carboxylated polymers are precipitated from aqueous solution by the addition of excess ethanol or glycerin.

6. Carboxylated polymers can be salted out by the addition of relatively high concentrations of salts of monovalent cations such as ammonium sulfate.

The two last phenomena are reversible; the polymers redissolve readily on dilution with water.

The incompatibilities of *tannic acids or tannins,* which are high molecular weight glycosides of polyhydroxylic phenols present in the wood, bark, leaves, and roots of many plants, are of special pharmaceutical interest. Tannins precipitate proteins from aqueous solution below the isoelectric point, forming complex coacervates. The reaction products of tannins with albumin and casein have found pharmaceutical use. Tanning, or the reaction of hide collagen with tannins to form insoluble tannates, is the basis for making leather.

The precipitation of basic drugs by tannins is a problem when the drugs are formulated in vehicles rich in tannins such as wild cherry syrup. On the other hand, this reaction provides a means for reducing the water solubility of amine drugs, and is the basis for long-acting oral dosage forms. The precipitated drug-tannin complexes slowly dissociate as they move through the gastrointestinal tract, releasing the amine drugs gradually. The dissociation of the tannates is enhanced by low pH values and by electrolytes. The following are examples of basic water-soluble drugs formulated as their salts or complexes with tannic acid which have low water solubility: Atropine (Atratan* Tablet), cryptenamine alkaloids (Unitensen* Tablet), phenylephrine with pyrilamine and chlorpheniramine (Rynatan* Tabule Durabonded), and dextroamphetamine (Synatan* Tabule). The termination *-tan* indicates complexation with tannic acids.

Another anionic polyelectrolyte used to prepare slightly soluble salts of basic drugs with high water solubility is polygalacturonic acid. An example is quinidine polygalacturonate (Cardioquin†).

The use of strong tea as an antidote for poisoning is probably related to its high content of tannic acid, which forms insoluble salts with alkaloids, complexes heavy metal ions, and is likely to precipitate toxins as well, since the latter are proteins.

Synthetic, Nonionic, Water-Soluble Polymers [9,40]

In this category are **Polyethylene Glycols** 300 and 1540, official in the N.F., and 400 and 4000, official in the U.S.P. These are polymers of ethylene oxide,

$$HO-(CH_2-CH_2-O)_n-H,$$

made by controlled ring-opening polymerization. The numbers indicate average molecular weights. Up to molecular weights of 600, the polyethylene glycols are viscous liquids at room temperature. Polyethylene glycols 1000 and 1540 are waxy solids; products with higher molecular weights are correspondingly harder at room temperature. The uses of these polymers as bases for ointments

* Trademark, Mallinckrodt Chemical Works.
† Trademark, The Purdue Frederick Co.

and vehicles for suppositories are discussed in Chapters 8 and 9.

Povidone, N. F., or *polyvinyl pyrrolidone*

$$\left(\!\!\begin{array}{c} CH_2-CH \\ | \\ N \\ H_2C \diagdown \diagup C=O \\ | \quad\quad | \\ H_2C\!-\!\!-\!\!-\!CH_2 \end{array}\!\!\right)_n$$

is used as a protective colloid and as a film former. It is soluble in water and in a wide variety of polar solvents. Commercial grades are available with weight-average molecular weights between 10,000 and 360,000. Polyvinyl pyrrolidone thickens aqueous solutions less than many other polymers of comparable molecular weight. As it does with starch, iodine forms a weak complex with polyvinyl pyrrolidone, Povidone-Iodine, N.F. It serves as a vehicle for iodine, combining the somewhat attenuated antiseptic action of iodine with the film-forming ability of the polymer. Its solution is also available as an aerosol.

Synthetic polymers have several advantages over natural polymers like gums. They can be obtained as uniform products with little variation in properties from batch to batch. The wide choice of functional groups, degrees of substitution, molecular weights, and other structural features such as the frequency and length of branches, in which synthetic polymers are available enables the pharmacist to select a product that is tailor-made for a given application. The disadvantages in all but topical applications are that the physiological properties, biochemical reactions, and metabolites of many synthetic polymers are not known, and many contain chemical linkages that cannot be broken down by the enzymes in the human body.

Proteins and Polypeptides. The polymer most widely employed in pharmacy is **Gelatin, U.S.P.** In solution, it is used as a protective colloid, a suspending and emulsifying agent, and as a binder in tableting. As a positively charged polyelectrolyte, it is used as a sensitizing or flocculating agent in the clarification of liquids, e.g., in the removal of tannins. Solid gelatin is used as the shell of hard gelatin capsules and for coating tablets and pills. Plasticized with glycerin, gelatin is employed to form soft elastic capsules, as a base for suppositories,

and, with zinc oxide and water in addition to glycerin, as a boot in topical applications (Zinc Gelatin, U.S.P.). Absorbable Gelatin Sponge, U.S.P., is a hemostatic for controlling bleeding.

Type A gelatin is manufactured from the collagen of porkskin. Porkskin is treated for 24 hours with dilute mineral acids at pH values of 1 to 3. After washing, the swollen stock is cooked with hot water, which hydrolyzes collagen to gelatin and extracts the latter. Type A gelatin, with an isoelectric point in the pH range of 7 to 9, results. Type B gelatin is manufactured by treating hide and decalcified bones with lime slurries at pH = 12.3 for several weeks. This removes impurities like soluble proteins and mucopolysaccharides, but also causes the collagen to lose ammonia through the hydrolysis of a few of the amide linkages. Washing, neutralization of the unremoved lime with acid, and cooking with water follow. The resultant Type B gelatin has a lower isoelectric point, in the pH range of 4.7 and 5.0.

Among relatively low molecular weight polypeptides are the following *antibiotics*: Bacitracin, U.S.P., ($\overline{M} = 1,460$); the three closely related cyclic decapeptides Colistin Sulfate, N.F., ($\overline{M} = 1,170$). Sodium Colistimethate, U.S.P., ($\overline{M} = 1,750$), and Polymyxin B Sulfate, U.S.P.; and the two related mixtures of cyclic polypeptides Gramicidin, N.F., and Tyrothricin, N.F., which consist chiefly of decapeptides. Dactinomycin, U.S.P., ($\overline{M} = 1,255$) is an antineoplastic drug.

Glucagon, U.S.P., a *hormone* and hyperglycemic factor produced by the pancreas, is a polypeptide with 29 amino acid residues and a $\overline{M}$ value of 3,464. Other polypeptidic hormones include oxytocin, available as Oxytocin Injection, U.S.P., and vasopressin, available as Vasopressin Injection, U.S.P. Both contain 9 amino acid residues and were originally isolated from the posterior lobe of the pituitary gland. These polypeptides and the proteins discussed below are monodisperse; $\overline{M}$ represents therefore the number-average as well as the weight-average molecular weight.

Official products based on high molecular weight proteins fall into many categories. *Insulin* is the pancreatic hormone which enables the body to utilize and store glucose. It is available in various official forms including Insulin Injection, U.S.P., and Insulin Zinc Suspension, U.S.P. Its molecular weight is 5,733, but association in solution produces the dimer or higher aggregates.

Many official proteinaceous medicaments are *enzymes.* Chymotrypsin, N.F., ($\overline{M} = 24,500$) and Trypsin Crystallized, N.F. ($\overline{M} = 23,800$) are proteolytic enzymes obtained from the bovine pancreas. Pancreatin, N.F., is a preparation from bovine or porcine pancreas containing amylase, protease, and lipase. Hyaluronidase for Injection, N.F., hydrolyzes the mucopolysaccharide hyaluronic acid (an integral part of the ground substance or cement between cells in connective and other tissues) and thereby accelerates the spreading of suspensions and solutions injected subcutaneously.

Among the official *biological products based on proteins* are the following: Bacterial vaccines (Cholera, Pertussis, Plague, and Typhoid Vaccines, U.S.P.); viral vaccines (Influenza, Poliomyelitis, Rabies, and Typhus Vaccines, U.S.P.); toxoids (Diphtheria and Tetanus Toxoids, U.S.P.); antitoxins (Botulism, Diphtheria, and Tetanus Antitoxins, U.S.P.); antivenins (Polyvalent Crotaline Antivenin, U.S.P.); immune serums (Antirabies, Measles, Tetanus, and Pertussis Immune Globulins, U.S.P.); and the diagnostic, Purified Protein Derivative of Tuberculin, U.S.P.

Proteinaceous biologics with official standing which promote the *clotting of blood* include Fibrinogen, U.S.P., ($\overline{M} = 330,000$) and Thrombin, N.F., an enzyme that transforms soluble fibrinogen into fibrin. Fibrin is a fibrous protein; it forms a sticky, 3-dimensional network to which blood cells and tissue adhere and holds the clotted blood together. Protamine Sulfate, U.S.P., a strongly basic protein of low molecular weight, is antagonistic to heparin. Heparin, which prolongs the clotting time of blood, is an anionic mucopolysaccharide containing sulfuric acid groups (p. 168). Protamine contains strongly basic guanidino groups belonging to arginine residues, through which it forms a complex coacervate with heparin and inactivates it.

Other *blood-related official biologics* of proteinaceous character include Plasma Protein Fraction, U.S.P., and Normal Human Serum Albumin, U.S.P., which are blood-volume supporters; and Iodinated I 125 and I 131 Serum Albumin, U.S.P., which are diagnostic aids used to measure blood volume and cardiac output. The molecular weight of the globular protein human serum albumin is 69,000.

OFFICIAL MILKS, MAGMAS, AND INORGANIC GELS AND JELLIES

Milks or magmas and inorganic gels are viscous aqueous dispersions containing gelatinous masses of flocculent inorganic precipitates or of other fine inorganic hydrated particles. If the disperse phase is present in sufficiently high concentrations to confer a yield value and viscoelasticity to the disperse system, it can be classified as a gel or jelly according to the rheological connotation of the word (p. 114).[34,79] Particle size does not seem to be a criterion for including a disperse system among the official milks, magmas, gels, and jellies because sodium bentonite and bismuth subcarbonate are both included. Bentonite has primary particles in the lower end of the colloidal range while bismuth subcarbonate consists of coarse primary particles. As can be seen from the descriptions below, the official inorganic gels, milks, and magmas belong to the group known as *gelatinous precipitates.* Bentonite magma may be classified as an inorganic jelly. Except for it, magmas and inorganic gels resemble each other in consistency and appearance to the naked eye and when viewed under the microscope.

Milks and gels are intended for oral administration. If the products have been prepared correctly, the particles remain uniformly dispersed throughout the system; however, a supernatant liquid develops in time. The uniformity of the mixtures is reestablished easily by shaking the container. Directions to "shake well before using" must be included on the labels of all magmas, milks, and gels. The size and range of sizes of the particles may be reduced by passing the product through the appropriate mill which breaks up flocs or aggregates into smaller aggregates or into primary particles.

Bentonite, U.S.P., is the sodium form of an aluminum silicate clay with a layer structure. Its primary particles are platelets only

9.4 Å thick. Solid bentonite consists of stacks of these platelets. Water penetrates between adjacent platelets and pries them apart, causing the clay to swell extensively. One gram of sodium bentonite can absorb as much as 11 cm.^{3} of water. In excess water, the clay breaks up into the individual platelets or into stacks consisting of a few platelets which are stuck together. Sodium bentonite has a cation exchange capacity of nearly one milliequivalent per gram, owing to silicate ions which impart a negative charge to the faces of the platelets. Details of its structure and properties are given in several monographs.[15,75]

Bentonite Magma, U.S.P., is a 5 percent w/v dispersion of sodium bentonite in water. It is a suspending medium for insoluble medicaments. For instance, Calamine Lotion, U.S.P., is a suspension of calamine and zinc oxide in bentonite magma; Phenolated Calamine Lotion, U.S.P., contains phenol as well. The thixotropic properties of bentonite magma (p. 116) contribute to the stability of the suspension. At rest, the magma sets to a gel, acquiring a yield value. This prevents settling of the suspended zinc oxide particles. Shaking destroys the gel structure, so that the suspension is poured readily from the bottle.

Sodium bentonite is incompatible with heavy metal ions and with water-soluble cationic drugs. Metathesis with soluble zinc salts, for instance, produces zinc bentonite, which possesses little of the gel-forming ability of sodium bentonite and precipitates as coarse lumps. Even potassium and calcium bentonite do not thicken water nearly as much as the sodium form. Chemisorption of cationic drugs (pp. 126–127) reduces the bioavailability of these drugs. Also, nonionic water-soluble drugs and surfactants become less available owing to physical adsorption by bentonite. Bentonite magma has a pH value of 9 and considerable buffering power; it should not be formulated with acids.

Several aqueous *suspensions of aluminum and/or magnesium hydroxide* are used as antacids. Aluminum Hydroxide Gel, U.S.P., is prepared by hydrolyzing ammonium alum with sodium carbonate. Alumina and Mag-nesia Oral Suspension, U.S.P. (Aludrox*), Magnesia and Alumina Oral Suspension, U.S.P. (Maalox†) and Milk of Magnesia, U.S.P., are prepared by treating aluminum and/or magnesium salts with sodium hydroxide. Magnesia has mild cathartic properties and counteracts the constipating effect of alumina. Magaldrate Oral Suspension, N.F., also contains magnesium and aluminum hydroxides; it is prepared by the reaction between sodium aluminate and a magnesium salt:

$$Na_2O.Al_2O_3 + MgSO_4 + 4H_2O \rightarrow$$
$$2Al(OH)_3 + Mg(OH)_2 + Na_2SO_4$$

Aluminum Phosphate Gel, N.F., $AlPO_4$, is precipitated by the reaction of aluminum salts with sodium phosphate. It possesses about one half of the acid-binding power of aluminum hydroxide. Dihydroxyaluminum Aminoacetate Magma, N.F., $H_2N–CH_2–COOAl(OH)_2$, precipitates when aluminum isopropoxide dissolved in isopropanol is added to an aqueous solution of glycine.

Milk of Bismuth, N.F., is an astringent, an antacid, and a protectant and adsorbent for coating ulcer craters and the lining of the intestines. It is used in the treatment of enteritis, diarrhea, dysentery, and ulcerative colitis. Milk of bismuth is an aqueous suspension of bismuth subcarbonate, $[(BiO)_2 CO_3]_2·H_2O$, precipitated by the reaction between bismuth nitrate and ammonium carbonate.

Official *hydrophilic inorganic powders* of small particle size include Kaolin, N.F., a laminar clay consisting of platelets about 0.1 μ thick which often have hexagonal shape. Kaolin is used as an adsorbent (p. 127). Titanium Dioxide, U.S.P., is a white pigment of 0.3 μ average particle size. Its exceptionally high refractive index of 2.55 to 2.70 gives it excellent covering or hiding power and makes it a useful ingredient in ointments and lotions as a protective agent against sunlight. Colloidal Silicon Dioxide, N.F., is described on page 163.

---

* Trademark, Wyeth Labs.
† Trademark, Wm. H. Rorer, Inc.

REFERENCES

1. Adam, N. K.: The Physics and Chemistry of Surfaces. ed. 3. London, Oxford University Press, 1941.
2. Adamson, A. W.: Physical Chemistry of Surfaces. ed. 2. New York, Wiley-Interscience, 1967.
3. Alexander, A. E., and Johnson, P.: Colloid Science. London, Oxford University Press, 1949.
4. Allen, P. W.: Techniques of Polymer Characterization. London. Butterworths, 1959.
5. Andrade, E. N. da C.: Viscosity and Plasticity. Cambridge (England), Heffer & Sons, 1947.
6. Barr, M., and Arnista, E. S.: J. Am. Pharm. A. (Sci. Ed.) *46*:493, 1957.
7. Battista, O. A.: Am. Sci. *53*:151, 1965.
8. Batuyios, N. H., and Brecht, E. A.: J. Am. Pharm. A. (Sci. Ed.) *46*:524, 1957.
9. Billmeyer, F. W.: Textbook of Polymer Science. ed. 2. New York, Wiley-Interscience, 1971.
10. Buechi, J.: Grundlagen der Arzneimittelforschung und der synthetischen Arzneimittel. Basel, Birkhaeuser Verlag, 1963.
11. Burton, A. C., *in* Ruch, T. C., and Patton, H. D. (eds.): Physiology and Biophysics. ed. 19, chap. 27. Philadelphia, W. B. Saunders, 1965.
12. Burton, E. F., *in* Alexander, J. (ed.): Colloid Chemistry. vol. 1, chap. 6. New York, Chemical Catalog Co., 1926.
13. Cross, M. M.: J. Colloid Interface Sci., *20*: 417, 1965; *33*:30, 1970.
14. Edmundson, I. C., *in* Bean, H. S., Beckett, A. H., and Carless, J. E. (eds.): Advances in Pharmaceutical Sciences. vol. 2, chap. 2. New York, Academic Press, 1967.
15. Eitel, W.: Silicate Science. vol. 1. New York, Academic Press, 1964.
16. Elworthy, P. H., Florence, A. T., and McFarlane, C. B.: Solubilization by Surface-Active Agents. London, Chapman & Hall, 1968.
17. Evcim, N., and Barr, M.: J. Am. Pharm. A. (Sci. Ed.) *44*:570, 1955.
18. Fischer, E. K.: Colloidal Dispersions. New York, Wiley, 1950.
19. Fowkes, F. M., *in* Shinoda, K. (ed.): Solvent Properties of Surfactant Solutions. chap. 3, New York, Marcel Dekker, 1967.
20. Gillespie, T.: J. Colloid Interface Sci., *15*: 219, 1960; *22*:554, 1966.
21. Goodeve, C. F.: Trans. Faraday Soc., *35*: 342, 1939.
22. Green, H.: Industrial Rheology and Rheological Structures. New York, Wiley, 1949.
23. Hermans, J. J.: Flow Properties of Disperse Systems. Amsterdam, North-Holland Publishing Co., 1953.
24. Houwink, R.: Elasticity, Plasticity and Structure of Matter. ed. 2. Washington, D.C., Harren Press, 1953.
25. Jaenicke, R.: Kolloid-Z. u. Z. Polymere, *212*: 36, 1966.
26. Jordan, J. W.: J. Phys. Colloid Chem., *53*: 294, 1949; *54*:1196, 1950.
27. Jungermann, E. (ed.): Cationic Surfactants. New York, Marcel Dekker, 1970.
28. Kaspar, H., Buechi, J., Schwarz, T. W., and Steiger-Trippi, K.: Pharm. Acta Helv., *37*:48, 1962.
29. Kipling, J. J.: Adsorption from Solutions of Non-Electrolytes. New York, Academic Press, 1965.
30. Kruyt, H. R.: Colloid Science. vol. 1. New York, Elsevier, 1952.
31. ———: Colloid Science. vol. 2. New York, Elsevier, 1949.
32. Kuhn, A. (ed.): Kolloidchemisches Taschenbuch. ed. 5. Leipzig, Akademische Verlagsgesellschaft Geest & Portig K.-G., 1960.
33. Lesshafft, C. T., and DeKay, H. G.: Drug Standards, *22*:155, 1954.
34. McBain, J. W.: Colloid Science. Boston, D. C. Heath & Co., 1950.
35. McBain, M. E. L., and Hutchinson, E.: Solubilization and Related Phenomena. New York, Academic Press, 1955.
36. Martin, A. N., Banker, G. S., and Chun, A. H. C., *in* Bean, H. S., Beckett, A. H., and Carless, J. E. (eds.): Advances in Pharmaceutical Sciences. vol. 1, chap. 1. New York, Academic Press, 1964.
37. Matthews, B. A., and Rhodes, C. T.: Pharm. Acta Helv., *45*:52, 1969.
38. Miller, M. L.: The Structure of Polymers. New York, Reinhold, 1966.
39. Moilliet, J. L., Collie, B., and Black, W.: Surface Activity. ed. 2. London, E. & F. N. Spon, 1961.
40. Muenzel, K., Buechi, J., and Schultz, O. E.: Galenisches Praktikum. Stuttgart, Wissenschaftliche Verlagsgesellschaft MBH, 1959.
41. Mulley, B. A., *in* Bean, H. S., Beckett, A. H., and Carless, J. E. (eds.): Advances in Pharmaceutical Sciences. vol. 1, chap. 2. New York, Academic Press, 1964.
42. Mysels, K. J.: Introduction to Colloid Chemistry. New York, Wiley-Interscience, 1959.
43. Nakagawa, T., *in* Schick, M. J. (ed.); Nonionic Surfactants. chap. 17. New York, Marcel Dekker, 1967.
44. Ostwald, Wo.: Die Welt der vernachlaessigten Dimensionen (The World of the Neglected Dimensions). ed. 10. Dresden, Steinkopff, 1927.
45. Ott, E., Spurlin, H. M., and Grafflin, M. W. (eds.): Cellulose and Cellulose Derivatives. ed. 2, vols. 1–3. New York, Wiley-Interscience, 1954.
46. Ottewill, R. H., in Schick, M. J. (ed.): Nonionic Surfactants. chap. 19. New York, Marcel Dekker, 1967.

47. Partington, J. R.: A Short History of Chemistry. ed. 3. New York, Harper & Brothers, 1960.

48. Perrin, J.: Les Atomes. Paris, Presses Universitaires de France, 1948.

49. Perrin, J. H., and Ishag, A.: J. Pharm. Pharmacol., *23*:770, 1971.

50. Philippoff, W.: Viskositaet der Kolloide. Dresden, Steinkopff, 1942.

51. Reier, G. E., and Shangraw, R. F.: J. Pharm. Sci., *55*:510, 1966.

52. Reinders, W., and Bendien, W. M.: Rec. Trav. Chim., *47*:977, 1928.

53. Reiner, M.: Deformation, Strain and Flow. ed. 2. New York, Wiley-Interscience, 1960.

54. Riegelman, S., Allawala, N. A., Hrenoff, M. K., and Strait, L. A.: J. Colloid Sci., *13*:208, 1958.

55. Rowland, F., Bulas, R., Rothstein, E., and Eirich, F.: Ind. Eng. Chem., *57* (9):46, 1965.

56. Schick, M. J. (ed.): Nonionic Surfactants. New York, Marcel Dekker, 1967.

57. Schmitz, R. E., and Hill, J. S.: J. Am. Pharm. A. (Pract. Ed.), *9*:493, 1948.

58. Schoenfeldt, N.: Oberflaechenaktive Anlagerungsprodukte des Aethylenoxyds. Stuttgart, Wissenschaftliche Verlagsgesellschaft MBH, 1959.

59. Scholtan, W.: Kolloid-Z., *142*:84, 1955.

60. Schott, H.: J. Phys. Chem. *70*:2966, 1966; *71*:3611, 1967.

61. ———: Kolloid-Z. u. Z. Polymere, *219*:42, 1967.

62. ———: J. Pharm. Sci., *58*:1443, 1969.

63. ———: J. Pharm. Sci., *60*:1893, 1971.

64. Schott, H., and Young, C. Y.: J. Pharm. Sci., *61*:182, 1972.

65. Schwartz, A. M., and Perry, J. W.: Surface Active Agents. vol. 1. New York, Interscience, 1949.

66. Schwartz, A. M., Perry, J. W., and Berch, J.: Surface Active Agents and Detergents. Vol. 2. New York, Interscience, 1958.

67. Shinoda, K., *in* Shinoda, K. (ed.): Solvent Properties of Surfactant Solutions. chaps. 1 and 2. New York, Marcel Dekker, 1967.

68. Shinoda, K., Nakagawa, T., Tamamushi, B.-I., and Isemura, T.: Colloidal Surfactants. New York, Academic Press, 1963.

69. Sjoeblom, L., *in* Shinoda, K. (ed.): Solvent Properties of Surfactant Solutions. chap. 5. New York, Marcel Dekker, 1967.

70. Smith, F., and Montgomery, R.: The Chemistry of Plant Gums and Mucilages. New York, Reinhold, 1959.

71. Stromberg, R. R., *in* Patrick, R. L. (ed.): Treatise on Adhesion and Adhesives. vol. 1, chap. 3. New York, Marcel Dekker, 1967.

72. Svedberg, T.: Colloid Chemistry. New York, Chemical Catalog Co., 1928.

73. Swarbrick, J.: J. Pharm. Sci., *54*:1229, 1965.

74. Tanford, C.: Physical Chemistry of Macromolecules. New York, Wiley, 1961.

75. Van Olphen, H.: Clay Colloid Chemistry. New York, Wiley-Interscience, 1963.

76. Van Wazer, J. R., Lyons, J. W., Kim, K. Y., and Colwell, R. E.: Viscosity and Flow Measurement. New York, Wiley-Interscience, 1963.

77. Vold, M. J., and Vold, R. D.: Colloid Chemistry. New York, Reinhold, 1964.

78. Von Weimarn, P. P., in Alexander, J. (ed.): Colloid Chemistry. vol. 1, chap. 2, New York, Chemical Catalog Co., 1926.

79. Weiser, H. B.: A Textbook of Colloid Chemistry. ed. 2. New York, Wiley, 1949.

80. Winsor, P. A.: Solvent Properties of Amphiphilic Compounds. London, Butterworths, 1954.

81. Zisman, W. A., *in* Contact Angle, Wettability, and Adhesion. Advances in Chemistry. Series 43, chap. 1. Washington, American Chemical Society, 1964.

7

James Swarbrick, D.Sc., Ph.D., *Director of Product Development,*
Sterling-Winthrop Research Institute

Coarse Dispersions: Suspensions, Emulsions, and Lotions

INTRODUCTION

Pharmaceutical dispersions are an important group of preparations, including as they do emulsions, suspensions, aerosols, creams, lotions, and ointments. In their simplest form, these preparations consist of a dispersed phase distributed throughout a second, a continuous phase, called also the dispersion medium. This terminology is comparable to that used in solutions, namely solute and solvent. However, the dispersed phase in pharmaceutical dispersions consists of discrete particles or globules containing many molecules—in contrast to solutions, in which the solute is dispersed as single molecules or ions throughout the solvent. It is not always possible to state unequivocally which phase is the dispersed one and which is the continuous one. In such cases, the phase present in excess is usually spoken of as the continuous phase.

Depending on the particle size of the dispersed phase, pharmaceutical dispersions are subdivided into colloidal and coarse dispersions. Colloidal dispersions are generally considered those dispersions in which the particle size is from less than 0.5 to 1 micron. Above this limit, which is chosen somewhat arbitrarily, the dispersion is referred to as a coarse one. Colloidal dispersions and their properties are described in Chapter 6. In this chapter we shall examine two of the several types of pharmaceutical coarse dispersions, namely, suspensions and emulsions. Other types of coarse dispersion are considered in Chapters 8 and 12.

Suspensions are dispersions of solid particles in a liquid continuous phase which most frequently is aqueous in nature. However, in some pharmaceutical suspensions the solid particles are dispersed in an oil. For convenience, suspensions are often referred to as "solid-liquid dispersions." The size of the particles normally range from 0.5 μ up to 100 μ, although some preparations may contain particles above 100 μ. Emulsions are liquid-liquid dispersions—that is, a mixture of two immiscible liquids such as an oil and water, one dispersed within the other. The particle size range commonly observed in preparations for pharmaceutical use is similar to that for suspensions.

Suspensions and emulsions have been used by the pharmacist for many years. Over the last two decades, the number of suspensions in use has increased significantly. This expansion is due, in large part, to the fact that many of the new drugs developed in the last three decades have a very low solubility in water or aqueous vehicles. Originally, suspensions were used only for drugs to be administered orally or those for topical use. Currently, they are also used for drugs to be administered parenterally and for ophthalmic drugs. Suspensions are frequently employed as an alternative to solid dosage forms such as tablets and capsules, especially when the drug is to be given to children or when the dose required would result in a tablet of a size difficult to swallow.

The medicinal use of emulsions dates back to the second half of the 17th century when Grew, a physician, described preparations containing egg yolk and oils to the Royal Society of Great Britain. A report published in 1757 referred to the use of acacia, syrups, honey, egg yolk, tragacanth, quince seed mucilage, and starch jelly for the emulsification of almond, linseed, olive, anise, and clove oils, and for beeswax, benzoin, and similar medicinal substances.

From the time of the early development of pharmaceutical emulsions in the 17th and 18th centuries, o/w emulsions were prepared by the gradual addition of oil to egg yolk, to acacia and tragacanth mucilages, or to an aqueous suspension of crushed almond seeds. This is frequently called the wet gum method, since the process involves wetting and dispersing the emulsifying agent, usually gum acacia, with water to form a mucilage and adding oil gradually to the aqueous phase with trituration.

In 1874, Wilder[63] described a method whereby acacia was dispersed in the oil contained in a dry mortar, after which the water was added all in one portion, and the mixture was then triturated until emulsification had occurred. This has become known as the dry gum method.

The synthesis of a large number of surface-active agents in recent years and the development of many new cosmetic and medicinal emulsions have led to the popularity of emulsified lotions and creams and have greatly stimulated research in this field.

Lotions, which are liquid preparations intended for external application to the skin, frequently contain suspended particles or emulsified liquid droplets. Depending, therefore, on whether they are solid-liquid or liquid-liquid dispersions, some lotions can also be classified as suspensions or emulsions. Medicinal lotions are antiseptic and germicidal and are used in the treatment of skin diseases and as cooling and mildly anesthetic applications for skin irritations.

A lotion which contains suspended or emulsified material is acceptable if the particles settle or rise only slowly and if solid particles do not form a hard cake at the bottom of the container. The material that separates on standing should be easily redispersed when the vessel is shaken. The lotion should pour freely from the bottle and apply evenly over the affected area, and should not run off the surface of the skin. A good product dries quickly and provides a protective film that will not rub off easily. The lotion should also have an acceptable color and odor, and it must remain physi-

cally and chemically stable and free of mold growth during storage.

Cosmetic lotions are applied to hair, scalp, face, and hands and are popular as sunscreen preparations. They may be oily or hydroalcoholic solutions or emulsions, and, frequently, they contain glycerin, perfumes, and preservatives.

Examples of official lotions are Benzyl Benzoate Lotion, N.F., Calamine Lotion, U.S.P., Hydrocortisone Lotion, N.F., and White Lotion, N.F. The first is an emulsified product; all the rest are examples of lotions containing suspended solids.

Common Features and Differences

Suspensions and emulsions contain particles, solid and liquid respectively, dispersed in a continuous phase. They are both subject, therefore, to sedimentation processes brought about by the effect of gravity on the dispersed particles. Accordingly, the factors that influence sedimentation rate, such as particle size and density, and the viscosity and density of the dispersion medium operate to the same extent in both types of system. Additionally, both systems require some input of energy to disperse the particles and effect preparation. Both have properties related to the presence of an extensive interface between the particles and the continuous phase. For example, the particles of both an emulsion and a suspension can be caused to come together (flocculate) by the addition of an agent that will reduce the net charge on the particles. Agents that impart a charge to the particles often work to disperse (deflocculate) the particles of an emulsion as well as of a suspension.

The major difference between emulsions and suspensions is that the particles of the former are liquid droplets, whereas those of the latter are solid. This means that the droplets of an emulsion can fuse or coalesce if they come together. Should this happen, the complete separation of the once-dispersed liquid phase can occur. When the solid particles of a suspension come together, they do not coalesce to form a larger particle but usually retain their original shape. In this sense, emulsions are metastable products whereas suspensions can be considered stable toward coalescence. The difference in the physical state of the dispersed phase also affects the biological availability of the drug if it constitutes or is present in the dispersed phase. For example, a drug dissolved in the dispersed droplets of an emulsion is already present as free molecules which are more readily available for absorption from the gastrointestinal tract. Drug present as a solid particle in a suspension must first undergo a dissolution process before it becomes available in a free molecular form that is suitable for absorption.

MICROMERITICS

A knowledge of the behavior of small particles is important for an understanding of the properties of coarse pharmaceutical dispersions. Accordingly, this topic is introduced prior to dealing with the specific pharmaceutical systems under consideration.

Not only are size, shape, and surface area of particles factors in affecting the physical stability of emulsions and suspensions, but these parameters also control the dissolution rate of solid drug particles. This, in turn, may affect the biological availability of the drug. The manufacturing and clinical aspects of micromeritics in pharmaceutical practice has been reviewed by Lees[42] and, more recently, by Fincher;[17] the reader should consult these papers for further information and references to other useful works. As may be seen from Table 7-1, particles found in pharmaceutical coarse dispersions such as emulsions, suspensions, and powdered dosage forms range from about 0.5 μ to 100 μ and can be observed with the optical microscope. Particles in this range are officially identified in the compendia as "fine" and "very fine"

powders. Particles in excess of 50 to 100 μ can normally be observed by the unaided eye. In the compendia the description "coarse" is the official term used for particles lying within the range of 150 to 1,000 μ.

Sedimentation and Creaming of Particles

If one prepares a dispersion of coarse solid or liquid particles in a liquid vehicle, a separation of these particles is normally seen within a period of time ranging from a few seconds to a few hours. Depending on the relative densities of the dispersed phase and the dispersion medium, one will observe either a downward or an upward movement of the particles. These processes are referred to as *sedimentation* and *creaming* (upward sedimentation), respectively. Sedimentation occurs when the dispersion contains particles whose density is greater than that of the liquid vehicle; creaming is observed when the density of the dispersed particles is less than that of the dispersion medium. Sedimentation usually occurs in suspensions; creaming is normally found in emulsions.

The rate of sedimentation or creaming can be determined by the application of Stokes' law (see below). For the sake of convenience, no differentiation will be made between sedimentation and creaming in most of the subsequent discussions. The term "sedimentation" will therefore be used to denote both downward and upward movement of particles relative to their dispersion medium.

Stokes' Law. The terminal velocity with which particles in a coarse dispersion settle may be expressed by Stokes' law:

TABLE 7-1. PARTICLE DIMENSIONS IN PHARMACEUTICAL SYSTEMS

PARTICLE SIZE (microns)	APPROXIMATE SIEVE SIZE	EXAMPLES
0.5–10	—	Fine suspensions and emulsions.
10–50	—	Ordinary suspensions and emulsions; upper limit of subsieve range.
50–100	325–140	Very fine powder range, lower limit of sieve range; lower limit of visibility.
150–1,000	100–18	Coarse powder range.
1,000–3,350	18–6	Average granule size.

$$V = \frac{d^2(\rho - \rho_0)g}{18\eta_0} \qquad (1)$$

where V is the terminal velocity of fall of an average particle in the dispersion, d is the mean particle diameter, ρ is the density of the particles, ρ_0 is the density of the dispersion medium, g is the acceleration constant associated with the force of gravity, and η_0 is the viscosity of the dispersion medium. Stokes' equation was derived for a very dilute dispersion comprised of rigid, perfectly spherical particles of uniform size, settling at a velocity that produced no turbulence in the dispersion medium. Under such conditions the particles do not interfere with one another, and so-called *free settling* occurs. In most pharmaceutical suspensions the particles are rigid, but they are not spheres. In most emulsions, the dispersed phase usually exists as spherical globules but, being liquid, these are not rigid. Furthermore, the particles are not of one size but exhibit a distribution of sizes. The concentration of particles is usually high, and the particles tend to interact with one another and with the suspending medium. Consequently, Stokes' law does not hold exactly for pharmaceutical dispersions. Nevertheless, Equation 1 can be used to give a good indication of those factors that contribute to settling and indicates what adjustments can be made to improve the product by reducing sedimentation.

Since the velocity of sedimentation is proportional to the square of the particle diameter, the rate of sedimentation may be decreased markedly by reducing the particle size of the dispersed phase to as fine a state of subdivision as possible. However, as will be seen later (p. 190) this does not always lead to formation of the best product. According to Equation 1, the sedimentation rate is inversely proportional to the viscosity of the dispersion medium when this is Newtonian (see Chap. 6). Physical stability can therefore be enhanced by increasing the Newtonian viscosity of the dispersion. In practice, too high a Newtonian viscosity is not desirable, since such a product is difficult to pour, and any material that does settle is difficult to redisperse. The sedimentation rate also depends on the difference between the densities of the dispersed particles and the dispersion medium. Since most oils have a density less than that of water, upward sedimentation (creaming) occurs when the oil is the dispersed phase. Most solids have a density greater than that of water; consequently, downward sedimentation occurs with suspensions. However, it must be reiterated that, regardless of whether sedimentation is downward or upward, the factors involved are identical and the rate, at least in ideal systems, can be quantitated by means of Stokes' equation. The reader should also realize that if the densities of the dispersed phase and the dispersion medium are identical no net movement (sedimentation) of the dispersed particles takes place. Attempts are sometimes made to adjust the density of the vehicle to that of the suspended particles in order to prevent sedimentation. However, this is not always possible or practical and is, accordingly, not often attempted.

In practice, pharmaceutical dispersions are not usually ideal in the sense of complying with all the criteria on which Stokes' law is based. Thus, most dispersions are fairly concentrated and polydisperse. This means that larger particles settling down past smaller ones cause the latter to move at a velocity that is in excess of that calculated according to Stokes' law. Furthermore, because of concentration, the particles do not fall independently of one another. Sedimentation under such conditions is termed "hindered settling." In the case of flocculated suspensions, settling of the total particle mass tends to occur, with the result that a sharp boundary exists between the sedimentation and the clear supernatant. The rate of fall of this boundary is sometimes referred to as the rate of subsidence.

Particle Size Measurement

A knowledge of the size range and average diameter of particles in a dry powder, a suspension, or an emulsion is necessary in order to be able to predict the degree of physical stability of a preparation in terms of its potential to resist sedimentation. Such information can, in turn, lead to an estimate of the surface area of the particles, a factor of importance in the dissolution rate of sparingly soluble drugs. Surface area of particles can also be determined directly, using methods to be described in detail later in this section.

The most widely used methods for measuring the size of coarse particles are microscopy, sieving, sedimentation, and electronic counting. The surface area can be computed by the techniques of permeation and adsorption. The method of choice for a particular analysis depends on the size range of the particles and the use for which the data are collected. For example, in order to relate the size of particles in a suspension or emulsion to the settling characteristics of the dispersed phase, it is best to employ a sedimentation technique that provides an estimate of the particle size distribution of the sample. This is superior to a microscopic method which would yield a mean diameter not closely related to the hydrodynamic properties of the particles in the liquid dispersion. However, if the material in suspension is used as a gastric adsorbent (e.g., kaolin or bismuth subnitrate), the surface area of the particles is the relevant property, since it relates directly to the use of the product. Consequently, a permeability or gas adsorption method should be employed in preference to one that measures particle diameters.

Particle Size Distribution. The many particles in a sample of material do not usually have identical diameters but, rather, exhibit a distribution of sizes. Therefore, it is convenient to group them for analysis into various size classes, as shown in Table 7-2.

In particle size analyses, the number of particles or the weight fraction of the sample occurring in a definite size range is obtained and plotted against the mean particle size of each range. Such a plot is termed a frequency distribution curve. Results for a sample of material with particle sizes ranging from 0.5 to 3.9 μ are presented in Table 7-2, and the data are plotted in Figure 7-1 both as a frequency distribution curve and as a bar graph or histogram. A figure of this type is very useful, for it depicts the relative amounts of particles that lie within the various size ranges. Furthermore, the contour of the bell-shaped frequency distribution curve is characteristic for each powder sample and provides a rapid estimation, not only of the average particle size, but also of the range of particle sizes within the sample. These characteristics are frequently important considerations in the manufacture, quality control, and bioavailability of the drug and the dosage form. Particle size distribution is, therefore, of considerable utility to the product development pharmacist.

The particle size data are often handled in another manner, whereby the number or weight of particles in each size range is added consecutively to those in the previous ranges to obtain what is termed a cumulative frequency. Data from Table 7-2 presented in this manner are shown in Table 7-3. The cumulative frequency expressed as a percentage of the whole may be plotted against the particle size to yield a graph as shown in Figure 7-2. The size in microns at 50 percent cumulative frequency may then be obtained from the graph to give a median diameter. For example, the result from Figure 7-2 is 2 microns. A number of other averages are used in particle size analysis, and these have been discussed in depth by

TABLE 7-2. DISTRIBUTION OF PARTICLE DIAMETERS IN A POWDER SAMPLE

SIZE RANGE (in microns)	MIDPOINT OF SIZE RANGE	FREQUENCY (number of particles)
0.5–0.9	0.7	2
1.0–1.4	1.2	10
1.5–1.9	1.7	22
2.0–2.4	2.2	54
2.5–2.9	2.7	17
3.0–3.4	3.2	8
3.5–3.9	3.7	5

TABLE 7-3. CUMULATIVE FREQUENCIES FOR SAMPLE OF POWDER*

SIZE RANGE (microns)	FREQUENCY	CUMULATIVE FREQUENCY (number)	CUMULATIVE FREQUENCY (percent)
0.5–0.9	2	2	1.7
1.0–1.4	10	12	10.1
1.5–1.9	22	34	28.8
2.0–2.4	54	88	74.6
2.5–2.9	17	105	89.0
3.0–3.4	8	113	95.8
3.5–3.9	5	118	100.0

* Data from Table 7-2.

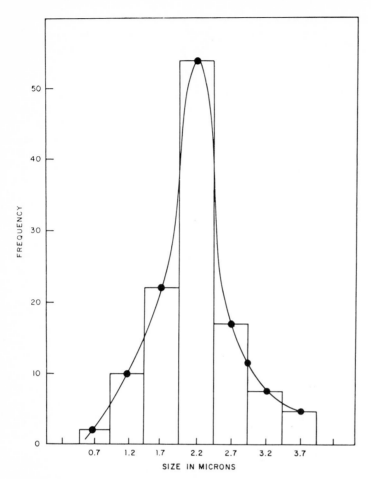

SIZE IN MICRONS

FIG. 7-1. Bar graph and frequency distribution curve, from the data given in Table 7-2. (Martin, A. N., Swarbrick, J., and Cammarata, A.: Physical Pharmacy, ed. 2, p. 471. Philadelphia, Lea and Febiger, 1969)

Edmundson.[16] Only two simple average diameters will be described here, namely the arithmetic mean diameter and the mean volume-surface diameter.

The arithmetic mean diameter is found frequently in expressions of particle dimensions, although it is not a particularly useful measure of size. It is defined as:

$$d_m = \frac{\Sigma \eta d}{\Sigma \eta} \qquad (2)$$

where η is the frequency or number of particles in each class and d is the mean of the size range of the class. The arithmetic mean diameter d_m for the particles of the sample in Table 7-4 is:

$$d_m = \frac{259.6}{118} = 2.2 \, \mu$$

A more useful diameter in particle size analysis is the mean volume-surface diameter, d_{vs}. Its formula and the calculation involved for the sample in Table 7-4 are as follows:

$$d_{vs} = \frac{\Sigma \eta d^3}{\Sigma \eta d^2} \qquad (3)$$

$$d_{vs} = \frac{1551.1}{614.7} = 2.5 \, \mu$$

The mean volume-surface diameter is a size parameter related to the surface area of the particles, and it may be derived from surface area measurements of powders, a topic discussed later.

Optical Microscopy. The ordinary optical microscope is used for the analysis of particles within the range of about 0.5 to 100 μ. The electron microscope is applicable for sizes ranging from 0.001 to 10 μ, and finds more use in the field of colloid dispersions

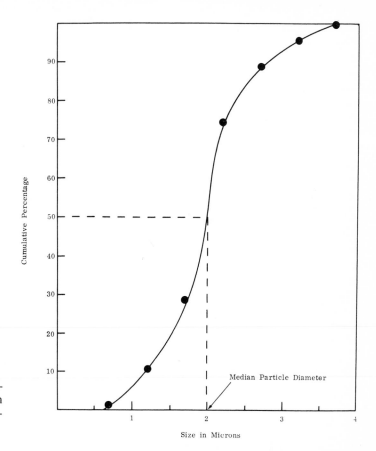

Fig. 7-2. Graphical method of obtaining the median diameter of a sample of particles.

(Chap. 6). In the microscopic method, the sample to be studied is dispersed in a suitable liquid, and the suspension is mounted on a slide or ruled cell. Dry powders may be placed directly on the slide and mixed with a drop of liquid by the use of a small glass rod. The eyepiece of the microscope is fitted with a calibrated micrometer or ruled scale; by matching the particle against the scale, its size may be obtained. In order to obtain statistically valid results, the diameters of at least 500 to 1,000 particles should be obtained. The data are grouped into particle size ranges as illustrated in Table 7-2, and the statistical diameters calculated. Modifications of this technique in-

TABLE 7-4. DERIVATION OF VALUES USED IN CALCULATION OF ARITHMETIC MEAN DIAMETER AND MEAN VOLUME-SURFACE DIAMETER*

SIZE RANGE (microns)	d	η	ηd	ηd^2	ηd^3
0.5–0.9	0.7	2	1.4	1.0	0.7
1.0–1.4	1.2	10	12.0	14.4	17.3
1.5–1.9	1.7	22	37.4	63.6	108.0
2.0–2.4	2.2	54	118.8	261.4	575.0
2.5–2.9	2.7	17	45.9	123.9	334.6
3.0–3.4	3.2	8	25.6	81.9	252.2
3.5–3.9	3.7	5	18.5	68.5	253.3
Totals		118 ($\Sigma\eta$)	259.6 ($\Sigma\eta d$)	614.7 ($\Sigma\eta d^2$)	1,551.1 ($\Sigma\eta d^3$)

* Data from Table 7-2.
d = Midpoint of size range (in microns).
η = Frequency.

volve photographing the particles and measuring the sizes from the film or projecting the microscope field onto a screen and measuring the enlarged particles directly.

The major disadvantage of the microscopic method is that only two dimensions (length and breadth) of each particle are measured. This can lead to significant errors in estimating the mean particle size, especially if the length and breadth of the particles are much greater than the depth.

Sieve Analysis. This method is applicable for particles in the size range of 50 to 5,000 μ. Several sieves are placed one on top of another to form what is known as a "nest" of sieves. The sieves are arranged in a series with the top sieve having the largest openings between the wires and the bottom sieve having the smallest. With 8-inch diameter sieves, approximately 50 to 100 grams of sample is placed on the top sieve; the nest is then attached to a mechanical shaker (Fig. 7-3). After agitation for a known period of time (usually 5 to 10 minutes), the mass of powder retained on each of the sieves is collected and weighed.

The results of such an analysis (Table 7-5) may be plotted as cumulative percentage by weight greater than each sieve size versus the size of the sieve openings in microns to yield a plot and a measure of the average diameter such as those shown in Figure 7-2.

Sieving can of course be used both as a method of particle size analysis and for separating a sample of powder into various size ranges. The method is simple, rapid, and reproducible—provided that the duration of sieving is not excessive, which would lead to attrition and an effective reduction in particle size. Sieving is widely used for sizing granules, a step involved in tablet manufacture.

Sedimentation. The size distribution of a sample of particles dispersed in a liquid may be determined by measuring the rate at which the particles settle in a cylinder. The method is applicable for particles lying in the size range 0.5 to 100 μ, although these limits depend in part on the density of the particles under examination.

The technique is based on the rate of fall of particles in a fluid, which, for noncolliding spheres in a dilute suspension, is given

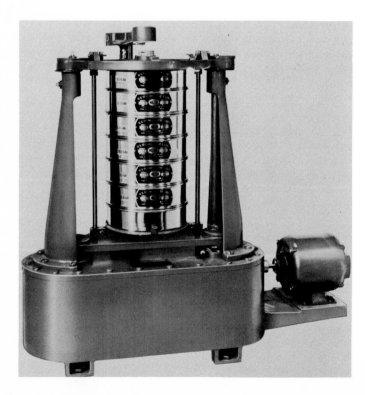

FIG. 7-3. Nested sieves on a power-driven agitator. (The W. S. Tyler Company, Cleveland, Ohio)

TABLE 7-5. RESULTS OF A SIEVE ANALYSIS

SIEVE OPENING (in microns)	SIEVE MESH	WEIGHT GREATER THAN THE SPECIFIED SIZE		CUMULATIVE PERCENTAGE RETAINED ON SIEVE
		g.	percent	
125	115	15	6	6
110	140	10	4	10
74	200	55	22	32
55	270	95	38	70
45	325	50	20	90

by Stokes' law (p. 177). Equation 1 can be rearranged to give the following equation, in which the terms have the same meanings as given previously:

$$d^2 = \frac{18V\ \eta_0}{(\rho - \rho_0)g} \qquad (4)$$

The mean diameter, d, is the diameter in cm. of the normally irregular particle taken as equivalent to the diameter of a perfect sphere of equal density which falls with the same velocity. Thus, the parameter obtained by the sedimentation method of analysis is that of a sphere that would settle at the same velocity as the particle being analyzed. For this reason, the diameter is often termed the Stokes equivalent diameter, d_{st}. When the particles undergoing sedimentation are spherical, d_{st} equals d as defined in Equations 1 and 4. Experimentally, the method measures the fall of a mass of particles; the results are therefore expressed in terms of the weight percentage of the sample which contains particles within a definite range of Stokes equivalent diameters.

The methodology for carrying out sedimentation analysis is fairly simple. Usually, a 1 to 2 percent dispersion of the particles is prepared in a vehicle of known density and viscosity. Frequently, a small amount of a suitable deflocculating agent (e.g., sodium hexametaphosphate) is added to prevent the particles from forming clumps. The dispersion is placed in a cylinder, and samples (usually 10 ml. volumes) are withdrawn from a definite level (10 or 20 cm.) below the surface of the dispersion at various known time intervals. From a knowledge of the time elapsed, the distance of fall (i.e., the sampling depth), the density of the particles, and the density and viscosity of the dispersion medium, the investigator can cal-culate the Stokes equivalent diameter. The actual weight of particles in the withdrawn sample is then determined by a suitable ana-lytical method, or the sample is simply evap-orated and weighed. The particles obtained at each time interval have a size equal to, or less than, the Stokes equivalent diameter calculated according to Stokes' law. The cu-mulative percent by weight and the equiv-alent diameter obtained at each time interval are then arranged as shown in Table 7-6. A plot, similar to that shown in Figure 7-2, is then constructed of cumulative weight versus particle size, and an average particle size is obtained.

More sophisticated instrumented and au-tomated devices are available commercially for sedimentation analyses. The majority of these instruments have an automatic record-ing balance at the bottom of the column which continuously records the weight of particles that have landed on the balance pan. From a knowledge of the weight de-posited versus time curve obtained, the cu-mulative percent by weight can be calculated and plotted against the computed equivalent diameter.

Particle Volume Measurements. A useful technique for determining particle size is based on the principle that a particle in sus-pension will displace a volume of dispersion medium equal to its own volume. If the par-ticle is between two electrodes and if the dis-persion medium is an electrical conductor, the presence of the particle will cause a change in resistance proportional to its vol-ume. In this way, an estimate of the diam-eter of the particle can be readily obtained.

Several instruments based on this principle are now available commercially, including the Coulter Counter (Fig. 7-4). A suspen-sion of particles is prepared in a solution of

TABLE 7-6.   DATA FOR SEDIMENTATION ANALYSIS OF A SAMPLE OF
MAGNESIUM OXIDE

TIME INTERVAL OF SAMPLING 20 CM. DEPTH (minutes)	SEDIMENTATION RATE (cm./min.)	STOKES' LAW DIAMETER d_{st} (in microns)	CUMULATIVE PERCENT BY WEIGHT OF PARTICLES BELOW STATED SIZE
1.3	15.0	96	94
4.0	5.0	53	81
28.6	0.7	20	32
100.0	0.2	10	12

sodium chloride or other conducting solution. The suspension is pumped through a minute hole of known size in a glass cell. If the suspension is sufficiently dilute, the particles pass through the hole essentially one at a time. The passage of each particle displaces a volume of electrolyte in the aperture, momentarily changing the resistance between the two electrodes situated on either side of the opening, and a voltage change having a magnitude proportional to the volume of the particle is produced. The number of particles within each size range is electronically counted and recorded in the instrument. A series of counts is made at various threshold settings for voltage pulse. When the threshold is exceeded, the particle is counted. Thus, each run registers the number of particles having a size larger than the selected threshold size. A fresh quantity of the suspension is pumped through the orifice for each counting run. The recorded results from the series of runs provide the data for plotting the cumulative frequency of particles larger than the stated particle volume. A frequency distribution curve and an average particle size

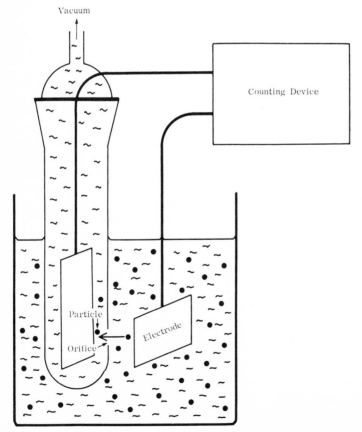

FIG. 7-4.   Diagram of the Coulter Counter, showing the glass cell, the electrodes, and the orifice through which the particles pass when a vacuum is applied to the dispersion.

are thus obtained. Since tens of thousands of particles are counted at each flow-through of suspension, the over-all accuracy of the measurement should be very good. The method is useful in the range of roughly 1 μ to 100 μ and has been used to measure the size of blood cells, emulsion globules, and powdered drugs in suspension. This approach has also been used to follow the dissolution rates of particles in suspension and the changes in particle size that sometimes occur when a suspension is stored over a period of time.[31] The method has also enabled the effect of antibacterial agents on the growth of microorganisms to be determined.[21]

Surface Area Measurement

Frequently, it is of value to know the surface area of the particles in a powder, a suspension, or an emulsion as well as to have a measure of the average particle diameter. This is particularly true when interfacial considerations, such as adsorption, rate of dissolution, and stability of the disperse system, are of importance in the design and the study of a pharmaceutical product.

The specific surface (see Chap. 6) may be obtained by adsorption of a gas on the particles, by adsorption of solutes from solution onto the particles, or by the rate of flow of a fluid* through a bed of the particles.

The specific surface, S_w, expressed as the area per unit mass, is related to the mean volume-surface diameter of the particles by the equation:

$$S_w = \frac{6}{\rho d_{vs}} \qquad (5)$$

where ρ is the density of the material. The equation applies to spheres, but it may also be used for particles that are not greatly different in shape from spheres.

Adsorption of Gases and Solutes. Adsorption at the solid-liquid and solid-gas interface has already been introduced in Chapter 6, together with a consideration of the Freundlich and Langmuir isotherms. Accordingly, the student should be familiar with the fact that if a mass of particles having a large

* The term fluid is used in this chapter to signify either a liquid or a gas.

specific surface is exposed to a gas, the gas is adsorbed on the surface of the particles depending on the pressure, p, of the gas. When the volume in ml of gas adsorbed per gram of powder is plotted against the pressure of the gas, p, relative to the saturation vapor pressure, p_0, of liquefied nitrogen at the temperature of the experiment, a plot of the form shown in Figure 7-5 is obtained. The gas is adsorbed as a layer one molecule thick at low pressures and it becomes multimolecular at higher pressures. The point V_m in the figure signifies the volume of gas in cm.[3] which 1 gram of powder can adsorb on its surface to form a completed layer of gas one molecule thick. The specific surface, S_w, of the particles is given in terms of the monolayer volume, V_m, of gas by the expression:

$$S_w = \frac{A_m N}{M/\rho_0} \times V_m \qquad (6)$$

where A_m is the area of a nitrogen molecule adsorbed on the surface of a particle, N is Avogadro's number, M is the molecular weight of the gas, and ρ_0 is its density at standard conditions of 0°C. and atmospheric pressure. The mean volume-surface diameter, d_{vs}, can then be calculated by the application of Equation 5. The values of monolayer volume, specific surface and mean volume-surface diameter for some pharmaceutical powders are given in Table 7-7.

Experimentally, the gas adsorption method is conducted as follows: Nitrogen or another

TABLE 7-7. SPECIFIC SURFACE MONO-
LAYER VOLUME FOR SOME PHARMACEUTICAL
POWDERS AS DETERMINED BY THE
NITROGEN ABSORPTION METHOD*

MATERIAL	V_m (ml.)	S_w (M²/g.)	d_{vs} (microns)
Ammoniated mercury	0.241	0.93	1.19
Bismuth subnitrate	0.136	0.59	1.93
Sulfadiazine, U.S.P.	0.360	1.57	2.55
Microcrystalline sulfadiazine	3.46	15.1	0.27
Sulfur	0.059	0.25	11.1

* From Swintosky, J. V. et al.: J. Am. Pharm. A. (Sci. Ed.) *38*:308, 1949.

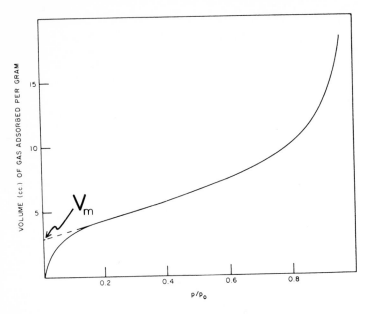

FIG. 7-5. Volume of nitrogen adsorbed on a powder at increasing pressure ratios. V_m represents the volume of adsorbed gas corresponding to the completion of a monomolecular film.

suitable gas is introduced into an evacuated vessel containing the powder, and the volume of gas adsorbed at various pressures is plotted as shown in Figure 7-5. An elaborate method, developed by Brunauer, Emmett, and Teller and known as the BET method, may be used to obtain a more accurate measure of V_m. The method has been used to study the influence of various pharmaceutical methods of comminution on the dimensions of particles in powder form.[52] Haines and Martin[26] used a technique of adsorption from solution to determine the amount of stearic acid required to form a monolayer on particles of sulfamerazine contained in a liquid suspension.

Permeation through Powder Beds. When a gas or a liquid flows through a carefully packed powder bed, the rate of flow of the fluid and the pressure drop across the bed can be measured and used to compute the surface area of the particles in the bed. This technique, which employs the principle of permeability, is known as permeametry. An instrument, the Fisher Sub-Sieve Sizer, is commercially available for measuring specific surface. Another apparatus, the Blaine permeameter, can be obtained from the Precision Scientific Company. The results of permeametry can be converted into a rough average particle size, but the nature of this average is not clearly understood. The in-struments are inexpensive and simple to operate, and give results rapidly; consequently, they are popular for routine measurements.

Bephenium hydroxynaphthoate, included in the 1968 edition of the *British Pharmaceutical Codex,* exemplifies the application of permeametry for the standardization of medicinal agents. The monograph of the *British Pharmaceutical Codex* states that bephenium hydroxynaphthoate must exhibit a surface area of not less than 7,000 sq. cm./g. as determined by an air permeability method. The drug is an anthelmintic which is administered as a suspension, and the activity of the product is reduced if the specific surface of the powder falls below the required value.

Density and Porosity of Particulate Matter

Density is considered ordinarily to be a well understood physical property and an easily determined quantity. However, in regard to particulate matter, it requires careful consideration; moreover, more than one kind of density is recognized in the field of micromeritics.

Density is defined as the mass, or weight, of a substance per unit volume. The weight of a powder or other solid material is determined easily and is unambiguous. The volume determination of nonporous material also is straightforward, but it is more difficult to obtain the volume of particles containing cracks and capillary spaces.

Particle Density. The volume of a nonporous solid is determined usually by immersing the body in a nonsolvent liquid (gases may also be used) and obtaining the weight of the fluid that the body displaces, i.e., the loss in weight of the immersed material. An ordinary weighing bottle or pycnometer may be used for the measurement. The problem of determining the volume of porous particles is more complicated. The displacing liquid or gas may merely surround the particles and not penetrate into the minute pores. For example, a liquid such as mercury normally does not wet the surfaces of solid particles and, therefore, does not enter the pores. Gases such as helium under pressure can be made to fill the crevices of porous particles, and the volume estimated will be smaller than the volume obtained by the use of mercury. Therefore, the computed density, being the mass divided by the measured volume, will be correspondingly greater. Experimental methods for determining the volumes of powdered materials have been described.[49]

Accordingly, the value obtained for the density of a porous solid depends on the ability of the fluid employed to penetrate into the small pores of the particles making up the powder. This phenomenon may be understood more clearly by reference to Figure 7-6, in which two particles of the same composition and approximately the same size and gross shape are shown. One (Fig. 7-6, *top*) is a particle with no cracks or pores, and special fluids need not be used to obtain the true volume of the particle. The density of such a particle is determined readily by the use of either a nonpenetrating medium, such as water or mercury, or a gas such as helium. The density thus obtained is referred to as the true or absolute density of the particle. In Figure 7-6 (*bottom*) is shown a particle with pores that can be penetrated only by a small atom, such as the helium atom, but not by mercury or by water. A smaller particle volume and, hence, a larger density is obtained for the porous particle when helium is employed than would be found if water were used as the displacing fluid. The use of water results in the inclusion of both the solid material and the pore spaces in the total particle volume. On the other hand, gases under pressure penetrate into the tiny pores of the particle, and only the solid material makes a contribution to the measured volume.

The density obtained by media that penetrate into the smaller crevices of porous particles is known as *true density,* and the volume measured is referred to as the *true volume.* The density obtained by media that do not penetrate into the crevices is called *granule density,* and the volume estimated by such means is known as the *granule volume.* Of course, it is possible that very tiny cracks will not be penetrated by even the smallest gas molecules under great pressure. Moreover, internal spaces sealed off from the outside sometimes exist in particles (Fig. 7-6, *bottom*). These cannot be penetrated by any fluid unless the particles are disintegrated so as to expose the hidden cavities. In such cases, true density is somewhat arbitrary and depends on the characteristics of the displacing fluid, the pressure under which it is used, and the possible presence of empty spaces sealed within porous particles. In the case of nonporous particles the true density is obtained by the use of either liquids or gases and does not change under variable gas pressure.

The variability of density and the inability to obtain the absolute density of some porous solids are facts of nature. Once this is recognized, the experimenter will not be startled to find a change in particle density when different displacement fluids are used under varying pressures or when particles are comminuted to expose cracks that may have been sealed deep within the solid.

Bulk Density. Another kind of density— *bulk density*—is often referred to in the literature and represents an important concept in micromeritics. It has no direct relationship to the true density or the granule density of the particles in a powder mass; rather, it deals with the bulkiness of a powder in a container.

Bulk density may be defined as the weight of a material divided by the volume of the powder bulk confined in a container. It depends on the extent to which the powder mass is compacted in the container. Bulk

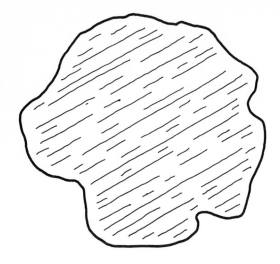

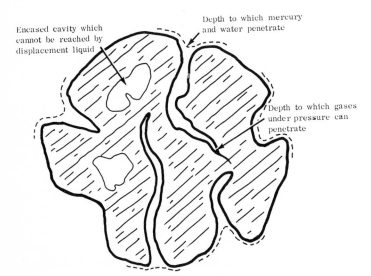

Encased cavity which cannot be reached by displacement liquid

Depth to which mercury and water penetrate

Depth to which gases under pressure can penetrate

FIG. 7-6. Diagram of (*top*) nonporous particles and (*bottom*) porous particle, showing the relationship of particle density to the penetration of the displacing liquid. The deep cracks in the porous particle are penetrated only by small gas molecules. Water and mercury penetrate only to the surface boundary of the particle (dotted line). Unshaded areas within particle represent internal cavities that cannot be reached by the dispersing liquid.

density, or its reciprocal, *bulk specific volume,* is sometimes given for both loosely packed powder and tightly packed powder. The method of measuring bulk density involves introducing a known weight of the material into a graduated cylinder and compacting the powder by a standardized procedure,[7,8] then reading the final volume in ml. occupied by the sample. Thus, the total volume used in expressing bulk density is the sum of the volumes of the solid particles, the pores within the particles, and the spaces between the particles in the cylinder. The more the particles adhere to one another and bridge and arch to form cavities within the

mass in the cylinder, the larger is the estimated bulk volume of a given mass of material. The arrangement of the particles packed in a container is shown schematically in Figure 7-7, in which large empty spaces between the particles as well as the pores within the particles may be observed. The bulk volume of the mass, as read on the graduated cylinder, is 135 ml.

Porosity. Theoretically, spheres of uniform size can pack into one of two arrangements: *close packing,* or *open packing.* The voids or open spaces between the particles in close packing occupy about 26 percent of the bulk and in open packing about 48 per-

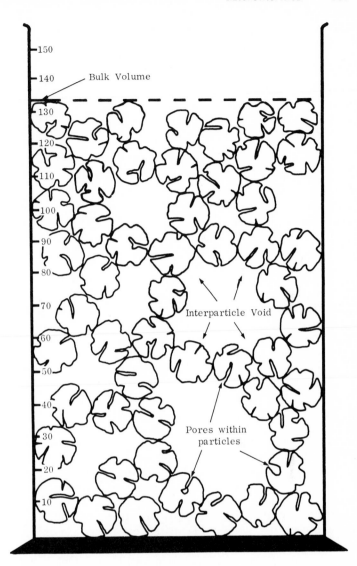

FIG. 7-7. Representation of the arrangement of particles in a container. The bulk volume of the powder is seen to be considerably greater than the total volume of the particles, for it includes interparticle voids and pores within the particles.

cent of the total volume. These figures are often referred to as the bulk porosity of the powder.

Bulk porosity is defined as the ratio of the void volume (the total volume of space between the particles) to the bulk volume of the packing. The void volume is obtained by taking the difference between the bulk volume of the powder mass and the true volume of the particles making up the powder. The powder shown in Figure 7-7 has a bulk volume of 135 ml. If the true volume of the solid particles is found to be 85 ml., the void volume is

$$135 \text{ ml.} - 85 \text{ ml.} = 50 \text{ ml.}$$

and the bulk porosity (expressed as %) is

$$\frac{50}{135} \times 100 = 37\%$$

The particles in real systems are neither spherical in shape nor uniform in size, and they may contain cracks and crevices. Therefore, the porosity can vary considerably from the theoretical limits of 26 percent and 48 percent. Most powders have porosities between 30 and 50 percent. However, in a powder composed of particles of widely different sizes, the smaller particles can become lodged between the larger ones so as to reduce the interparticle void or bulk porosity.

In powders containing aggregates which lead to arches or bridges in the mass (as in Fig. 7-7) the bulk porosity may be considerably larger than the theoretical value of 48 percent.

Stability and inversion of emulsions are related to a similar quantity, namely the volume of globules relative to the total volume of the emulsion. This will be discussed in more detail later in this chapter. The loose and the compact natures of particles in sediments also will be considered later relative to caking and redispersion of materials in suspension.

SUSPENSIONS

Suspensions are a class of official preparations that includes both powders in dry form to be placed in suspension and drugs suspended in liquid vehicles by means of appropriate suspending agents.

Accordingly, a pharmaceutical suspension may be defined as a coarse dispersion containing finely divided insoluble material suspended in a liquid medium or available in dry form to be distributed in the liquid when desired. Sterile suspensions are intended for injection or for ophthalmic use (see Chap. 14).

An acceptable suspension for oral use should possess certain qualities, among which are the following. The material must be composed of small, uniformly sized particles that do not settle rapidly; the particles that do settle to the bottom of the container should not pack into a hard cake and should be redispersed completely and evenly with a minimum amount of agitation; the suspension should not be too viscous to pour freely from the orifice of the bottle; the product should have an agreeable odor, color, and taste and must not decompose or support mold growth during storage. In short, an oral suspension must provide the patient with a uniform, therapeutically active dose of the drug in a preparation that is pleasant and convenient to take.

The particles in a suspension have diameters for the most part greater than 0.1μ. The individual particles range in size from about 0.5 to 5μ; aggregates of particles may attain sizes of 50μ or larger.

Particles with diameters less than 5μ show Brownian movement and remain distributed uniformly throughout the suspension, provided that the collisions do not result in agglomeration, i.e., grouping together in clumps. The small particles that settle may pack into a dense sediment which may set into a rigid cake or clay that is difficult to redisperse. Caking may result from slow chemical reactions or dissolution and recrystallization which may occur between the particles as sedimentation progresses. On the other hand, because of their size, particles that tend to flocculate, i.e., to group together in the form of light, fluffy clumps, settle more rapidly than do individual particles, but they form loosely packed sediments that do not cake and, therefore, are redispersed easily.

Suspensions intended for injection must contain particles of a size such that they can pass freely through the syringe needle. In this regard, the shape of the particle is important. Thus, needle-shaped crystals are frequently desirable in order to produce suspensions that are thixotropic (see p. 116) for use in depot therapy and in sustained release preparations that are given intramuscularly. It is then the length of the long axis of the needle-shaped crystal that is important if one is to avoid blockage of the syringe needle. Crystal growth in suspension, often brought about by temperature fluctuations during storage, is undesirable in all pharmaceutical suspensions, and particularly so in the case of suspensions for parenteral administration.

Ophthalmic suspensions should be formulated such that the particles do not exceed 10μ. Below this size, the patient experiences no pain when the suspension is instilled into the eye. Should the particles greatly exceed this size the patient becomes aware of their presence and experiences pain or a degree of discomfort.

Somewhat similar criteria apply to suspensions formulated for topical use, since they should not feel gritty when applied to the skin. Furthermore, the smaller the particle size the greater the covering and protective power of the preparation. With topical suspensions containing an active ingredient that must undergo dissolution prior to penetration into the skin, particle size affects the rate of dissolution and this may control the rate of penetration.

Formation of Suspensions

Compared to many other types of dosage form used today, suspensions are relatively easy to manufacture. The primary process involved is one of mixing. The major problems arise with the physical stability of the product following manufacture (see p. 201). In the great majority of cases, the process starts with the dry powder which has to be dispersed in the vehicle of choice. Occasionally, the powder is prepared in situ by taking a solution of the drug in a suitable solvent and then causing precipitation by a change of solvent, a change of pH, or a double decomposition reaction to form an insoluble product. The aim in forming a suspension is to make a product that will produce a uniform dispersion of particles immediately prior to and during use of the suspension by the patient. As a consequence, the powder used should be of a relatively small size, e.g., within the range of 1 to 50 microns. Generally, a thickening agent is used in the formulation to reduce sedimentation of the particles or any flocs that might be formed, and a wetting agent is added to assist in the initial dispersion of the particles. Frequently, flavoring and coloring agents and preservatives are also present in the formulation if the suspension is intended for oral administration.

The following section deals with the mechanics of mixing involved in the formation of suspensions and the types of processing equipment used in large and small scale operations. The theoretical aspects of the preparation and formulation of suspensions from the point of view of maximizing physical stability of the product are examined in the section on physical stability (p. 201). Therefore, justification of the presence of additives such as wetting and flocculating agents is treated under that heading rather than in the following section.

Principles of Mixing

To achieve the proper degree of dispersion of solid particles in a liquid vehicle, it is necessary to ensure that adequate mixing is being achieved. Mixing is a combination of two factors. First, there must be an adequate flow of vehicle within the container so that the solid particles are entrained and distributed uniformly throughout the vehicle. Second, sufficient shear should be set up within the system to achieve dispersion of individual particles, rather than agglomerates of particles. These two factors are affected by several variables, including the size and location of the impeller in relation to the container, the speed at which the impeller is operated, and the absence or presence of baffles in the container. The effect of impeller location and the presence of baffles on the flow pattern of the vehicle is shown in Figure 7-8. Slightly different flow patterns are observed if a flat blade turbine impeller is used, rather than the propeller type illustrated. With a relatively large impeller operating at a low speed, the fluid flow is large but the shear set up is low. At the other end

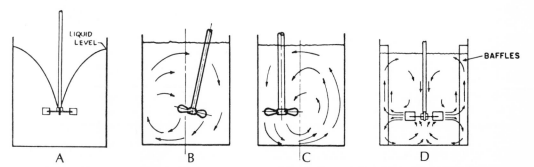

Fig. 7-8. Flow patterns produced by propeller located (A) in center of unbaffled tank, (B) inclined and off center in unbaffled tank, (C) off center in unbaffled tank, and (D) in center of baffled tank. (Oldshue, J. Y.: J. Pharm. Sci., *50*:523, 1961. Reproduced with permission of the copyright owner.)

of the scale, a small impeller operating at a high speed results in a low fluid flow, but with a high level of fluid shear.

Several other factors are involved in efficient mixing, and include viscosity of the vehicle, impeller shape, and the properties of the solid phase. For a detailed discussion of the physical principles involved in the mixing of solid-liquid suspensions, the reader is referred to the article by Oldshue.[48]

Small Scale Processing

For the production of small batches of a suspension, such as might be involved in the extemporaneous preparation of a prescription, a mortar and pestle is most frequently used. The insoluble drug (or drugs) is levigated with a portion of the suspending agent previously dispersed in water to form a mucilage. If the formulation does not call for the use of viscosity-imparting agents, dispersion of the particles may be undertaken by the use of a nontoxic surface-active agent or a levigating agent such as propylene glycol or glycerin. When a smooth paste has been formed, the rest of the vehicle is added in divided portions. Any soluble drugs, flavoring agents, and coloring materials are added to this portion of the vehicle. Instead of preparing a mucilage of the suspending agent, it is sometimes possible to mix the latter as a dry powder along with the other powders in the formula prior to the formation of the smooth paste. Yet another alternative is to wet the suspending agent with a nonabsorbing liquid such as alcohol, glycerin, or propylene glycol. When water is added, it penetrates between the individual particles of the suspending agent, wets them, and ultimately forms a mucilage without producing lumps. The suspension is then transferred to a graduate, and final portions of the vehicle are used to rinse the mortar and pestle. The product is then brought to the desired volume.

Methylcellulose, a commonly used suspending agent, is unique in that it is soluble in cold water and insoluble in hot water. A mucilage of this material is therefore prepared by adding hot water to distribute the particles of the powder. The mixture is cooled or ice-water is added to dissolve the dispersed methylcellulose. The mucilage is then made up to volume.

The degree of dispersion of the final product can sometimes be improved by passing the suspension through a hand homogenizer (Fig. 7-9). The small model has a capacity of about one pint. The suspension is placed in the bowl of the homogenizer and the operator uses a pumping action on the lever arm to force the suspension through an orifice in the bottom of the bowl and against a spring-loaded plate. Care must be taken not to do this too vigorously, especially if a wetting agent has been used, otherwise an excessive amount of air may be introduced into the product, resulting in the formation of a foam. The hand homogenizer is also useful for the bench preparation of emulsions (see p. 214).

Large Scale Processing

Suspensions are prepared on the industrial scale by the use of large mixing tanks fitted with a variable speed stirring device, such as a propeller or a turbine impeller (Fig. 7-10). Invariably, the product is then passed through a homogenizer or colloid mill, which operates on a continuous flow basis.

The homogenizer for large-scale manufacturing is operated electrically rather than by hand. The principle of operation is, however, the same—passage of the suspension through a narrow orifice under pressure to achieve shearing and particle dispersion. Frequently, with the use of high pressures, particles that have undergone homogenization tend to clump together to form floccules. This may be undesirable. It then becomes

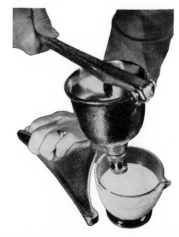

Fig. 7-9. Small hand homogenizer.

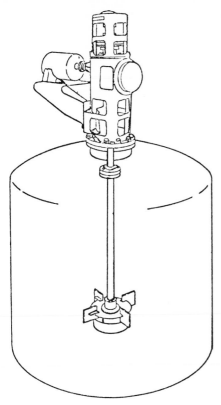

FIG. 7-10. Mixing tank fitted with variable speed turbine impeller. (From Perry's Chemical Engineers' Handbook. Ed. 4, p. 19-7. New York, McGraw-Hill, 1963. Copyright 1963, McGraw-Hill. Reproduced with permission of McGraw-Hill Book Company.)

on the shear produced between cone-shaped discs, one of which is stationary while the other rotates at a high velocity. The distance between the two discs is on the order of thousandths of an inch and can be varied, thereby affecting the amount of shear applied to a particular system. A typical colloid mill is shown in Figure 7-11. The rotor and stator discs are shown in Figure 7-12. The suspension is gravity-fed into the hopper; by means of the auger, the suspended particles are forced through the adjustable gap between the stationary and rotating discs; the sheared, homogenized particles are then passed out through the bottom of the mill. The product can be recycled if needed; alternatively, two such mills can be set up in series. In this way, continuous operation can be maintained. The operation of impellers, homogenizers, and colloid mills has been reviewed.[35]

PHYSICAL PROPERTIES OF DISPERSED PARTICLES

As mentioned earlier in this chapter, the main problem associated with the successful formulation of suspensions is achieving a uniform dispersion of particles at the time the patient uses the product, whether it be oral, topical, or administered parenterally by the physician or nurse. It is therefore necessary to consider those factors affecting physical stability, namely particle-vehicle and particle-particle interactions and the rheological properties of the suspension. Particle-vehicle interactions are significant in wetting and dispersion of particles; particle-particle interactions play an important role in flocculation/deflocculation mechanisms. An appreciation of the various types of flow is necessary in order to understand the contribution rheology can make to the successful formulation of pharmaceutical suspensions.

Particle-Vehicle Interactions

When a solid is reduced to small particles by comminution, the surface area is greatly increased and the free energy associated with the surface becomes correspondingly larger. The particles are now highly energetic and tend to agglomerate into larger masses in order to obtain a minimum surface free energy. This agglomeration is commonly re-

necessary to employ a two-step homogenization process in which the pressure of the second homogenization is considerably less than that of the first step. The second pass breaks down the floccules formed as a result of the first, high pressure, step. For example, the pressure employed in the first step of two-stage homogenization might be from 2,500 to 5,000 pounds per square inch while a pressure of 500 to 1,000 pounds per square inch might be used in the second step.

The colloid mill is used frequently as an in-line process for suspension preparation. The term "colloid mill" is really a misnomer —the process produces only a very low percentage of particles in the colloidal size range. The action of the colloid mill is based

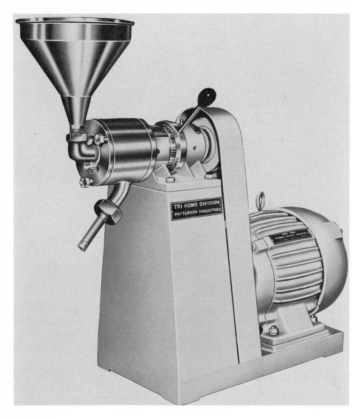

FIG. 7-11. Colloid mill. (Tri Homo Division, Patterson Industries, East Liverpool, Ohio)

ferred to as *flocculation*. This phenomenon occurs both in air and in liquid media and is responsible for the clumping of solid particles in suspensions. The situation also occurs in emulsions. Because of this tendency, systems of finely dispersed particles are unstable from a thermodynamic point of view. They attempt to achieve thermodynamic stability by adhering to each other and reducing the free energy at the particle surfaces.

The increase in surface free energy, ΔF, which results from dividing a substance into fine particles and dispersing it in a liquid medium has already been discussed in the previous chapter. The relevant expression is:

$$\Delta F = \gamma_{sl} \cdot \Delta A \qquad (7)$$

where γ_{sl} is the interfacial tension between the liquid medium and the particles, and ΔA is the increase in surface area resulting from the decrease in particle size. This simplified expression disregards the electrical potential at the surface of the particles, which will be treated at another point in the discussion.

The suspension approaches a thermodynamically stable condition as ΔF approaches zero. As seen in Equation 7, this state may be reached either by lowering the interfacial tension or by reducing the interfacial area. The interfacial tension can be reduced by the addition of surface active agents, but it cannot ordinarily be made equal to zero. However, the use of such agents is desirable because they can reduce the excess surface free energy primarily through surface tension reduction, rather than decreasing the interfacial area. Accordingly, dispersion of the particles within a vehicle is promoted. Such materials are termed wetting agents. While they serve to disperse the particles in the medium they also reduce the tendency of the material to flocculate.

The initial dispersion of the particles in a suspension constitutes the first important step in the manufacturing process. Powders that are wetted with difficulty by the vehicle are called lyophobic. The particles of lyophobic powders tend to clump and float on the surface of the vehicle as, for example,

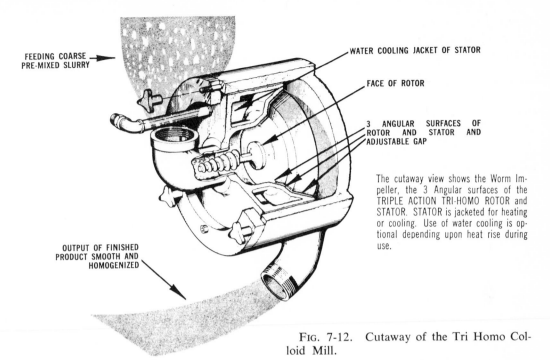

FEEDING COARSE
PRE-MIXED SLURRY

WATER COOLING JACKET OF STATOR

FACE OF ROTOR

3 ANGULAR SURFACES OF
ROTOR AND STATOR AND
ADJUSTABLE GAP

The cutaway view shows the Worm Impeller, the 3 Angular surfaces of the TRIPLE ACTION TRI-HOMO ROTOR and STATOR. STATOR is jacketed for heating or cooling. Use of water cooling is optional depending upon heat rise during use.

OUTPUT OF FINISHED
PRODUCT SMOOTH AND
HOMOGENIZED

FIG. 7-12.   Cutaway of the Tri Homo Colloid Mill.

sulfur or magnesium stearate do in water. Layers of air and other contaminants may adhere to the particles, making them even more difficult to wet and disperse in the medium. Lyophilic or solvent-attracting powders are easily wetted by the vehicle and present no great difficulty in the initial dispersion stage. Examples are talc and magnesium carbonate in water.

The wettability of lyophobic powders may be increased by passing the material through a colloid mill in the presence of a wetting agent. Alcohol, glycerin, and other hygroscopic liquids frequently are used in the initial wetting stage to displace the air, disperse the particles, and allow penetration of the vehicle into the powder mass.

Hiestand[29] has suggested a useful test for choosing the best surfactant for the wetting and the initial dispersion of powders in aqueous media. He uses a trough several inches long, coated with Teflon or paraffin, at one end of which is placed the powder and at the other the solution of the wetting agent. The rates of penetration of various detergent solutions into the powder mass can be observed directly.

As will be discussed in a later section dealing with formulation, although good dispersion through the use of wetting agents is desirable, it can lead to caking within any sediment formed subsequently.

Particle-Particle Interactions

Attraction and repulsion between particles result from forces that reside at the particle surfaces. Equation 7 accounted only for the surface energy arising from the interfacial tension and the extension of the surface area. Of prime importance in considering flocculation and deflocculation is the presence of surface electrical charges and the distribution of ions around the particles. This phenomenon has been detailed in the previous chapter (p. 155 et seq.). As was described, the source of the charge on particles may arise because of ionizable groups on their surfaces or because of adsorption of ions from the surrounding solution. Regardless of the specific mechanism, the particles will all bear either a negative or a positive charge. The electrostatic repulsion thereby set up between adjacent particles prevents them from adhering to one another.

The surfaces of the particles can also become solvated, which, in turn, helps to prevent particles coming together. In the presence of a suitable vehicle, a surface charge or the possession of a solvated sheath around the particles results in the dispersion of primary particles rather than aggregates. Accordingly, deflocculation occurs.

Flocculation results from the collision and combination of primary particles in a suspension. If the particles are protected by a barrier of electrical charge or adsorbed molecules, not all collisions will result in binding. The greater the protective barrier the slower will be the rate of combination of the particles; when the electrical or molecular barrier is very large, flocculation will be negligible.

Brownian motion is sufficient to bring about the collision of small particles, from less than 1 to 5 μ, but is relatively ineffective in producing the contact of larger particles in a suspension. The large particles may be brought into contact by mild agitation to increase the rate of flocculation, but mechanical agitation and the motion caused by thermal convection can also deflocculate a system. Thus, initial flocculation of particles is usually rapid, followed by a long period before an equilibrium is finally reached. Vigorous agitation and the addition of certain protective polymers may lead to a deflocculated system. The properties of flocculated and deflocculated particles in suspension are summarized in Table 7-8.

Sedimentation Parameters

The protective effect of the electrical double layer against flocculation has been described previously (Chap. 6). Agents that can be added to the medium to promote flocculation by counteracting the effect of the protective layer are termed flocculating agents. The three types of flocculating agents commonly used are electrolytes, detergents, and polymers. However, before discussing their mode of action in any detail, it is necessary to introduce two so-called sedimentation parameters that are used as semiquantitative measurements of flocculation in a suspension. These are the sedimentation volume, F, and the degree of flocculation, β.

Sedimentation Volume. This parameter, given the symbol F, is defined as the ultimate volume of the sediment, V_u, divided by the original volume, V_o, of the suspension before settling:

$$F = \frac{V_u}{V_o} \qquad (8)$$

The sedimentation volume, F, of a product may have a value of less than 1, more than 1, or equal to 1. When F is less than 1, we have the ordinary case in which the sediment settles to some ultimate volume that is less than the original volume of the

TABLE 7-8.   PROPERTIES OF FLOCCULATED AND DEFLOCCULATED PARTICLES
IN SUSPENSION*

DEFLOCCULATED	FLOCCULATED
1. Particles exist in suspension as separate entities.	Particles form loose aggregates.
2. Rate of sedimentation is slow, since each particle settles separately and particle size is minimal.	Rate of sedimentation is high, since particles settle as a floc, which is a collection of particles.
3. A sediment is formed slowly.	A sediment is formed rapidly.
4. The sediment eventually becomes very closely packed, owing to weight of upper layers of sedimenting material. Repulsive forces between particles are overcome and a hard cake is formed which is difficult, if not impossible, to redisperse.	The sediment is loosely packed and possesses a scaffoldlike structure. Particles do not bond tightly to each other and a hard, dense cake does not form. The sediment is easy to redisperse, so as to reform the original suspension.
5. The suspension has a pleasing appearance, since the suspended material remains suspended for a relatively long time. The supernatant also remains cloudy, even when settling is apparent.	The suspension is somewhat unsightly, due to rapid sedimentation and the presence of an obvious, clear supernatant region. This can be minimized if the volume of sediment is made large. Ideally, volume of sediment should encompass the volume of the suspension.

* Swarbrick, J.: *In* Remington's Pharmaceutical Sciences. ed. 14, p. 331. Easton, Pa., Mack Publishing Co., 1970.

suspension. In those cases in which F is greater than 1, the ultimate sediment volume is greater than the original volume of the suspension. This result at first appears to be an impossibility, but it is readily understood when one realizes that as the particles form a loose fluffy network in the vehicle the final volume of the sediment may swell sufficiently to become greater than the total volume of the original suspension.[15] When F = 1, the sediment is equal to the total volume of the suspension and the product is said to be in a state of "flocculation equilibrium." Such a product is quite acceptable from a pharmaceutical standpoint because, on standing, it shows no sediment or clear supernatant.

Degree of Flocculation. A better parameter for evaluating flocculation in a suspension is the degree of flocculation, β, which describes the relationship between the sedimentation volume of the flocculated suspension, F, to the sedimentation volume of the same suspension when deflocculated, F_{inf}. A completely deflocculated or peptized suspension will have a relatively small ultimate volume of sediment, and this can be designated as V_{∞}. The sedimentation volume of such a suspension, F_{∞}, is written thus:

$$F_{\infty} = \frac{V_{\infty}}{V_0} \qquad (9)$$

The ratio of F to F_{∞} is the degree of flocculation, β:

$$\beta = \frac{F}{F_{\infty}} \qquad (10)$$

Substituting for F and F_{∞} in Equations 9 and 10, the significance of β becomes apparent:

$$\beta = \frac{V_u/V_0}{V_{\infty}/V_0} = \frac{V}{V_{\infty}} \frac{\text{(Ultimate sediment volume of flocculated suspension)}}{\text{(Ultimate sediment volume of deflocculated suspension)}} \qquad (11)$$

Thus, β is observed to be a measure of the degree of flocculation of a system. A suspension consisting of floccules held loosely in an open scaffoldlike arrangement will be

characterized by a large β value. Conversely, a suspension containing a highly condensed sediment has a small β value. The lower limiting value of β is 1. Under such conditions F = F_{∞}, i.e., there is no flocculation in the system.

Studies have shown that the shape and the size of the suspension particles and the distribution of sizes can influence β.[29] The temperature, the density, and the viscosity of the medium are less influential factors.

In Figure 7-13 are shown a deflocculated and a flocculated suspension of a material, together with the sedimentation volume ratios and the β value.

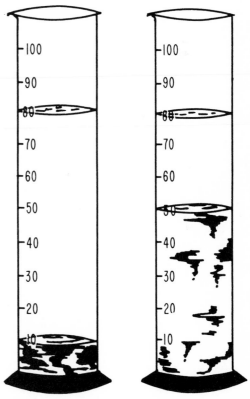

Deflocculated

$$F_{\infty} = \frac{V_u}{V_0} = \frac{10}{80} = 0.125$$

Flocculated

$$F = \frac{V_u}{V_0} = \frac{50}{80} = 0.625$$

$$\beta = \frac{F}{F_{\infty}} = \frac{0.625}{0.125} = 5.0$$

FIG. 7-13. Deflocculated and flocculated suspensions of a material, illustrating the calculations of the sedimentation volume ratios, F_{∞} and F, and the β value.

Flocculating Agents

Particles in suspension that have acquired a surface charge will tend to repel one another, resulting in the formation of a deflocculated dispersion. This can be reversed by the use of flocculating agents which include electrolytes, detergents, and polymers. The mode of action of each of these types is described briefly here and can be studied in more detail in the paper by Hiestand.[29]

Electrolytes as Flocculating Agents. Electrolytes are frequently used for flocculating the particles of suspensions to obtain a product of large sedimentation volume. The ions probably reduce the electrical barrier between the particles and, also, form a bridge between particles so as to link them together.[26,44,46,64] Thus, the particles are held in a loosely arranged structure in suspension. Although these large aggregates settle rapidly, they yield an open cell-like structure and are easily resuspended by agitation.

The use of an electrolyte may be illustrated by the addition of monobasic potassium phosphate, a negative flocculating agent, to a suspension of bismuth subnitrate, the particles of which are positively charged (Fig. 7-14). Initially, the bismuth subnitrate particles have a large positive charge, as shown in Figure 7-14. With the addition of monobasic potassium phosphate, the apparent zeta potential ζ, a measure of the charge on the particles, decreases to the point at which the system is observed under the microscope to exhibit maximum flocculation. Sedimentation studies were made on the bismuth subnitrate suspension with increasing concentrations of the flocculating agent, monobasic potassium phosphate. V_u/V_o (F) was found to be low initially,

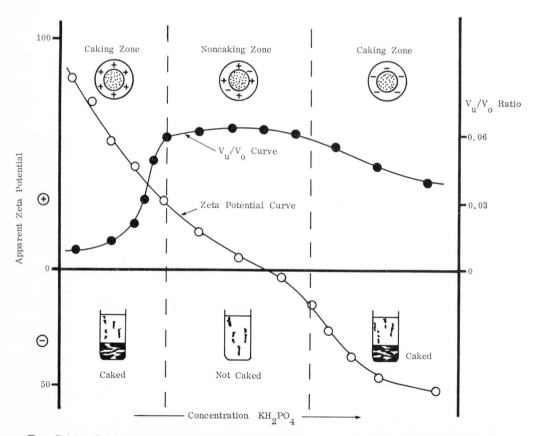

FIG. 7-14. Caking diagram, showing the flocculation of a bismuth subnitrate suspension in which monobasic potassium phosphate was employed as the flocculating agent.

a condition that suggests a close-packed sediment of bismuth subnitrate particles. Flocculation by KH_2PO_4 increases the sediment volume relative to the initial value until V_u/V_o reaches a maximum value. This is referred to as the "noncaking zone" in Figure 7-14. Additional flocculating agent neutralizes the charge on the particles and can eventually reverse the charge from positive to negative and again yield a caked suspension. Similarly, a negatively charged product, such as a sufamerazine suspension, can be flocculated with a positively charged agent such as aluminum chloride. Wilson and Ecanow[64] presented evidence to show that flocculation can be accounted for by the formation of chemical bonds between the particles of the suspension and the ions of the flocculating agent. They consider the bridging action of the flocculating ions to be more important than the neutralization of surface charge on the particles. The formation of chemical bonds perhaps leads to a decrease in the apparent zeta potential, such as may be observed in Figure 7-14. Whatever the reason for the electrokinetic changes, the results of zeta potential measurements correlate well with sedimentation volume ratios; and both ζ and F may be used as indices of caking.

Detergents as Flocculating Agents. Both ionic and nonionic surfactants have been used to bring about flocculation of the particles in suspension. Hiestand[30] demonstrated the use of an ionic surface-active agent to increase the sedimentation volume. Nonionic detergents such as polyoxyethylated nonylphenols also may be adsorbed onto suspended particles and can produce flocculated systems at the appropriate concentration.

Polymers as Flocculating Agents. Lyophilic polymers are commonly used as suspending agents in pharmaceutical products. According to Silberberg,[59] the polymer molecules contain active groups spaced along their chains. Part of the long molecules may be adsorbed on the particles, leaving extended segments projecting out from the particle surfaces. The ends of the polymer may be adsorbed, and loops of the intervening chain segments may protrude into the medium. These ends or loops are available for bridging across to adjacent particles and, thus, produce a flocculated system.

A number of hydrocolloids are polyelectrolytes. Their flocculating action is dependent on the pH and the ionic strength of the medium, and an optimum pH is observed for sedimentation. Gelatin, a natural hydrocolloidal material, may be used to bring about flocculation and prevent caking.[5] In this process, soluble sodium sulfathiazole was precipitated from acid solution in the presence of gelatin. The powder, "Microform" sulfathiazole, thus prepared was found to flow freely in the dry state and did not cake in suspension. Although sulfathiazole itself was negatively charged, the "Microform" sulfathiazole powder was found to be positively charged, presumably owing to the fact that in an acid medium gelatin bears a positive charge.[44] Haines and Martin[26] proposed the use of fatty acid amines and quaternary amines to render the particles in suspension positively charged and, thus, to produce free-flowing powders with anticaking characteristics.

In the preparation of suitable suspensions, the suspending agent may act both as a protective colloid to keep the settled particles from caking and as a flocculating agent to produce the loose cell-like structure in the liquid medium. Through its rheological properties the suspending agent itself may provide a certain consistency to assist in supporting the particles. It is therefore appropriate at this point to consider the rheological properties of suspensions.

Rheological Properties of Dispersed Particles

The reader has been introduced to the various types of flow in Chapter 6. A knowledge of the flow, or rheological, properties of particulate dispersions is valuable to the pharmacist engaged in the development and production of pharmaceutical suspensions. Thus, prevention of sedimentation, ease of particle redispersion, and the development of a product that either pours readily from its container or spreads evenly over the skin are all factors that depend in large part on the rheological characteristics of the product.

In a deflocculated suspension (or emulsion, for that matter) where the concentration of dispersed particles is relatively low (less than 10%), the viscosity is essentially Newtonian. In a more concentrated dispersion, non-Newtonian flow occurs, owing to the attractive forces between the particles becoming sufficiently large that flocculation takes place. Analysis of these structured dispersions in a rotational viscometer yields flow curves that are ordinarily recognized as being either plastic, pseudoplastic, or dilatant. Frequently, thixotropy is associated with these flow patterns. All of this has been discussed in detail in Chapter 6.

The characteristics of plastic flow are believed to be determined by the latticelike structure of floccules and larger aggregates in the dispersion. A definite force equivalent to the yield value must be exceeded in order to overcome the attractive force between the particles before the material will begin to flow. The relationship of suspension stability to yield value of the product has been investigated[47] using a carboxyvinyl polymer. In the studies, permanent suspensions of several powdered materials were prepared when sufficient polymer was added to provide a critical minimum yield value.

Thixotropy, the time-dependent sol-gel reversible transition, is found frequently to be associated with systems exhibiting plastic flow. In describing such systems quantitatively it is necessary to specify their thixotropy, yield value, and plastic viscosity. A statement of any one of these parameters alone is not sufficient to describe the overall consistency of a complex material. The yield value, plastic viscosity, and qualitative estimation of thixotropy of some products are included in Table 7-9. Foernzler et al.[19] studied the role of thixotropy in suspension stability. Zinc oxide was suspended in an aqueous vehicle containing an activated attapulgite as the thixotropic suspending agent. The velocity of sedimentation of the powder was found to be approximately inversely proportional to the thixotropy of the suspension.

Pseudoplastic flow is frequently exhibited by liquid dispersions of high molecular weight polymers. The characteristic bowed curve of a pseudoplastic material results from the shearing of the long polymer molecules. At rest, these molecules are entangled and in disorder. As the shearing stress is increased, the molecules become aligned in the direction of flow and tend toward an ordered arrangement. The internal resistance of the material decreases and, thus, the viscosity is reduced. As the shearing stress is lowered, the molecules return to their former matted arrangement and the viscosity increases.

When a viscous suspending agent is added to the product, as is a common practice in commercial suspensions, the plastic viscosity of the simple particle-vehicle system can be modified considerably by the pseudoplastic character of the suspending agent. The various factors that influence the rheological properties of suspending agents are discussed in the article by Martin et al.[45]

Dilatancy is another phenomenon which involves changes in consistency of a product with agitation. As described in Chapter 6, dilatant systems thicken with an increase of shear—the opposite of what is found with pseudoplastic products. Dilatancy is found in deflocculated suspensions containing 50 percent or more of solid particles. When

TABLE 7-9.   RHEOLOGICAL PROPERTIES OF SOME NON-NEWTONIAN MATERIALS*

MATERIAL	PLASTIC VISCOSITY (poises)	YIELD VALUE (dynes/sq.cm.)	THIXOTROPY
Lotions, emulsions, oil base paints, ketchup	low 0.1–5	low to medium 0–500	low
Creams, mayonnaise	low 1–10	medium 100–5,000	medium
Ointments	medium 5–50	high 1,000–10,000	medium to high
Resins, asphalt	high 1,000–10,000,000	high —	—

* Modified from Fischer, E. K.: Colloidal Dispersions. p. 156. New York, Wiley, 1950.

agitated, the particles crowd against one another, displacing the medium. As a result, the resistance to flow increases markedly. When the shearing force is removed, the liquid medium can return to coat the particles once more, and the resistance to flow is reduced. Dilatant materials are potentially hazardous if unrecognized, since they can jam and overload high speed roller and colloid mills.

FORMULATION OF SUSPENSIONS

We must now turn our attention to the formulation of suspensions, with a view to optimizing the physical stability of the product, its utility to the patient, and the bioavailability of the drug. There are several criteria with which a suspension should comply if it is correctly formulated. These may be summarized as follows:

(1) A uniform dispersion of particles must be obtained immediately prior to, and during, the use of the product.

(2) The flow characteristics must be such that the product can function correctly. For example, if it is an oral suspension, it must flow readily from the container. If for topical use, the product must spread evenly and easily on the skin, yet should remain confined to the area of application.

(3) The particle size must be such that the release characteristics of the drug comply with the proposed use of the product. Thus, the size of the primary particles in an oral suspension containing a systemically active drug must be such that optimum bioavailability is achieved. If an ophthalmic product, the particles must be of a size that does not cause pain to the patient when placed in the eye.

Physical Stability of Suspensions

The degree of success in achieving a uniform dispersion of particles when a pharmaceutical suspension is being used hinges on the ability of the formulator to promote the physical stability of the particles present. Thus, at first sight it would appear adequate to ensure that (a) the particles settle as slowly as possible, and (b) when a sediment is formed, it should be readily redispersed by shaking. However, as the following discussion will seek to demonstrate, the problem of physical instability is not solved that easily, and frequently the formulator has to compromise between slow sedimentation and facilitated redispersion.

Up until perhaps ten or fifteen years ago, physical stability of suspensions was most commonly achieved by reducing the particle size and/or increasing the viscosity of the dispersion medium in accord with Stokes' law (p. 178). There are, however, limits to these approaches. For example, processing of solids by comminution down to particles on the border between the coarse and the colloidal size range can be time-consuming and involve the use of expensive equipment. Furthermore, the increase in total surface area frequently may cause uncontrolled clumping of the particles, owing to the high surface free energies generated. Coupled with these considerations, the formulator must take into account the relationship between particle size and drug dissolution. Thus, with orally administered drugs, it may be eminently desirable to reduce the particle size in order to increase the specific surface and potentiate drug dissolution. This reduction in particle size would be compatible with increased physical stability due to a decreased sedimentation rate. However, if the product is a suspension for intramuscular use, a reduced particle size could be a distinct disadvantage if the product is designed to elicit a sustained effect brought about by slow dissolution. Biopharmaceutical considerations would obviously outweigh physical stability considerations in this instance.

An additional complication can arise with suspensions formulated solely on the basis of particle size reduction. Invariably, in such suspensions, the particles are deflocculated because of the presence of a common surface charge. If a sediment does form during the shelf life of the product, it is often virtually impossible to achieve redispersion because of a slow fusion of the discrete particles that originally form the densely packed sediment. This phenomenon of particle fusion is termed "caking." As we have already seen (p. 156), whether there is a net energy of attraction or repulsion between two particles depends on their distance of separation. As one particle approaches another there is, at a certain distance, a small net energy of attraction. It is in this attractive energy "well" that the particles lie when flocculated. They are prevented from coming any closer and developing stronger attractions by the presence of a high energy of repulsion. If, however, this energy barrier can be overcome, a very strong attraction is set up between the particles, causing them to fuse with one another and form a "cake." In a sediment of deflocculated particles, this large energy barrier is thought to be overcome by the mass of the high density sediment bearing down on the bottom particles. This forces the particles together and effectively "pushes" them over the energy barrier into the region of strong attraction. The cake so formed progresses upward through the sediment as a function of time and the packing of the sediment. The process cannot be reversed by shaking, as can flocculation, and it is thus impossible to obtain a uniform dispersion of the drug. Caking does not occur in the sediment of a flocculated suspension because the density of the sediment is low, owing to the very open porous structure of the flocs.

In conjunction with a reduction in particle size, the other traditional approach has been to raise the viscosity of the dispersion medium to the point at which sedimentation is very slow. Two major disadvantages accrue from this approach. First, it frequently becomes extremely difficult to remove a dose from the bottle, vial, or other container in which the product is packaged. Second, although it is possible to reduce significantly the rate of sedimentation by raising viscosity, it is not generally possible to *halt* sedimentation. As a result, when particles do reach the bottom of the container, thereby producing an unequal distribution of drug, it is difficult to redisperse the particles adequately prior to use. This is because the high viscosity vehicle which served to slow down sedimentation now serves to drastically hinder redispersion. This can be overcome in part by the use of shear-thinning vehicles (see p. 200).

Although an undesirable degree of sedimentation and/or caking does not arise in all instances of suspensions containing deflocculated particles, increasing numbers of formulators have felt the need to utilize another approach when developing products. This involves the deliberate flocculation of the particles and the subsequent suspension of the floccules in a moderately viscous vehicle that possesses shear-thinning properties. As presented in the next section, this results in a product in which, even though sedimentation is fairly rapid, caking is absent, and redispersion is accomplished usually with mild shaking. Thus, although the appearance of the suspension may be thought by some to have suffered, the utility and physical shelf life of the product have been enhanced.

Controlled Flocculation. The mode of action of flocculating agents was discussed on page 198. The relationship between zeta potential, sedimentation volume, and presence or absence of caking as a function of flocculating agent concentration shown in Figure 7-14, forms the basis for preparing flocculated suspensions. Thus, the formulator prepares a deflocculated dispersion of particles, generally using a wetting agent to aid dispersion; controlled flocculation is then attempted by the use of a flocculating agent (p. 198). The aim is to add that concentration which results in the maximum sedimentation volume, for under these conditions caking is minimized. This can be achieved in the laboratory by setting up a series of dispersions to which increasing amounts of various flocculating agents are added. Confirmation of data can be obtained if zeta potential determinations are carried out simultaneously and the test suspensions are checked periodically for any tendency toward caking or poor redispersibility. The approach has been illustrated (p. 198) using a model system of bismuth subnitrate, which bears a net positive charge in water, flocculated with monobasic potassium phosphate, the anion of which acts as the flocculating agent by reducing the positive zeta potential of the bismuth subnitrate particle. In the more usual case of negatively charged particles, such as sulfonamides, flocculation can be readily achieved by the addition of polyvalent cations, such as Ca^{++} and Al^{+++}.

It is not necessary for the zeta potential to reach zero before flocculation occurs, because there are always forces of attraction between particles. Thus, when the zeta potential is lowered to a particular value, which depends on the material in question, the attractive forces just exceed the repulsive forces, owing to common charge effects, and flocculation takes place. There is, accordingly, a range of zeta potential, extending on both sides of zero, within which flocculation will occur under a given set of conditions. The approach of controlled flocculation is summarized in Figure 7-15, under (B).

Controlled Flocculation in Structured Vehicles. This represents perhaps the ultimate in suspension formulation, since it results in a noncaking and readily dispersible suspension that does not settle readily.

In practice, the approach described above and designated (B) in Figure 7-15 is not widely used as such because the flocs settle rapidly and leave an unsightly supernatant layer. Consequently, a suspending agent with the appropriate rheological properties, such as carboxymethylcellulose, bentonite,

Carbopol 934, or a combination of these is added to produce a final product with sufficient structure to support the particle flocs but not so rigid as to prevent flow when the material is agitated and poured from the vessel. Most suspending agents belong to the class of negatively charged hydrophilic colloids; when added to suspensions containing positively charged flocculating agents, they tend to produce an unsightly stringy mass of coagulated suspending agent which settles rapidly and fails in its suspending action.

Phosphate ions and other negatively charged agents which are used to flocculate positively charged particles are compatible with the commonly used suspending agents, and they pose no serious problems. The scheme is shown in Figure 7-15, under (C).

The difficulty with negatively charged drugs mentioned above may be overcome by adsorbing onto the drug particles certain agents that will reverse the surface charge from negative to positive. This may be accomplished by the use of fatty acid amines, gelatin at a pH below its isoelectric point, or other positively charged molecules. Then

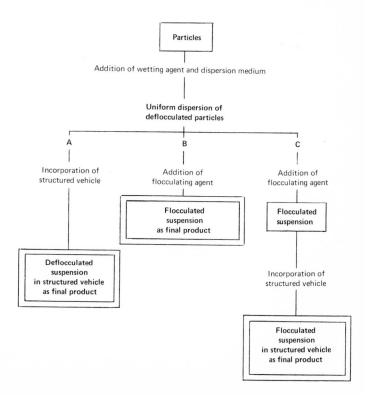

FIG. 7-15. Alternative approaches to the formulation of suspensions (Swarbrick, J.: *In* Remington's Pharmaceutical Sciences. Ed. 14, p. 333. Easton, Pa., Mack Publishing Co., 1970)

KH_2PO_4 or another anionic agent can bring about the appropriate flocculation. These flocculating agents are not incompatible with the commonly used suspending agents.

The technique of adsorbing a positively charged substance on suspension particles followed by flocculation with a negative ion and, finally, stabilization of the product with a negatively charged suspending agent is illustrated in Figure 7-16. The steps in this scheme are summarized as follows:

1. The particles, irrespective of their charge, are coated with a positively charged agent (which of course must be checked for lack of toxicity before use). Flavoring,

coloring and other ingredients are added in the ordinary manner.

2. The particles are flocculated by use of a negatively charged agent to bring the product into the noncaking zone (see Fig. 7-14).

3. Finally, a minimum amount of the desired suspending agent or mixture of suspending agents is added, and the suspension is again observed for optimum flocculation and freedom from caking.

Both a good and a poor product are illustrated in Figure 7-17: On the right is the kind of product that can be prepared by the application of the principles discussed in

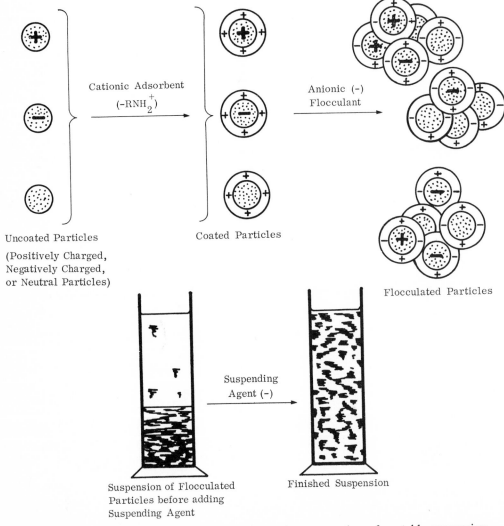

FIG. 7-16. The sequence of steps involved in the preparation of a stable suspension.

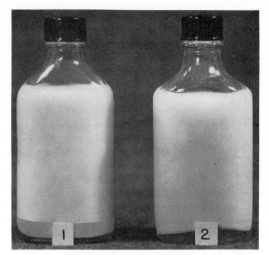

FIG. 7-17. Suspensions of sulfamerazine. (*Left*) A deflocculated product that shows a caked sediment. (*Right*) A well flocculated suspension, with a viscous suspending agent. (Haines, Bernard: Ph.D. Thesis, Purdue University, 1960. *In* Martin, A. N.: J. Pharm. Sci., *50*:516, 1961)

the preceding paragraphs. The suspension on the left was prepared with the particles in the deflocculated state, to which a viscous suspending agent was added. The particles in this product were well suspended for some time by the viscous agent; however,

when they eventually settled, they formed a compact cake, which can be seen in the bottom of the container (Fig. 7-17, *left*). The sediment could not be redispersed even by vigorous agitation of the bottle. The product shown in Figure 7-17, *right,* contained just sufficient suspending agent to support the small flocs and allow their rapid redistribution on agitation. This method should be applicable for positively charged or neutral particles as well as negative particles. Any of these charge types of powders, or a mixture of charge types, may be coated with the positively charged agent and treated as outlined in this section to produce stable noncaked suspensions.

Flocculated suspensions can be differentiated from deflocculated ones by microscopic examination if one is careful to wait a sufficient time for flocculation to develop. Flocs appear under the microscope as large clumps of loosely arranged particles (Fig. 7-18, *left*). The individual particles in a deflocculated suspension fall more slowly, but, after settling, they may form a cake of strongly aggregated particles. Particles from such a caked sediment removed from a sulfamerazine suspension are shown in Figure 7-18, *right*.

As indicated here, rate of sedimentation

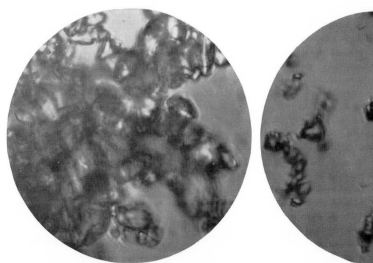

FIG. 7-18. Photomicrograph of sulfamerazine particles. (*Left*) A clump of particles from a flocculated suspension. (*Right*) Particles from the caked region of a deflocculated suspension. (Haines, Bernard: Ph.D. Thesis, Purdue University, 1960. *In* Martin, A. N.: J. Pharm. Sci., *50*:516, 1961)

is less important to the suspension technologist than is a knowledge of the structural properties of the particles and the suspending medium in a system that has reached a state of equilibrium.

Rheological Considerations

Regardless of whether the formulation of a particular suspension is treated in accord with (A) or (B) in Figure 7-15, the flow properties of the structured vehicle and the final product must be taken into account. This is important with respect to prevention of settling of the dispersed particles, promotion of resuspension of the material when the container is shaken, and provision of proper flow properties of the product for ease of pouring from the bottle and, in the case of products for external application, ease of spreading over the affected area.

When a suspension remains at rest on the shelf, only a negligible shear is produced in the product as the particles slowly settle. But when the container is shaken and the product is poured from it, a high rate of shear is produced. When the product is passed through a colloid mill or forced through a syringe, the shear is also large.

Kostenbauder and Martin[39] estimated the rate of shear created in spreading a layer of ointment on the surface of the skin. Henderson et al.[28] also determined the approximate rates of shear encountered in certain processes. The results are recorded in Table 7-10.

In selecting a rheological instrument for

the analysis of a pharmaceutical product, it is desirable to choose a viscometer that operates within a shear range roughly comparable to that produced by the treatment that the product will undergo in practice. A number of rheological instruments and their ranges of speed have been reviewed by Martin et al.[45] Further, the components of a product should be chosen on the basis of the rheological properties that they exhibit under various conditions of flow. For example, a suspending agent should have a high viscosity at negligible shear when the suspension remains at rest during storage, and it should exhibit low viscosity at high shear rates when it is being agitated, poured from its container, or spread on an affected area.

Pseudoplastic materials such as tragacanth, sodium alginate, and sodium carboxymethylcellulose show those properties. The flow curves of these agents, together with the curve for glycerin, are shown in Figure 7-19. Glycerin and other Newtonian liquids do not exhibit the desirable change in viscosity with shear rate that is characteristic of

TABLE 7-10.   APPROXIMATE RATES OF SHEAR FOR VARIOUS PHARMACEUTICAL OPERATIONS

OPERATION	RATE OF SHEAR*
Spreading ointment on skin	400–900 sec.$^{-1}$
Rubbing on ointment tile	500 sec.$^{-1}$
Colloid mill processing	100,000 sec.$^{-1}$
Hypodermic needle passage	Up to 10,000 sec.$^{-1}$
Nasal spray from plastic squeeze bottle	2,000 sec.$^{-1}$
Pouring from bottle	Less than 100 sec.$^{-1}$

* The rate of shear, G, is given in reciprocal seconds, sec.$^{-1}$ or 1/sec., because $dv/dr = G$ can be expressed in the units of (cm./sec.)/cm. or 1/sec.

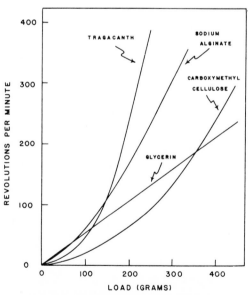

FIG. 7-19.   Rheological flow diagrams of pseudoplastic suspending agents. The flow curve of glycerin, a Newtonian liquid, is included for comparison. (Martin, A. N., Swarbrick, J., and Cammarata, A.: Physical Pharmacy. ed. 2, p. 525. Philadelphia, Lea and Febiger, 1969)

pseudoplastic materials. The consistency of glycerin is not sufficient to support the particles in a suspension; thus, glycerin does not yield a product that redisperses, pours easily, and spreads smoothly on the skin.

Hiestand[29] suggested that the particles could perhaps be supported in liquid suspension by the use of a vehicle, the molecular aggregates of which exhibit a cell-like structure in which the particles would become entrapped. He called such a medium a *structured vehicle*. The use by Meyer and Cohen[47] of Carbopol 934, a structured vehicle of high yield value, has already been mentioned.

Haines and Martin[26,44] have stated that adequate suspension could be attained by flocculating the particles to be supported and then adding just enough suspending agent to help support the flocs, yet allow rapid redispersion of the drug on agitation and pouring from the container. A vehicle of high consistency is not desired, since it may not permit rapid resuspension of settled material, may not pour well from the container, and may leave a thick tenacious film on the skin and the mucous membrane which is unpleasant and difficult to remove.

For the suspending agent, Martin[46] has suggested that a combination of gums, one exhibiting pseudoplasticity and the other thixotropy, might provide a desirable vehicle for the support of particles in liquid suspension. Samyn[53] has tested this possibility. He found that the best formulation could easily be determined for a new suspension by preparing a series of samples in which the ratio of thixotropic and pseudoplastic materials was varied until optimal flow properties for permanent particle suspension was attained. The advantage of the vehicle combination is that the system remains in a gelled state at rest but pours freely after the container is agitated. The combined thixotropic and pseudoplastic nature of the vehicle may be observed in Figure 7-20, in which the flow curve is shown. Note the very high viscosity at low r.p.m. and the low viscosity (steep slope of the line) at high r.p.m. The thixotropy of the vehicle is evidenced by the area of the hysteresis loop.

Probably the best solution to the problem

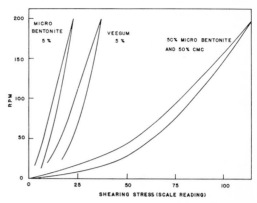

FIG. 7-20. Flow curves for the individual suspending vehicles, bentonite and Veegum, and for the combined suspending agent consisting of a mixture of bentonite and carboxymethylcellulose. The combined agent shows both thixotropy and pseudoplasticity. (Martin, A. N., Swarbrick, J., and Cammarata, A.: Physical Pharmacy, ed. 2, p. 526. Philadelphia, Lea and Febiger, 1969)

of suspension of particles in a liquid vehicle may be achieved by combining the use of structured vehicles and particle flocculation. However, the structure associated with the vehicle may prove to be insignificant relative to the flocculation structure which, according to Heistand,[29] probably makes the major contribution to the support of the particles in the medium.

It should be apparent to the reader that the successful formulation of suspensions involves the principles of rheology, micromeritics, physical chemistry, and electrokinetics. Only when these concepts have been properly applied will the final product be both therapeutically effective and aesthetically pleasing to the patient.

Biopharmaceutical Considerations

Suspensions are a highly effective dosage form in terms of bioavailability, ranking second only to solutions when administered orally.[22] It is easy to see why suspensions are normally more effective than tablets or capsules, even though the particle size of the material used in both may have been identical at the start. Drug particles formulated in a tablet invariably undergo some enlargement as a result of compression, and the tablet must undergo disintegration to achieve an increase in surface area that even approaches that of particles or floccules in a suspension. Rupture of the capsule shell is usually regarded as a prerequisite for dissolution and availability from capsule dosage forms. Consequently, although the particles released from the capsule might be of the same size range as those in a suspension, at least some delay may be expected before absorption from the capsule form took place. No such delay would be expected from a suspension formulation.

With poorly absorbed drugs it is reasonable to assume on the basis of available surface area that deflocculated dispersions might be better absorbed than flocculated ones. However, one must be careful to consider the physical state (i.e., flocculated versus deflocculated) of the suspension in vivo. The presence of endogenous materials in the gastrointestinal tract may markedly change the in-vitro physical state of the suspension following its administration.

Particle size and shape, the presence of polymorphic forms, and the addition of complexing agents are some of the factors that can be expected to affect the dissolution and bioavailability of drugs whose absorption is dissolution-rate limited. The reader is referred to Chapters 10 and 11 for a discussion of these factors as they are involved in tablet and capsule dosage forms. The possible consequences of some of these factors in regard to drug bioavailability from suspensions will be considered here.

Brief mention has already been made of some of the aspects of particle size control that can influence the bioavailability of oral suspensions, the release rate of parenteral products, and the patient-acceptability of ophthalmic suspensions. However, the alert formulator must be aware that other physical properties of the total suspension can modify the anticipated effect of a change in particle size and, therefore, specific surface. Two such properties are viscosity and polymorphism.

A slowing down in the rate of drug dissolution from suspensions for intramuscular injection is normally obtained by increasing particle size. Surprisingly, however, when a highly thixotropic nonaqueous gel was used as the vehicle for such a product of procaine penicillin, the effect (as indicated by blood levels) was prolonged as the particle size was reduced below 5 μ.[6] It was postulated that this effect was due to these very small particles being actually trapped in the pore-like structure of the gel. The larger particles used, it was assumed, did not enter the pores of the gel to the same extent and were therefore unable to undergo the same degree of entrapment. The dissolution rate of the larger particles was accordingly more rapid than that of the finer, but entrapped, particles.

In recent years an increasing number of pharmaceutical substances have been shown to exhibit polymorphism, which may be defined as the existence of one or more crystalline forms of a single chemical entity. The polymorph or polymorphs produced depend on such factors as the choice of solvent used for crystallization and the time-temperature sequence used in dissolving and subsequently recrystallizing the solid. Polymorphs are chemically indistinguishable from one another, but they possess different x-ray diffraction patterns, melting points, and other physical properties. The pharmaceutical significance of the potential existence of polymorphs of a drug lies in the different solubilities possessed by different polymorphs and the effect this has on dissolution rate and bioavailability. The pharmaceutical applications of polymorphism have been discussed.[27]

Under a given set of environmental conditions, one polymorph will be stable and all other polymorphs present will be converted to the stable form. The rate of conversion, which either may be very rapid or may take place over a span of years, is the important factor which determines, in large part, whether polymorphism in that compound will be an advantage or a disadvantage in the formulation. As a general rule, the polymorph that is most stable at a given temperature and pressure is the least soluble and the least stable is the most soluble. Therefore, if the rate of conversion to the stable polymorph is slow or can be effectively retarded, it may well be worth using the unstable polymorph in the formulation because of its greater solubility. On the other hand, a fairly rapid conversion frequently requires that steps be taken to ensure that all of the drug is in the stable form prior to making the suspension. Cortisone, sulfathiazole, riboflavin, chlormaphenicol palmitate, and methylprednisolone are all examples of contemporary drugs whose biological availability and therapeutic efficacy have been found to vary because of the formation of different polymorphs. Biopharmaceutical differences have also been observed between crystalline and amorphous forms of penicillin G, insulin, and novobiocin. For a more detailed discussion on these drugs, and other physical factors that can affect bioavailability, the reader is referred to papers by Macek[43] and Gibaldi.[22]

Polymorphism can also lead to undesirable changes in the physical state of the suspension. Frequently, if the drug in suspension is composed of more than one polymorph, conversion of all the unstable forms to the stable polymorph can result in an increase in particle size and the formation of a cake in the sediment.

OFFICIAL SUSPENSIONS

The suspensions for oral administration and external application in the *U.S.P. XVIII* and *N.F. XIII* represent two types: (1) suspensions of the drugs together with other agents in an aqueous or nonaqueous medium, and (2) dry powder mixtures containing the drug, the suspending agent, and other adjuncts, all to be dispersed in water when required. Examples are contained in Table 7-11. The individual monographs of the U.S.P. and N.F. should be consulted for specific information concerning these and other official suspensions. Sterile and ophthalmic suspensions are dealt with elsewhere in this book (Chaps. 8 and 14).

EMULSIONS

An emulsion may be defined as a preparation consisting of two immiscible liquids, usually water and oil, one of which is dispersed as small globules in the other. Unless a third component—the emulsifying agent—is present the dispersion is unstable, and the globules undergo coalescence to form two separate layers of water and oil.

The aqueous phase may contain water-soluble drugs, preservatives, and coloring and flavoring agents. It is desirable to use distilled or deionized water, since calcium and magnesium ions, found in hard water, can have an adverse effect on the stability of some emulsions, particularly those containing fatty acid soaps as the emulsifying

TABLE 7-11.   TYPES OF OFFICIAL SUSPENSIONS FOR ORAL ADMINISTRATION AND EXTERNAL APPLICATION

TYPE OF SUSPENSION	GENERAL DESCRIPTION	EXAMPLES
For oral administration in aqueous vehicle	The active ingredient, or ingredients, suspended in a suitable suspending or dispersing agent. The oral suspensions frequently contain flavoring agents, coloring and preservatives, and some of them are also buffered.	Calcium Novobiocin Oral Suspension, N.F.; Kaolin Mixture with Pectin, N.F.; Primidone Oral Suspension, U.S.P.; Tetracycline Oral Suspension, U.S.P.
For oral administration in nonaqueous vehicle	In the only example, particles are suspended in a vegetable oil.	Methenamine Mandelate Oral Suspension, U.S.P.
For oral administration following the addition of vehicle	Dry mixtures of the active ingredient, together with suitable suspending agents, flavors, colors, preservatives and, occasionally, buffers. The product is dispersed in water when required.	Demeclocycline for Oral Suspension, N.F.; Nystatin for Oral Suspension, U.S.P.; Phenoxymethyl Penicillin for Oral Suspension, U.S.P.
External application	An aqueous stabilized suspension (of selenium sulfide) containing a suitable dispersing agent, a buffer, and a detergent.	Selenium Sulfide Detergent Suspension, N.F.

agent. Care must be taken to ensure that flavors and preservatives which may have some oil solubility are present in the aqueous phase in a concentration sufficient to elicit their desired effect. The oil phase of an emulsion frequently consists of fixed or volatile oils and drugs that exist as oils, such as oil-soluble vitamins and antiseptics. It is frequently necessary to add an antioxidant to prevent autoxidation of the oil and consequent rancidity and/or destruction of any vitamin present. Oils used in the preparation of emulsions should also be kept free of microorganisms, since these too can cause rancidity. The emulsifying agent is the most important component of the emulsion in terms of achieving stability. At one time, natural emulsifying agents were used almost exclusively in pharmacy. However, they are being continually replaced by synthetic emulsifying agents that are highly surface active. Solid particles have also been used, although their pharmaceutical applications have been somewhat limited. As will be discussed in detail later, all emulsifying agents act by forming a film around the dispersed globule. This film acts to prevent coalescence and separation of the dispersed liquid as a separate phase.

Two types of emulsion can exist; a product in which oil is dispersed as globules in water (an oil-in-water or o/w emulsion), and one in which water is dispersed as globules in the oil phase (a water-in-oil or w/o emulsion). In an o/w emulsion, the oil is sometimes referred to as the "internal phase," the water being the "external phase." With w/o emulsions, water is the internal phase and oil is the external phase. A photomicrograph of an o/w emulsion is shown in Figure 7-21. Currently, there are only two "official" emulsions, Sterile Phytonadione Emulsion, *U.S.P. XVIII* and Mineral Oil Emulsion, *N.F. XIII*. However, the number of emulsified products commercially available and of interest to the pharmacist is quite large, especially among cosmetic and dermatologic preparations. In addition, certain emulsified products for external use appear in both the *U.S.P.* and the *N.F.*, although these are not given the title Emulsion. These include some liniments, lotions, creams, and ointments.

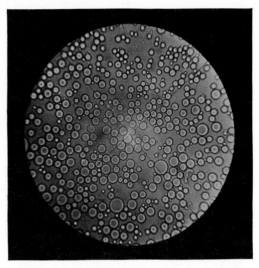

FIG. 7-21. Photomicrograph of an oil-in-water emulsion, showing the globules of oil dispersed throughout the continuous aqueous phase. (Atlas Surface-Active Agents, Wilmington, Del., Atlas Chemical Co.)

USES OF EMULSIONS

Based on the use to which they are put, emulsions are divided into two groups—emulsions for internal use, and emulsions for external application. Emulsions for internal use may be administered orally or by intravenous injection. Emulsions used externally are applied to the skin or the mucous membranes.

Orally Administered Emulsions

Pharmaceutical emulsions which are given orally are of the oil-in-water type. The enveloping of the medicinal oil in a film of emulsifying agent aids in masking the disagreeable taste and the "oily" sensation which often accompany the oral administration of such a drug. Flavoring agents may be added to the external aqueous phase of the emulsion to increase the palatability.

The distribution of drugs and flavors between the oil and the water phases is an important consideration in disguising unpleasant tastes. According to the distribution principle, a substance will be found in both phases of an emulsion but will concentrate predominantly in the liquid in which it is more soluble. The attempt to mask a distasteful drug by oil-in-water emulsification may be defeated if the drug possesses some water-solubility and passes partially into the external phase, and if the flavor and the masking agent are predominantly oil-soluble and concentrate primarily in the internal phase.

Emulsification is also useful for increasing the absorption of fats through the intestinal walls. It is first necessary to consider briefly the stages of fat digestion and assimilation. When fats and oils are ingested, they are emulsified in the duodenum by the bile salts. Then the emulsified fats are partially hydrolyzed by the pancreatic juice and are finally absorbed through the intestinal wall. That portion of fat which is not broken down to fatty acids and lower glycerides may be absorbed in the emulsified form and passed into the bloodstream if the emulsion globules are less than about 1 μ in diameter.

Olive oil and mineral oil in emulsified form are assimilated rapidly when the particles are sufficiently small.[34,56,57] Consequently, the most efficient absorption is attained by dispersing the oil by homogenization into globules preferably of about 0.5 μ diameter.

Intravenous Injection of Emulsions

Parenteral emulsions have been studied for administration of food and medicinal oils in both animals and human beings. Vitamin A is taken up rapidly by the tissues when injected in the form of an emulsion.[25] Emulsified chaulmoogra oil, vitamin K, and some sex hormones have also been injected, and rats have been protected from rickets by injections of a cod liver oil emulsion.[38] Emulsified oils also have been injected as diagnostic aids in the study of the function of the liver and other organs. Hom et al.[32] studied the emulsification of a radiopaque substance to be administered intravenously for visualization of the liver and the spleen.

Parenterally administered emulsions require special care during manufacture. The choice of the emulsifying agent and the size and the uniformity of the globules are critical in preparations for intravenous use. Egg lecithin was used in the early work, but later investigations showed it to be hemolytic. A sterile form of gelatin, serum albumin, purified soybean phosphatides, and combinations

of sorbitan esters of fatty acids and their polyoxyethylene derivatives have been used. However, as a result of preliminary clinical trials,[41] untoward physiologic effects were found in man which militated against the widespread use of such emulsifiers.

The preparation of emulsions for injection involves the formation of a coarse emulsion, which is then homogenized, collected and sealed in sterile flasks, and autoclaved. Finally, the product is tested for sterility and for globule size.

Emulsions for External Application

Both o/w and w/o emulsions may be applied to the surface of the skin and the mucous membranes. By the process of emulsification, it is possible to produce a lotion or a cream that has the proper consistency, spreads well over an affected area, is washed from the surface easily, does not stain clothing, and is appealing to the patient from the standpoint of general appearance, odor, color, and "feel." When one contrasts the well-formulated emulsion base of today with the greasy product of earlier times, it is not difficult to realize why the physician and the patient demand the modern dermatologic preparation.

Emulsification of a drug in a base may lead to a decrease in the rate and the extent of absorption through the skin and the mucous membranes. This principle is employed in the use of an o/w emulsion of ephedrine which, when applied to the nasal mucosa, is absorbed more slowly than an oil solution of the drug. The presence of the medication is thus prolonged in the desired area.

However, emulsification sometimes increases the rate of *percutaneous absorption*, i.e., absorption into and through the skin. Water-soluble antiseptics are absorbed through the skin more readily when incorporated in the aqueous phase of o/w bases than when administered in greasy vehicles. Coal tar is absorbed more effectively from an emulsified base, and the physician should reduce the concentration of coal tar below that which ordinarily is specified when the drug is administered in a grease base. The degree to which the concentration of coal tar should be reduced has not yet been established, but usually it is safe to lower it to about one half of the original strength.

Other factors influencing the percutaneous absorption of drugs and the selection of appropriate ointment bases (including emulsified bases) are discussed in Chapter 8.

FORMATION OF EMULSIONS

The preparation of stable emulsions depends on how well the formulator can (a) disperse one liquid as droplets in another and (b) stabilize this dispersion against coalescence or fusion of the droplets, which ultimately would result in the return of the system to its original state, i.e., two separate liquid phases. A successful formulation is one in which dispersion is optimized and maintained, while any coalescence is minimized.

Dispersion and Coalescence of Droplets

If two immiscible liquids in contact with each other are shaken vigorously, the interface between them first becomes distorted. "Fingers" of liquid penetrate the opposing phase from which droplets break off and are dispersed in the other liquid. Thus, in a mixture of oil and water, there are formed simultaneously oil droplets in water and water droplets in oil. Which of these dispersions ultimately predominates in a stable emulsion is discussed later in a consideration of emulsion type (p. 214). The size of the dispersed droplets is a function of several parameters, among which is the rate of shear applied to the system. Generally, the higher the rate of shear, the finer the dispersion produced. At some point in time, no further reduction in size takes place, because the number of new droplets formed is offset by the increased number of collisions resulting in coalescence and a resultant decrease in the number of total particles. It is obviously uneconomical to continue agitation beyond this point, which is often reached within 1 to 5 minutes depending on the degree of agitation employed. In actuality, the most dramatic reduction in particle size occurs within the first few seconds following the initiation of agitation.

From Equation 7 (p. 194), the reader is aware that a reduction in particle size, with a concomitant increase in surface area, raises the free energy of the system. A thermodynamically unstable dispersion has been produced from what was a thermodynamically stable system comprised of two separate bulk phases. As a result, once agitation ceases, the process of coalescence becomes the significant process, for this works to reduce the excess free energy created in the system during dispersion.

Coalescence is the actual fusion of two or more liquid droplets to form a larger droplet. It is preceded by flocculation, or the coming together of two or more particles. The phenomenon of flocculation and the factors that govern it has been described earlier, under *Suspensions* (p. 194). The coalescence of droplets dispersed in a liquid is usually quite rapid because of the relatively small energy barrier opposing their fusion. As a consequence, even though an excellent dispersion may be readily prepared by the use of equipment generating an adequate rate of shear, reformation of the original bulk phases is rapid unless steps are taken to stabilize the dispersion. Stabilization is achieved by the addition of an effective emulsifying agent which is adsorbed at the interface between the dispersed droplet and the dispersion medium. In this way, a "barrier" to coalescence is introduced into the system. As will become apparent in the next section, this "barrier" can be an energy barrier and/or a mechanical barrier. As a result, even if flocculation of the stabilized droplets occurs (i.e., by reduction of the energy barrier), there still exists a mechanical barrier opposing coalescence. This is because the flocculated droplets are still separated by a "sandwich" consisting of a thin layer of continuous phase between the two interfacial layers of emulsifying agent surrounding the droplets. Thus, whereas in an unstabilized dispersion (i.e., no emulsifying agent present) flocculation necessarily precedes coalescence, coalescence is not a necessary consequence of flocculation in a stabilized system (i.e., one containing an adequate concentration of an effective emulsifying agent). A more detailed description of the role of emulsifying agents in stabilizing emulsions is given in the next section.

Stabilization of Dispersions

Emulsions are stabilized by the presence of a film that is formed at the interface between the oil and water phases. The material that is adsorbed to form this film is referred to as the emulsifying agent. The type of film produced falls into one of three classifications, namely monomolecular, multilayer, and solid particle (Table 7-12).

The emulsifying agents, obviously, must have a degree of affinity for the interface between the two phases. With the monomolecular and multilayer films, the emulsifying agent must be soluble in both phases to some extent. However, it should not be too soluble in any one phase, otherwise it will not be adsorbed to the interface but will remain instead in the bulk of that phase. A similar balance must exist for solid particles to function as emulsifying agents. If wetted too strongly by either phase, the particles will move into that bulk phase rather than remain at the interface.

The emulsifying agents that form monomolecular films are highly surface active and lower surface tension in proportion to their tendency to be adsorbed at the oil/water interface. This relationship is expressed in quantitative terms by Gibbs' equation (see Chap. 6). Coalescence is prevented by the presence of a coherent yet flexible film, and the stability is enhanced by the reduction in excess surface free energy brought about by the usually marked reduction in interfacial tension. If the emulsifying agent is ionic, additional stability is present owing to the mutual electrical repulsion between adjacent droplets. However, the most frequently used examples of this type of emulsifying agent are the nonionic surfactants. The manner in

which these agents stabilize emulsions has recently been the subject of review.[18]

Multilayer films are formed by naturally occurring hydrophilic colloids, such as acacia. These compounds function as emulsifying agents primarily because of the mechanical strength of the films formed rather than their negligible ability to lower interfacial tension. Although widely used in the past, especially for the extemporaneous preparation of emulsions, they have been largely replaced by synthetic surfactants which form monomolecular films of the type described above.

Friberg and Wilton[20] have suggested that, under certain conditions, the approach of two droplets stabilized by a monomolecular film can result in the emulsifier concentration between the oil droplets being increased and the water content reduced to the point where liquid crystalline phases are formed. These highly ordered multilayer structures would be expected to confer upon the system a high degree of resistance to coalescence.

The use of solid particles as emulsifying agents in pharmaceutical preparations has also declined with the advent of synthetic agents whose structures can be chemically manipulated far more readily to produce a range of compounds with differing physical properties. When solids are used, the particles must be wetted by both the oil and the water phase. The phase that preferentially wets the particles will become the continuous phase. Additionally, the particles must be small in relation to the size of the droplets they are to stabilize.

TABLE 7-12.   MECHANISM OF ACTION OF EMULSIFYING AGENTS

TYPE OF FILM	EXAMPLE	MECHANISM
Monomolecular	Potassium laurate Polyoxyethylene sorbitan monooleate	Coherent, flexible film formed by surface-active agents. These agents also lower interfacial tension markedly, and thus contributes to stability of emulsion. Are widely used, especially the nonionic type. Depending on the particular agent(s) chosen, can prepare O/W or W/O emulsions.
Multimolecular	Acacia Gelatin	Strong, rigid film formed, mostly by hydrocolloids which produce O/W emulsions. Interfacial tension is not reduced to any degree; stability due mainly to strength of interfacial film.
Solid Particle	Bentonite Graphite Magnesium hydroxide	Film formed by solid particles that are small in size compared to the droplet of dispersed phase. Particles must be wetted by both phases to some extent in order to remain at the interface and form a stable film. Can form either O/W or W/O emulsions, depending on method of preparation.

* Swarbrick, J.: *In* Remington's Pharmaceutical Sciences. ed. 14, p. 339 Easton, Pa., Mack Publishing Co., 1970.

The mode of action of these three types of emulsifying agent is illustrated in Figure 7-22.

Emulsion Type

Whether the emulsion formed is of the o/w or w/o type depends on such factors as the relative amounts of each phase present (often expressed in terms of the phase volume ratio), the properties of the emulsifying agent used, and the sequence in which the various components are added during preparation.

Intuitively, one might suppose that the larger of the two phases present will become the continuous phase. This tends to be so, although of more significance is the emulsifying power of the agent employed to bring about a particular type of emulsion. For example, an emulsifying agent with a well-developed capability to form stable o/w emulsions can often cause the formation of an o/w emulsion composed of 80 percent oil dispersed as droplets in 20 percent water.

When phase volumes are similar, the order of mixing may be the most important factor affecting the type of emulsion formed. This is discussed on page 215.

The reader will recall from page 212 that when oil and water are shaken together, water droplets will be dispersed in oil and oil droplets will be dispersed in water simultaneously. According to Davies,[13,14] the type of emulsion formed in the presence of an emulsifying agent depends on the relative rates of coalescence of these o/w and w/o dispersions. Thus, if the w/o dispersion is transient and coalesces rapidly, while the o/w dispersion is stabilized by the emulsifier added, the final product is a stable o/w emulsion. The interested reader should consult the original papers of Davies for complete details of this interesting concept.

Methods of Achieving Emulsification

A number of different pieces of emulsifying equipment are used to achieve optimal dispersion of droplets. These include both hand-operated and power-driven machines.

Small Scale Processing. The Wedgwood or porcelain mortar and pestle are used most frequently in the laboratory or prescription department for the emulsification of fixed, and sometimes volatile, oils. The glass mortar and pestle is often unsatisfactory for this purpose, since the surfaces are not sufficiently rough to create adequate shear. However, it is possible, when using many of the highly active synthetic emulsifying agents (p. 218), to obtain excellent preparations by simply adding the warmed phases to a beaker and stirring until cool. In place of a beaker, the phases can sometimes be placed into a bottle, which is then shaken.

Kitchen-type mixers and blenders have also been used for the preparation of small batches of emulsions. Care must be taken to ensure that excessive amounts of air are not whipped into the product. A widely used device is the hand homogenizer whose operation has been outlined earlier in the section dealing with suspensions (p. 192). Hand homogenizers are particularly useful for further reducing the droplet size of relatively coarse emulsions that have been pre-

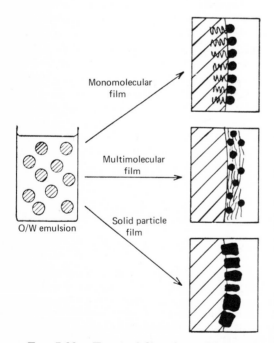

FIG. 7-22. Types of films formed by emulsifying agents at the oil/water interface. Orientations are shown for o/w emulsions. ▨: oil; □: water. (Swarbrick, J.: *In* Remington's Pharmaceutical Sciences. ed. 14, p. 338. Easton, Pa., Mack Publishing, 1970)

pared by another method, such as the mortar and pestle.

Large Scale Processing. The equipment used in the preparation of large batches of emulsions parallels that described earlier for suspensions (p. 192). Thus, emulsions are prepared using large tanks or vessels provided with jackets that permit heating and cooling of the ingredients and a high speed propeller or turbine impeller. The relatively coarse emulsion is then passed through a homogenizer (generally of the 2-stage type) or a colloid mill. The latter is favored when the emulsion is too viscous for homogenization or when suspended solids are present in the mixture.

Another type of homogenizer is commercially available which utilizes high frequency (ultrasonic) radiation to disrupt the liquids and achieve droplet dispersion. The apparatus can operate at an ultrasonic frequency of about 20,000 cycles per second, equivalent to a homogenization pressure of 30,000 p.s.i. It is not used to any great extent by the pharmaceutical industry.

Order of Mixing

Of considerable importance to the ease of preparation of an emulsion and the stability and type of the final product is the order in which the separate phases are mixed. Whether the emulsifying agent is added initially to the oil phase or the water phase is an additional factor.

There is no single order of mixing that universally produces the best emulsion. This is because the same component added at different times can result in either an o/w or a w/o emulsion. In addition, one sequence may be more desirable than another, depending on whether a small-scale process (using the mortar and pestle) or a large-scale process is being employed. The type of emulsifying agent can also dictate the order of mixing. For example, preparation of an emulsion using a natural gum, such as acacia or tragacanth, invariably requires greater attention to the sequence of addition than does the use of a synthetic nonionic emulsifier. With the latter it is almost impossible not to make a satisfactory product irrespective of the order of mixing!

With this in mind, some broad approaches will be outlined, with specific details included where appropriate.

Addition of Internal Phase to External Phase. With the widespread use of synthetic emulsifying agents today, the easiest and most frequently used sequence for emulsion preparation is by the gradual addition of the internal phase to the external phase. Prior to mixing, all water-soluble ingredients are dissolved in the aqueous phase and all oil-soluble components are dissolved in the oil. In the case of an o/w emulsion, the emulsifier will be predominantly water-soluble and so should be dissolved in this phase. If a blend of hydrophilic and lipophilic emulsifiers is used, as is frequently the case with nonionic emulsifiers, these are dissolved in the water and oil phases, respectively. Finally, when all soluble components have been dissolved in their respective phases, the oil phase is added gradually to the aqueous phase which is stirred continually. In this way, the external phase, water, is always in excess, and the ratio of the volume of the two liquids is such as to favor formation of an o/w emulsion. If a w/o emulsion is being prepared, the reverse procedure is adopted—the aqueous phase being gradually added to the oil phase.

On a small scale, such emulsions can be readily prepared in a beaker equipped with a variable speed stirrer, or the components can be added to a bottle and then shaken.

If fats, waxes, or surfactants that are solid or semisolid at room temperature are used in the formulation, it will be necessary to warm the two phases so that, before mixing, two homogeneous liquid phases are produced. Invariably, the aqueous phase is raised to a temperature that is 2 to 3° above that of the oil phase, irrespective of whether it is the internal or external phase. This ensures that no local crystallization of waxes takes place from the oil when the phases are mixed, since this could produce a coarse-grained product of low stability and poor appearance. If the formulation of an o/w emulsion calls for strong electrolytes, these are often not added to the aqueous phase until after the emulsion has been formed. In this way, any possibility of their interacting with the emulsifier and preventing emulsification is minimized.

When a hydrophilic gum, such as acacia

or tragacanth, is used as the emulsifying agent, a slightly different procedure must be adopted, otherwise it may not be possible to prepare a reasonable product. Thus, a primary, or concentrated, emulsion is first prepared using a set ratio of oil, water, and gum (Table 7-13). Although acacia is used most frequently in the two methods, particularly for the small-scale preparation of emulsions, other primary and auxiliary emulsifying agents such as egg yolk, gelatin, pectin, tragacanth, and chondrus may be employed. The 4:2:1 ratio is applicable only to emulsions prepared with acacia. When tragacanth is used as the emulsifying agent, for example, the ratio is 40:20:1, since only about one tenth as much tragacanth as acacia is necessary in either method. The mortar and pestle is most frequently used for small scale preparation.

Suppose we wish to make 60 ml. of the following o/w emulsion, containing 50 percent cod liver oil:

Cod liver oil......................... 30 ml.
Acacia, powder, a sufficient quantity
Purified water, a sufficient quantity to make 60 ml.

From Table 7-13, it is seen that a ratio of oil:water:gum equal to 4:2:1 should be employed to prepare the primary emulsion. Thus, two parts of water (15 ml.) are added *all at once* to 7.5 g. of acacia in a mortar and the mixture triturated with the pestle to produce a smooth dispersion. The oil (30 ml.) is then added slowly in small increments of 1 to 5 ml., with continuous trituration so that each portion is distributed and emulsified in the mucilage before the next quantity is added. The primary emulsion, once formed, is triturated for at least 5 minutes to ensure complete dispersion of the oil and

is then diluted with the required amount of water to bring the product to the final volume. This process, when a gum is used as the emulsifier, has been variously termed the Wet Gum, English, or American Method.

Addition of External Phase to Internal Phase. Another approach to the preparation of emulsions is the reverse of that just described, namely, the external phase is added to the internal phase. In the case of emulsions stabilized with synthetic emulsifying agents, a potential problem is that phase inversion (see p. 228), necessary for formation of the final emulsion type, may not occur. On the other hand, with the hydrophilic gums, the order of mixing now to be described readily results in very good emulsions and is frequently preferred to the previous procedure (internal phase added to external phase), at least insofar as gum emulsifiers are concerned.

Let us assume that one wishes to prepare an o/w emulsion and, as is more common these days, that a synthetic nonionic surfactant is to be employed as the emulsifying agent. A portion of the aqueous (external) phase is added to the whole of the oil (internal) phase. This invariably leads to the formation of a w/o emulsion, primarily because at this stage the oil phase is present in excess of the aqueous phase. The next step involves the addition of a sufficient quantity of water which, with adequate agitation, should invert the w/o emulsion to form an o/w product. Finally, the remaining water is added with stirring to bring the product up to the final volume. The main risk with this method of mixing is that inversion may not take place. However, this can be minimized by adding an adequate amount of water at one time to the initially formed w/o emulsion.

As with the method outlined in the previous section, waxy materials in the oil phase must be melted and dispersed prior to mixing; and the temperature of the aqueous phase should be a few degrees higher than that of the oil phase. Once the sequence of additions has been completed, the emulsion is allowed to cool while being stirred continuously. Often, phase inversion occurs during cooling to give the required emulsion type.

TABLE 7-13. OIL, WATER, AND
EMULSIFIER RATIOS

| | RATIOS OF OIL:WATER:EMULSIFIER | |
EMULSIFYING AGENT	Fixed Oils, Except Liquid Petrolatum and Linseed Oil	Linseed Oil and Liquid Petrolatum, Volatile Oils
Acacia	4:2:1	3:2:1 or 2:2:1
Tragacanth	40:20:1	30:20:1 or 20:20:1

The above process can be utilized with equal facility for the preparation of small batches in the laboratory or dispensary and for large industrial batches. The method can also be adapted readily for the preparation of w/o emulsions. Here, oil (the external phase) is added to an excess of water (the internal phase). The o/w emulsion is subsequently inverted by the addition of oil to form the desired w/o emulsion.

If small batches are to be prepared using hydrophilic gums as emulsifiers, the general procedure is as follows: The oil and powdered acacia are mixed in a dry mortar until the powder is distributed uniformly throughout the oil. A measured portion of water is added all at one time and, immediately, the whole is triturated to form a primary emulsion. Finally, the remaining water and other water-soluble components are added to complete the product. As before, the primary emulsion in the case of a fixed oil is prepared from 4 parts by volume of fixed oil, 2 parts by volume of water, and 1 part by weight of acacia, as listed in Table 7-13.

Using the same example as given in the earlier section describing the addition of the internal phase to the external phase, let us consider the specific steps involved using the present method of mixing. The 4 parts of oil (30 ml.) are mixed in a dry mortar with 1 part of powdered acacia (7.5 g.). One or two minutes may be required to distribute the gum evenly throughout the oil. To the oil and the well-dispersed emulsifying agent, 2 parts of purified water (15 ml.) are added *all at once*, and the primary emulsion is formed by light rapid trituration. At this stage, the oil is present in a large enough excess to favor a water-in-oil emulsion; if insufficient water is added, or if the water is added too slowly, a w/o primary emulsion will form in spite of the presence of the predominantly hydrophilic emulsifying agent. When more water is added to recover the o/w product, the emulsion usually breaks. An excessive amount of water added during the primary emulsification stage also results in a poor or a broken emulsion, since the viscosity of the continuous phase is reduced to a point at which the oil is no longer sheared into small globules. Although a w/o emulsion may be favored momentarily when

2 parts of water are added as required in this procedure, the well-dispersed acacia particles leave the bulk of the oil phase and are adsorbed rapidly at the interface where, following wetting and hydration by the water, they tend to produce a stable o/w emulsion. A few seconds after the addition of the 2 volumes of water, a creamy white primary emulsion is formed; a crackling sound is heard as the oil is extended into filaments and dispersed as globules in the viscous mucilage by the rapid movement of the pestle.

The primary emulsion should be triturated for at least 5 minutes before dilution in order to produce a fine-grained product. Additional water, containing flavoring ingredients, preservatives, and water-soluble drugs, may then be incorporated. Oil-soluble ingredients should be added to the oil phase before emulsification is begun. The emulsion is transferred to a graduate, and portions of water are used to rinse the mortar and the pestle and to bring the product to the final volume. This method of mixing has been referred to as the Dry Gum or Continental Method.

Nascent Soap Method. According to this procedure, an oil containing sufficient free fatty acid, such as linseed or olive oil, is placed in a suitable container, and an equal volume of alkali, such as calcium hydroxide solution, is added. When the mixture is agitated, the fatty acid of the oil reacts with the alkali to form a calcium soap which, in turn, promotes a w/o emulsion. Lime Liniment, which was official in *N.F. VIII*, was prepared extemporaneously in this manner. The soap is formed in situ (i.e., at the time of mixing); when formed in this manner, it is said to be a "nascent soap." The method may be used to prepare either o/w or w/o emulsions, depending on whether sodium hydroxide or calcium hydroxide solution is used. Other monovalent and polyvalent hydroxides also may be employed.

EMULSIFYING AGENTS

Desirable Properties of Emulsifying Agents

The mode of action of emulsifiers has been outlined on page 213. From this, it should be apparent that an emulsifying agent must possess at least some, and preferably all, of the following properties:

1. It should be surface active, at least to the extent that the interfacial tension is reduced to less than 10 dynes/cm.

2. It should be rapidly adsorbed around the dispersed droplets and form a coherent film capable of preventing coalescence.

3. It should result in the formation of an electrical potential at the droplet surface adequate to ensure repulsion between approaching droplets.

4. It should increase the viscosity of the emulsion as a means of enhancing stability.

5. It should be effective in a fairly low concentration.

The classification of these agents, now to be described, closely parallels the three ways in which emulsions are stabilized. Thus, the synthetic emulsifiers tend to form monomolecular films while the majority of naturally-occurring agents form multilayer films. Solid particles, of course, form solid particle films.

Types of Emulsifying Agents

The synthetic agents are classified as nonionic, anionic, and cationic, depending on whether the entire undissociated molecule, the anion (negative portion), or the cation (positive portion) provides the emulsifying action. Ampholytic emulsifying agents, containing both anionic and cationic groups in a single molecule, are now also known, an example being triethanolamine lauryl alanine. Some common synthetic emulsifying agents and their HLB values (see p. 223) are found in Table 7-14; emulsifying agents from natural sources are listed in Table 7-15.

It is convenient to make a distinction between true or primary emulsifying agents, which are capable of forming and stabilizing emulsions, and auxiliary agents, which are not capable of forming acceptable emulsions when used alone but assist the primary emulsifier in enhancing the stability of the product. A number of auxiliary agents are listed in Table 7-16.

Synthetic Emulsifying Agents

Synthetic emulsifiers are superior to natural gums and proteins in that they are not susceptible to decomposition by micro-

TABLE 7-14.   SYNTHETIC EMULSIFYING
AGENTS

IONIC CLASSES AND CHEMICAL COMPOUNDS	HLB*
Anionic	
Glyceryl monostearate—self emulsifying (Tegin)†	11
Triethanolamine oleate	12
Sodium oleate	18
Potassium oleate	20
Sodium lauryl sulfate	40 (approx.)
Cationic	
N-cetyl N-ethyl morpholinium ethosulfate (Atlas G-263)‡	25–30
Benzalkonium chloride (Zephiran Chloride)§	—
Nonionic	
Sorbitan monooleate (Span 80)‡	4.3
Sorbitan monolaurate (Span 20)‡	8.6
Polyoxyethylene monostearate (Myrj 45)‡	11.1
Polyoxyethylene monolaurate (Atlas G-2127)‡	12.8
Polyethyleneglycol 400 monolaurate‖	13.1
Polyoxyethylene vegetable oil (Emulphor El-719)#	13.3
Polyoxyethylene sorbitan monooleate (Tween 80)‡	15.0
Polyoxyethylene sorbitan monolaurate (Tween 20)‡	16.7

* Griffin, W. C.: J. Soc. Cosmet. Chem. 5:249, 1954.
† Goldschmidt Chemical Corporation, New York, N.Y.
‡ Atlas Chemical Company, Wilmington, Del.
§ Winthrop Labs., New York, N.Y.
‖ Kessler Chemical Co., Philadelphia, Pa.
General Aniline and Film Corporation, New York, N.Y.

organisms. Furthermore, being of synthetic origin, the ratio of hydrophilic to lipophilic groups in the molecule may be altered to supply a wide range of emulsifying agents. This versatility is advantageous in externally applied emulsions, among which the w/o type and the o/w class are of equal importance. Only a limited number of synthetic agents are safe for internal use. Among these are the sorbitan esters (Spans), the polyoxyethylene sorbitan esters (Tweens), and purified glyceryl monostearate.

Nonionic Emulsifying Agents. The entire undissociated molecule of certain chemicals containing hydrophilic and lipophilic groups in proper balance may act as an emulsifying agent. Included in this group are glyceryl esters, fatty acid esters of sorbitan and

TABLE 7-15. EMULSIFYING AGENTS
OF NATURAL ORIGIN

NAME	SOURCE AND COMPOSITION	EMULSION TYPE
Acacia	Potassium, calcium and magnesium salts of *d*-glucuronic acid	O/W
Egg yolk	Lecithin, cholesterol, proteins	O/W
Gelatin	Polypeptides, aminoacids	O/W
Malt extract	Proteins, dextrin	O/W
Lecithin	Phospholipid from egg yolk, soya bean and nerve tissue	O/W
Saponin	Nitrogen-free glycoside from quillaja and senega root	O/W
Cholesterol	A sterol found in nerve tissue and wool fat	W/O
Wool fat	A complex mixture of alcohols and fatty acids from the wool of the sheep	W/O

their polyoxyethylene derivatives, and polyethylene glycol esters and ethers. By combining hydrophilic radicals, such as hydroxyl (–OH) and polyoxyethylene $(-CH_2CH_2O)_n$ groups, with lipophilic substances, such as straight chain hydrocarbons, a wide range of hydrophil-lipophil character may be obtained in any series of nonionic emulsifying agents.

An important group of nonionic agents are obtained by partially esterifying the anhydrides derived from sorbitol and other sugar alcohols with various fatty acids. Sorbitan laurate, palmitate, stearate, and oleate constitute the series of Spans (see Chap. 6). Since they are lipophilic in nature, they tend to form w/o emulsions and to stabilize o/w emulsions. The polyoxyethylene derivatives of the Spans, known as the Tweens, are water-soluble or dispersible and favor o/w emulsions.

Polyethylene glycol esters, such as the monostearate, may be used to prepare emulsified lotions and creams. The formula for a representative member of this class is:

$$C_{17}H_{35}COO(CH_2CH_2O)_nH,$$

polyethylene glycol 400 monostearate in which n varies from 8 to 10.

Glyceryl monostearate, $C_{17}H_{35}COOCH_2$-$CHOHCH_2OH$, is too lipophilic to serve as an effective emulsifier, but it may be used as an auxiliary agent. When mixed with a small amount of an o/w emulsifier such as sodium stearate or sodium lauryl sulfate, it possesses the desired characteristics of an emulsifying mixture and is known as "glyceryl monostearate—self-emulsifying."

Nonionic surfactants have an advantage over anionic and cationic surfactants used as emulsifying agents in that they are not susceptible to pH changes and the presence of electrolytes. With nonionic emulsifiers the best results are often obtained by using a combination of a predominantly lipophilic agent (e.g., a Span) with a predominantly hydrophilic agent (e.g., a Tween). This use of blends is based on the HLB concept, which is discussed, with examples, on page 224.

The following formula can be used to prepare an o/w emulsion of mineral oil:

Tween 40	3.5 g.
Span 40	3.5 g.
Sodium benzoate	0.2 g.
Mineral oil	40.0 g.
Purified water, to	100.0 ml.

The emulsion is prepared by dissolving the Span 40 in the mineral oil which is warmed to 60°. The sodium benzoate and Tween are dissolved in the water which is warmed to around 62 to 65° and then added to the oil phase. The product is stirred until cold.

Anionic Emulsifying Agents. This class includes monovalent, polyvalent, and organic soaps, sulfates, and sulfonates (see Table 7-14).

Soaps are salts of long chain fatty acids in which the alkyl chain usually contains from 12 to 18 carbon atoms. They have a disagreeable taste and produce an irritating and laxative action in the intestinal tract; consequently, they are not used in orally administered emulsions.

The alkali soaps, including the sodium, potassium, and ammonium salts of lauric, myristic, palmitic, stearic, and oleic acids, are hydrophilic and form o/w emulsions. The metallic soaps, including the calcium, magnesium, zinc, lead, and aluminum salts of fatty acids, are water-insoluble and tend to promote w/o emulsions. Both types are used for the preparation of some phar-

TABLE 7-16.   AUXILIARY EMULSIFYING AGENTS

PRODUCT	SOURCE AND COMPOSITION	PRINCIPAL USE
Agar	Dried colloid substance from certain algae containing a polygalactose sulfate and other constituents	Hydrophilic thickening agent and stabilizer for o/w emulsions
Bentonite	Colloidal hydrated aluminum silicate	Hydrophilic thickening agent and stabilizer for o/w and w/o lotions and creams
Cetyl alcohol	Chiefly $C_{16}H_{33}OH$	Lipophilic thickening agent and stabilizer for o/w lotions and ointments
Chondrus	Dried bleached seaweed	Hydrophilic thickening agent and stabilizer for o/w emulsions; weak o/w emulsifier
Glyceryl monostearate	$C_{17}H_{35}COOCH_2CHOHCH_2OH$	Lipophilic thickening agent and stabilizer for o/w lotions and ointments
Magnesium hydroxide	$Mg(OH)_2$	Hydrophilic stabilizer for o/w emulsions
Methylcellulose	Series of methyl esters of cellulose	Hydrophilic thickening agent and stabilizer for o/w emulsions; weak o/w emulsifier
Pectin	Purified carbohydrate extracted from the inner rind of citrus fruits and apple pomace	Hydrophilic thickening agent and stabilizer for o/w emulsions; weak o/w emulsifier
Silica gel	Hydrous oxide of silica	Hydrophilic stabilizer used in the preparation of ointments
Sodium alginate	The sodium salt of alginic acid, a purified carbohydrate extracted from giant kelp	Hydrophilic thickening agent and stabilizer for o/w emulsions
Sodium carboxy-methylcellulose	Sodium salt of the carboxymethyl esters of cellulose	Hydrophilic thickening agent and stabilizer for o/w emulsions
Spermaceti	Waxy substance from the head of the sperm whale, containing cetyl palmitate	Lipophilic thickening agent and stabilizer for o/w and w/o ointments
Stearic acid	A mixture of solid acids from fats, chiefly stearic and palmitic	Lipophilic thickening agent and stabilizer for o/w lotions and ointments. Forms a true emulsifier when reacted with an alkali
Stearyl alcohol	Chiefly $C_{17}H_{35}OH$	Lipophilic thickening agent and stabilizer for o/w lotions and ointments
Tragacanth	Dried gummy exudation from species of *Astragalus,* containing a soluble portion and an insoluble portion that swells in water	Hydrophilic thickening agent and stabilizer for o/w emulsions; weak o/w emulsifier
Veegum	Colloidal magnesium aluminum silicate	Hydrophilic thickening agent and stabilizer for o/w lotions and creams

maceutical liniments and cosmetic creams. The nascent soap method is used frequently for these preparations; about 2 to 10 percent of soap is required to prepare the emulsion. In an emulsion prepared by reacting the fatty acids of the oil with an alkali, sufficient fatty acid should be present so that some remains unneutralized after the soap is formed. The excess free fatty acid improves the hydrophil-lipophil balance of the soap and acts as an auxiliary emulsifier. Although a soap alone forms a fairly stable emulsion, usually the product is improved by the addition of an auxiliary stabilizing agent such as cetyl alcohol, stearyl alcohol, or glyceryl monostearate.

Organic soaps, which are known also as amino soaps, are prepared by reacting aminohydroxy compounds with fatty acids. Triethanolamine oleate is prepared according to the following reaction:

$$(HOCH_2CH_2)_3N + C_{17}H_{33}COOH =$$

triethanolamine   oleic acid

$$(HOCH_2CH_2)_3N^+H^-OOCC_{17}H_{33}$$

triethanolamine oleate

Soaps formed from 2-methyl-2-amino-1,3-propanediol also have been suggested for pharmaceutical emulsions.[4] The formula of the stearate is:

$$CH_3-\overset{\overset{\displaystyle CH_2OH}{|}}{\underset{\underset{\displaystyle CH_2OH}{|}}{C}}-\overset{+}{N}H_3{}^-OOCC_{17}H_{35}$$

2-Methyl-2-amino-1,3-propanediol stearate

Organic soaps produce o/w emulsions. They have the advantage over inorganic soaps in that they represent a better balance between hydrophilic and lipophilic groups and are practically neutral in reaction (pH 8). The soap ordinarily is formed in situ during mixing and emulsification, and the final emulsion is fine-grained and stable.

Some amines, such as morpholine,

$$HN\underset{CH_2-CH_2}{\overset{CH_2-CH_2}{\big\langle}}O$$

are volatile and, consequently, are useful for preparing horticultural sprays and polishing waxes. The volatile amine evaporates after the emulsion is applied, leaving a water-resistant film of oil or wax.

The following formulae illustrate the use of organic soaps in emulsions.

Liquid petrolatum	20 g.
Stearic acid	3 g.
Triethanolamine	1 g.
Purified water	76 g.

The stearic acid and the mineral oil are heated on a water bath to 75°C. to melt the acid. The triethanolamine is dissolved in the water, and the solution is heated to 78°C. and added slowly, with stirring, to the oil phase. The emulsion is allowed to cool, with occasional mixing. The cream has a pH of about 8.

Liquid petrolatum, heavy	30 g.
Paraffin	7 g.
Ceresin	2 g.
Stearic acid	8 g.
2-Amino-2-methyl-1,3-propanediol ..	3 g.
Purified water	50 g.

The first 4 ingredients, constituting the oil phase, are heated at 75°C. until fused; the last 2 ingredients are mixed and heated to 78°C. and then are added slowly, with stirring, to the oil phase. The mixture is agitated until it has cooled.

Other types of anionic surfactants occasionally used as emulsifying agents are *sulfated alcohols* and *sulfonates*. Sulfated alcohols, such as sodium lauryl alcohol,

$$C_{12}H_{25}OSO_3{}^-Na^+$$

are used as o/w emulsifying agents, particularly with an auxiliary agent. Sulfonates are sometimes preferred because they have a higher tolerance to calcium ions and do not hydrolyze as readily as the sulfates. A frequently used sulfonate is sodium dioctyl sulfosuccinate:

$$\underset{C_8H_{17}-OOC-CH_2}{\overset{C_8H_{17}-OOC-CH-SO_3{}^-\ Na^+}{|}}$$

Cationic Emulsifying Agents. Benzalkonium Chloride is an important member of this class and has the formula $C_6H_5CH_2-N(CH_3)_2RCl$, in which R represents a mixture of alkyl radicals from C_8H_{17} to $C_{18}H_{37}$.

Cationic agents have marked bactericidal properties and are used primarily as local anti-infectives rather than as emulsifying agents. They must not come in contact with anionic chemicals such as soaps, since the two types are incompatible. The active group of the cationic agent combines with the anion, and, although precipitation may not be evident immediately when the substances are used in low concentration, the germicidal action of the cationic agent is destroyed. The emulsifying property of the anionic emulsifier may also be impaired or nullified.

Natural Emulsifying Agents

Acacia is probably the only true emulsifying agent of the natural gum class; the other gums produce viscous but coarse emulsions and are used principally as stabilizers. Acacia is particularly useful for preparing emulsions in a mortar, since it provides a mucilage of ample consistency to allow the oil to be sheared into finely divided particles. However, acacia is not viscous enough to prevent rapid rise of the globules, with subsequent formation of a cream layer on the surface of the emulsion. Thickening agents such as agar and tragacanth sometimes are added to acacia emulsions to minimize the creaming effect.

Emulsions prepared with acacia are stable over a pH range of 2 to 10.[40] However, preparations containing acacia are not resistant to attack by microorganisms and require the presence of a preservative. About 6 percent by volume of alcohol, 0.2 percent of benzoic acid, or 0.2 percent of methyl para-hydroxybenzoate may be used for this purpose.

Gelatin is a negatively charged colloid at pH values above its isoelectric point and is positively charged at pH values below its isoelectric point. Since the oil globules in an o/w emulsion are negatively charged, gelatin is readily adsorbed on the surface of the particles if the pH is below the isoelectric point.

The isoelectric point of gelatin varies with the origin of the product. Gelatin that is obtained from an acid-treated precursor (Type A) has an isoelectric point between pH 7 and pH 9 and acts best as an emulsifying agent at about pH 3.2, at which it is positively charged. Gelatin from an alkali-treated precursor (Type B) has an isoelectric point between pH 4.7 and pH 5 and is used at about pH 8, at which it is negatively charged.

Since gums such as acacia, tragacanth, and agar are negatively charged, they cannot be combined with a positively charged gelatin; two oppositely charged hydrophilic colloids, such as acid-treated gelatin and acacia, may be incompatible in certain proportions, since they tend to form a coacervate. However, gelatin having an isoelectric point between pH 4.7 and pH 5 may be combined with gums if the preparation is maintained at a high pH value at which the gelatin has a negative charge.

Gelatin is available as Type A for use in acid solution and as Type B for use in the alkaline range. The characteristics of the gelatins, Types A and B, are summarized in Table 7-17.

Although gelatin emulsions cannot be formed in a mortar, fine-grained products are prepared by use of the homogenizer.

Cholesterol, wool fat, and certain wool-fat concentrates and derivatives form stable w/o emulsions and are used primarily for the

TABLE 7-17. CHARACTERISTICS OF GELATINS TYPE A AND B

PRODUCT	ISO-ELECTRIC POINT	OPTIMUM pH FOR USE	ELECTRIC CHARGE IN THE USEFUL pH RANGE
Gelatin A	7–9	3.2	+
Gelatin B	4.7–5	8	−

preparation of ointments.[10] The reader is referred to the chapter on Semisolid Dosage Forms for a detailed discussion of this group.

Most of the natural emulsifying agents which form oil-in-water emulsions are nontoxic and are used in the preparation of oral and parenteral emulsions.

Finely Divided Solids as Emulsifying Agents

Colloidal clays such as bentonite, Veegum, Pharmasorb Colloidal, magnesium hydroxide, aluminum hydroxide, magnesium oxide, and silica gel are some of the insoluble substances that have been used as emulsifying agents. As early as 1907, Pickering[50] undertook an extensive study of insoluble emulsifying agents and showed that powders that were easily wetted by water formed o/w emulsions, whereas those that were wetted preferentially by oil tended to produce w/o emulsions. The clays represent the first type, and carbon black the second type, of solid emulsifiers. It is believed that, like other emulsifying agents, the finely divided solids form and stabilize emulsions by concentrating at the interface where they produce a coherent film around the globules and prevent coalescence of the internal phase.

Bentonite may be used to form either an o/w or a w/o emulsion, depending on the order of mixing. If a bentonite magma is placed in a mortar and the oil phase is added gradually with trituration, an o/w emulsion is produced, since the aqueous phase is always in excess during the preparation. However, if bentonite is dispersed in oil and water is added gradually, it is possible to form a w/o emulsion. The following formula demonstrates the use of bentonite in o/w and w/o emulsions.[33]

| Camphor ⎱ aa | 0.6 |
| Menthol ⎰ | |

Phenol 1.2

| Calamine   ⎱ aa | 7.2 |
| Zinc oxide ⎰ | |

Boric acid 3.6

Olive oil 48.0

Bentonite (6%) in lime water, q.s. ad. 120.0

The bentonite suspension is placed in an electric mixing apparatus; a uniform mixture of camphor, menthol, phenol, calamine, zinc oxide, and boric acid is added and, finally, the olive oil is incorporated. An oil-in-water emulsion is formed. If a water-in-oil product is wanted, the oil containing the menthol, the camphor, and the phenol is placed in the mixer, and the mixture of powders is added. The bentonite in lime water is added last.

Veegum may be used to prepare stable o/w emulsions of mineral and vegetable oils; however, it is employed more frequently as a stabilizer for lotions and creams containing soap or nonionic emulsifying agents. Pharmasorb Colloidal serves as a secondary emulsifier. Magnesia magma and kaolin are sometimes added to mineral-oil emulsions to serve as stabilizing agents. Silica gel has been recommended as a solid emulsifier for the preparation of ointments.[51]

Auxiliary Emulsifying Agents

The compounds listed in Table 7-16 are normally incapable themselves of forming stable emulsions. Their utility is generally based on their thickening action which helps the primary emulsifying agent in achieving a highly stable emulsion.

SELECTION OF EMULSIFYING AGENTS

The selection of an emulsifying agent, or agents, for a particular emulsion is probably the most important step involved in achieving a successful product. There are several factors that have to be kept in mind when deciding which agent, or agents, to employ. These include the following: chemical stability of the emulsifier under the conditions of pH, electrolyte concentration, and temperature to be employed; likelihood of an interaction with other components such as drugs and preservatives; intended use of the product—oral, parenteral, or topical—and what this entails in terms of toxicity requirements; whether the emulsifier is synthetic or natural; and maintenance of the quality of the emulsifier from batch to batch. However, the single most important requirement is to achieve a physically stable emulsion of the required type, and the initial selecton of potential emulsifiers is based on their ability to fill this need. Unfortunately, the formulator will be confronted with a list of literally thousands of emulsifying agents. Although many emulsifiers can be discarded because of failure to comply with specific aspects of the intended product such as those mentioned above, the development pharmacist must still make his choice from a large number of emulsifiers. An approach to this problem which is especially useful for selecting relative amounts of nonionic surfactants in combinations designed to give optimum emulsifying properties is the HLB system developed in the 1950's by Griffin. Mixtures of emulsifying agents are also used to enhance the stability of the interfacial film and can often improve the consistency and feel of the emulsion.

The HLB System

One of the desirable properties of an emulsifying agent is that it undergo strong adsorption at the interface between the oil and water phases. This requires a proper balance between the hydrophilic and the lipophilic tendencies of the surfactant. If an emulsifying agent is predominantly hydrophilic, it tends to form an o/w emulsion; if it is predominantly lipophilic, it favors the formation of a w/o emulsion. Sodium oleate has the characteristics of a good o/w emulsifying agent, since it possesses a hydrophilic carboxyl group ($-COO^-$) that predominates over the lipophilic hydrocarbon group ($C_{17}H_{33}-$).

Lipophile   Hydrophile

On the other hand, calcium oleate and other polyvalent soaps are predominantly lipophilic and form w/o emulsions.

The hydrophil-lipophil balance of surface-active agents has been expressed empirically by Griffin[23,24] in terms of a numerical HLB scale that extends, roughly, from 1 to 50. An agent with a low HLB (i.e., with a value of about 1 to 10) is primarily lipophilic, whereas a surfactant having a higher HLB is hydrophilic.

For the preparation of a w/o emulsion, the emulsifying agent should have an HLB of about 3 to 8. An o/w emulsion, on the other hand, is favored by an emulsifying agent with a HLB of about 8 to 18. The HLB values for a number of synthetic emulsifying agents are found in Table 7-14. The most favorable range for various classes of surfactants is shown in the HLB scale illustrated in Figure 7-23.

In practice, a Span and a Tween usually are mixed to provide an emulsifier combination that has the HLB necessary to produce a stable emulsion of the desired type. Knowing the required HLB of the oil phase as listed in Table 7-18, one may calculate the quantities of any Span and Tween, several of which are found in Table 7-14, that are necessary to produce the proper balance for a stable emulsion. For example, if one desired to prepare 100 ml. of a mineral oil emulsion (required HLB 12) emulsified with a 5-g. mixture of Span 20 (HLB 8.6) and Tween 20 (HLB 16.7), the product would require about 60 percent or 3 g. of Span 20 and 40 percent or 2 g. of Tween 20 in the emulsifier phase. These figures are easily checked, since the percentage contributions of the 2 emulsifiers to the over-all HLB must be additive, or:

$$(8.6 \times 0.6) + (16.7 \times 0.4) = 11.8$$

The details of the method are given in the booklet of the Atlas Chemical Co.[1]

The optimum HLB ranges for the formation of stable w/o and o/w emulsions depend, in part, on the particular oil or mixture of oils involved. That is to say, each oil re-

TABLE 7-18. "REQUIRED HLB" VALUES FOR OIL-PHASE INGREDIENTS (approx., ±1)*

	W/O EMULSION	O/W EMULSION†
Acid, stearic	—	17
Alcohol, cetyl	—	15
Lanolin, anhydrous	8	12
Oil, cottonseed	—	6
mineral, heavy	4	10
mineral, light	4	12
Petrolatum	4	7–8
Wax, bees	5	9
paraffin	4	10

* The Atlas HLB System. Ed. 2 (revised), p. 6. Atlas Chemical Co., Wilmington, Del., 1963.
† Refers to fluid o/w emulsions. O/W emulsions of a thicker texture or creaminess require a somewhat lower HLB.

quires an emulsifying agent of a specific HLB value for the formation of an o/w emulsion and another value for the formation of a w/o product. These are known as the "required HLB" values of the oil. The "required HLB" values for a number of oil-phase ingredients are found in Table 7-18. The "required HLB" of any material is likely to vary slightly with the source of the material, the concentration desired, and the method of preparation.[1]

Mixed Emulsifying Agents

An emulsifying agent frequently consists of a blend of emulsifiers rather than a single agent. Auxiliary agents may be mixed with primary emulsifiers for various purposes. Furthermore, primary emulsifying agents that tend to form water-in-oil emulsions may be combined with true oil-in-water emulsifying agents to provide a blend which is more efficient than either agent alone.

The mixture contributes one or several actions: (1) it provides the proper hydrophil-

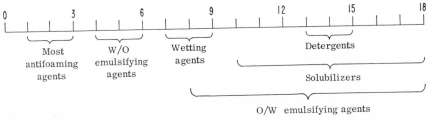

FIG. 7-23. The Atlas HLB System. (ed. 2, rev., p. 4. Atlas Chemical Co., Wilmington, Del., 1963)

lipophil nature, (2) it establishes a stable film at the interface, and (3) it supplies the desired consistency to the product and contributes certain other properties such as emolliency, spreading, and deflocculation.

1. As explained previously, the type of emulsion which is formed depends on the relative proportion of hydrophilic and lipophilic character that the emulsifying agent or mixture of agents exhibits.

Lecithin is an o/w emulsifying agent, and cholesterol is a w/o emulsifier. However, when mixed together in the proper proportions, they are capable of forming a stable emulsion of either type. The data in Table 7-19 show that when the ratio of lecithin to cholesterol is greater than 10 to 1, an o/w emulsion is produced; when the ratio is less than 6 to 1, a w/o emulsion is formed; finally, when an intermediate ratio of about 8 to 1 is chosen, an unstable product results.[11]

The HLB system of Griffin[23,24] is based on a similar principle. When Span 80, which is lipophilic (HLB = 4.3), is combined with Tween 80, which is hydrophilic (HLB = 15.0), the emulsifier mixture is capable of producing either an o/w or a w/o emulsion, depending on the ratio of the two agents. Chun et al.[9] attribute the action of tragacanth in acacia emulsions to HLB. They found the HLB of acacia to be 8.0 and that of tragacanth to be 13.2. A mixture of the 2 agents in the proper ratio yields the desired HLB for the formation of a stable o/w emulsion. Since these agents are complex natural emulsifiers, other factors are no doubt also important.

2. According to Schulman and Cockbain,[54] some emulsifying agents tend to form weak compounds or "interfacial complexes" at the surface of the globules. For example, the o/w emulsifying action of sodium oleate is improved by combination with cetyl alcohol, cholesterol, and similar lipophilic agents, through a tendency of the molecules to form a complex.

Schulman and Cockbain suggest that a complex favors the formation and the stabilization of an o/w emulsion by lowering the interfacial tension to a greater extent than is accomplished by either agent alone; by forming a compact yet flexible film at the interface; and by increasing the electric charge on the surface of the globules owing to the increased concentration of emulsifier ions at the interface. On the other hand, a complex that promotes a w/o emulsion forms a rigid, electrically uncharged interfacial film, according to these investigators.

3. Tragacanth, agar, and chondrus frequently are combined with acacia to thicken the external phase of an o/w emulsion and to reduce the rate of creaming. Pectin, alginates, and cellulose esters also are used for this purpose. Cetyl alcohol, stearyl alcohol, glyceryl monostearate, and certain waxes such as spermaceti and beeswax serve as "bodying agents" to improve the consistency of the oil phase of lotions, creams, and ointments and to supply emollient properties to these bases.

Serrallach et al.[55] proposed another hypothesis to explain the exceptional efficiency of mixtures of emulsifying agents. They observed that tragacanth tended to increase the rapidity of film formation, acacia imparted strength to the film, and agar increased the consistency of a cod liver oil emulsion that was stabilized with a combination of these 3 agents.

TABLE 7-19.   EFFECT OF LECITHIN:CHOLESTEROL RATIOS ON THE TYPE OF EMULSION FORMED*

VOLUME OF OIL PHASE (in ml.)	VOLUME OF AQUEOUS PHASE (in ml.)	LECITHIN (percent)	CHOLESTEROL (percent)	RATIO OF LECITHIN: CHOLESTEROL	TYPE OF EMULSION FORMED
5	6.0	0.33	0.017	19.4:1	O/W
5	5.5	0.18	0.018	10:1	O/W
5	5.4	0.148	0.0185	8:1	Indefinite
5	5.3	0.113	0.019	6:1	W/O
5	5.2	0.077	0.019	4.1:1	W/O
5	5.1	0.04	0.02	2:1	W/O

* Corran, J. W., and Lewis, W. C.: Biochem. J., *18*:1368, 1924.

It should be noted that some emulsifying agents are incompatible and cannot be used in combination. For example, colloids that possess electric charges of opposite sign are likely to coagulate when combined.

The older view held that all lipophilic and hydrophilic emulsifiers are necessarily "antagonistic" because they tend to form emulsions of opposite types. However, in light of the arguments presented in paragraph (1), this idea has been replaced by the principle of hydrophil-lipophil balance. The findings of Schulman and Cockbain as discussed in paragraph (2) and those of Serrallach et al. under (3) also justify the practice of mixing emulsifiers of opposite types.

EMULSION STABILITY

One of the most important properties of pharmaceutical and cosmetic emulsions is the stability of the finished product. A stable emulsion is characterized by absence of flocculation and creaming; absence of coalescence of the globules and separation of the internal phase from the emulsion; absence of deterioration by microorganisms; and maintenance of elegance with respect to general appearance, odor, color, and consistency. Accordingly, the types of instability in a pharmaceutical emulsion may be classified as follows: (1) flocculation and creaming, (2) coalescence and breaking, (3) deterioration by microorganisms, and (4) miscellaneous physical and chemical changes.

The factors contributing to these forms of instability, as well as the methods of stabilizing and preserving emulsions against degradation, are discussed in this section.

Flocculation and Creaming

Flocculation is the joining together of globules to form large clumps or floccules which rise or settle in the emulsion more rapidly than do the individual particles. As previously mentioned under homogenization, the passage of an emulsion through an orifice at a high pressure sometimes results in flocculation.

Creaming is the rising ("upward creaming") or settling ("downward creaming") of globules or floccules to form a concentrated layer at the surface or at the bottom of the emulsion. The term has been derived from the well-known process of cream formation which occurs in milk when it is allowed to stand for some time.

Although the formation of a thick cream layer is sometimes desirable in milk, it is regarded as a mark of *instability* in pharmaceutical emulsions. Creaming results in a lack of uniformity of the product, and, unless the container is agitated thoroughly before each dose is removed, it may lead to variations in the amount of drug administered. Furthermore, the appearance of the emulsion is affected by creaming, and this is as real a problem to the pharmaceutical compounder as is separation of the internal phase.

Stokes' equation (Equation 1, p. 178) includes the various factors involved in the creaming process. Equation (1) shows first that the diameter of the globules (d) is a major consideration; doubling the diameter increases the velocity of settling or creaming by a factor of 4. Reducing the particle size by passing the emulsion through a homogenizer decreases the velocity of creaming considerably. The result of homogenization of milk is well known. However, as previously noted, homogenization under high pressure sometimes leads to flocculation, and the large clumps which are formed may cream more rapidly than the individual globules in the unhomogenized emulsion.

The density difference ($\rho - \rho_0$) in Equation (1) shows that, when the density of the internal and the external phases are equal (i.e., when $\rho = \rho_0$), the velocity of creaming is zero. When the internal phase is less dense than the continuous liquid, which generally is the case in o/w emulsions, $\rho - \rho_0$ takes on a negative value and thus V is also negative. A negative velocity expresses the fact that creaming occurs in an *upward* direction. When the dispersed liquid is denser than the dispersion medium, the density difference ($\rho - \rho_0$) is positive and V likewise is positive. This condition, which generally occurs in w/o emulsions, results in a settling of the globules, or, as it is sometimes expressed, in *downward* creaming.

The gravity factor in the numerator of the equation is essentially constant under ordinary circumstances. However, creaming may be accelerated, as is often done in the dairy industry, by centrifugation.

The velocity of creaming is inversely proportional to the Newtonian viscosity of the external phase of the emulsion; that is, the creaming velocity is reduced by an increase in viscosity of the continuous medium. If the viscosity is non-Newtonian, which may be the case for concentrated emulsions containing high concentrations of emulsifying agents, it is not clear what value for viscosity should be used to satisfy the Stokes' law equation. Auxiliary emulsifiers, such as agar and methylcellulose, sometimes are added to improve the consistency of the emulsion. However, the use of an unsuitable thickening agent may result in clumping, with a subsequent increase in effective particle size and a corresponding increased rate of creaming.

Coalescence and Breaking

Unlike creaming, the coalescence of globules and the subsequent breaking of an emulsion are irreversible processes. Under the conditions of creaming, the globules are still surrounded by a protective sheath of emulsifying agent and may be redispersed simply by agitating the product. However, in an emulsion which has broken, i.e., in which the phases have separated as distinct layers, simple mixing fails to re-establish the stable emulsion. The emulsion may be reconstituted only by incorporating more emulsifying agent and passing the product through the proper emulsifying machinery.

Any system containing finely divided particles is unstable, owing to the excess energy of the dispersed phase. Accordingly, the conditions of equilibrium in an emulsion are satisfied only when the immiscible liquids have separated into 2 layers. The globules coalesce slowly or rapidly, depending on the strength of the emulsifier film and, to a less extent, on other factors, until the product is completely "cracked." Although many properties, such as electric charges on the particles, low interfacial tension, and increased viscosity, have been suggested as stabilizing factors, it generally is agreed today that the most significant element in stabilizing an emulsion against breaking is the emulsifier film surrounding the dispersed particles. If the emulsifying agent or combination of agents is adsorbed and oriented at the interface in a manner such as to form a tough, coherent barrier, the film will withstand the tendency of the globules to coalesce, and the emulsion will remain stable for the desired period of time.

According to King,[36] the only precise method for quantitating the rate of emulsion breaking involves a microscopic analysis in which the average globule size is determined from time to time as the emulsion ages. The degree of coarsening of the emulsion at each time indicates the rate of breaking. In the case of rapidly breaking emulsions, of course, it is possible to observe the separation visually. Microscopic methods, while more accurate, require the measurement of several hundred to several thousand globules for each analysis and, therefore, are tedious and time-consuming.

Deterioration by Microorganisms

Molds, yeasts, and bacteria may bring about the decomposition of the emulsifying agents, contaminate the aqueous phase, produce rancidity in the oil, and destroy oil-soluble vitamins. White[62] states that a preservative should be a powerful fungistatic rather than bacteriostatic agent, since it is more likely that fungi (molds and yeasts) may contaminate emulsions. The presence of certain drugs, such as benzoic and salicylic acid, or high concentrations of alcohol may provide adequate protection against microorganisms; however, it is usually desirable to add an agent that will act specifically as a preservative. Combinations of parahydroxybenzoates—0.1 to 0.2 percent of the methyl ester and 0.02 to 0.05 percent of the propyl ester—frequently are used; the combination of these agents is particularly effective against molds, yeasts, and bacteria as long as the emulsifying agent and other ingredients do not complex with the preservative agents to nullify their action.

Since most preservatives are partially soluble in oil, some of the agent tends to pass into the oil, where it becomes ineffective as a protective agent for the aqueous phase. Consequently, one must be certain that the preservatives are added in adequate amounts to protect the product.

Wedderburn[61] has reviewed the preservation of emulsions against microbial attack.

Miscellaneous Physical and Chemical Changes

Care must be taken to protect emulsions against deterioration caused by light, extreme temperatures, and oxidative and hydrolytic rancidity of the oil. Freezing and thawing result in a coarsening and, sometimes, in the breaking of an emulsion; high temperatures produce the same effects. However, some emulsions, particularly those that are stabilized with synthetic emulsifying agents, are unusually resistant to extreme heat and cold. Benerito and Singleton[2,3] reviewed the effect of heat on the stability of emulsions. Hom et al.[32] employed heat tests in the evaluation of the stability of emulsions for injection. Light and rancidity affect the color and the odor of oils and may destroy their vitamin activity. Antioxidants are necessary if the oils are likely to become rancid. Emulsions should be kept in tight containers and stored at moderate temperatures; if affected by light, they should be stored in dark bottles.

Inversion is a physical process whereby an o/w emulsion changes to a w/o product, or vice versa. Although little quantitative work has been carried out on emulsion inversion, it is known that phase volume ratio, the addition of electrolytes, and temperature changes can bring about this phenomenon. Apart from its deliberate use in the preparation of emulsions by the method of adding the external phase to the internal phase (p. 216), inversion is generally regarded as a manifestation of physical instability in an emulsion.

RHEOLOGY OF EMULSIONS

Emulsions show non-Newtonian flow properties except at low concentrations of the dispersed phase. They may show plastic or pseudoplastic flow, and these characteristics may be accompanied by thixotropy. Simple emulsions that do not contain appreciable quantities of viscous emulsifying agents do not develop a lattice-like structure and, consequently, may not show thixotropy.

Emulsions, like suspensions, should possess rheological characteristics that are appropriate to the intended topical or internal use of the product. Thus, any creamed layer in an emulsion must be redispersible with agitation; the product must pour readily from the container; it must spread smoothly on the skin or, in the case of an oral preparation, it must be capable of being administered conveniently with a spoon. A product that shows shear-thinning, i.e., one that is highly viscous at rest and flows readily at high shear, is needed to meet these requirements.

The factors involved in the formulation of an acceptable emulsion may have significant influence on the rheological properties of the final product. These factors have been summarized by Sherman and are listed in Table 7-20. The increase in the concentration of the internal phase of an emulsion causes a gradual rise in the viscosity of the system up to the point at which the globules

TABLE 7-20. FACTORS INFLUENCING
EMULSION VISCOSITY*

Internal phase

A. Volume concentration (ϕ): hydrodynamic interaction between globules; flocculation, leading to formation of globule aggregates.
B. Viscosity (η_1): deformation of globules in shear.
C. Globule size, and size distribution, technique used to prepare emulsion: interfacial tension between the two liquid phases: globule behavior in shear; interaction with continuous phase; globule interaction.
D. Chemical constitution.

Continuous phase

A. Viscosity (η_0), and other rheological properties.
B. Chemical constitution, polarity, pH: potential energy of interaction between globules.
C. Electrolyte concentration if polar medium.

Emulsifying agent

A. Chemical constitution: potential energy of interaction between globules.
B. Concentration, and solubility in internal and continuous phases: emulsion type; emulsion inversion; solubilization of liquid phases in micelles.
C. Thickness of film adsorbed around globules, and its rheological properties: deformation of globules in shear; fluid circulation within globules.
D. Electroviscous effect.

Additional stabilizing agents

Pigments, hydrocolloids, hydrous oxides: effect on rheologic properties of liquid phases, and interfacial boundary region.

* Sherman, P.: *Emulsion Science*, p. 286. 1968, Academic Press, London and New York.

are packed in as close an arrangement as possible ("close-packing"—see discussion on micromeritics). When the ratio between the internal and the external phases is approximately 74/26, the emulsion may invert and break, and the viscosity drops precipitously. Concentrated emulsions exhibit plastic flow, and the ratio of the phases determines the magnitude of the yield value. The increase in consistency of an o/w emulsion with an increase in the oil phase concentration is well demonstrated in Figure 7-24. The limiting concentration of the internal phase should be 74 percent if the globules are uniform spheres and not distorted. In reality, the ratio can go much higher when both large and very small globules are present in the emulsion and when the particles are not perfect spheres but are irregularly shaped. A photomicrograph of such a highly concentrated emulsion is shown in Figure 7-25. Note that the smaller globules fit into the spaces between the larger ones, and some of the large globules are distorted to permit very close packing.

The hydrocolloids ordinarily used as emulsifying agents in pharmaceutical emulsions impart non-Newtonian flow properties

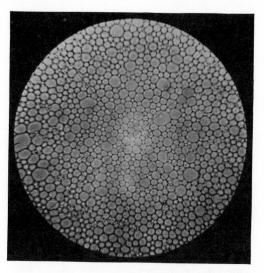

FIG. 7-25. Photomicrograph of a close-packed emulsion. The smaller globules lie between the larger globules, and some of the larger globules are irregular in shape. In such a case ϕ can be considerably larger than 0.74. (Atlas Surface-Active Agents. Atlas Chemical Co., Wilmington, Del.)

to the product, and, if the volume ratio of the phases is held constant, different emulsifying agents can provide markedly different viscosities. Knoeckel and Wurster[37] used various viscosity types of methylcellulose to prepare a number of emulsions. The over-all viscosity of the emulsions was found to follow the change in viscosity grades of methylcellulose.

The viscosity of the internal phase, i.e., the oil in an o/w emulsion, has little influence on the over-all viscosity of the product. However, different oils can produce products with very different viscosities. The interfacial film surrounding the oil droplets can be affected by the physical and the chemical properties of the internal phase and, thus, may produce a significant effect on the viscosity of the emulsion.[58]

Although the particle size of the dispersed phase does not have a marked influence on viscosity of an emulsion below the concentration at which close packing occurs, a decrease in particle size usually leads to an increased viscosity. Particle size distribution also has an influence on viscosity. Emulsions having particles of uniform size are

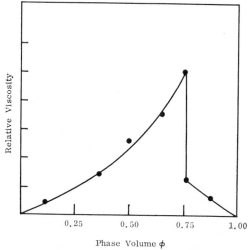

FIG. 7-24. The effect of concentration on the viscosity of an emulsion. The emulsion inverts at $\phi = 0.74$, and the viscosity drops sharply. Beyond the inversion point the curve represents the viscosity of the inverted emulsion. (After Becher, P.: Emulsions: Theory and Practice. p. 73. New York, Reinhold, 1965)

more viscous than products with a wide range in particle sizes.

Thus, it is seen that many factors, including the characteristics of the internal phase, the external continuous phase, and the emulsifying agent, must be taken into consideration in studying the flow properties of emulsions. The performance of emulsions, lotions, and creams depends in part on their rheology. Consequently, the flow properties of dispersions must be understood by the pharmacist if he is to design these dosage forms to meet the multiple specifications required in their application.

Biopharmaceutical Considerations

Unfortunately, little published work has appeared on the availability of drugs when formulated in emulsion dosage forms. However, it is possible to make some generalizations as to the potential effects brought about by this formulation approach.

It may be theorized that the oral administration of drugs in an oil solution will result in a slower, perhaps lower, bioavailability than administration of the same drug as an aqueous solution. This would result if the rate-limiting step in absorption was the rate at which drug partitions from the oil to the aqueous contents of the gastrointestinal tract. Emulsification could be expected to enhance this transfer from oil to aqueous phase because of the large increase in specific area. However, two other factors must be taken into account. First, what is the likely effect of the emulsifying agent per se, especially if it is a synthetic surfactant? At the present time, there are conflicting reports in the literature as to whether the addition of surfactant enhances or retards absorption. Consequently, any increase in availability on emulsification might be offset by the emulsifier, if it worked to retard availability. Second, what will be the effect of the interfacial film of emulsifying agent on the partitioning of the drug from the oil phase into the surrounding aqueous medium? It is possible that the presence of a dense interfacial film could slow down this process by providing a mechanical barrier to diffusion.

In comparing the rate and extent of bioavailability of a drug from the oil phase of an emulsion with that from an aqueous suspension, bioavailability might be adversely affected if partitioning is slow compared to

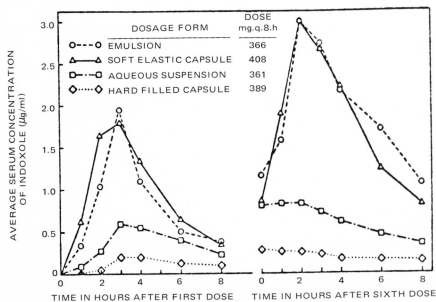

FIG. 7-26.   Average serum concentrations of indoxole following the first and sixth low doses of indoxole in four different dosage forms. (Wagner, J. G., Gerard, E. S., and Kaiser, D. G.: The effect of the dosage form on serum levels of indoxole. Clin. Pharmacol. Ther., 7:610-619, 1966)

absorption. On the other hand, with solid particles of drug suspended in water, dissolution is frequently the rate-limiting step in the absorption process. If partitioning from the oil phase of the emulsion across the interfacial film is more rapid than dissolution from the solid particle, it can be anticipated that the emulsified dosage form will be superior to an aqueous suspension from the biopharmaceutical point of view.

Two studies show the potential advantage to the use of emulsified dosage forms. When comparing the effect of dosage forms on the serum levels of indoxole, a nonsteroidal anti-inflammatory agent, Wagner and co-workers[60] found the oral emulsion to be as good as or superior to three other types of dosage forms tested. The drug was dissolved in the oil phase of the emulsion, which consisted of a vegetable oil and was present in an oil-to-water phase volume ratio of approximately 0.67. The average serum concentrations of indoxole following the first and the sixth dose of indoxole when administered as an emulsion, a soft elastic capsule, an aqueous suspension, and a hard capsule are shown in Figure 7-26. Enhanced bioavailability of sulfonamides was observed by Daeschner et al.[12] when administered orally in an emulsion, as compared to an aqueous suspension.

BIBLIOGRAPHY

Becher, P.: Emulsions; Theory and Practice, New York, Reinhold, 1965.

Berkman, S., and Egloff, G.: Emulsions and Foams. New York, Reinhold, 1941.

Carter, P. J.: Basic emulsion technology. Am. Perfumer Aromat., *71*:43, 1958.

Chen, J. L., Cyr, G. N., and Langlykke, A. F.: Pharmaceutical emulsions. Drug Cosmetic Ind., *81*:596, 1957.

Sherman, P.: Emulsion Science. London, Academic Press, 1968.

Sumner, C. G.: Clayton's Theory of Emulsions, and Their Technical Treatment. Ed. 5. New York, Blakiston, 1954.

White, R. F.: Pharmaceutical emulsions and emulsifying agents. London, Chemist and Druggist, 1964.

REFERENCES

1. The Atlas HLB System. Ed. 2 (revised). Atlas Chemical Co., Wilmington, Del., 1963.
2. Benerito, R. R., and Singleton, W. S.: J. Am. Oil Chem. Soc., *33*:364, 1956.
3. ———: Am. Perfumer Aromat., *69*:37, 1957 (March).
4. Bergy, G. A.: J. Am. Pharm. A. (Pract. Ed.), *3*:358, 1942.
5. Blythe, R. H.: U.S. Patent No. 2,369,711, 1945.
6. Buckwalter, F. H., and Dickison, H. L.: J. Am. Pharm. A. (Sci. Ed.), 47:661, 1958.
7. Butler, A. Q., and Ramsey, J. C., Jr.: Drug Std., 20:217, 1952.
8. Carr, R. L., Jr.: Chem. Eng., 72:163, 1965 (Jan. 18).
9. Chun, A. H. C., Joslin, R. S., and Martin, A. N.: Drug Cosmet. Ind., 82:164, 1958.
10. Conrad, L. I.: Am. Perfumer Aromat., 71:70, 1958 (June).
11. Corran, J. W., and Lewis, W. C. McC.: Biochem. J., *18*:1364, 1924.
12. Daescher, C. W., Bell, W. R., Stivrins, P. C., Yow, E. M., and Townsend, E.: Am. J. Dis. Child., *93*:370, 1957.
13. Davies, J. T.: Proc. Second Internat. Congr. Surface Activity, *1*:426, 1957.
14. Davies, J. T., and Rideal, E. K.: Interfacial Phenomena. New York, Academic Press, 1963.
15. Dintenfass, L.: Kolloid-Z., *163*:48, 1959.
16. Edmundson, I. C.: *In* Bean, H. S., Beckett, A. H., and Carless, J. E. (eds.): Advances in Pharmaceutical Sciences. Vol. 2, p. 95. New York, Academic Press, 1967.
17. Fincher, J. H.: J. Pharm. Sci., 57:1825, 1968.
18. Florence, A. T., and Rogers, J. A.: J. Pharm. Pharmacol., *23*:153, 1971.
19. Foernzler, E. C., Martin, A. N., and Banker, G. S.: J. Am. Pharm. A. (Sci. Ed.), *49*:249, 1960.
20. Friberg, S., and Wilton, I.: Am. Perfum. Cosmet., *85*:27, 1970 (December).
21. Garrett, E. R., Miller, G. H., and Brown, M. R. W.: J. Pharm. Sci., 55:593, 1966.
22. Gibaldi, M.: Introduction to Biopharmaceutics. Philadelphia, Lea and Febiger, 1971.
23. Griffin, W. C.: J. Soc. Cosmet. Chem. *1*:311, 1949.
24. ———: J. Soc. Cosmet. Chem. 5:249, 1954.
25. Groth, H., and Skurnik, L.: Acta med. scand., *101*:333, 1939.
26. Haines, B. A., and Martin, A. N.: J. Pharm. Sci., 50:756, 1961.
27. Haleblian, J., and McCrone, W.: J. Pharm. Sci., 58:911, 1969.
28. Henderson, N. L., Meer, P. M., and Kostenbauder, H. B.: J. Pharm. Sci., 50:788, 1961.
29. Hiestand, E. N.: J. Pharm. Sci., 53:10, 1964.
30. ———: Proc. Am. A. Coll. Pharm. (Teacher's Seminar), *13*:125, 1961.
31. Higuchi, W. I., *et al.:* J. Pharm. Sci., *51*: 1081, 1962; 52:162, 1963; 53:405, 1964; *54*: 74, 1205, 1303, 1965.
32. Hom, F. S., Autian, J., Martin, A. N., Berk, J. E., and Teplick, J. G.: J. Am. Pharm. A. (Sci. Ed.), 46:254, 1957.
33. Hubbard, D. G., and Freeman, L. G.: J. Am. Pharm. A. (Pract. Ed.), 2:78, 1941.

34. Jones, C. M., Culver, P. J., Drummey, G. D., and Ryan, A. E.: Ann. Int. Med., *29*:1, 1948.
35. Kempson-Jones, G.: Am. Perfum. Aromat., *71*:88, 1958 (June).
36. King, A.: Trans. Faraday Soc., *37*:168, 1941.
37. Knoeckel, E. L., and Wurster, D. E.: J. Am. Pharm. A. (Sci. Ed.), *48*:1, 1959.
38. Koehne, M., and Mendel, L. B.: J. Nutr., *1*:399, 1929.
39. Kostenbauder, H. B., and Martin, A. N.: J. Am. Pharm. A. (Sci. Ed.), *43*:401, 1954.
40. Krantz, J. C., Jr., and Gordon, N. E.: J. Am. Pharm. A., *15*:83, 1926.
41. Lambert, G. F., Miller, J. P., and Frost, D. V.: J. Am. Pharm. A. (Sci. Ed.), *45*:685, 1956.
42. Lees, K. A.: J. Pharm. Pharmacol., *15*:43T, 1963.
43. Macek, T. J.: *In* Remington's Pharmaceutical Sciences, Ed. 14. Chap. 79. Easton, Pa., Mack Publishing Co., 1970.
44. Martin, A. N.: J. Pharm. Sci., *50*:513, 1961.
45. Martin, A. N., Banker, G. S., and Chun, A. H. C.: *In* Bean, H. S. Beckett, A. H., and Carless, J. E. (eds.): Advances in Pharmaceutical Sciences. Vol. 1, p. 1. New York, Academic Press, 1964.
46. Martin, A. N., Swarbrick, J., and Cammarata, A.: Physical Pharmacy. Philadelphia, Lea and Febiger, 1969.
47. Meyer, R. J., and Cohen, L.: J. Soc. Cosmet. Chem., *10*:143, 1959.
48. Oldshue, J. Y.: J. Pharm. Sci., *50*:523, 1961.
49. Orr, C., Jr., and DallaValle, J. M.: Fine Particle Measurement. Chap. 10. New York, Macmillan, 1959.
50. Pickering, S. U.: J. Chem. Soc., *91*:2001, 1907.
51. Prout, W. A., and Harris, R. G.: J. Am. Pharm. A. (Pract. Ed.), *2*:431, 1941.
52. Riegelman, S., Swintosky, J. V., Higuchi, T., and Busse, L. W.: J. Am. Pharm. A. (Sci. Ed.), *39*:44, 1950.
53. Samyn, J. C.: J. Pharm. Sci., *50*:517, 1961.
54. Schulman, J. H., and Cockbain, E. G.: Trans. Faraday Soc., *36*:651, 661, 960, 1940.
55. Serrallach, J. A., Jones, G., and Owen, R. J.: Ind. Eng. Chem., *25*:816, 1933.
56. Shoskes, M., Geyer, R. P., and Stare, F. J.: Proc. Soc. Exp. Biol. Med., *75*:680, 1950.
57. Shoskes, M., Van Itallie, T. B., Geyer, R. P., and Stare, F. J.: Am. Dietet. A., *27*:191, 1951.
58. Shotton, E., and White, R. F.: J. Pharm. Pharmacol., *12*:108T, 1960.
59. Silberberg, A.: J. Phys. Chem., *66*:1884, 1962.
60. Wagner, J. G., Gerard, E. S., and Kaiser, D. G.: Clin. Pharmacol. Ther., *7*:610, 1966.
61. Wedderburn, D. L.: *In* Bean, H. S., Beckett, A. H., and Carless, J. E. (eds.): Advances in Phamaceutical Sciences. Vol. 1, p. 195. New York, Academic Press, 1964.
62. White, R. F.: Pharmaceutical emulsions and emulsifying agents. Chemist and Druggist p. 116, London, 1964.
63. Wilder, H.: Druggist Circ., December, 1874.
64. Wilson, R. G., and Ecanow, B.: J. Pharm. Sci., *52*:757, 1031, 1963.

8

Louis C. Zopf, D.Sc., *Dean Emeritus, College of Pharmacy,*
University of Iowa
and
Seymour M. Blaug, Ph.D., *Professor of Pharmacy, College of Pharmacy*
University of Iowa

Semisolid Dosage Forms:
Ointments, Creams and Pastes

OINTMENTS

GENERAL CONSIDERATIONS

Semisolid dosage forms for external application include ointments (unguents), pastes and creams. An ointment for use in the eye is called an ophthalmic ointment or oculentum. Other semisolid preparations for external use are cerates and poultices (cataplasms); however, they are seldom prescribed in modern dermatologic practice. Cerates were used as dressings and protectives for inflamed areas of the skin, and poultices were used to reduce inflammation or, in some instances, to act as counterirritants.

For centuries, the word ointment implied a semisolid preparation containing medicinal agents uniformly dispersed in a fatty base. The modern concept of an ointment is much broader and includes semisolid preparations entirely free of oleaginous materials. The following definition is offered as consistent with modern thinking: Ointments are semisolid preparations intended for application to the skin with or without inunction. They may be oleaginous (e.g., White Ointment); they may be entirely free of oleaginous substances (e.g., Polyethylene Glycol Ointment), or they may be emulsions of fatty or waxlike materials containing relatively high proportions of water (e.g., Hydrophilic Ointment). Besides serving as vehicles for topical application of medicinal substances they also function as lubricating agents (emollients) for the skin and as protectives to prevent contact of the skin surface with aqueous solutions and skin irritants.

Lane and Blank[58] reviewed ways in which a therapeutic agent may act when applied to the skin after incorporation in a topical vehicle. For example, it may react chemically with the skin by direct chemical combination, oxidation or reduction. The exact chemical reactions of many drugs with the skin are not well defined; however, clinical experience has taught the physician how to use many drugs topically. The vehicle is not thought to react chemically with the skin.

If a drug penetrates the skin it may alter the physiologic activity of the skin. Again, the vehicle itself seldom alters the physiology of the skin. However, insofar as it may affect the penetration of the drug, the vehicle may indirectly influence the physiologic activity of the skin.

Finally, a topically applied preparation may produce a physicochemical effect. Almost all medicated and nonmedicated topical vehicles influence the skin in one way or another by virtue of their physical and physicochemical properties. Vehicles containing constituents with low boiling points will cool the skin, through evaporation; an occlusive covering such as an oil will warm the skin by preventing normal evaporation of the sweat and retarding radiation of heat; the same type of covering will make the skin more supple, due to hydration of dry skin; an organic solvent will make the skin less supple, due to defatting and/or dehydration.

In dermatologic therapy, the vehicle rarely undergoes a specific biochemical reaction with the skin, and physiologic and allergic reactions to the vehicle are rare. However, physicochemical changes which depend to a large extent on the vehicle do occur. These changes may be an important part of the over-all action of the therapeutic agent.

According to Beeler,[8] various authors have described the ideal ointment base in terms of its physicochemical properties as follows: (1) stable; (2) neutral in reaction; (3) nongreasy; (4) not degreasing in action; (5) nonirritating; (6) nondehydrating; (7) nonhygroscopic; (8) water removable; (9) compatible with all medication; (10) free from objectionable odor; (11) nonstaining; (12) capable of serving as a medium for medicaments soluble in either fat or water; (13) efficient on dry, oily or moist skins; (14) capable of stock preparation for extemporaneous use; (15) composed of readily available ingredients of known chemical composition; (16) capable of holding at least 50 percent of water; (17) easily compounded by the pharmacist, and (18) melting or softening at body temperature.

An ointment base may possess several of these properties, depending on the type of base and its end-use. For example, an anhydrous absorption base is capable of absorbing a large quantity of water but is not readily removed from the skin with water. It is a stable base, neutral in reaction and nonhygroscopic. When a water-containing absorption base is used as a skin emollient, the lack of ease of removal with water is a desirable property, since the base forms an occlusive film on the skin and thus prevents water loss through evaporation. On the other hand, this would be an undesirable property if the ointment were to be used on a hairy region such as the scalp.

HISTORY

Fats from every available source and mixtures of these with active and inert materials were among the earliest substances employed by man for medicinal purposes. Our earliest records of the use of various fats and oils (Ointments-Unguents) date back to the Babylon-Assyria era, about 3,000–5,000 B.C. Examination of remains of such ointments found in the excavated tombs of Egyptian kings supports the view that the fats of ointment bases of olden times were taken almost exclusively from the animal kingdom.

The concept of Ointment in the modern sense was long in developing. In ancient times, there was no special terminology differentiating between liquid and semisolid preparations used as an anointment. The Greeks had terms classifying the different anointments: (1) partly according to use, e.g., "malagma," softening ointment (*malasso,* soften) and (2) partly according to some important ingredient, e.g., "keroma," wax ointment (*keros,* wax), which was the predecessor of cerates.

The great Greco-Roman physician Claudius Galenus (A.D. 2nd century) formulated an ointment consisting of olive oil, rose oil, white wax and a small quantity of water. This was the prototype for all the cosmetic ointments which later were known as cold cream. In the form as given by a mysterious 13th century author who wrote under the name of Mesuë Jr., this cold cream has found its way, with minor modifications, into all of the pharmacopeias of the world up to and including the present. At about that time (13th century) the distinctions between oils, ointments and plasters became general: Olea being liquid oily ointments, Unguenta semisolid smears, and Emplastra masses sticking firmly to the skin.

The above concept of ointments remained unchanged for almost half a millennium. The following definition from the first *U.S.P.,* published in 1820, shows that the concept of Mesuë Jr. still prevailed in the early 19th century:

Ointments are prepared from lard or oil rendered of the consistence of butter by the addition of suet, wax or spermaceti, so as to suspend the dry powders and more ponderous articles, with which they are frequently incorporated. As they are to be applied to the skin, they should be soft or fluid at the temperature of the body. The following formulas are calculated for a temperature not exceeding 60° Fahr. In higher temperature, more suet or wax may be added.

From the middle of the 19th century on, we encounter several attempts at a broadening of the concept of the term ointment. The ointment bases offered by nature were purified, augmented and partly replaced by artificial ones, introduced with special regard for the purposes they were intended to serve. These new ointment bases appeared in the following sequence:

1858: Glycerin and Starch. The apothecary Schacht found that glycerin and starch, if heated in certain proportions and to a certain temperature, combined to a translucent jelly, which he called *plasma* and recommended as a good ointment base. This mixture appeared in continental pharmacopeias as Unguentum Glycerini, in the *British Pharmacopœia* as Glycerinum Amyli and in the *U.S.P.* as Glyceritum Amyli.

1873: Cosmolin and Paraffin Ointment. Dr. A. W. Miller published a paper on "Cosmolin and Paraffin Ointment," which later was to be known as petrolatum.

1876: Stearic Acid. Herman Hager wrote in his handbook that "stearic acid is used as a substitute for white wax in the preparation of ointments to be sold over the counter."

1885: Wool Fat, "Oesypus," Rediscovered. The pharmacologist Oscar Liebreich rediscovered the therapeutic value of wool fat, the "œsypus" of the ancient Greeks, which he called *lanolin.*

1895–98: Wool Fat Alcohols. The Russian chemist Lifschuetz discovered and proved that the ease with which wool fat (lanolin) is taken up by water depends, not as formerly was supposed, on the cholestrin ethers it contains but on the free alcohols which he had isolated as a group.

1907: Eucerin. The great dermatologist Unna, on the basis of his research, introduced "Eucerin," a new base for ointments consisting of a part of Lifschuetz's alcohols with 20 parts of paraffin ointment and 20 parts of water. This was the forerunner of the American counterpart, "Aquaphor."

1920–44: Numerous contributions appeared, among which hydrogenated oils, sulfated and sulfonated hydrogenated oils, stearic acid, sodium stearate, glyceryl stearate mixtures possessing self-emulsifying properties, polymers of glycols, such as polyethylene glycol 4,000, and esters of these glycols such as polyethylene glycol monostearate, became of foremost importance.

1945–59: Surface-active agents, Plastibase (a hydrocarbon base), attapulgite, silicones, Veegum, guar gum, Carbopol, etc.,

were introduced. These are useful as adjuncts to ointment bases or as bases themselves.

1960–: The popularity of emulsion bases, especially of o/w emulsion bases, increased. One of the outstanding advantages of o/w emulsion bases is the ease with which they can be removed from skin and clothing with water. Oil-in-water emulsion vehicles deserve special mention because of the claims that they promote percutaneous absorption of drugs, due to the presence of surfactants.[60] Zeutlin and Fox[121] and Strakosch and Clark[106] supported with their experiments the theory of superiority of emulsion type vehicles over oleaginous vehicles. However, it should be noted that contradictory results may be found in percutaneous absorption studies of ointment bases because of many types of test subjects and the different medicaments used in each study.[35]

Creams, which are usually described as semisolid preparations less viscid than ointments, also increased in popularity in the sixties. In addition to Cold Cream, *U.S.P. XVIII* contains monographs for 6 official creams, and 13 creams are official in *N.F. XIII.* There were only 2 creams official in each of the previous editions of the *U.S.P.* and the *N.F.*

Ointments to soften the skin, i.e., emollient ointments, and ointments to protect the skin against moisture, air and chemicals increased in usage in the early sixties.

Medicated tapes were introduced in the sixties. These are plastic surgical tapes impregnated with an active ingredient, such as flurandrenolide.* The pressure-sensitive tape serves as both a vehicle and an occlusive dressing. Retention of perspiration by the tape results in hydration of the stratum corneum and improved diffusion of the medicament.

In summary, we may note that the term *ointment* has passed from the Greco-Roman times when it was used in its broadest sense (to include anything used as a "smear," whether it be aqueous or oily) through a period of more restricted use (from the time of Mesuë Jr.) when it was applied to only soft unctuous preparations, to the modern

---

* Cordan Tape, Eli Lilly and Co., Indianapolis, Ind.

tendency toward a broader use of the term to again include aqueous as well as fatty and hydrocarbon bases; e.g., the designation of vanishing creams and bentonite pastes as ointments.

CLASSIFICATION OF BASES

Ointments can be classified best according to type (based on composition):

I. OLEAGINOUS OINTMENT BASE

1. Anhydrous
2. Does not absorb water readily (hydrophobic)
3. Insoluble in water
4. Not water removable

II. ABSORPTION OINTMENT BASE

1. Anhydrous
2. Will absorb water (hydrophilic)
3. Insoluble in water
4. Most are not water removable

III. EMULSION OINTMENT BASE

A. Emulsion Ointment Base w/o
   1. Hydrous
   2. Will absorb water
   3. Insoluble in water
   4. Not water removable
   5. Water-in-oil emulsion
B. Emulsion Ointment Base o/w
   1. Hydrous
   2. Will absorb water
   3. Insoluble in water
   4. Water removable
   5. Oil-in-water emulsion

IV. WATER-SOLUBLE OINTMENT BASE

1. Anhydrous
2. Will absorb water
3. Soluble in water
4. Water removable
5. Greaseless

Lane and Blank[58] classified topical vehicles (including ointments, creams and pastes) according to the physicochemical action of the vehicle on the skin, i.e., according to whether the vehicle acted on the skin primarily as an aqueous vehicle, an oily vehicle, a powder or an organic solvent.

1. Vehicles which act as aqueous mixtures:
   A. Water
   B. Shake lotions: e.g., a mixture of zinc oxide and water
   C. Gels of hydrophilic colloids: e.g., bentonite jelly or surgical lubricant
2. Vehicles which act as oils:
   A. Water-immiscible oils: e.g., petrolatum or olive oil
   B. Water-miscible oils: e.g., anhydrous lanolin
   C. Oil-in-water emulsions: e.g., vanishing creams
   D. Water-in-oil emulsions: e.g., lanolin
   E. Pastes: e.g., a mixture of starch and petrolatum
   F. Collodions
3. Vehicles which act as powders:
   A. Hydrophilic powders: e.g., starch
   B. Hydrophobic powders: e.g., talc or zinc stearate
4. Vehicles which act as organic solvents:
   A. Water-miscible solvents: e.g., alcohol or acetone
   B. Water-immiscible solvents: e.g., ether

At one time it was believed that the primary factor influencing penetration through the skin was the vehicle itself. Thus, Goodman[36] classified ointments according to penetration or penetrability, as follows:

1. **Epidermic ointments** are those which demonstrate no, or at the most very slight, power of penetration into the skin. These are indicated especially when it is intended that a therapeutic effect shall be exerted chiefly on the diseased epithelium. In this group are placed the bases which contain petrolatum, waxes and their combinations.

2. **Endodermic ointments** are those which possess some power of penetration into the deeper layers of the skin. In this group are placed the softer bases which liquefy at body temperature, such as the vegetable oils, lard, lanolin, anhydrous lanolin and/or combinations of these.

3. **Diadermic ointments** are those which penetrate the skin, thus offering a better opportunity for absorption of the medicament. Ointments of the emulsion type and the water-soluble bases belong to this group.

In the light of more recent evidence on the process of absorption through the skin and the liberation of substances from ointment bases, we must look on the above therapeutic classification with some degree of skepticism.

PERCUTANEOUS ABSORPTION

Ointments, creams and pastes may be employed as (1) protectives, (2) agents to soften or render the skin more pliable and (3) vehicles or carriers for medicaments. In the last-mentioned case, they may serve as vehicles for drugs having as their chief purpose a local action, i.e., topical anesthetics, steroids, etc., or they may serve as vehicles for drugs from which absorption and systemic effects are desired. The term *percutaneous absorption* is used when referring to the passage of medicinal substances through the skin. Rothman[87] defines percutaneous absorption as the penetration of substances from the outside into the skin and through the skin into the bloodstream. However, it should be noted that, in general, localized action is desired for cosmetics and medicaments. Systemic absorption should be kept to a minimum, both to prolong the contact of the drug with the skin tissues and to reduce undesirable side-effects produced by systemic absorption.

The skin is composed of many different tissues, including blood vessels, sebaceous glands, sweat glands, sense organs and nerves, connective tissues, smooth muscle and fat. In the average human, the skin surface area has been estimated at approximately 18 square feet. Excluding fat, the weight of this skin is about 8 pounds.[118]

The human skin (Fig. 8-1) consists of three distinct layers, the epidermis, the dermis and the subcutaneous fat tissue.

The epidermis is the external layer of the skin, varying in thickness from 0.16 mm. on the eyelids to 0.8 mm. on the palms and soles. Histologists have subdivided the epidermis into five layers; starting from the outermost, they are as follows:

1. Stratum corneum (horny layer)
2. Stratum lucidum; "barrier zone"
3. Stratum granulosum (granular layer)
4. Stratum spinosum (prickle cell layer)
5. Stratum germinativum; basal cell layer

The epidermis functions as a protective barrier against bacteria, chemical irritants, allergens, etc.

The horny layer, or stratum corneum, is thickest on the soles of the feet and is much thinner on the eyelids, cheeks and forehead. There is a microscopic surface film of emulsified lipids covering the stratum corneum. This protective film usually has a pH on the acid side, from about 4.5 to 6.5. This so-called acid mantle of the skin is derived from the lactic acid and dicarboxylic amino acids in the sweat secretions, mixed with the sebaceous lipoidal substance. Drastic changes in the pH of this mantle may give rise to bacterial invasion and various dermatoses.[28]

The stratum corneum consists of layers of flattened, stratified and fully keratinized dead cells. The superficial dead cells are shed or scraped off and are continually renewed by the cornification of other cells that are evolved by the basal cell layer and pushed up from below.

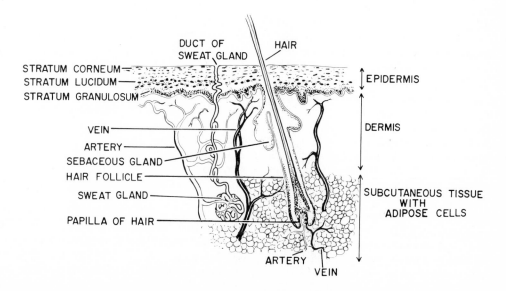

FIG. 8-1. Cross section of human skin.

The stratum corneum probably represents the principal skin barrier to water loss. The several layers of the dead, keratinized cells are strongly hydrophilic and swell considerably when immersed in water. This water-holding capacity of keratin, a sulfur-containing fibrous protein, tends to keep the skin's surface supple and soft. The skin becomes dry and scaly when the water content of the stratum corneum falls. The surface film of emulsified lipids on the skin surface does help retain the water in the skin, although the lipid film is not an occlusive water-repellant coat.[48]

The stratum lucidum is the intermediate region between the stratum corneum and the granular layer. It has been referred to as a "barrier area," since it is clearly demonstrable only in the sole of the foot and the palm of the hand.

The stratum granulosum actively participates in the keratinization process, although the exact mechanism remains obscure. This layer consists of flattened, coarsely granular cells which started out in the germinal layer as columnar, nucleated cells. As they move toward the surface, the germinal or basal cells start losing their columnar shape and become polyhedral in the lower level of the stratum spinosum and increasingly flattened at the higher levels. The stratum spinosum and stratum germinativum are together called the malpighian layer.

The basal cell layer is the innermost layer of the epidermis and consists of regularly outlined columnar cells which form the imaginary base line separating the epidermis from the corium. The function of the basal cells is to reproduce and to form the layers that constitute the epidermis.

The dermis, or corium, is 3 to 5 mm. thick. Its surface projects into the undersurface of the epidermis and helps connect the two layers of the skin. The dermis is mainly a network of collagen and elastin fibers which form a network that is responsible for many of the important properties of the skin. The dermis contains blood vessels, lymph vessels, hair follicles, sebaceous glands, sweat glands, muscle and nerve fibers and pacinian corpuscles. In the uppermost region of the corium there are many conelike ridges, or papillae, which form the papillary layer projecting into the epidermis. The papillary layer contains the nerve endings which are affected by changes of temperature and by the application of local anesthetics, as well as by irritants.

The subcutaneous fatty tissue is a specialized layer of the corium which acts as a cushion and heat insulator.

The intact skin is an effective barrier to penetration. The absorption of drugs depends primarily on the physiologic state of the skin and the physicochemical properties of the drug and, to a lesser degree, the vehicle in which the drug is incorporated.

Despite the vast amount of literature in the field, there is little agreement on the basic mechanism responsible for percutaneous absorption through intact skin. Percutaneous absorption can occur through the anatomic zones shown in Figure 8-2, i.e., directly through the intact epidermis, either between or through the cells of the stratum corneum or through the appendages of the skin such as the sweat glands, sebaceous glands and the hair follicles (or both). Griesemer[37] and Katz and Paulsen[55] consider in more detail these various anatomic zones as they affect permeability of the skin.

Acording to Tregear,[111] it appears that the route of entry is through the epidermis itself rather than through the appendages and that the resistance to this entry is a physical property of dead cells uncomplicated by "active processes." The resistance does not appear to be a function of a specialized membrane but is a property of the keratinized cell matrix of the stratum corneum, assisted by the surface lipids. Penetration probably occurs through this cornified system rather than down the hair shafts or sweat glands, but whether through or around the keratinized cells is unknown. Penetration reaches practical proportions when the penetrant is a very small molecule which is present in very high concentration or is highly active locally or systemically.[112] Scheuplein[92] considers the entire stratum corneum to function as the rate-limiting barrier to penetration in the skin, and not a "barrier layer" at the base of the tissue. Once through the stratum corneum, diffusion increases rapidly in the dermis.

The hair follicles and sweat glands of skin

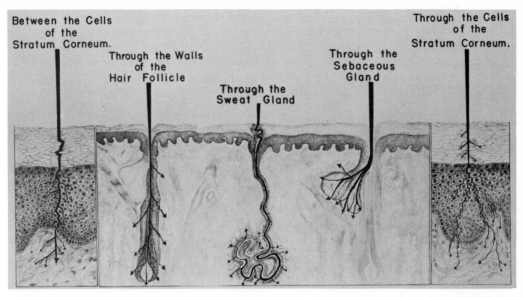

FIG. 8-2.   Possible avenues of penetration into and through the unbroken skin. (Griesemer, R. D.: J. Soc. Cosmetic Chem., *11*:81, 1960)

represent potential parallel paths, or shunts, through which materials may penetrate the skin. According to Tregear[112] there is no preferred pathway through the pilosebaceous apparatus, for in man the hair follicles are probably not important as a means of penetration. However, Sheuplein et al.[93] feel that percutaneous absorption of the steroids and probably other large molecules occur via appendages as well as through the intact stratum corneum.

Treherne[113] studied the permeability of excised rabbit skin to some nonelectrolytes. He concluded that the barrier to diffusion through the skin is situated in the epidermis and that the rate of penetration is related to the ether/water partition coefficient of the penetrant, the compounds with a high partition coefficient penetrating more rapidly than those with a lower value. He concluded that the barrier is lipid in character and that diffusion through the dermis resembles that through a large-pored membrane, with diffusion probably occurring through the liquid-filled extracellular spaces.

According to Mali,[71] the main avenue of penetration for medicaments is through the epidermis rather than the sebaceous glands or the sweat glands, simply because the epidermis presents a surface area 100 or 1,000 times greater than the other two. Under special conditions the sweat glands or the sebaceous glands may be preferential pathways, as during sweating or for lipid-soluble substances. However, for most conditions and substances the direct path through the epidermis is probably the important one.[37]

OTHER FACTORS AFFECTING PERCUTANEOUS ABSORPTION

According to Higuchi[41] and Wagner[116] chemical and physical relationships between the base and the medicament incorporated therein are of greater significance than the penetrating properties of the base itself in influencing percutaneous absorption. More precisely, whether the medicament itself can be absorbed is the important consideration.

Based on diffusion coefficients determined for sodium radioiodide in several ointment bases,[44] the skin presents a formidable barrier to the diffusion of drug molecules. Thus, the rate-determining step in percutaneous absorption through intact skin must be the diffusion across the stratum corneum. Only when the drug reaching the stratum corneum is immediately absorbed and carried away, i.e., sink conditions, can one ignore the properties of the skin as far as percutaneous absorption is concerned. Under these conditions, the rate-determining step for the absorption process would be the release rate of the drug from the vehicle. The latter depends on the properties of the drug and of the vehicle in which the drug is incorporated. Sink conditions might occur when the epidermis has been traumatized or diseased, thereby reducing or eliminating the stratum corneum as a diffusion barrier.

Diffusion through the skin is usually a passive process governed by Fick's Law of Diffusion. Higuchi[42] developed the basic equations, based on Fick's general law, which are useful in describing the variables affecting the release rate of drugs in solution and uniformly distributed throughout a vehicle or the release rate of solid drugs suspended in a topical vehicle. In either case, the rate-controlling step is diffusion within the vehicle phase.

When a drug is in solution in the vehicle, its release rate can be altered by changing either the drug concentration or its diffusion coefficient, provided that certain conditions are met—i.e., only a single drug species is important in the vehicle, the components of the vehicle cannot diffuse out, the diffusion constant of the drug in the vehicle is constant with respect to both time and position in the vehicle, and the drug reaching the receptor phase (skin) is removed rapidly. The release rate can be altered more readily by changing the concentration of the drug than by attempting to vary its diffusion coefficient.

For drug particles suspended in a topical vehicle such as a homogeneous ointment (e.g., petrolatum) or in the external phase of an emulsion type base, Higuchi[42] showed that the release rate of the drug, when its solubility in the base is very small, may be described by the following simple equation:

$$\frac{dQ}{dt} \simeq \left[\frac{ADC_s}{2t}\right]^{1/2}$$

where A is the drug concentration in units per cm.^{3}, D is the diffusion coefficient of the drug in the vehicle, and C_s is the solubility of the drug in units per cm.^{3}. The release rate can be controlled by changing the diffusion coefficient, the total drug concentration, and the solubility of the drug in the vehicle.[42]

For most drugs, the percutaneous absorption is limited by the impermeability of the skin; i.e., the rate-limiting step is diffusion across the stratum corneum or skin barrier. Diffusion through the skin is almost always a passive process. The rate of diffusion $\left(\frac{dQ}{dt}\right)$, as defined by Fick, depends on the magnitude of the concentration gradient (Δc) across the membrane whose area is A, and the permeability coefficient (P). The permeability coefficient depends on the diffusivity of the molecule through the skin barrier, the effective partition coefficient of the drug between skin barrier and vehicle, and the effective thickness of the skin barrier.

$$\frac{dQ}{dt} = - PA\, \Delta_c$$

In essence, the driving force or the rate of transfer across the membrane is the concentration of the applied drug.

The activity of the drug in the vehicle is the product of the drug concentration and the activity coefficient of the drug in the vehicle. Since, for most drugs, the rate-limiting step in percutaneous absorption is the diffusion across the skin barrier, the highest activity of the drug in the vehicle is needed to obtain the maximum rate of penetration. At a given drug concentration, the activity coefficient of the drug and its thermodynamic activity in the vehicle at that concentration may vary manyfold from one vehicle to another. A drug that has a strong affinity for a vehicle shows a low activity coefficient. Therefore, the thermodynamic activity of the drug in that vehicle is low, and its rate of release from the vehicle will be slow. Drugs that have a low affinity for a vehicle exhibit high activity coefficients; therefore, their rates of release from the vehicle are higher.

Treherne[113] found a direct relation between the ether/water partition coefficient of an aqueous solute and its permeability constant through rabbit skin. Other investigators[56,73] also recognized the relation between the partition coefficient of a compound and its ability to penetrate through human skin.

The partition coefficient can be defined as:

$$PC = \frac{C_s}{C_v}$$

where C_s and C_v are the drug concentrations found at equilibrium in the stratum corneum and the vehicle, respectively. The lipid/water partition coefficient of a compound is not as significant as the stratum corneum/vehicle partition coefficient. A low partition coefficient value indicates a high degree of affinity between the drug and vehicle and reflects the tendency of the drug to remain in the vehicle.[41] If the drug is much more soluble in the stratum corneum than in the vehicle in which it is dissolved, a large partition coefficient value would indicate that the concentration of drug in the initial layers of the stratum corneum at equilibrium may be much higher than the concentration in the vehicle. Drug concentration in the lower regions of the stratum corneum will remain near zero, since these regions are in contact with a fluid through which diffusion is relatively fast. Therefore, the amount of drug which penetrates per unit area in unit time is more closely related to the concentration gradient between the upper and lower layers of the stratum corneum. The concentration of drug in the top layer of the stratum corneum is related to the solubility of the drug in the stratum corneum and the vehicle, i.e., its partition coefficient (PC), as shown in the expanded form of Fick's law:

$$\frac{dQ}{dt} = \frac{D(PC)\Delta c}{h}$$

where D is the diffusion constant of the drug in the skin barrier, h is the thickness of the skin barrier, and the permeability coefficient (P) now becomes:

$$P = \frac{(PC)D}{h}$$

D can be calculated when PC and P have been determined experimentally and h is known. It should be kept in mind that this equation applies only to simple diffusion and then only to the "steady state" period of diffusion. When true steady-state diffusion is reached, the permeability coefficient is independent of concentration. Changes in the diffusion constant may occur if the diffusing drug interacts with the skin or the skin interacts with the vehicle, resulting in deviations from the expanded form of Fick's law.

The expanded form of Fick's law shows that the diffusion rate of a drug through the skin barrier is directly dependent upon the partition coefficient and on the concentration of drug dissolved in the vehicle. To relate diffusion rate through the skin to the partition coefficient requires the use of partition coefficient values determined for the equilibrium distribution of the drug between the vehicle and the skin rather than the values determined in an arbitrarily selected two-phase system, such as ether/water or chloroform/water.

The partition coefficient of a drug is roughly proportional to the drug's solubility in the two immiscible phases, i.e., the skin and the vehicle. Since the diffusion rate of a drug through the skin barrier is directly dependent on its partition coefficient and on the concentration of drug in the vehicle, the percutaneous absorption of a drug can be more easily altered by modifying the solubility of a particular drug in the vehicle, by altering the composition of the vehicle, or by modifying the structure of the drug rather than by attempting to improve the solubility of the drug in the skin barrier. The positive effects of such modifications on percutaneous absorption have been illustrated with the corticosteroids. Triamcinolone has only one tenth the topical activity of hydrocortisone. Converting the triamcinolone to its acetone increases its lipid solubility, yielding a more favorable partition coefficient and a much enhanced topical activity.[67] Similarly, the conversion of betamethasone to betamethasone-17-valerate increased topical activity over tenfold.[68]

Dempski et al.[25] and Poulsen and coworkers[82] demonstrated the effects of altering vehicle composition on the release of dexamethasone and fluocinolone acetonide and its acetate ester, respectively. Their results indicated that the important factors influencing the release of the steroids into the receptor phase, in vitro, were the solubility in the vehicle and the partition coefficient of the steroid between the vehicle and the receptor phase. For example, Poulsen's study showed that optimal release was obtained from vehicles containing the minimum concentration of propylene glycol required for complete solubilization of the steroid while maintaining a high partition coefficient. When propylene glycol in excess of that required to solubilize the steroid was present, release from the base was decreased because the partition coefficient decreases at higher propylene glycol concentrations.

The availability of a drug applied to the skin in a semisolid vehicle depends on the rate of release of the drug from the vehicle and on the permeability through the skin barrier. For many years it was believed that the primary factor influencing penetration through the skin was the vehicle itself—thus, the classification of ointments according to penetration rather than to type based on composition.[36] Absorption can and does occur from any ointment base, depending not only on the composition of the base but on many other factors such as the condition of the skin, the site of application, the hydration state of the stratum corneum, skin temperature, the presence of solvents which can combine with or dissolve in the stratum corneum, plus the factors already discussed, such as concentration of active ingredient, solubility characteristics of the penetrating drug, and the vehicle-skin barrier partition coefficient of the penetrant.

The influence of the vehicle on percutaneous absorption has been reviewed by many investigators.[4,7,80] The percutaneous absorption of some drugs, particularly the corticosteroids, is markedly affected by changes in vehicle composition.[28,82] However, the influence of vehicle composition on percutaneous absorption is usually related to an effect on the solubility of the drug in the vehicle, on the activity coefficient of the drug, and on the vehicle/skin partition coefficient of the drug rather than on the effect of the vehicle on the skin itself.

A vehicle that affects the hydration state of the skin can have a marked influence on percutaneous absorption. Hydration of the stratum corneum is probably the most important factor influencing percutaneous absorption.[100] Hydration results from water diffusing from lower epidermal layers and from the accumulation of perspiration after the application of an occlusive vehicle or covering on the skin surface.

Wurster and Kramer[120] studied the absorption of three salicylate esters under hydrous and anhydrous skin conditions. The absorption rate of the three salicylates increased markedly under hydrous conditions. The absorption rates were related to the distribution coefficients and the solubilities of the three drugs in water. Fritsch and Stoughton[34] showed the importance of both temperature and humidity on the penetration of acetylsalicylic acid through excised human skin. Full hydration dramatically increased the penetration when compared to the penetration obtained under conditions of lower humidity.

Powers and Fox[84] showed that water-insoluble materials such as petrolatum and lanolin retarded the rate of loss of water from the skin, while some emulsifiers and humectants increased the rate of water loss. Dempski et al.[24] compared the effect of petrolatum, an isopropyl myristate gel, three oil-in-water corticosteroid creams, and an occlusive covering (Saran wrap) on moisture retention in vitro. The three creams were permeable to water and the petrolatum and isopropyl myristate were about equal to Saran wrap in their resistance to water loss.

Sulzberger and Witten[108] and McKenzie and Stoughton[69] have shown that the topical efficacy of corticosteroids can be improved and their penetration through the skin barrier enhanced by occluding the site of application with a thin plastic film which aids in hydrating the stratum corneum.

Although the intact skin acts as a formidable barrier to skin penetration, diseased or traumatized skin usually becomes permeable to almost any substance. If the skin barrier is destroyed by trauma, as in cuts, chapping, ruptured blisters, or eczema, all substances pass freely into the dermis.[37]

Very little work has been published on the variations in percutaneous absorption from one skin site to another. Furthermore, reports[72,91] in the literature present conflicting views, i.e., there are wide variations in the reported absorption of a specific substance through the same skin site. However, variations in absorption rates from different sites is probably proportional to the thickness of the area to which the substance is applied, the rate of penetration being inversely proportional to the thickness.

The resistance of skin to penetration by drugs is reduced by increases in temperature.[13] Although there is a direct relationship between temperature and the permeability of skin, it is probably of minor importance, since the effect of solvents and vehicles on skin temperature is transitory. Occlusive coverings such as Saran wrap probably increase the skin temperature by a few degrees, but the effect is probably slight when compared to that produced by the increase in skin hydration.

Idson[47] discussed the role of organic liquids used to increase the penetration of topically applied drugs. Such penetration enhancers or accelerants[1] apparently have a direct effect on the permeability of the skin barrier. The best known of the accelerants are dimethyl sulfoxide (DMSO), dimethyl formamide (DMF), and surface active agents. DMSO and DMF are strongly hygroscopic, and their presence in the stratum corneum probably increases its hydration. Kligman[57] reviewed the role of DMSO as a penetration enhancer.

DMSO is an unusually effective solvent. In addition to solvating the stratum corneum (human skin is highly permeable to DMSO), DMSO may bring about configurational changes in skin protein structure, with resultant swelling. Swelling may open channels within the stratum corneum, thereby lowering its effectiveness as a barrier to certain drugs. Also, DMSO can leach out soluble fractions from the stratum corneum, increasing its permeability.[29] DMSO has been shown to enhance the penetration of many drugs.[105,107] No drug product containing DMSO is marketed in the United States at the present time, owing to FDA restrictions.

Many nonpolar solvents increase the permeability of the skin, probably through removal of lipids from the stratum corneum. Such delipidization reportedly lowers the activation energies for water through the stratum corneum.[13]

High concentrations of nonpolar solvents such as heptane, chloroform, etc., or of polar solvents such as DMSO, are required to produce a marked increase in the permeability of the skin. In contrast to this is the reported effectiveness of dilute solutions of anionic surfactants in increasing the permeability of the skin to water.[12] Scheuplein and Ross,[94] using a diffusion cell, determined the permeability of human abdominal epidermis to aqueous solutions of sodium lauryl sulfate in order to measure the effect on the permeability of the epidermal membrane. Dilute solutions of sodium lauryl sulfate produced large increases in water permeation. The permeability constant for water increased with increasing concentrations of the surfactant. Partial recovery of the barrier function of the skin was observed after removal of the surfactant. The effect of the surfactant on stratum corneum permeability was attributed to reversible denaturation of the epidermal protein caused by the laurate anion, accompanied by a gross expansion of the tissue and possible hole formation.

Drawing our conclusions from the more recent evidence in regard to the part that ointment bases play in the absorption of substances through the skin, we may postulate that:

1. Ointment bases in general tend to slow or delay absorption through the intact epidermis and from mucous surfaces.

2. It is not the penetration of the base in a direct sense which determines whether absorption will occur through the intact skin or not, but the chemical and the physical (solubility) relations between the drug and the base and the drug and the skin which determine whether absorption will occur and in what amounts it will occur.

3. Petroleum ether, benzene and chloroform are efficient substances for preparing the skin for absorption and they carry substances dissolved in them through the skin much more efficiently than if these same substances were incorporated in ointment bases. Polar solvents such as dimethyl sulfoxide (DMSO) are also penetration enhancers.

4. The degree of hydration of the skin is of greater significance in influencing percutaneous absorption than is the vehicle itself.

5. The amount of damage to the epidermis and the degree of loss of normal skin barriers to absorption are more important than the vehicle in determining penetration through the epidermis.

6. Vehicle composition is important in

topical therapy, since the vehicle can and does exert its own effect on the skin because of its soothing, emollient, and protective action. As discussed previously, the vehicle can exert a profound effect on the release of the active ingredient.

Much study also has been devoted to the field of ointment bases as carriers for antiseptics. These studies also reveal a conflict of opinion as to the value of aqueous ointment bases and anhydrous bases as carriers for antiseptics. Some authors have reported the increased effectiveness of antiseptics in aqueous bases, while others have reported that the antiseptic action was not greatly increased over that with the anhydrous base. In summarizing and analyzing the results of these reports, one may make the following general statements:

1. There is as yet no ointment base reported which can serve as a universal ointment base.

2. The conclusion by G. F. Reddish, "that the antiseptic value of an ointment could not be told by the antiseptic value of its constituents" still holds true.

3. Claims for water-containing ointment bases as vehicles for antiseptics over that of the greasy type bases are not justified unless on an individual basis.

4. The chemical and the physical nature of the antiseptic which is incorporated in the base has as much or, perhaps, more to do in determining the final bactericidal action of the product than the composition of the vehicle in which it has been incorporated.

CHEMICAL AND PHYSICAL CLASSIFICATION

The following is a classification of those substances which, at this time, are used to a greater or lesser extent as ointment bases in themselves or contribute some pharmaceutical property to the base as a whole.

I. HYDROCARBONS

Liquid petrolatum
White petrolatum
Yellow petrolatum
Paraffin
Ceresin
Microcrystalline wax
Plastibase (Jelene)

II. ALCOHOLS
A. Aliphatic
  1. Monohydroxy
    Lauryl
    Myristyl
    Cetyl
    Oleyl
    Stearyl
  2. Polyhydroxy
    Ethylene glycol
      a. Polyethylene glycols 200 to 700 are liquids
      Polyethylene glycols 1,000 to 6,000 are solids and are known as Carbowaxes
    Diethylene glycol
    Propylene glycol
    Glycerol
B. Cyclic
  Cholesterol
  Isocholesterol
  Oxycholesterol
  Anhydrous lanolin ⎫ Mixtures, the
  Lanolin   ⎬ hydrophilic property of which is due, in part, to these alcohols

III. ACIDS
A. Aliphatic
  Lauric
  Myristic
  Palmitic
  Oleic
  Stearic
B. Cyclic
  None commonly used in ointments

IV. ESTERS
A. Monohydroxy alcohols
  1. Aliphatic
    Beeswax white
    Beeswax yellow
    Carnauba wax
    Spermaceti
  2. Cyclic
    Cholesterol palmitate
    Cholesterol stearate
B. Polyhydroxy alcohols
  1. Dihydroxy (glycols)
    a. Mono-esters
      Ethylene glycol laurate, oleate, ricinoleate, stearate
      Propylene glycol laurate, oleate, ricinoleate, stearate
      Diethylene glycol laurate, myristate, oleate, palmitate, ricinoleate, stearate
      (1) Polyethylene glycol 400 monolaureate, monostearate

b. Di-esters
 Ethylene glycol dilaurate, distearate
 Diethylene glycol dilaurate, distearate
  (2) Polyethylene glycol 300 di-oleate, polyethylene glycol 1,000 di-oleate

2. Trihydroxy (glycerol)
 a. Mono-esters
  Glycerol monomyristate, oleate, palmitate, ricinoleate, stearate
 b. Di-esters
  None commercially prepared
 c. Tri-esters (fats)
  Synthetic
   Glyceryl tristearate
  Natural (animal)
   Lard
   Lard, benzoinated
  Natural (vegetable)
   Almond oil, expressed
   Cacao butter
   Castor oil
   Coconut oil
   Corn oil
   Cottonseed oil
   Linseed oil
   Olive oil
   Soybean oil
  Modified natural fats
   Hydrogenated castor oil
   Hydrogenated corn oil
   Hydrogenated cottonseed oil
   Hydrogenated soybean oil
   Sulfated-hydrogenated castor oil
   Sulfonated (sulfated) castor oil

3. Hexa-hydroxy (mannitol, sorbitol, dulcitol)
 a. Mono-esters
  Mannitol monolaureate, oleate, stearate
  Sorbitol monolaurate, oleate, stearate
 b. Di-esters
  Sorbitol dilaurate, dioleate, distearate
  Mannitol distearate
 c. Tri-esters
  Mannitol triricinoleate, tristearate
  Sorbitol triricinoleate

4. Hexahydroxy anhydrides (sorbitan and hexitan)
 Sorbitan monolaurate, oleate, stearate
 Polyoxyethylene (20) sorbitan mono-oleate (Polysorbate 80, U.S.P.) also known as Tween 80

5. Fatty acid esters
 Polyoxyethylene stearate (Polyoxyl 40 Stearate, U.S.P.) also known as Myrj 52

V. SOAPS

Oleates (sodium, potassium, ammonium, calcium, magnesium)
Stearates (sodium, potassium, ammonium, calcium, magnesium)
Vanishing creams (sodium, potassium, ammonium, triethanolamine soaps)

VI. MISCELLANEOUS

A. Silicon derivatives
  Colloidal clays
   1. Bentonite
   2. Hectorite
   3. Veegum
  Silicones
B. Cellulose derivatives (see chapter on Emulsions)
C. Gelatin (see chapter on Emulsions)
D. Sodium alginate (see chapter on Emulsions)
E. Glycerite of starch (see under History)

VII. PHYSICAL CLASSIFICATION (BASED ON COMPOSITION)

A. Oleaginous-hydrocarbon (see under chemical classification)
B. Absorption
C. Emulsion, w/o & o/w
D. Water-soluble

VIII. OPHTHALMIC OINTMENTS

HYDROCARBONS

This group represents the most inert of chemical compounds. It comprises a group of substances with a wide range of melting points, so that a mixture of any desired consistency and melting point may be prepared with representatives of this group. These substances are stated to possess the least power of penetration and, therefore, are used chiefly as protectives and emollients in topical application.

The liquid paraffins are used chiefly as agents in which powders are incorporated (triturated, rubbed) before they are mixed with the bases of a higher consistency. This aids in reducing the particle size of the powder. These are also mixed with petrolatum to make it less viscous.

White Petrolatum U.S.P. and Petrolatum N.F. are frequently used as ointment bases or as constituents of emulsion bases. White petrolatum is petrolatum wholly or nearly decolorized. Both are composed of microcrystalline, solid hydrocarbons suspended in liquid and semisolid hydrocarbons.

The advantages of the petrolatums lie in their consistency, stability, blandness and chemical inertness, which allow almost any medicinal substances to be incorporated in them. Their disadvantages lie in their greasiness and inability to absorb or mix with water. However, this can be remedied by mixing 15 percent of anhydrous lanolin with them; this mixture will absorb up to 50 percent of water.

Petrolatums are used as vehicles for most types of medicaments, particularly those that are unstable in the presence of water, i.e., antibiotics (penicillins, bacitracin, tetracyclines). They are used also as emollient, protective coverings for the skin, since they form an occlusive film on the skin which retards moisture evaporation. Large amounts of powder added to petrolatum form a stiff ointment referred to as a paste.

In order to keep the skin supple, a certain water content must be maintained (probably between 10 and 20% of water). At a low water content, the stratum corneum usually becomes dry and brittle. This may occur when the water diffusing into the stratum corneum from the lower tissue layers is insufficient to replace the water lost by evaporation when the relative humidity is low. While hydrocarbons and other oil materials do not lubricate dry skin, probably because of inability to penetrate the stratum corneum, they are sufficiently occlusive to reduce the loss of water from the skin. Their action as simple emollients is primarily a surface phenomenon, in that they help the stratum corneum maintain an adequate water content. Oil-in-water and water-in-oil emulsions can be formulated to be occlusive or nonocclusive; however, water-in-oil emulsions are usually more occlusive than the oil-in-water type, since the oil phase in water-in-oil emulsions is continuous (see Chap. 7).

The use of white and yellow wax to stiffen white and yellow petrolatum yields two official hydrocarbon bases, White Ointment U.S.P. and Yellow Ointment N.F. The official compendia permit variations in the amounts of petrolatum and wax to maintain a suitable consistency under various climatic conditions.

Paraffin and ceresin are of a higher melting point and are used chiefly as stiffening agents. Paraffin melts between 50° to 57°C. and ceresin melts between 61° to 78°C. Their advantages lie in their homogeneous structure. They do not crystallize on cooling after having been melted, and for this reason they are preferred to beeswax in cosmetic ointments. Ceresin is also known as ozokerite, earth wax and mineral wax. It is composed of hydrocarbons of complex composition and frequently is adulterated by the addition of paraffin.

Microcrystalline wax is an extremely complex mixture of saturated hydrocarbons. It does not include waxes showing gross crystalline structure such as paraffin wax. It is obtained from petrolatum by removal of a large percentage of the oil by solvent treatment, leaving a hard microcrystalline wax. Waxes varying widely in melting point or consistency can be prepared by varying the dilution ratio of solvent to petrolatum and the temperature of de-oiling. Microcrystalline waxes are used in cosmetic and dermatologic formulations to modify the crystal structure of other waxes present, particularly paraffin waxes, so that the mixture does not exhibit the change in crystal structure usually exhibited by paraffin wax alone over an extended time period. They also tend to minimize the seepage of oils from blends of waxes and oils. For dermatologic purposes, microcrystalline waxes fall between petrolatum and paraffin waxes. They generally have higher melting points than the paraffin waxes.

Plastibase (Jelene)* is a combination of mineral oils and heavy hydrocarbon waxes having a mol. wt. of about 1,300; the large part, which is liquid, is retained in what is believed to be a matrix of submicroscopic interstices. The base is a soft, unctuous, colorless, jellylike material which melts at 90° to 91°C. and maintains a desirable consistency over a wide temperature range (−15° to 60°).

Some precautions must be observed in the compounding of Plastibase ointments, since

---

* Product of **E. R. Squibb & Co.**

substances such as menthol, methyl salicylate and camphor are dissolved by Plastibase, with the result that ointments containing these chemicals become too soft. Likewise, coal tar produces an ointment too soft to prevent separation. Plastibase does not lend itself to the incorporation of waxes as stiffening agents because it is difficult to cool the resulting mixture to a smooth consistency. Plastibase ointments are best prepared by levigating the medicinal agent with a small portion of the base, then incorporating this with the remainder of the base.[51]

Plastibase is used as a vehicle for a dental protective paste, Orabase Emollient.† Orabase combines gelatin, pectin, and sodium carboxymethylcellulose in Plastibase. The emollient paste provides a protective, soothing covering for minor mouth irritations, and, because it adheres well to oral mucous membranes, it helps to protect minor irritated areas of the mouth and gums against further irritation from chewing, swallowing, and other normal mouth activity. Orabase Emollient contains no antibiotic, analgesic, or antiseptic and is nonirritating and nontoxic if swallowed.

ALCOHOLS

Aliphatic: MONOATOMIC. This group is made up of the fatty alcohols chiefly from C_{12} through C_{18}. They are used in some cases as stiffening agents but chiefly for their emollient and emulsion-stabilizing properties. They are greaseless, forming water-absorbent emulsions, and render the skin velvety rather than smooth and slippery. Cetyl alcohol is the most commonly used of this group, athough stearyl alcohol has been recommended for use in several bases. These may be used as additives in 1 to 5 percent concentration of from 5 to 20 percent as the principal wax. Beeler's Base[9] and the University of California Hospital Base illustrate their use:

BEELER'S BASE

Cetyl alcohol	15.0
White wax	1.0
Propylene glycol	10.0
Sodium lauryl sulfate	2.0
Water	72.0

† Product of Davies Rose Hoyt, Needham Heights, Mass.

U. C. H. BASE

Cetyl alcohol	6.4
Stearyl alcohol	6.4
Sodium lauryl sulfate	1.5
White petrolatum	14.3
Mineral oil	21.4
Water	50.0

Ointments that are made with these alcohols must be stirred thoroughly during their preparation.

POLYATOMIC. This group, which includes substances such as diethylene glycol, propylene glycol and glycerol, is used chiefly in ointments containing water—particularly when the emulsion is of the oil-in-water type. Due to hygroscopicity, they absorb and retain moisture from the air, thus acting as humectants in the emulsion. Propylene glycol has been recommended as a substitute for glycerol not only because of shortages during war but also because it assists in obtaining a more intimate dispersion of soaps, oils, greases and other such substances in water.

The application of this group of compounds developed greatly with the introduction of polymers of these substances into pharmacy. Various polymers of ethylene glycol of the general formula $HOCH_2(CH_2OCH_2)_nCH_2OH$ having molecular weights from 200 to 6,000 have been utilized in many formulas. Polyethylene glycols are liquids when the molecular weight is below 700 and are waxlike and increasingly solid in consistency as the molecular weight increases to 6,000. The compounds with molecular weights of 1,000 or more are unctuous but water-soluble; they are inert and may be recommended as major ingredients of water-removable ointment bases.

Cyclic. Cholesterol and the cholesterol alcohols, oxy and iso, together with the mixture of these alcohols and of their esters in their natural proportions as in lanolin or in a purified and concentrated form dispersed in a suitable mineral hydrocarbon vehicle (Aquaphor,* Hydrophilic Petrolatum U.S.P.) are the chief representatives of this group. The latter mixtures are included here because their hydrophilic properties and the beneficial softening effect on the skin are reported to be due to the

* Duke Laboratories, Norwalk, Conn.

lanolin alcohols and esters present in these mixtures. Dryness or oiliness of the skin is attributed to a combination of several factors such as the nature and the amount of sebum secreted, sweating, the degree of hydration of the stratum corneum, etc. The emolliency of human sebum is due in part to the presence of cholesterol, which is the chief sterol in human sebum[37] (see also Rothman[87]). Calvery et al.[17] attributed the emollient effect of cholesterol to its hydrophilic properties in the unesterified form.

The modern use of lanolin (Anhydrous Lanolin U.S.P.) began with the rediscovery of its properties by Liebreich. Hartman (1860) and Schulze (1872) proved that lanolin contained cholesterol and oxycholesterol, and O. Braun discovered the hydrophilic properties of this same material. In 1886, Liebreich assigned the hydrophilic properties of lanolin to the cholesterol esters. Lifschuetz discovered in lanolin the free alcohols isocholesterol and oxycholesterol. Unna realized the medical and the pharmaceutical value of Lifschuetz's discovery and, in 1907, introduced Eucerin, a mixture of 5 percent of Lifschuetz's alcohols in petrolatum. This base possessed the property of absorbing up to 700 percent of water.

There is still disagreement as to which lanolin fraction endows lanolin with the ability to absorb water. Tiedt and Truter[110] attribute this ability to the free alcohols in lanolin, mixtures of the alcohols being better emulsifiers than a single alcohol. However, Bertram[11] claims that it is the high-molecular-weight diesters of hydroxy acids that endow lanolin with the ability to absorb water.

Many lanolin derivatives and fluid lanolins were developed in order to overcome some of the disadvantages of lanolin such as its stickiness, poor solubility in mineral oil, water and alcohol, its inability to penetrate into the stratum corneum and its sensitizing potential. Modification of the lanolin structure has resulted in the preparation of lanolin derivatives such as acylated lanolins, ethoxylated lanolins, hydrogenated lanolins, transesterified lanolins, etc. Wagner[115] and Sagarin[89] give examples of commercial products in each of these categories. Lanolin derivatives have varying solubility

characteristics, i.e., they may be alcohol-soluble, water-soluble, soluble in mineral and vegetable oils, etc. The lanolin derivatives generally are less sensitizing than lanolin. However, it should be noted that allergic reactions to the use of lanolin are very few in number; compared with the amount of lanolin used, they are negligible. A study of the incidence of allergic skin reaction to lanolin and its components revealed that 1.04 percent of 1,430 persons tested responded with positive patch test reactions.[117] This incidence was observed in a selected group of persons suffering from various dermatologic disorders, and a much lower incidence may be expected among the general population.

Lantrol,*[59] a clear, light amber liquid lanolin produced by a solvent crystallization process that separates the higher, "waxy," sticky esters from the oil-soluble liquid esters, possesses some unusual characteristics. It is a chemically unchanged lanolin that is soluble in mineral oil and a wide variety of oils and solvents. It is mutually soluble with the human skin lipids[15] and forms water-in-oil emulsions that release their moisture content very slowly to soften desiccated keratin.[78] Lantrol has been shown to be effective in retarding the rate of moisture loss through human skin without completely occluding the skin surface.[83]

An emollient ointment containing Lantrol was developed in the Dermatology Research Laboratory at the University of Iowa, College of Pharmacy.

University of Iowa Emollient Ointment

White petrolatum	41.0
Microcrystalline wax	3.0
Lantrol	10.0
Span 80*	4.75
Tween 80† (Polysorbate 80, U.S.P.)	0.25
Purified water	41.0

Warm the aqueous dispersion of Span 80 and Tween 80 to 75°C. and add it to the melted wax, white petrolatum, Lantrol phase slowly, with stirring. Stir until congealed.

Clark[21] has published a comprehensive

* Malmstrom Chemical Corp., Newark, N.J.
* Sorbitan monooleate, Atlas Chemical Industries, Inc., Wilmington, Del.
† Polyoxyethylene sorbitan monooleate, Atlas Chemical Industries, Inc., Wilmington, Del.

report on liquid lanolin, its development, production, properties and uses. The report includes a list of liquid lanolin trade names with their producers or suppliers.

The foregoing facts do not in themselves reveal the tireless efforts of workers to prepare a satisfactory ointment base. The introduction of lanolin in 1885 was hailed because it was thought that at last a base was available that did not possess the undesirable properties of the others—namely, immiscibility with water, alcohol and glycerin— and yet possessed the advantages of stability, blandness and unctuousness.

The disadvantages of anhydrous lanolin were soon to be discovered: (1) tendency toward rancidity, (2) disagreeable odor, (3) water-absorbing capacity less than desirable for cooling ointments, and (4) pitchlike consistency. While the introduction of hydrous lanolin reduced the above objections somewhat, they still remain to a certain degree; therefore, these two bases are generally mixed with the hydrocarbon bases.

Hydrophilic Petrolatum, U.S.P., contains cholesterol. This formula differs from the one which was introduced in *U.S.P. XIII* in that the original formula contained less cholesterol and 15 percent of anhydrous lanolin. Anhydrous lanolin was deleted because of its potential sensitizing effect on the skin; however, apprehension on the part of practitioners in regard to the use of anhydrous lanolin in dermatologic preparations has been decreasing. The increase in cholesterol in the *U.S.P. XIV* and *XV* formulas gives a product that is capable of absorbing large quantities of water.

The *British Pharmacopœia* contains a Wool Alcohols Ointment:

WOOL ALCOHOLS OINTMENT, B.P.

Wool alcohols*	60.0
Hard paraffin	240.0
White or yellow soft paraffin	100.0
Liquid paraffin	600.0

ACIDS

The acids of this group which are used in the ointment field are generally from 12 to

* Wool alcohol is a crude mixture of sterols and triterpene alcohols prepared by treating wool fat with alkali and separating the fraction containing cholesterol and other alcohols.

18 carbon atoms in length. They are used generally as a source of free acid in order to react with alkali and form a soap either in cold or vanishing cream ointment bases. Sometimes stearic acid is used as a stiffening agent, but this use is not general.

The following formula illustrates the use of a fatty acid which is reacted with an alkali to form a soap.

VANISHING CREAM

Lanolin	2.0
Cetyl alcohol	1.0
Mineral oil	5.0
Stearic acid	9.0
Potassium hydroxide	0.5
Propylene glycol	5.0
Purified water	77.5

Warm the lanolin, cetyl alcohol and mineral oil until blended. Dissolve the potassium hydroxide and propylene glycol in the water and heat to approximately the same temperature as the oil mixture. Add the aqueous phase to the oil phase, with constant stirring. Stir until the mixture congeals.

As these acids generally are used to form a soap and this, in turn, is to act as the emulsifying agent, the acid of choice, of course, is the one that will make the most stable emulsion. In this respect, it has been shown that there is an increase in emulsifying power of soaps from C_{12} to C_{18} and that, above C_{18}, we again have a continual decrease in this property. Therefore, it follows that stearic acid is probably the most frequently used acid of the group and explains why vanishing creams are almost always known as stearate creams.

ESTERS

Esters of Monoatomic Alcohols: ALIPHATIC. This group includes chiefly beeswax (yellow and white), carnauba wax and spermaceti. The melting point ranges are from 42° to 50°C. for spermaceti to 84° to 86°C. for carnauba wax. Beeswax is intermediate, with a melting point of 62° to 65°C. These substances are used chiefly to increase the consistency of ointments, particularly those that are distributed in the warmer southern areas. They are used generally in amounts up to 5 percent.

These compounds consist chiefly of esters of the higher fatty alcohols and acids such as cetyl palmitate, myricyl cerotinate and melissyl palmitate. However, beeswax and carnauba wax contain, in addition to the esters, free fatty acids such as cerotic acid, carnaubic acid and melissic acid. It is this free fatty acid content that is desired in beeswax for use in cold creams. For this purpose, beeswax should possess an acid number of 18 to 23 in order that enough soap may be formed by reaction with the alkali to stabilize the emulsion formed. Spermaceti, while chiefly ester, contains a small amount of free cetyl alcohol and very small amounts of free acid. Hence, it is used only for its hardening effect and the free cetyl alcohol it contains.

While comparatively stable, these substances will turn somewhat rancid on long standing if exposed to air.

CYCLIC. These consist chiefly of the fatty acid esters of cholesterol, oxycholesterol and isocholesterol. They are used with the cyclic alcohols in amounts up to 3 and 5 percent to confer hydrophilic properties on petrolatum. Petrolatum containing cyclic alcohols with and without cyclic esters absorb and emulsify water, forming water-in-oil emulsions.

Esters of Polyhydric Alcohols. This group is comprised of the fatty acids (C_{12}–C_{18}) esters of the polyhydroxy alcohols from glycol to mannitol. It also includes the esters of such compounds as glycol ethers. Of the many compounds of this type already known, it is interesting to note that, up to the present, the only polyhydric alcohol fatty acid esters occurring naturally have been the triglycerides of various animal, vegetable and fish oils and fats. All of the others are prepared synthetically, generally by reacting the chlorhydrin with the sodium salt of the acid; e.g., glycerochlorhydrin or propylene glycol chlorhydrin and sodium stearate.

Because of their similar properties, all of the synthetically prepared compounds are discussed together, and the following comments hold for all of the groups under Esters of Polyhydric Alcohols, except the naturally occurring triglycerides.

SYNTHETIC COMPOUNDS. It should be made clear that the usual commercial products available are not single chemical compounds but are mixtures of the mono-, the di- and in some cases the tri-fatty acid

esters, with perhaps a small percentage of free fatty acids. In addition, because these compounds in themselves are poor emulsifying agents, small amounts of soap, wetting agent or other surface-tension reducing agents are necessary to give these compounds emulsifying properties. Thus, glyceryl monostearate is available as glyceryl monostearate, nonemulsifying and glyceryl monostearate, self-emulsifying. Glyceryl monostearate is admixed with soap (usually sodium stearate), which lends it the self-emulsifying properties.

In themselves, these mixtures do not possess the necessary properties of an ointment base. They do not melt or soften at body temperature. However, they are excellent emulsifying agents and are useful in preparing ointment bases of the cold and the vanishing cream types. The type of emulsion formed is determined generally by the ratio of free hydroxyl groups to esterified ones and the percentage of free fatty acid. Thus, glyceryl monostearate will make an o/w emulsion whereas glyceryl tristearate will make a w/o emulsion. Sorbitol distearate is used to prepare o/w emulsions and sorbitol tetrastearate to prepare w/o emulsions. The ratio of free hydroxyl groups to esterified ones determines whether the agent is more water-miscible or more oil-miscible, and this, in turn, determines which phase, oil or water, will be the external phase. (The phase with which the emulsifying agent is most miscible will generally be the external phase.)

Glyceryl monostearate, glyceryl monostearate self-emulsifying, diglycol stearate and other similar compounds are widely used in the cosmetic and the pharmaceutical industries. The following formula serves as illustration:

OINTMENT BASE

White petrolatum 25.0
Cetyl alcohol 5.0
Lanolin 5.0
Glyceryl monostearate S.E. 15.0
Glycerin 5.0
Water 45.0

The general procedure for preparing emulsions containing polyhydric alcohol esters is to mix the oil miscible ingredients and warm to 80°C. Heat the water phase to about 85°C. and add the oil phase to the water phase with constant stirring.

Diglycol stearate or polyethylene glycol esters may often be used as the emulsifier in place of glyceryl monostearate, self-emulsifying.

Polyhydric alcohol esters confer on petrolatum, when mixed with it, the property of absorbing or emulsifying water; e.g., petrolatum when incorporated with small amounts of sorbitol oleate or laurate will absorb high percentages of water. The following formulae will serve to illustrate the use of these compounds:

Glyceryl monostearate, self-emulsifying	15.0
Mineral oil	5.0
Lanolin	1.0
Stearyl alcohol	1.0
Propylene glycol	5.0
Purified water	73.0

Warm the first four ingredients on a water bath and stir until blended. Dissolve the propylene glycol in the water and heat to approximately the same temperature as the oil phase. Add the aqueous phase to the oil phase, with constant stirring. Stir until congealed.

Diglycol stearate S*	15.0
Mineral oil	30.0
Lanolin	5.0
Water	50.0

Warm the first 3 ingredients on a water bath and stir until blended. Heat the water approximately the same temperature as the oil phase and add to the oil phase, with stirring. Stir until the base congeals.

NATURAL TRIGLYCERIDES OR ESTERS. This group, which comprises the natural animal and vegetable fats, served as the chief source of ointment bases until the middle of the 19th century. Among these fats, mutton suet and lard have played the most important roles. Of the animal fats, lard has always been preferred.

These fats, while similar chemically in that they are mixtures of the glycerides of palmitic, stearic and oleic acids, vary in the percentage of unsaturated acids (oleic, linoleic, linolenic) as esters and, thereby, differ in consistency. The consistency of these fats is in a direct ratio to the iodine number or degree of unsaturation of the glycerides. The glycerides of unsaturated fatty acids have lower melting points than those of the saturated acids. Thus, lard is softer and blander

* Glyco Products Co., Inc., Brooklyn, N.Y.

in consistency than mutton suet because of its higher percentage of triolein.

The vegetable and the animal fats have two disadvantages as ointment bases: (1) the water-absorbing capacity is low; (2) a pronounced tendency toward rancidity is present.

The property of water absorption is desirable in order that crystalline substances may be dissolved in water and the solution then incorporated into the base. This makes for smoother and more uniform ointments. Also, high percentages of water are desirable in ointments because of cooling and soothing effects. The property of water absorption also makes bases easier to wash off the skin.

The development of rancidity in ointments is definitely undesirable because of the irritating properties of the oxidized fats. Also, rancid fats possess a nauseating odor which is undesirable from a psychological standpoint. This disadvantage of animal and vegetable fats was recognized very early in the use of these compounds. In 1843 Deschamps discovered the preservative action of benzoin on lard. Since that time, benzoinated lard has become official in many of the leading pharmacopeias of the world. However, the true mechanism of the preservative action of benzoin on fats was not reported until 1933, when Husa and Riley[46] proved conclusively that coniferyl benzoate was the constituent of Siam benzoin responsible for the preservative effect on lard.

It has been shown also that air, light and metal containers hasten the development of rancidity in these fats.

VEGETABLE OILS. Olive oil, cottonseed oil, expressed almond oil, sesame oil and corn oil are used in ointments chiefly to lower the melting point or soften bases of a higher consistency and, also, as an adjunct to hydrocarbon bases to increase their emollient effects and decrease their drying effects. These oils can be used as ointment bases in themselves when a high percentage of powder is incorporated in a small amount of oil so that the resulting consistency is quite viscous. Thus, zinc oxide in castor oil is prescribed occasionally.

Vegetable oils are used extensively in cosmetic preparations such as cold and cleansing creams, dry skin creams and hand lotions.

Galen's original cold cream containing olive oil and the older pharmacopeia formulae containing almond oil were essentially emollient creams. The use of mineral oil in place of the vegetable oils gives a cream with enhanced spreading properties but less emolliency. Such creams are more suitable as cleansing creams, since the mineral oil is not absorbed as readily as vegetable oils. The uses and the formulation of various cosmetic ointments, creams and lotions are discussed by Harry.[39]

Castor oil differs from the other oils in that it contains hydroxy fatty acids and, therefore, has slightly different solubility properties. It is soluble in 95 percent alcohol, whereas the other oils are not. It is miscible with such substances as Peruvian balsam, whereas the other oils are not and will separate on standing.

HYDROGENATED OILS. Two of the three disadvantages of vegetable oils for use in ointment bases, i.e., consistency and development of rancidity, apparently are overcome for the most part through the process of hydrogenation. This is true because consistency and development of rancidity are both directly dependent on the degree of unsaturation. The immiscibility with water still remains as a disadvantage.

By hydrogenation under controlled conditions, such oils as cottonseed, soybean, corn oil and castor oil can be converted into white, semisolid, lardlike fats, or into hard, almost brittle, waxes. A completely hydrogenated oil is brittle and waxlike and is not satisfactory for use as an ointment base (unless it is mixed with a base of a much softer consistency). Conversely, an oil hydrogenated to an ointmentlike consistency is not completely hydrogenated and, therefore, contains unsaturated acids or esters. These are subject to oxidation and the development of rancidity; therefore, these bases can never reach the stability of petrolatum bases, although they are much more stable than the natural fats and can be used satisfactorily in prescription work. They have been the subject of much research as to their value as ointment bases.

Hydrogenated oils never achieved great popularity in dermatologic practice and are seldom used in prescription work. Fiero[32] gives an extensive treatment of these bases.

Hydrogenated Sulfated Oils. With the application of the process of sulfonation to hydrogenated oils, it appears that, for the most part, the disadvantages of vegetable fats as ointment bases have been overcome.

The consistency is satisfactory, the development of rancidity is very slow, the miscibility with liquids of an aqueous nature is sufficient for all pharmaceutic as well as most therapeutic needs.

Up to the present, the only sulfated hydrogenated oil recommended for ointment use has been castor oil. This oil, when hydrogenated to an iodine number of less than 10, is still capable of sulfation, because of the presence of the hydroxyl radical. It has the consistency of an ointment, whereas other sulfated oils are liquid. The consistency varies with the extent of sulfation. It has a pH of 6, and this is considered valuable because this is approximately the pH of the skin. It readily incorporates water, alcohol, glycerin, glycol and liquid petrolatum, as well as other bases such as petrolatum, spermaceti and wax. Hydrogenated sulfated castor oil is not subject to rancidity because it is completely hydrogenated and free from unsaturated acids.

The oil, according to Fiero,[33] possesses a peculiar stickiness which is advantageous when it is desired to produce an ointment that will adhere to the skin. For ointments in which a smooth, less adhesive property is desired, this stickiness can be removed by the addition of substances such as petrolatum, fats, glycerin, glycols or water. If the resulting ointment is too soft, the consistency may be increased by the addition of spermaceti, hydrogenated castor oil, stearic acid and other substances.

Hydrogenated sulfated oils are seldom, if ever, used in dermatologic prescriptions. However, sulfated oils, usually castor or soya, were used in shampoo formulations and in water-softening bath oil preparations. They have largely been replaced by synthetic detergents.

POLYOXYETHYLENE SORBITAN ESTERS. Polysorbate 80, U.S.P., chemically is polyoxyethylene sorbitan monooleate and is one of a series of compounds characterized by the partial fatty acid esterification of the anhydrides of sorbitol, with the addition of a polyalkalene oxide molecule through one of the hydroxy groups. This increases its water miscibility and, therefore, influences these products to form oil-in-water emulsions. This group of compounds is known commercially as Tweens. The Spans compounds are the partial fatty acid esters of sorbitan. This makes these compounds less water-miscible; therefore, they tend to form water-in-oil emulsions.

The compounds are utilized most effectively when formulated on the basis of their hydrophil-lipophil balance values (HLB) and on a knowledge of the required HLB values of the ingredients to be emulsified. The HLB value seems to be an expression of the relative simultaneous attraction of an emulsifier for oil and for water. In this way, the oil-loving Spans* have low HLB values (1.8 to 8.6) while the water-loving Tweens† have high values (9.6 to 16.7). The following formulae[3] will serve to illustrate the use of these compounds:

W/O ABSORPTION BASE

Petrolatum 90.0
Arlacel 83 sorbitan sesquioleate 10.0
Melt the ingredients and mix.

Arlacels are the same as Spans but are processed to provide unusually light color. The above formula can be used as an ointment base, or, if desired, water can be added to it to form a w/o ointment base.

O/W OINTMENT BASE

Cetyl alcohol 20.0
Mineral oil 20.0
Arlacel 80 sorbitan monooleate 0.5
Tween 80 (Polysorbate 80, U.S.P.) 4.5
Purified water 55.0

Heat the first four ingredients on a water bath to 70°C. Heat the water to 72°C. and add to the oil phase slowly, with agitation. Continue agitation until the ointment has cooled.

POLYOXYETHYLENE FATTY ACID ESTERS. Polyoxyl 40 Stearate, U.S.P., chemically is polyoxyethylene stearate, a reaction product of stearic acid and ethylene oxide. Polyoxyethylene derivatives of fatty acids are known commercially as Myrjs (Atlas Chemical Industries).

---

* Sorbitan fatty acid esters, Atlas Chemical Industries Inc., Wilmington, Del.
† Polyoxyethylene sorbitan fatty acid esters, Atlas Chemical Industries Inc., Wilmington, Del.

Like Polysorbate 80, Polyoxyl 40 Stearate is dispersible in water. This water miscibility influences Polyoxyl 40 Stearate and the other polyoxyethylene fatty acid derivatives to form oil-in-water emulsions. Since the polyoxyethylene fatty acid derivatives are nonionic in nature, they possess the advantages characteristic of this type product. They are particularly useful for emulsification in the presence of astringent salts.

Polyoxyl 40 Stearate was used as the emulsifying agent in Hydrophilic Ointment U.S.P. XV. Certain medicaments, phenolic compounds, carboxylic acids, etc., had to be incorporated with care in Hydrophilic Ointment U.S.P. XV, since it was shown that Polyoxyl 40 Stearate interacted with some pharmaceuticals to form soluble and insoluble molecular complexes.[20] This interaction was evidenced by a marked softening of the finished product. The formula for Hydrophilic Ointment U.S.P. now contains sodium lauryl sulfate as the emulsifying agent in place of Polyoxyl 40 Stearate, thereby eliminating this particular difficulty.

POLYOXYETHYLENE FATTY ALCOHOL ESTERS. A series of compounds closely related to the Myrj surfactants are the Brij group of surfactants (Atlas Chemical Industries). These compounds are polyoxyethylene fatty ethers while the Myrjs are esters. The ether type of product, since no ester linkages are present, is stable to many acids and alkalis beyond the usual pH ranges which emulsifiers might be expected to withstand. Therefore, they are useful for emulsifying oils and waxes in unusually acid or alkaline media. Like the polyoxyethylene fatty esters, the Brijs are nonionic and can be used in the presence of anionic and cationic materials.

SOAPS

While there are many soaps that may be used as ointment bases, the sodium, the ammonium and the potassium salts of oleic or stearic acid are used most commonly. The calcium and the magnesium salts are used sometimes, but not so frequently as the above.

Soaps may be used as such (preformed), e.g., as sodium stearate, and satisfactory ointment bases may be prepared by mixing water with the powdered soap (generally in concentrations of from 20 to 30%), after which other ingredients may be incorporated.

Soaps may serve as ointment bases or contribute some property to the base and be formed as a reaction product during the preparation. Ammonium oleate, when formed by the reaction between oleic acid and ammonium hydroxide in light liquid petrolatum and wax, yields the class of bases known as petroxolins. Sodium stearate, when formed by the reaction between stearic acid and a sodium base in the presence of oils, water and waxes, yields the vanishing cream bases. Calcium oleate, when formed by mixing olive oil and lime water in correct proportions and adding calamine and zinc oxide, yields the frequently used calamine cream. In slightly different proportions, this mixture yields calamine liniment.

Although soaps are used generally in ointment bases for their emulsifying properties, they were introduced initially into the ointment field to increase the penetrating properties of the preparations in use at that time. For instance, it generally is believed that the class of preparations known as oleates (e.g., mercury oleate), were advocated not only for their pharmaceutical value, but also because of their supposedly increased penetrating properties. The use of soap as an emulsifier is illustrated in the following formula:

Mineral oil	50.0
Beeswax	16.0
Borax	1.0
Purified water	33.0

Heat the beeswax and mineral oil to 70°C. Dissolve the borax in water at 75°C. and add to the melted oil phase, with continuous stirring. Stir until cool.

In this cold cream formula the soap is formed by the reaction of borax with the wax acids contained in beeswax. Other alkalies instead of borax can be used, e.g., potassium hydroxide.

The class of preparations known as petroxolins (chiefly ammonium oleate) were introduced because of their miscibility with water and their power of penetration. In addition to ammonium oleate, they contained mineral oil and wax to form a solid petroxolin.

Solid petroxolin N.F. IX was recommended as a base for Peru balsam, resins and all other balsams, since these ingredients do not separate out as they do when they are incorporated in hydrocarbon or fatty bases. Petroxolins are no longer used in dermatologic practice.

VANISHING CREAMS. The emulsifying properties of soaps are exhibited best in the group of ointment bases classed as vanishing creams. Here we have a comparatively small amount of soap emulsifying up to 80 percent of water, forming o/w emulsions. Vanishing creams have been in use as a cosmetic for many years and, more recently, as carriers of medicinal agents.

The advantage of these preparations as carriers of medicinal agents supposedly lies in their high water content. This, it is claimed, leads to more rapid release of the medicament from the base, thereby favoring absorption by the skin and more rapid and satisfactory antiseptic action on the surface of the skin. These claims must be discounted to some extent in the light of more recent evidence (see p. 244).

Soaps formed by the reaction between a fatty acid such as stearic acid and an amine such as triethanolamine are widely used as emulsifying agents in modern dermatologic formulations. In contrast with metallic soaps, amine soaps are less alkaline; hence, they are less likely to be irritating to injured epidermis. Emulsions prepared with amine soaps are more stable in the presence of divalent and trivalent metal ions than are those prepared with monovalent metal soaps like sodium oleate.

Vanishing creams usually consist of from 10 to 25 percent of stearic acid, a portion of which (15 to 25%) is saponified, and from 60 to 80 percent of water. The following formula is basic.

Stearic acid triple pressed	200.0
Potassium hydroxide	14.0
Water	800.0
Perfume q.s.	

In the preparation of vanishing creams, one of the important considerations is the choice of saponifying agent. Each possesses properties which, in some cases, might be considered an advantage and in others, a disadvantage.

Carbonates may be used successfully in

the hands of the skilled operator but should not be used by the novice. There is always the possibility of entrapping the CO_2 formed by the interaction of stearic acid and the carbonate. Generally, after the cream has thickened and set, it will be found to be impregnated with numerous bubbles.

Both sodium and potassium hydroxides are good and possess no serious disadvantages. The chief difference between them lies in the fact that the potassium soap generally produces a softer cream with a higher degree of pearliness than does a sodium soap.

Sodium borate produces a very white cream. However, it is said to have the disadvantage in that creams emulsified with it have a tendency to grain.

Ammonia water has a tendency to discolor creams made with it. It has also been stated that it is difficult to stabilize the perfume in these creams.

The ethanolamines, di- and tri-, have been recommended as alkalis for creams and are used frequently. The advantages claimed are their mild alkalinity, the good texture of the resulting creams and their pearly appearance. The di- or triethanolamine may be reacted with the stearic acid in the preparation of the cream, or di- and triethanolamine stearate may be purchased and used as such.

Vanishing Cream Base

Stearic acid	15.0
White wax	2.0
White petrolatum	8.0
Triethanolamine	1.5
Propylene glycol	8.0
Purified water	65.5

The emulsifier, triethanolamine stearate, is prepared in situ. Melt the white wax, stearic acid and white petrolatum on a water bath. Disperse the T.E.A. in water containing propylene glycol, and heat to approximately the same temperature as the oil phase. Add the aqueous phase to the oil phase, with stirring. Stir until congealed.

This base can be used as a carrier for many medicinal substances. It is easily removed from the skin and hair with water and, hence, can be used on the scalp or on other hairy regions. The following formula illustrates this use:

Sulfur	2.0
Ammoniated mercury	5.0
Coal tar solution	2.0
Vanishing cream base	qs. 60.0

Levigate the sulfur and ammoniated mercury with a small quantity of vanishing cream base. Gradually incorporate the remaining base and the coal tar solution.

Glycerin in the past was a constituent of most vanishing creams. Its chief use was as a hygroscopic agent to prevent the creams from drying through evaporation of water.

When included in the formula, it should not exceed 10 percent, and generally 5 percent is sufficient. The objection to too much glycerin is its tendency to absorb moisture after application to the skin. Propylene glycol has largely replaced glycerin in these formulas.

The general methods of manufacture are as follows: The stearic acid is melted on a water bath and heated up to 85°C. If any other oil-miscible or oil-soluble ingredients are included in the formula, these are added to the stearic acid and heated with it. The water, containing the alkali and any other water-soluble ingredients of the formula, is also heated to 85°C. Then the hot alkaline solution is added to the hot oil solution slowly and with stirring. The temperature should be maintained for 10 to 15 minutes to ensure complete reaction between the stearic acid and the alkali. Then the cream is allowed to cool slowly with stirring. However, the stirring must not be so vigorous as to beat air into the product. After standing for 24 hours, the cream is perfumed and run through an ointment mill. If an ointment mill is not available, it is very important that the temperatures mentioned above be adhered to and that the cream cool very slowly to prevent the crystallizing out of the waxes and the free stearic acid. If these directions are adhered to rigidly, a fairly satisfactory cream can be made without the use of a mill.

When vanishing creams are to be used as ointment bases, one must keep in mind that they are essentially soaps and, therefore, are incompatible with acids or acidic substances. Therefore, their use is limited.

Silicon Derivatives

This group includes products that are related to each other mineralogically. The products referred to are the bentonites, hectorite and Veegum.* All of these possess active constituents which are members of the montmorillonite group of clays. Montmorillonite is used as a group name for a series of clays with related properties and also a specific mineral name.

The mineral is a hydrous aluminum silicate with a silicon:metallic oxide ratio of about 4 and with a small content of alkalies and alkali earths. An essential characteristic of montmorillonite and of all clay minerals is an expanding lattice structure, enabling the clay to hydrate extensively.[5] Another common property of clay minerals which makes them of value in external and internal preparations is their lack of irritating and sensitizing potential.[103]

The bentonites are the chief representatives of this group. They may be divided into two general classes: the sodium bentonites, which absorb large quantities of water, swelling enormously in the process, and the calcium bentonites, which absorb very little water and do not swell noticeably. Sodium bentonite has properties that make it of particular interest in pharmaceuticals as a suspending agent (see Chap. 7) and a hydrophilic thickener.

The *U.S.P.* describes bentonite as a native, colloidal, hydrated aluminum silicate. It is insoluble in water but swells to approximately 12 times its volume when added to water. When mixed with 8 to 10 parts of water, a base of ointment consistency is formed. The consistency of the base can be controlled by increasing or decreasing the amount of water in the formula. Medicinal agents can be incorporated into the already formed base.

Much work has been carried out to determine the value of bentonite as an ointment base,[6,23,45] because an aqueous preparation of it possesses many of the qualities a dermatologist desires from a nongreasy base, i.e., it is water-removable, hydrophilic, nonirritating, nondehydrating, compatible with many medicaments, etc. However, in actual use, some disadvantages have been discovered. Ointments prepared from bentonite and water alone are slightly drying and unstable on standing. Addition of a

humectant (glycerin, propylene glycol) in amounts up to 10 percent will retard this action. Bentonite ointments are subject to mold growth, which, however, can be prevented by methylparaben (0.15%) and propylparaben (0.05%).

Darlington and Guth[23] prepared several bentonite bases, including a vanishing cream base, an anhydrous absorption base and a water-in-oil emulsion base.

BENTONITE BASE

Bentonite	20.0
Glycerin	10.0
Purified water	70.0

BENTONITE BASE WITH SURFACE ACTIVE AGENTS

Bentonite	28.0
Tween 20 (polyoxyethylene sorbitan monolaurate)	4.0
Tween 80 (Polysorbate 80, U.S.P.)	8.0
Propylene glycol	10.0
Methylparaben	0.15
Propylparaben	0.05
Purified water	44.8

All bases were prepared by sprinkling the bentonite on the liquid portion of the base and stirring at a low rate of speed in a mechanical mixer.

Darlington and Guth also reported that the pH of bentonite bases can be adjusted by means of buffer mixtures. The in-vitro activity of ammoniated mercury was enhanced by incorporation in acid-buffered bentonite bases.

Hectorite is a member of the montmorillonite clay minerals and, therefore, has an expanding lattice structure. It is sometimes referred to as magnesium bentonite, since it differs from bentonite in the almost complete substitution of aluminum in the lattice structure of bentonite by magnesium in hectorite. The lattice structure of hectorite also contains lithium and fluorine.

Malcaloid,* a purified hectorite, swells to from 35 to 40 times its volume in water—substantially more than bentonites. It is nontoxic and has been cleared by the F.D.A. for use in internal and external preparations.[70]

Colloidal Magnesium Aluminum Silicate. Veegum† is an inorganic emulsifier, thickener, suspending agent and film former and

---

* R. T. Vanderbilt Co., Inc., New York, N.Y.

* The Inerto Co., San Francisco, California.
† R. T. Vanderbilt Co., New York City.

is described by its manufacturer as a complex colloidal magnesium aluminum silicate. It is derived from the minerals montmorillonite and hectorite and is refined by a special process. Because it is a blended product, it is more uniform in its properties from lot to lot than are most other montmorillonite clay minerals. It is whiter in color and swells more extensively in water than do the bentonites.[114] It is dispersed readily in water by adding it to the water slowly with continuous agitation. Usually 1 to 4 percent of Veegum is employed to stabilize emulsions and suspend insoluble material. However, firm preparations of ointment consistency can be prepared, using 10 percent Veegum. The viscosity of a Veegum Dispersion containing more than 3 percent of solids is decreased by simple agitation. The apparent viscosity increases again when the material is allowed to remain at rest. This increase and decrease in viscosity is known as *thixotropy.*

Aqueous dispersions of Veegum are slightly alkaline, as are aqueous dispersions of other montmorillonite clays.

Kariya et al.[54] prepared several Veegum ointments, using Veegum HV. Veegum HV is a small flake Veegum which produces more viscous aqueous dispersions than does Veegum. It is used in pharmaceuticals when high viscosity is desired.

VEEGUM BASE
Veegum HV 8.2
Sodium Lauryl sulfate 0.1
Hot water (97–99°C.) 91.7

Dissolve the sodium lauryl sulfate in the hot water. Agitate the solution vigorously by means of a high speed electric mixer. Add the Veegum HV in divided portions and continue the agitation for 5 minutes after all of the Veegum has been added.

Commonly used dermatologic ingredients such as Peru balsam, salicylic and benzoic acids, zinc oxide, coal tar, ammoniated mercury, etc., were compatible with the Veegum HV base.

Silicones. The silicones are a series of synthetic polymers in which the basic structure is not carbon but a chain of alternating silicon and oxygen atoms (e.g., —O—Si—O—Si—). Each silicon atom has one or more organic groups, generally methyl or methylphenyl groups, attached to it.

Dimethylpolysiloxanes* are the most commonly known silicones. They are clear fluids and are available in a wide range of viscosities. The viscosities normally employed in ointment and cosmetic formulations are between 50 and 1,000 centistokes. Water repellency is their outstanding feature, and this property, combined with their resistance to change due to heat or oxidation, makes them very useful in preparations for the management of dermatologic disorders in which protection from moisture is indicated. Talbot et al.[109] found that a silicone ointment containing 30 percent of Dow Corning 200 centistoke viscosity fluid in a petrolatum base† was effective in the management of dermatologic conditions such as diaper rash, irritation from colostomies, intertrigo, decubitus ulcers and others in which protection from moisture was indicated. Shaw and Crowe[98] compared the effectiveness of several protective ointments and found that two that contained silicones gave the best results. They concluded that the vehicle in which the silicone was incorporated influenced to a marked degree the efficacy of the test ointments. The most effective protection was provided by the mixture of 30 percent silicones in petrolatum. Lubowe[65] has reported on the uses of silicones in dermatology and cosmetics.

Steigleder and Raab[104] compared the protective action of a petrolatum ointment containing 25 percent silicone with the protective action of a variety of ointments such as Hydrophilic Petrolatum, U.S.P., Hydrophilic Ointment, U.S.P., White Petrolatum, U.S.P., Olive Oil, U.S.P., etc. The best protective effect against contact with water was afforded by the white petrolatum.

Methylphenylpolysiloxane available from Dow Corning as DC 556 Cosmetic Grade Fluid has all the characteristics typical of silicone fluids but, in addition, it is soluble in 95 percent ethanol and has somewhat greater compatibility with organic ingredients. It is used in protective creams and lotions, suntan lotions, aerosol hair sprays and shaving lotions.

* DC 200 Fluid, Dow Corning Corp., Midland, Michigan.
† Silicote Ointment, Arnar-Stone Labs., Inc.

A stearyl ester of dimethylpolysiloxane is available from Dow Corning as DC F-157. It is a straw-colored waxy semisolid. The stearyl groups improve compatibility with some organic substances. It is suitable for use in semisolid or stick preparations such as lipsticks and lip pomades.[77]

Tests on laboratory animals and on humans demonstrate that dimethyl- and methylphenylpolysiloxanes are essentially nontoxic, nonirritating and nonsensitizing.[50,63,88]

Plein and Plein[80,81] studied the compatibility of dimethylpolysiloxanes with other substances used in the formulating of ointments and also prepared a number of silicone ointment bases. They found that, although silicone fluids were practically immiscible with vegetable oils and mineral oil, stable mixtures could be prepared if other substances were added to stabilize the mixture. They prepared a number of silicone ointment bases, using silicone fluids in place of petrolatum. The following are examples of such formulae:

Silicone Absorption Base

Arlacel C*	6.0
Carnauba wax	20.0
DC 200: 200,000 cts.	24.0
DC 200: 1,000 cts.	40.0
Anhydrous lanolin	10.0

Melt the carnauba wax over a hot water bath. Add the other ingredients, with stirring. Remove from the water bath and stir until congealed.

Silicone Emulsion Base

Cetyl alcohol	10.0
DC 200: 1,000 cts.	25.0
Sodium lauryl sulfate	1.0
Distilled water	64.0
Methylparaben	0.025
Propylparaben	0.015

Warm the cetyl alcohol-DC 200 mixture to 75°C. on a water bath. Add an aqueous mixture of the sodium lauryl sulfate and the parabens, previously warmed to 75°C. Stir until the base congeals.

Physical Classification

Oleaginous and Hydrocarbon Bases

These are discussed in the sections headed Hydrocarbons, Natural Triglycerides and Vegetable Oils.

* Sorbitan sesquioleate, Atlas Chemical Industries, Wilmington, Del.

Absorption Bases

Absorption bases usually are anhydrous bases which have the property of absorbing several times their weight of water, forming emulsions; the word absorption does not refer to the action of these bases when applied to the skin. Hydrophilic Petrolatum U.S.P. and Anhydrous Lanolin U.S.P. are examples of anhydrous absorption bases. On the addition of water to these bases a water-in-oil emulsion is formed. Hydrous water-in-oil emulsion bases also may be classified as absorption bases, since additional quantities of water or aqueous solutions can be incorporated in them. These are discussed under emulsion bases. Lanolin U.S.P. and Cold Cream U.S.P. are examples of such bases.

Absorption bases vary in their composition, but, for the greater part, they are mixtures of cyclic alcohols (cholesterol and cholesterol alcohols) with petrolatum.

Aquabase*

Cholesterol	30.0
Cottonseed oil	30.0
White petrolatum	940.0

The water number[38] of petrolatum can be increased by the addition of ingredients other than cyclic alcohols. Casparis and Meyer[19] reported that fatty alcohols such as cetyl and stearyl alcohol increased the water number of petrolatum, the increase depending on the concentration of fatty alcohol and the water number of the vehicle.

Anhydrous absorption bases also can be formed by the addition of lipophilic surfactants to petrolatum. The following illustrate such bases:[3]

Petrolatum Absorption Base (BF-16)

Petrolatum	90.0
Arlacel 83 sorbitan sesquioleate	10.0

Melt the ingredients and mix. Add water as desired.

Petrolatum Absorption Base (BF-17)

Beeswax	5.0
Petrolatum	60.0
Mineral oil	25.0
Arlacel 83 sorbitan sesquioleate	10.0

Melt the ingredients and mix. For use in preparing a w/o emulsion, heat the base to 65°C. Add water which has been heated to 67°C., agitating thor-

* From the Formulary of the University of Iowa Hospitals, 1972.

oughly during the addition. About 40 percent of water can be added.

Anhydrous water removable bases can be formulated by the addition of hydrophilic surfactants to petrolatum. The following illustrates such bases:[3]

WASHABLE ANHYDROUS PETROLATUM (BF-21)

	a	b	c
Petrolatum	95	95	95
Tween 61[†]	5	–	–
Tween 81[‡]	–	5	–
Myrj 52 (Polyoxyl 40 Stearate U.S.P.)	–	–	5

Melt the ingredients and mix, continuing agitation as the mixture cools.

Mendes et al.[74] studied the effect of various surfactants on the water number of white petrolatum. They found that the lower the hydrophil-lipophil balance of the surfactant, the greater the water number, or water-absorbing capacity of the base.

Absorption bases were developed because it was desirable to have a product to which water or an aqueous solution of medicinal substances could be added easily. They generally have a high degree of compatibility with the majority of medicaments used topically. As a class, they are relatively heat-stable and can be utilized in their anhydrous form or emulsified with the addition of water. However, absorption bases still possess the undesirable property of greasiness, but they are more readily removable from the skin than are the oleaginous bases. The *British Pharmacopoeia* contains an absorption base under the title Wool Alcohols Ointment (see page 249).

Emulsion Bases

Bases coming under this classification are water-in-oil or oil-in-water type emulsion bases. Lanolin and Cold Cream or cold cream type emulsion bases are classified as water-in-oil emulsions. They are used as emollients, the aqueous phase hydrating the skin and the oil phase forming an occlusive covering which prevents water loss due to evaporation. These bases are used also as

vehicles for medicinal agents such as sulfur, ammoniated mercury, Peru balsam, zinc oxide, etc.

Oil-in-water type emulsion bases such as Hydrophilic Ointment and vanishing creams (described under soaps) are used as vehicles for medicinal agents. They are water-removable and, hence, can be removed readily from skin and clothing with water alone. This is one of the outstanding advantages of these bases, particularly when an ointment is to be applied to a hairy region such as the scalp. Vanishing creams are used also as a cosmetic. Although they contain a significant amount of oil phase, the residue left on the skin is soft in appearance and does not feel greasy. Vanishing creams are sometimes used as hand creams and as foundations to provide a suitable substrate for powder and other make-up.

Cold creams were defined as emulsions made up of oil (40 to 70%), wax or spermaceti (5 to 15%) and water (20 to 35%). A characteristic feature of these cold creams was the presence of a relatively large amount of water loosely held in the water-in-oil mixture. The name cold cream referred to the cooling effect produced by the slow evaporation of water when these creams were applied to the skin. It was not until the latter part of the 19th century that these creams were rendered more stable by the inclusion of borax which reacted with the fatty acids present in the beeswax to form the sodium soap. The soap contributed to the stability of the cream. However, the development of the present multitude of emulsifying agents, particularly the nonionics, led to the formulation of cold creams made with nonionic emulsifiers alone or in combination with beeswax-borax. Some of the compounds used give oil-in-water creams similar in character to the classic cold creams.[39]

O/W COLD CREAM BASE

Beeswax	15.0
Mineral oil	50.0
G-1431* (polyoxyethylene sorbitol lanolin)	3.0
Borax	1.0
Water	31.0

Heat the oil, beeswax and G-1431 to 80°C. Dissolve the borax in the water and heat to 85°C. Add

---

† Polyoxyethylene (4) sorbitan monostearate, Atlas Chemical Industries Inc., Wilmington, Del.

‡ Polyoxyethylene (5) sorbitan monooleate, Atlas Chemical Industries Inc., Wilmington, Del.

* Atlas Chemical Industries, Wilmington, Del.

the aqueous phase to the oil phase, with gentle agitation. Agitate until congealed.

Manufacture. In the past cold creams generally were prepared with vegetable oils, such as almond oil, olive oil or expressed almond oil (Rose Water Ointment), and waxes and spermaceti. However, in later years, the vegetable oils were replaced largely by mineral oils, as in the official Cold Cream (petrolatum rose water ointment), because of the greater stability of mineral oil. This eliminated the problem of preservation, which is always a complication in the use of vegetable oils. However, vegetable oils and lanolin are sometimes added in small quantities when more emolliency is desired.

In preparing cold creams, the same general rule applies as for vanishing creams, i.e., the oil-miscible or -soluble ingredients are mixed and heated to approximately 75°C. The water-miscible or -soluble ingredients are added together and heated to the same temperature. Then the water solution is added to the oil phase slowly and with stirring. The temperature should be maintained for about 10 minutes and allowed to decrease slowly, to prevent crystallizing of the waxes. Stirring should be slow and continuous, using care not to whip air into the product. The following is a typical formula:

Mineral oil 50.0
Beeswax 14.0
Borax 0.7
Purified water 35.3

In most cold cream formulas, the emulsifying agent is the soap formed by the reaction between the alkaline sodium borate and the free acids in the beeswax. The amount of borax required for complete neutralization of the wax acids depends on the acid number of the beeswax. The acid number of the white wax which is specified in the *U.S.P.* for Cold Cream is 17 to 24. The amount of borax usually recommended to give a stable cream is 5 to 7 percent of the weight of beeswax. It should be noted that no correlation has ever been established between the emulsifying characteristics of a particular beeswax sample and its acid number.

The amount of beeswax used in cold creams varies from about 5 to 15 percent.

Creams with the lower amount of beeswax are softer than the *U.S.P.* product which contains 12 percent of white wax. However, soft creams can be stiffened by the incorporating of other waxes such as microcrystalline wax, spermaceti, etc. In addition to the white wax, Cold Cream U.S.P. contains 12.5 percent of spermaceti.

One peculiarity of the beeswax-borax system is that both water-in-oil and oil-in-water creams may be produced without the aid of secondary emulsifiers. Salisbury et al.[90] studied a 3-component system of mineral oil, water and beeswax fully neutralized with borax. They found that creams containing less than 45 percent of water were water-in-oil creams, and those containing more than 45 percent of water were oil-in-water creams. This critical level of 45 percent water does not apply to all cold cream formulations, but it does indicate that there is a critical water level below which a water-in-oil cream will be formed preferentially.

The use of synthetic emulsifiers, particularly the nonionics, alone or in conjunction with beeswax, produces cold creams whose properties are less dependent on processing conditions and critical levels of water. The following formulation illustrates the use of such compounds:

W/O COLD CREAM BASE

Mineral oil 45.0
Beeswax 10.0
Lanolin 2.0
Span 80 sorbitan monooleate 1.0
Borax 8.0
Water 41.2

Heat the first four ingredients on a water bath to 70°C. Dissolve the borax in water and heat to 72°C. Add the aqueous phase to the oil phase, with stirring. Stir until congealed.

A water-in-oil emulsion base entirely free of soap also can be formulated. These preparations are more stable to acids or substances having acidic properties.

W/O OINTMENT BASE

Petrolatum 54.0
Arlacel 83 sorbitan sesquioleate 6.0
Water 40.0

Heat the petrolatum and Arlacel 83 to 65°C. Add the water which has been heated to 67°C., agitating thoroughly during the addition.

Water-removable ointment bases contain an aqueous phase, an emulsifying agent and an oleaginous phase. The water phase may vary from 10 to 80 percent of the total base. These bases are referred to as hydrophilic ointment bases; however, since they are oil-in-water emulsions, the incorporation of additional water may produce a loss of ointment consistency. Due to the high water-content of the external phase, water-removable bases must be protected from evaporation and therefore must be dispensed in tubes or tightly closed jars. Humectants such as glycerin or propylene glycol generally are included with the aqueous phase to reduce water loss through evaporation.

Many emulsion bases contain cetyl and/or stearyl alcohol. These fatty alcohols add stability to the emulsion, impart a smooth feel to the skin and assist in water retention of emulsion bases. Stearyl alcohol, in particular, causes the greatest potentiation of the water number of petrolatum.[19] The water number[38] is defined as the largest amount of water which 100 g. of an ointment base will hold at normal temperature. A typical oil-in-water emulsion base containing fatty alcohols is illustrated by the following formula:

Cetyl alcohol 5.0
Stearyl alcohol 5.0
White petrolatum 20.0
Sodium lauryl sulfate 1.0
Propylene glycol 8.0
Purified water 61.0

Melt the alcohols and the white petrolatum on a water bath. Dissolve the sodium lauryl sulfate and the propylene glycol in the water and heat to approximately the same temperature as the oil phase. Add the aqueous phase to the oil phase and stir until congealed.

The availability of a number of newer organic compounds, the surface-active agents, has given a much greater degree of flexibility to ointment formulation, particularly of emulsion bases. In the field of surface-active agents which perform such functions as wetting, emulsifying, dispersing and solubilizing agents, we have a multiple choice. Surface-active agents may be ionic or nonionic. The ionic types are either anionic or cationic, depending on whether the characteristically surface-active portion of the compound lies

in the anion or the cation. For example, in soap the anion (oleate) is the effective portion of the molecule; therefore, soap is classified as anionic.

Nonionic surfactants depend chiefly on hydroxyl groups and ether linkages (polyhydric alcohol anhydrides and polyoxyethylene chains) to create the hydrophilic action. Polysorbate 80* and Polyoxyl 40 Stearate† official in the *U.S.P.* represent such surface-active agents.

Generally, nonionic agents may be used more widely in ointment formulation. Ionic surface-active agents exhibit a particle charge, hence are sensitive to the presence of other ions. Thus, soaps (anionic agents) are ineffective in hard water and undergo hydrolysis at pH's much below 6. Cationic agents, on the other hand, are not stable in the presence of anionic agents or soap. Since nonionic agents do not ionize, they are comparatively insensitive to hard water, electrolytes and ionic surface-active agents. Furthermore, nonionic surfactants are generally less toxic and less irritating than ionic agents.[61]

Polysorbate 80 and Polyoxyl 40 Stearate have been shown to interact with preservatives and active ingredients used in ointments.[14,20] Medicaments such as phenol and benzoic and salicylic acids incorporated in a base prepared with Polyoxyl 40 Stearate produced a marked softening of the base. This was attributed to the interaction between medicament and emulsifying agent to produce a molecular complex. Little is known about the effect of such interactions on the therapeutic efficacy of the medicament.

Hydrophilic Ointment, U.S.P., contains sodium lauryl sulfate, an anionic surfactant, as the emulsifying agent. Medicaments that produced a marked softening of the base prepared with Polyoxyl 40 Stearate can be incorporated successfully in a hydrophilic emulsion base prepared with sodium lauryl sulfate.

The British Pharmacopoeia and the British Pharmaceutical Codex contain formulas for emulsifying bases that produce oil-in-water

* Tween 80, Atlas Chemical Industries, Wilmington, Del.
† Myrj 52, Atlas Chemical Industries, Wilmington, Del.

emulsions on the addition of water. Emulsifying Wax, B.P., and Emulsifying Ointment, B.P., Cetrimide Emulsifying Wax, B.P.C., and Cetrimide Emulsifying Ointment, B.P.C., Cetomacrogol Emulsifying Wax, B.P.C., and Cetomacrogol Emulsifying Ointment, B.P.C., are examples of such emulsifying bases. Cetrimide is chiefly tetradecyl trimethylammonium bromide, a cationic surfactant. Cetomacrogol is polyethylene glycol 1000 monocetyl ether, a nonionic surfactant.

EMULSIFYING WAX, B.P.

Cetostearyl alcohol	90
Sodium lauryl sulfate	10
Purified water	4

Melt the cetostearyl alcohol and heat to about 95°. Add the sodium lauryl sulfate, mix, add the purified water, heat to 115°, and maintain at this temperature, stirring vigorously, until frothing ceases and the product is translucent. Cool quickly.

EMULSIFYING OINTMENT, B.P.

Emulsifying wax	300
White soft paraffin	500
Liquid paraffin	200

Melt together and stir until cold.

Emulsifying Ointment is used to prepare Aqueous Cream, B.P., which contains almost 70 percent of water.

There are several factors which must be considered in the preparation of emulsion bases (see Chap. 7). The quality and the quantity of ingredients, the order of mixing, the speed and the type of mixing, the temperature at which the emulsion is made, the choice of the emulsifier—all are important. The usual method of preparation involves melting the grease-like materials and waxes in one container, heating the water with the water-soluble components in another container and mixing both at the same temperature, 75°C. Stirring is continued until a smooth cream results.

Water-Soluble Bases

Water-soluble ointment bases include those bases prepared from Carbowax* polyethylene glycols. Carbowax polyethylene gly-

* Union Carbide Chemicals Co., New York, N.Y.

cols are polymers of ethylene oxide with the generalized formula $HOCH_2(CH_2OCH_2)_n$ CH_2OH, n representing the average number of oxyethylene groups. Products in this series are designated by a number which roughly represents their average molecular weight, i.e., 200, 300, 400, 600, 1000, 1540, 4000, and 6000. Carbowax 1500 is a blend of equal parts of Carbowaxes 300 and 1540 and has the consistency of petrolatum. At 25°C. Carbowaxes 200 through 600 are clear liquids and Carbowaxes 1000 through 6000 are white, waxy solids. They are nonionic, water-soluble, nongreasy and do not hydrolyze or deteriorate.[18]

Carbowax polyethylene glycols can be blended to form a variety of water-removable ointment bases with consistencies varying from semisolid to hard. Polyethylene Glycol Ointment U.S.P. is a blend of Carbowaxes 4000 and 400. The high degree of solubility of this base precludes the addition of aqueous solutions much in excess of 5 percent of the total formula. The following formula is recommended when larger amounts of aqueous solution are to be incorporated:

Carbowax polyethylene glycol 4000	47.5
Carbowax polyethylene glycol 400	47.5
Cetyl alcohol	5.0

Heat and mix the components on a water bath until blended, remove heat and stir until congealed.

Certain medicaments, e.g., benzoic and salicylic acids, tannic acid, phenol, bacitracin, etc., have a solubilizing effect on bases containing the high-molecular-weight Carbowax polyethylene glycols. Medicaments containing an acidic hydrogen have been shown to interact with high molecular weight Carbowax polyethylene glycols forming molecular complexes having solubility characteristics different from those of the parent compounds.[43] The effect of such interactions on the physiologic activity of the medicament has not been reported.

Although medicaments diffuse readily from Carbowax polyethylene glycol bases,[64,75] very little percutaneous absorption is reported to occur from such bases.[76,99]

Collins and Zopf[22] prepared a Carbowax polyethylene glycol ointment base containing 1,2,6-hexanetriol. The modified ointment base was reported to be more compatible with dermatologic medicaments than the unmodified base.

MODIFIED POLYETHYLENE GLYCOL OINTMENT

Carbowax polyethylene glycol 4000 .... 42.5
Carbowax polyethylene glycol 400 .... 37.5
1,2,6-Hexanetriol 20.0

Heat Carbowax polyethylene glycol 4000 with the 1,2,6-hexanetriol on a water bath at 60 to 70°C. Add this melt to Carbowax polyethylene glycol 400 at room temperature, with vigorous stirring. Stir occasionally until solidification takes place.

Smyth et al.[101,102] reported that the acute oral and dermal toxicity and irritating potential of Carbowax polyethylene glycols is very low. They reported that in human patch tests the compounds were no more irritating than lanolin, petrolatum and simple ointment.

The *British Pharmaceutical Codex* contains a monograph for a water-soluble ointment base, Macrogol Ointment.

MACROGOL OINTMENT

Hard Macrogol 500
Liquid Macrogol 500

Melt the hard macrogol, add the liquid macrogol, and stir until cold.

Hard Macrogol is polyethylene glycol 4000 and Liquid Macrogol is polyethylene glycol 300.

OPHTHALMIC OINTMENTS

Vehicles for ophthalmic ointments should be nonirritating and sterile. Absorption bases and emulsions may be irritating, due to the surfactant emulsifier in the base. Petrolatum, petrolatum–mineral oil and petrolatum–anhydrous lanolin bases are often used in ophthalmic ointments because of their low irritating potential. The petrolatum–anhydrous-lanolin base is used when an aqueous solution of a medicament is to be incorporated.

Petrolatum bases may be sterilized in a hot-air oven at 175°C. for 2 hours. After sterilization the active ingredient is aseptically incorporated in the base by using sterile utensils, i.e., mortar and pestle, spatula, ointment slab, graduates, etc. Most utensils may be autoclaved in a pressure cooker and the ointment slab washed with an antiseptic solution. The finished ointment should be dispensed in sterile ophthalmic-tipped tubes to reduce the possibility of contaminating the ointment. Ointment tubes may be sterilized by storage in 70 percent ethanol for 24 hours prior to use.

The active ingredient should be finely powdered, and, if possible, it should be sterile, although bulk chemicals usually do not support bacterial growth within the lattice structure of the dry material.

The pharmacist is seldom called on to prepare an extemporaneous ophthalmic ointment. However, a nonsterile ointment applied to an eye in which the corneal epithelium has been damaged may cause infection and even loss of the eye.

PREPARATION

Since ointments are applied primarily to irritated areas, it is an unbreakable rule that these preparations must not contain granular or gritty particles which might cause further irritation.

Regardless of the condition of the skin, ointments must be smooth and free from granular or gritty particles. Therefore, all techniques in the preparation of ointments should be carried out with the express purpose of having the substances incorporated therein in the finest state of subdivision it is possible to achieve.

In compounding ointments, the following rules should be observed:

1. Insoluble substances to be incorporated in ointment bases should always be in the impalpable powder form.

2. Insoluble substances are best incorporated when first levigated with a small portion of the base to form a smooth nucleus and then incorporated into the remainder of the base.

3. Water-soluble salts should be incorporated by dissolving them in a small amount of water and incorporating with the base, using anhydrous lanolin, if necessary, to absorb the aqueous solution. This method produces a smooth ointment with a minimum of levigation. The following formulation illustrates this technique:

Merbromin 0.6
Petrolatum qs. 30.0

Dissolve the merbromin in 1 ml. of water. Incorporate in 2 g. of anhydrous lanolin and then incorporate 26.4 g. of petrolatum.

When substances incorporated into ointment bases must be reduced to a fine state of subdivision, three methods are generally available: (1) use of an ointment slab and spatula, (2) use of the mortar and pestle, (3) use of an ointment mill.

These methods may or may not involve fusion, depending on the nature of the medicament to be incorporated into the base and the base itself. Fusion is necessary when waxes, paraffins, fatty alcohols, fatty acids or any hard waxlike materials are included in the formula. Fusion is used also when a medicament is soluble in the melted base. Most emulsion and absorption bases are prepared by fusion.

In preparing ointments by fusion the substance having the highest melting point is placed in an evaporating dish or beaker on a water bath and melted at the lowest temperature possible. Other substances are added in order of decreasing melting points. In this way the entire base is not heated to the highest temperature. According to Price and Osborne,[85] if the order of mixing is reversed, i.e., melting the substance with the lowest melting point first, then adding the remaining substances in ascending order of melting points, or if all the constituents of the base are melted together, the substance with the highest melting point can be incorporated at a temperature below its melting point. The mixture must be stirred until the base congeals to prevent separation and the crystallization of the higher melting point substances.

Medicaments soluble in the melted base should be added to the base just before it congeals. Insoluble medicaments should be levigated with a small quantity of the melted base. After the remainder of the base has congealed, it can be incorporated with the levigated medicament.

Water and water-soluble ingredients such as glycerin or propylene glycol must be heated to approximately the same temperature as the melted oleaginous phase before mixing the two phases. If cold water is added to the melted oleaginous phase, separation and crystallization of the higher melting substances will occur.

Ointment Slab. The usual technique consists of rubbing the powder with a small amount of base until it is thoroughly distributed in a finely subdivided state, then incorporating this concentrated ointment into the remainder of the base. Mineral oil or a vegetable oil can be used as a levigating agent if small quantities of medicaments are to be incorporated in the base. The use of large amounts of levigating agents may result in undue softening of the finished ointment.

A stainless-steel spatula with a long, broad, flexible blade is essential to the preparation of good ointments. Two spatulas usually are used, one to levigate the ointment, the other to remove accumulating ointment from the levigating spatula. Where danger of chemical reaction between the steel spatula and active ingredients such as iodine, mercury salts, salicylic acid, etc. is a possibility, a hard rubber spatula or wooden tongue depressor should be used.

Mortar and Pestle. It is the general consensus that the mortar and pestle should be used when large quantities of liquid are to be incorporated into a base or when exceptionally large quantities of ointment are to be made. The use of mortar and pestle is considered not as efficient as the spatula in reducing the size of particles incorporated in or protected by an ointment base because of the small surface area under levigation at any one time. Then, too, the particles have a tendency to "ride" out from under the pestle, and the grinding effect is limited. Nevertheless, according to experiments by L. Rosenthaler,[86] the products obtained in either way differ very slightly as to their homogeneity, provided that the same accuracy has been employed. In these same experiments, he found that 5 minutes of actual rubbing time was necessary to produce homogeneity in products prepared by either method. However, he does not give any information as to which method is most effective in the breaking down of agglomerate particles.

Ointment Mill. The ointment mill is convenient and ideal for making ointments in lots of 5 lbs. or more, although small mills (Fig. 8-3) are available for use in the community pharmacy. With the small ointment mill favorite ointment prescriptions of skin specialists and general practitioners can be prepared in 1 lb. or smaller batches for stock

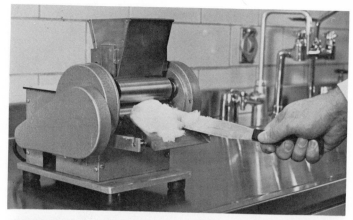

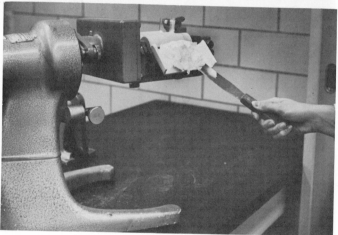

FIG. 8-3. (*Top*) ASRA three-roller ointment mill. (Industrial Pharmacy Laboratory, Univ. of Iowa, College of Pharmacy) (*Bottom*) Erweka all purpose motor drive wtih three roller mill. (Industrial Pharmacy Lab., Univ. of Iowa, College of Pharmacy)

use. The ointment is prepared in the usual manner and then run through the mill until smooth and free from gritty particles.

Small roller mills are available with stainless steel rollers or the more chemically resistant clay rollers.

When making ointments on a larger scale, the powdered medicaments are sifted into the softened or melted base which is contained in a "change can mixer" (Fig. 8-4). The mixture is stirred until it has congealed and then it is run through an ointment mill until smooth. In some instances, the powdered medicament is mixed with a small portion of the base to make a concentrate which is run through an ointment mill several times. Then the concentrate is mixed with the remainder of the base in a change can mixer or a Hobart mixer (Fig. 8-5).

There are two types of ointment mills, one known as the "paint mill" type, which consists essentially of a steel disk revolving on a stationary steel surface and the other known as the three-roller ink mill (Fig. 8-6). In the latter, the 3 rollers operate at different speeds. The roller having the highest speed takes the ointment off the slower roller, and, since the speed of each of the 3 rollers is different, a shearing action, which smooths out the ointment, is secured. The rollers are usually water-jacketed to prevent excessive rise in temperature due to the heat of friction. The variable-speed 3-roller mill is faster than the paint mill; hence, it is used more often in the manufacture of ointments on a large scale. The small ointment mill shown in Figure 8-3 is also a 3-roller mill and operates on the same principle.

PACKAGING, STORAGE AND LABELING

Packaging. Ointments are dispensed in either ointment jars or collapsible tin tubes. Jars of brown, green or opaque white glass

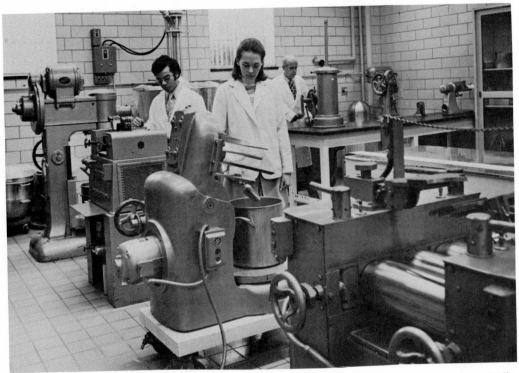

Fig. 8-4. Active ingredient being added to ointment in J. H. Day change can mixer. Roller mills on either side of the mixer. (Industrial Pharmacy Lab., Univ. of Iowa, College of Pharmacy)

are used most frequently by the community pharmacist when dispensing ointment prescriptions.

When using ointment jars, the container size should be such that the ointment fills the container but does not come in contact with the closure liner. Ointments are prepared by weight, hence, a 1-ounce ointment may or may not completely fill a 1-ounce ointment jar, depending on the density of the ointment ingredients. Ointments should be packed in jars with a spatula, tapping the jar against the palm of the hand during the filling procedure to ensure that air spaces are filled by the ointment. To give the product a finished appearance the spatula should be used to smooth the surface of the ointment.

If an ointment is made by fusion, it usually can be packed while the ointment is still warm enough to be poured directly into the ointment jar. This technique is particularly useful when one has to package a large quantity of ointment.

Ointment jars should be closed tightly when not in use, particularly if the ointment contains water. Evaporation of water may change the physical characteristics of the preparation.

Collapsible Tubes. For dispensing in small quantities in prescription work, collapsible tin tubes are the containers of choice. These containers reduce oxidation to a minimum, since they present a very small ointment surface to air and light. Also, they are more sanitary, since the ointment is not contaminated by the applicant's fingers, as is the case in removing ointments from jars.

Ointment tubes are available with special tips, i.e., eye tips, nasal tips, vaginal and rectal tips.

Ointment tubes can be filled easily by the pharmacist without the use of special equipment. The finished ointment is rolled into a cylinder in a piece of powder paper, the ointment cylinder being shorter than the tube and slightly smaller in diameter. After inserting the paper-wrapped cylinder in the tube, the paper is removed by carefully flattening about 1/8 inch of the open end of the tube with a spatula, then withdrawing the

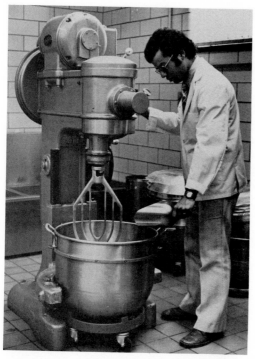

FIG. 8-5. Active ingredient being added to Hobart mixer containing an ointment. (Industrial Pharmacy Lab., Univ. of Iowa, College of Pharmacy)

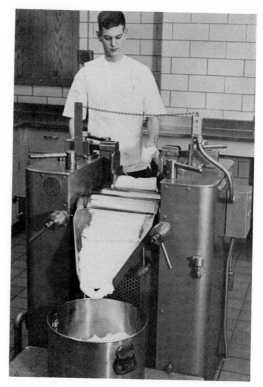

FIG. 8-6. Ointment passing through a Kent 3-roller ointment mill. (Industrial Pharmacy Lab., Univ. of Iowa, College of Pharmacy)

protruding paper while holding the flattened end of the tube together with the spatula. Two folds should be made at the flattened end of the tube by holding the spatula firmly on the bottom ⅛ inch of the flattened end then raising the tube, laying it over on itself. Flatten this fold with the spatula and repeat the operation. The cap on the top of the tube should be removed during the filling and folding procedure.

Hand-operated equipment is available for small-scale packaging of ointments and creams. Figures 8-7 and 8-8 show a paste and cream filler capable of filling 25 to 30 tubes a minute and a tube closer with a capacity of 20 tubes per minute, in the Industrial Pharmacy Laboratory at the University of Iowa College of Pharmacy.

In addition to filling tubes, the paste and cream filler can be used to fill jars, cans and bottles. A maximum of 10 pounds of air pressure may be used to facilitate the flow of materials such as pastes and stiff ointments which do not respond to gravity satisfactorily.

The hand-operated tube closer produces a quadruple-fold closure. The foot-operated crimper (Fig. 8-9) is used to produce the final corrugation on the folded ends of the tubes. It locks the folds, provides a decorative appearance and creates greater rigidity in the closed tube. The depth of the corrugation on the tube end can be regulated. The date or lot number can be stamped on the fold by using a special crimping jaw. The foot-operated crimper has a capacity of 30 tubes per minute.

Packaging of ointments on a large scale is carried out with automatic filling and crimping machines capable of filling and crimping 50 to 100 tubes per minute. Figure 8-10 shows the Arenco tube filling machine used in the Industrial Pharmacy Laboratory at the University of Iowa College of Pharmacy. This machine will fill up to 72 tubes per minute and will fill tubes ranging in capacity from ⅛ fluid ounce to 6 fluid ounces. Tubes are vacuum-cleaned automatically to remove

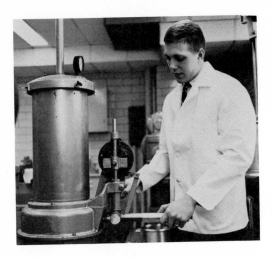

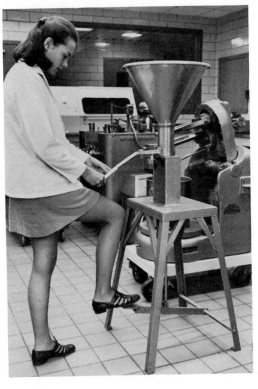

Fig. 8-7. (*Left*) Ointment tube being filled with a hand-operated Colton paste and cream filler. (Industrial Pharmacy Lab., Univ. of Iowa, (College of Pharmacy) (*Right*) Ointment tube being filled with a foot-operated Anderson paste and cream filler. (Industrial Pharmacy Lab., Univ. of Iowa, College of Pharmacy)

dust before being filled under the steam-jacketed ointment hopper. The ends of the tubes are automatically folded, corrugated and code-marked. From the machine, the tubes move by conveyor belt to the labeling and inspection station. The F. J. Stokes Machine Company of Philadelphia and the Cherry-Burrell Corporation of Cedar Rapids, Iowa, also make automatic tube fillers.

Storage and Labeling. Ointments should be stored in a cool place to prevent softening and eventual liquefaction of the base. Excessive heat or cold may cause an emulsion base to separate into two phases. Insoluble medicaments may settle to the bottom of the container if the ointment is permitted to liquefy.

No difficulty is encountered in labeling ointment jars. However, labels do not adhere well to collapsible tin tubes unless the area to be labeled is first coated with compound benzoin tincture or a lacquer and allowed to dry. It is desirable to use strip labels, so as to encircle the tube completely and, thus, help to prevent their coming off. Labels should be attached at the very top of the tube so that they will not be destroyed until the tube is almost empty.

PRESERVATION

Semisolid preparations have been considered microbiologically acceptable if they exhibit no visible or olfactory evidence of deterioration. However, recent studies indicate that gross contamination may be present in topical preparations, even though these preparations contain antimicrobial substances. The Food and Drug Administration reported[27,28] the presence of microbial contaminants in various topical pharmaceutical and cosmetic preparations. Wolven and Levenstein[119] reported that about 25 percent of the cosmetic preparations they examined were contaminated. Organisms found included *Pseudomonas aeruginosa* and other gram-negative rods and Salmonella species. In a survey conducted in Sweden of microbial flora present in nonsterile preparations, Kallings et al.[52,53] found appreciable levels of contamination in ointments, pastes, creams, liniments, powders, tablets, and mucilages.

The official compendia do not give microbiological standards for semisolid formulations, although microbiological standards may be designated for some of the raw ma-

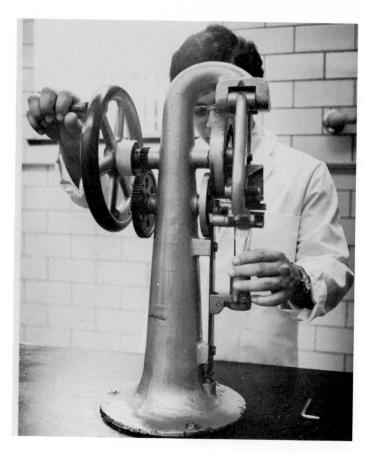

FIG. 8-8. Closing an ointment tube with a Colton tube closer. (Industrial Pharmacy Lab., Univ. of Iowa, College of Pharmacy)

terials used in the formulations. The U.S.P. and the FDA are considering microbiological standards for nonsterile pharmaceuticals. Semisolid formulations are usually intended for use in nonsterile situations, hence acceptable microbiological standards should include a listing of organisms that must be excluded from the formulation and should establish a limit on the total microbial count tolerable in a semisolid formulation. *U.S.P. XVIII* does contain a section on the microbial attributes of nonsterile pharmaceutical products. Among the desirable attributes of a suitable product is freedom from viable harmful microorganisms, examples of which are Salmonella species, *Escherichia coli,* certain species of Pseudomonas, including *Pseudomonas aeruginosa,* and *Staphylococcus aureus.*

A chemical preservative is a substance that inhibits or destroys microorganisms causing spoilage under normal conditions of manufacture, storage, handling, and use. Usually, the agent is simply inhibitory, although given

sufficient concentration and time, it may be germicidal.[26] Some of the most commonly used preservatives are benzoic acid, *p*-hydroxybenzoates, phenols, halogenated phenols, sorbic acid, sulfites, alcohol, quater-

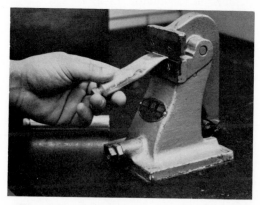

FIG. 8-9. Crimping an ointment tube with the Colton foot-operated crimper. (Industrial Pharmacy Lab., Univ. of Iowa, College of Pharmacy)

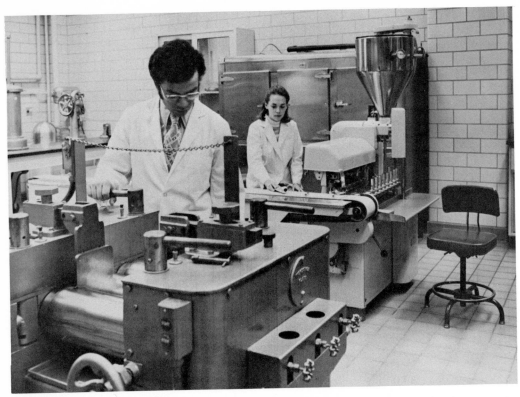

Fig. 8-10. In background, the filling and sealing of ointment tubes on the Arenco automatic filling and closing machine. In foreground, Kent 3-roller mill. (Industrial Pharmacy Lab., Univ. of Iowa, College of Pharmacy)

naries, and mercurials. Gemall, a new family of substituted imidazolidinyl urea compounds which have broad-spectrum antimicrobial activity, were discussed by Berke and Rosen.[10] Henley and Sonntag[40] discussed the use of formaldehyde and its donors as preservatives in cosmetic formulations. Schwarz[97] discussed the problems encountered in the preparation of sterile ointments and mentions several new preservatives.

The properties prerequisite for an ideal preservative for use in the cosmetic and pharmaceutical industries are postulated by Wells and Lubowe.[118] Although none of the prerequisites should be ignored, particular emphasis should be placed on the following properties: The preservative should have few physical and chemical incompatibilities, and it should be nontoxic and nonirritant in the concentrations employed. Many of the problems encountered with preservatives relate to their solubility, the effect of surfactants on preservative solubility, the partition coefficient of a preservative in emulsion formulations, and interactions between the preservative and many of the ingredients used in dermatologic preparations. Allergic skin reactions from preservatives have been reviewed by Schorr.[96] Finally, essential though it may be that preservative capacity be capable of arresting the growth of the organisms that cause contamination and infection, it should not convert a bland, soothing topical preparation into an antimicrobial preparation which upsets the equilibrium of the biozone created by microflora of the skin.

INGREDIENTS REQUIRING SPECIAL CONSIDERATION

Ingredients requiring special consideration when incorporated in ointments include alcoholic solutions, aqueous solutions, alkaloids, antibiotics, coal tar and Peruvian balsam.

Alcoholic Solutions. Small quantities of

TABLE 8-1. OINTMENTS OF THE U.S.P.

OINTMENT	PERCENTAGE OF ACTIVE INGREDIENT	BASE
Ammoniated Mercury	Ammoniated Mercury 5%	Mineral Oil, White Ointment
Bacitracin	Bacitracin 500 units/g.	Mineral Oil, White Petrolatum
Chloramphenicol	Chloramphenicol 0.85%	. . . .
Coal Tar	Coal Tar 1%	Zinc Oxide Paste, Polysorbate 80
Gentamicin Sulfate	Gentamicin Sulfate 1 mg./g.	. . . .
Hydrocortisone	Hydrocortisone 0.125–2.5%	Suitable Ointment Base
Hydrocortisone Acetate Ophthalmic	Hydrocortisone Acetate 0.5–2.5%	Suitable Ophthalmic Ointment Base
Hydrophilic	. . . .	Methylparaben, Propylparaben, Sodium Lauryl Sulfate, Propylene Glycol, Stearyl Alcohol, White Petrolatum, Purified Water
Hydrophilic Petrolatum		Cholesterol, Stearyl Alcohol, White Wax, White Petrolatum
Idoxuridine Ophthalmic	Idoxuridine 0.50%	Petrolatum Base
Iodochlorhydroxyquin	Iodochlorhydroxyquin 3%	Suitable Ointment Base
Lidocaine	Lidocaine 2.5–5%	Suitable Hydrophilic Ointment Base
Neomycin Sulfate	Neomycin Base 3.5 mg./g.	. . . .
Nystatin	Nystatin 100,000 units/g.	Suitable Ointment Base
Polyethylene Glycol	. . . .	Polyethylene Glycol 4000 and 400
Polymyxin B Sulfate	Polymyxin B Sulfate 20,000 units/g.	Anhydrous Petrolatum Base
Sodium Sulfacetamide Ophthalmic	Sodium Sulfacetamide 10%	. . . .
Sulfur	Precipitated Sulfur 10%	Mineral Oil, White Ointment, White Petrolatum
Triamcinolone Acetonide	Triamcinolone Acetonide 0.025 and 0.1%	Suitable Ointment Base
White	. . . .	White Wax, White Petrolatum
White Petrolatum	. . . .	White Petrolatum
Zinc Oxide	Zinc Oxide 20%	Mineral Oil, White Ointment

a highly alcoholic solution such as coal tar solution can be incorporated directly in many water-containing emulsion bases. However, it is advisable to evaporate most of the alcohol before incorporating in oleaginous bases.

Aqueous Solutions. Aqueous solutions can be incorporated readily in absorption bases such as Hydrophilic Petrolatum, U.S.P., and Aquaphor, using a mortar and pestle. Oleaginous bases will absorb very little water, and it is necessary to replace part of the base with anhydrous lanolin or Aquaphor if aqueous solutions are to be incorporated.

Burow's solution 5.0
Petrolatum q.s. 30.0

Replace 5 g. of petrolatum by 5 g. of anhydrous lanolin. Incorporate the Burow's solution in the anhydrous lanolin, using a mortar and pestle, and then incorporate 20 g. of petrolatum.

Iodine 2%
Petrolatum q.s. 30.0

Dissolve the iodine in 2 to 3 ml. of water containing 0.6 g. of potassium iodide. Incorporate the solution in 5 g. of anhydrous lanolin and then incorporate the petrolatum.

Alkaloids. Alkaloidal salts can be incorporated in absorption or emulsion bases by first dissolving the salt in a small quantity of water and then incorporating the solution directly in the base by levigation. If an oleaginous base is prescribed, the aqueous solution can be picked up with anhydrous lanolin and then added to the base. An alkaloidal salt or the free alkaloid can be incorporated directly in an ointment base by first powdering the salt or free alkaloid, then levigating it on an ointment slab with a small portion of the base to form a smooth nucleus which is incorporated with the remaining base.

Antibiotics. Anhydrous bases such as petrolatum and white ointment are employed extensively as vehicles for antibiotics such as the penicillins, bacitracin, chloramphenicol and the tetracyclines. These antibiotics are inactivated rapidly in water-containing

TABLE 8-2. OINTMENTS OF THE N.F.

OINTMENT	PERCENTAGE OF ACTIVE INGREDIENT	BASE
Anthralin	Anthralin 0.1 to 1.0%	Petrolatum or Suitable Base
Benzocaine	Benzocaine 1–20%	Suitable Ointment Base
Candicidin	Candicidin 0.06%	Suitable Ointment Base
Compound Resorcinol	Resorcinol 6%, Zinc Oxide 6%, Bismuth Subnitrate 6%, Juniper Tar 2%	Yellow Wax, Petrolatum, Anhydrous Lanolin, Glycerin
Compound Undecylenic Acid	Undecylenic Acid 5%, Zinc Undecylenate 20%	Polyethylene Glycol Ointment
Dexamethasone Sodium Phosphate Ophthalmic	Dexamethasone Sodium Phosphate 0.05%	. . . .
Dibucaine Ophthalmic	Dibucaine 1.0%	Suitable Ointment Base
Dimethisoquin	Dimethisoquin Hydrochloride 0.5%	. . . .
Flurandrenolide	Flurandrenolide 0.025 and 0.05%	. . . .
Hydroquinone	Hydroquinone 2%	. . . .
Ichthammol	Ichthammol 10%	Anhydrous Lanolin, Petrolatum
Iodochlorhydroxyquin and Hydrocortisone	Iodochlorhydroxyquin 3%, Hydrocortisone 0.5–1%	. . . .
Isoflurophate Ophthalmic	Isoflurophate 0.025%	Suitable Anhydrous Base
Monobenzone	Monobenzone 20%	. . . .
Neomycin Sulfate, Polymyxin B Sulfate & Zinc Bacitracin	Neomycin Base 3.5 mg./g., Polymyxin B Sulfate 5000 units/g., and Zinc Bacitracin 400 units/g., or Neomycin Base 3 mg./g., Polymyxin B Sulfate 8000 units/g., and Zinc Bacitracin 400 units/g.	. . . .
Nitrofurazone	Nitrofurazone 0.2%	Suitable Water-Miscible Base
Rose Water	. . . .	Spermaceti, White Wax, Almond Oil, Sodium Borate, Purified Water, Rose Oil
Tetracaine Ophthalmic	Tetracaine 0.5%	White Petrolatum
Triclobisonium Chloride	Triclobisonium Chloride 0.1%	. . . .
Yellow	. . . .	Yellow Wax, Petrolatum
Yellow Mercuric Oxide Ophthalmic	Yellow Mercuric Oxide 1%	Mineral Oil, White Ointment

ointment bases, due to hydrolysis and/or interaction with ointment base constituents.[16] Plaxco and Husa[79] showed that many surfactants inactivated bacitracin slowly, whereas water, water-containing bases, glycerin, propylene glycol and polyethylene glycol 400 inactivated bacitracin rapidly in ointments. Neomycin sulfate[95] and tyrothricin[2] are stable in aqueous solutions and in many types of ointment bases such as the water-miscible or polyethylene glycol type, the oleaginous type and the emulsion base. Aqueous solutions of polymyxin B sulfate will keep for many months at room temperature, and the antibiotic is stable in petrolatum and polyethylene glycol bases.[16]

Coal Tar. This substance is obtained as a by-product during the destructive distillation of coal. Among its numerous constituents are aromatic hydrocarbons such as benzene, toluene, naphthalene, anthracene, xylene, etc.; phenol, cresol and other phenols; ammonia, pyridine and other organic bases.

Although some coal tars used in ointments are prepared from anthracite (hard) coal, coal tars in the eastern part of the United States are obtained from bituminous (soft) coal and coal tars on the west coast are derived from oils of natural gas.[62]

Zetar,* a standardized commercial coal tar, is obtained from a particular type of anthracite coal. It is irradiated with ultraviolet light and the product is processed with a small amount of a surfactant to make it water-removable.

The physical characteristics of coal tar ointments are influenced primarily by: (1) the type, the source and the viscosity of the tar employed and (2) the order of incorporating the ingredients. There are 3 methods used in the preparation of prescriptions containing the well known combination of coal tar, zinc oxide, starch and petrolatum.

1. Incorporate the zinc oxide with the coal tar, then incorporate the petrolatum and the starch. A black or dark brown ointment is obtained, depending on the coal tar used. This technique does not permit good levigation of the zinc oxide.

2. Incorporate the coal tar in the petrolatum, then add the zinc oxide and the starch. A grayish green ointment results from this order of mixing.

3. Incorporate the zinc oxide in the petrolatum, add the starch, then incorporate the coal tar. A uniform, gray ointment is obtained with this, the preferred method of the three for compounding a coal tar ointment.

Coal Tar Ointment, U.S.P., contains a

* Dermik Laboratories, Inc., N.Y.

nonionic surfactant, polysorbate 80, which serves a dual purpose. It functions as a dispersing agent and aids in the removal of the ointment from the skin. The coal tar is mixed with the polysorbate 80 before incorporating it into the vehicle, zinc oxide paste.

Coal tar can be incorporated readily in emulsion bases such as Hydrophilic Ointment, U.S.P.

Peru Balsam. Balsams are resinous substances containing benzoic and cinnamic acids or their esters. Peru balsam and other resinous substances separate from ointments when the base is composed solely of a nonpolar substance such as petrolatum. Castor oil will prevent this separation if used as a levigating agent for Peru balsam before incorporating the balsam. Generally, it is desirable to use castor oil in an amount equal to that of the balsam. Castor oil is useful in this respect in that it contains the triglyceride of ricinoleic acid (12-hydroxyolic acid). The presence of the –OH group enables it to associate through hydrogen bonding with the acidic constituents of the resins to solubilize them. No special levigating agent is required when Peru balsam is incorporated in emulsion bases such as Hydrophilic Ointment, U.S.P. A small portion of the emulsion base can be used to levigate the balsam which is then incorporated in the remaining base.

CREAMS

HISTORY

Variations in the composition of ointment bases resulted in the designation of some semi-solid preparations as creams and others as paste. The term *cream* is loosely used, e.g., milk of magnesia is often referred to as a cream. Many cosmetic preparations are called creams, e.g., cold cream, hand cream, night cream, vanishing cream, etc. The *British Pharmacopoeia* uses the term as a synonym for zinc and castor oil ointment and also classifies as creams medicated liquid emulsions consisting of a mixture of anhydrous lanolin, olive oil (or other fixed oil) and lime water. Apparently, consistency and appearance have been responsible for the nomenclature of these preparations, since creams are thought of usually as opaque, soft semisolids or thick liquids intended for external use. If the term *cream* is accepted as a designation of a pharmaceutical dosage form, it should be defined more precisely. The following is offered as a definition: Creams are semisolid emulsions, usually medicated, intended for external application. This definition eliminates thick liquids (which are usually termed lotions or emulsion lotions) and suspensions of medicaments in petrolatum or water-soluble bases. In *U.S.P. XVIII* creams are described as "semisolid emulsions of either the oil-in-water or the water-in-oil type."

Creams became official with the introduction of the formula for Sun Cream in *N.F. VIII*. Sun cream was designed to prevent sunburn but, at the same time, to permit tanning. It contained 2 chemical sunscreening agents, benzocaine and phenyl salicylate, incorporated in an oil-water emulsion base.

Cosmetic creams, which usually are not medicated, include preparations classified as all-purpose creams, baby creams, barrier creams, bleaching creams, cleansing creams, cold creams, deodorant creams, foundation creams, hair creams, hand creams, etc. Modern cosmetic creams are discussed by Harry.[39]

The number of creams has increased dramatically in the official compendia. There were four creams official in 1960; the nineteen creams listed in Table 8-3 are now official. Creams are pharmaceutically and cosmetically appealing. They are soft, easy to apply, cooling to the skin, and many are water-removable.

PASTES

HISTORY

The introduction of the use of so-called pastes into the dermatologic field is comparatively recent when one thinks in terms of the length of time ointments have been in use. This class or group of preparations was introduced by the noted dermatologists Unna and Lassar about 1900. Up to that time, the term "paste" (Latin, *pasta*; French, *pata*) was used exclusively for internal preparations, the majority of which were of gum-like consistency—e.g., Pasta Althaeae and Pasta Glycyrrhizae. Pastes are now defined as ointmentlike preparations for external application. They are usually stiffer than ointments, less greasy and more absorptive, because of their high proportion of powdered medicaments such as starch, zinc oxide, calcium carbonate, etc. Zinc Oxide Paste, U.S.P., contains 50 percent of powdered medicament.

Pastes comprise two classes of ointmentlike preparations: One class is made from some hydrogel such as hydrated pectin or hydrated tragacanth; The other class, the fatty pastes, e.g., Zinc Oxide Paste, U.S.P., are thick, stiff ointments that usually do not flow at body temperature; hence, they serve as protective coatings over the areas to which they are applied.

USE

Because they are absorptive, pastes are used on acute lesions, especially those which are oozing. They are more difficult to apply and remove than ointments, but they adhere well to the skin and do not interfere appreciably with perspiration. Pastes have a heavy consistency, and, when covered with dressings, they provide a protective layer through which it is difficult for the patient to scratch and excoriate his skin.

The term *paste* for external medicaments, like the term *ointment,* seems to be an all-inclusive term. It has been applied to 2 entirely different types of preparations; (1) to ointmentlike mixtures of starch, zinc oxide or calcium carbonate with light liquid petrolatum, white petrolatum, anhydrous lanolin, white wax, benzoinated lard, etc., (2) to jellies containing glycerin with starch, and (3) glycerogelatins or other water-soluble gels containing pectin and tragacanth, glycerin, etc.

Some pastes contain as much as 50 percent of powder with petrolatum, or as much as 70 percent of powder with less viscous oils as the vehicle. Pastes containing these large amounts of powder differ from ointments by having a slight drying action, due to adsorption or capillarity. Medicaments incorporated in these bases are absorbed less readily than from ointments and, therefore, have a more superficial action, but they give better protection.[62] They are used chiefly as vehicles for astringent and antiseptic agents.

Thus Fantus[30] states:

Pastes are especially indicated when it is in-

TABLE 8-3.   CREAMS OF THE U.S.P. AND N.F.

OINTMENT	PERCENTAGE OF ACTIVE INGREDIENT	BASE
Cold, U.S.P.	....	Spermaceti, White Wax, Mineral Oil, Sodium Borate, Purified Water
Gamma Benzene Hexachloride, U.S.P.	Gamma Benzene Hexachloride 1%	Suitable Cream Base
Gentamicin Sulfate, U.S.P.	Gentamicin Sulfate 1 mg./g.	Suitable Semisolid Base
Hydrocortisone, U.S.P.	Hydrocortisone 0.125 to 2.5%	Mineral Oil, Hydrophilic Ointment
Iodochlorhydroxyquin, U.S.P.	Iodochlorhydroxyquin 3%	Suitable Cream Base
Tolnaftate, U.S.P.	Tolnaftate 1%	....
Triamcinolone Acetonide, U.S.P.	Triamcinolone Acetonide 0.025 to 0.5%	....
Betamethasone, N.F.	Betamethasone 0.2%	Suitable Water-Miscible Base
Dexamethasone Sodium Phosphate, N.F.	Dexamethasone Phosphate 0.1%	....
Dibucaine, N.F.	Dibucaine 0.5%	Suitable Cream Base
Dienestrol, N.F.	Dienestrol 0.01%	Suitable Water-Miscible Base
Fluorometholone, N.F.	Fluorometholone 0.025%	....
Iodochlorhydroxyquin and Hydrocortisone, N.F.	Iodochlorhydroxyquin 3%, Hydrocortisone 0.5 to 1%	....
Neomycin Sulfate and Dexamethasone Sodium Phosphate, N.F.	Neomycin Base 0.35%, Dexamethasone Phosphate 0.1%	....
Nitrofurazone, N.F.	Nitrofurazone 0.2%	Suitable Emulsified Water-Miscible Base
Pramoxine Hydrochloride, N.F.	Pramoxine Hydrochloride 1%	Suitable Water-Miscible Base
Triacetin, N.F.	Triacetin 25%	....
Triclobisonium Chloride	Triclobisonium Chloride 0.1%	....

tended that a therapeutic effect shall be exerted chiefly on the diseased epithelium (epidermatic action).

Pastes are not suitable for application to hairy parts such as the scalp, as they will form a densely matted mass.

Since pastes contain large amounts of powder and are stiff preparations, levigating agents such as mineral oil should not be used. The amount of mineral oil required to levigate the powdered medicaments would result in a soft product. Instead, a portion of the base should be melted and used as a levigating agent.

Starch	15.0
Zinc oxide	15.0
White Petrolatum qs.	60.0

Melt a portion of the white petrolatum and use it to levigate the powders. Incorporate the remaining base.

The water-soluble gels, such as glycerin with starch and pectins, are useful when

TABLE 8-4.   PASTES OF THE U.S.P. AND THE N.F.

PASTE	PERCENTAGE OF ACTIVE INGREDIENT	BASE
Zinc Oxide, U.S.P.	Zinc Oxide 25%, Starch 25%	White Petrolatum
Zinc Oxide with Salicylic Acid, N.F.	Salicylic Acid 2%	Zinc Oxide Paste

fatty bases are undesirable. According to Fantus,[30] fatty preparations are unsuited for application to wet or moist surfaces. He states:

Whenever an ointment does not stick to the site of application it not only does no good, but is liable to do harm by causing the retention of secretion, which forms a culture medium, and thus favors the proliferation of microorganisms and the consequent irritation of the surface by their poisonous products. In conditions that border on the prohibitive type, pastes, by reason of their slight drying action, may still be useful.

The water-soluble gels of about the consistency of ointments are advantageous when applied to moist surfaces, because of their miscibility with the aqueous fluids. Also, they have the advantages of easy removal from the skin.

Pectin and tragacanth pastes were introduced by Fantus and Dyniewicz[31] for the treatment of ulcers and bedsores. The cavity was first filled with the paste and then was covered with a piece of waterproof cellophane considerably larger than the sore. In modern dermatologic therapy, pectin and tragacanth pastes are seldom used to treat bedsores and ulcers. The pastes have been replaced by ointments, creams, and jellies containing enzymes such as trypsin,* chymotrypsin,† papain,‡ and streptodornase,§ and vitamins A and D, lanolin fractions, silicones, etc.

Pectin paste and thin pectin paste were official in *N.F. IX.* They contained pectin, glycerin and Ringer's solution. The pastes were prepared by mixing the pectin with the glycerin, then hot Ringer's solution was added to hydrate the pectin.

Pastes prepared with glycerogelatin as the base soften at body temperature and may be applied after softening by warming. When harder glycerogelatin pastes are prescribed, generally the jar is placed in warm water to melt the paste, which is then painted on with a brush. Zinc Gelatin, U.S.P., is an example of a firm glycerogelatin paste.

PREPARATION

For all practical purposes, the oily or fatty pastes containing insoluble powder are prepared in the same manner as ointments. Levigating agents should be used more cautiously when preparing pastes, since large quantities of levigating agents such as mineral oil will produce undue softening of the paste.

The water-soluble gels, such as pectin and tragacanth, generally are prepared by first wetting the pectin or the tragacanth with a small amount of glycerin and then adding a sufficient quantity of hot water. Starch and glycerin are simply mixed and heated together, while starch "paste" is made by mixing starch with cold water and then adding this to boiling water, with stirring. For practical purposes, the method of compounding prescribed in *N.F. IX* will serve as a guide in the extemporaneous preparation of this type of preparation.

STORAGE AND PACKAGING

Oily and fatty pastes may be packaged in glass ointment jars. However, pastes containing large amounts of water, such as pectin and tragacanth pastes and glycerogelatin pastes, must be stored in tightly closed containers to prevent the drying which occurs on exposure to air.

Pectin and tragacanth pastes are very liable to mold growth. They can be protected by the addition of preservatives like benzoic acid, 0.2 percent, or the parabens. Enzymatic hydrolysis of pectin caused by the growth of certain types of mold may cause liquefaction of pectin pastes.

* Trypsigel Creme, Bruce.
† Biozyme Ointment, Armour Pharm. Co. (Trypsin and Chymotrypsin).
‡ Panafil Ointment, Rystan Co.
§ Varidase Jelly, Lederle Labs.

REFERENCES

1. Allenby, A. C., Fletcher, J., Schock, C., and Lees, T. F. S.: Brit. J. Derm., *81*:31, 1969.
2. Antibiotics Brochure, Antibiotics Div., S. B. Penick and Co., New York, N.Y. 1955.
3. Atlas Cosmetic Formulary. Emulsification of Basic Cosmetic Ingredients. Atlas Chemical Industries, 1969.
4. Barr, M.: J. Pharm. Sci., *51*:395, 1962.
5. ———: Am. Perfumer and Cosmetics, *78*: 37, 1963.
6. Barr, M., and Guth, E. P.: J. Am. Pharm. A. (Sci. Ed.), *40*:13, 1951.
7. Barrett, C. W.: J. Soc. Cosmetic Chem., *20*:487, 1969.
8. Beeler, E. C.: J. Am. Pharm. A. (Pract. Ed.), *3*:231, 1942.
9. ———: Bull. Nat. Formulary Comm., *11*: 27, 1943.
10. Berke, P. A., and Rosen, W. E.: Am. Perfumer Cosmet., *85*:55, 1970.
11. Bertram, S. H.: J. Am. Oil Chem. Soc., *26*:454, 1954.
12. Bettley, F. R., and Donoghue, E.: Nature, *185*:17, 1960.
13. Blank, I. H., and MacFarlane, D. J.: J. Invest. Derm., *49*:582, 1967.
14. Blaug, S. M., and Ahsan, S. S.: Drug Standards, *28*:95, 1960.
15. Bradshaw, M.: Histochemical Demonstration of the Permeability of Lantrol Through Normal Human Skin, Clinical Report to Malmstrom Chem. Corp., 1959.
16. Buckwalter, F. H.: J. Am. Pharm. A. (Pract. Ed.), *15*:694, 1954.
17. Calvery, H. O., Draize, J. H., and Laug, E. P.: Physiol. Rev., *26*:495, 1946.
18. Carbowax Polyethylene Glycols for Pharmaceuticals and Cosmetics. Union Carbide Chemicals Co., 1959.
19. Casparis, P., and Myer, E. W.: Pharm. acta Helv. *10*:163, 1935.
20. Chakravarty, D., Lach, J. L., and Blaug, S. M.: Drug Standards, *25*:137, 1957.
21. Clark, E. W.: Am. Perfumer Cosmet., *77*: 10, 89, 1962.
22. Collins, A. D., and Zopf, L. C.: Am. Prof. Pharm., *691*, 1956.
23. Darlington, R. C., and Guth, E. P.: J. Am. Pharm. A. (Pract. Ed.), *11*:82, 1950.
24. Dempski, R. E., Demarco, J. D., and Marcus, A. D.: J. Invest. Derm., *44*:361, 1965.
25. Dempski, R. E., Portnoff, J. B., and Wase, A. W.: J. Pharm. Sci., *58*:579, 1969.
26. de Navarre, M. G.: The Chemistry and Manufacture of Cosmetics. Vol. 1. New Jersey, Van Nostrand, 1962, p. 862.
27. Dunnigan, A. P.: Soap, Perf. and Cosmet., *41* (No. 11):815, 1968.
28. ———: Drug Cosmet. Ind., *106* (No. 1): 48, 1970.
29. Elfbaum, S. G., and Laden, K.: J. Soc. Cosmet. Chem., *19*:119, 841, 1968.
30. Fantus, B.: Technic of Medication. p. 68. Am. Med. A., Chicago, 1938.
31. Fantus, B., and Dyniewicz, H.: J. Am. Pharm. A., *28*:299, 1939.
32. Fiero, G.: J. Am. Pharm. A. (Sci. Ed.), *29*:18, 187, 458, 502, 1940.
33. ———: J. Am. Pharm. A., *30*:145, 1941.
34. Fritsch, W. F., and Stoughton, R. B.: J. Invest. Derm., *82*:24, 1960.
35. Gemmell, D. H. O., and Morrison, J. C.: J. Pharm. Pharmacol., *10*:167, 1958.
36. Goodman, H. J.: J. Am. Pharm. A. (Pract. Ed.), *3*:7, 1942.
37. Griesemer, R. D.: J. Soc. Cosmetic Chem., *11*:79, 1960.
38. Halpern, A., and Zopf, L. C.: J. Am. Pharm. A. (Sci. Ed.), *36*:101, 1947.
39. Harry, R. G.: Modern Cosmeticology. Vol. 1. New York, Chemical Publishing, 1962.
40. Henley, W. O., and Sonntag, N. O.: Am. Perfumer Cosmet., *85*:95, 1970.
41. Higuchi, T.: J. Soc. Cosmetic Chem., *11*:85, 1960.
42. ———: J. Am. Pharm. A. (Sci. Ed.), *49*: 598, 1960.
43. Higuchi, T., and Lach, J. L.: J. Am. Pharm. A. (Sci. Ed.), *43*:465, 1954.
44. Higuchi, W. I.: J. Pharm. Sci., *51*:802, 1962.
45. Hollander, L., and McClanahan, W. S.: J. Invest. Derm., *11*:127, 1948.
46. Husa, W. J., and Riley, D. E.: J. Am. Pharm. A., *23*:544, 1934.
47. Idson, B.: J. Soc. Cosmet. Chem., *22*:615, 1971.
48. Jacobi, O.: J. Soc. Cosmet. Chem., *18*:149, 1967.
49. Jacobi, O., and Heinrich, H.: Proc. Sci. Sect. T.G.A., No. 21, May 1954.
50. Jarmecke, H.: Deut. med. Wschr., *80*:755, 1955.
51. Jones, E. R., and Lewicki, B.: J. Am. Pharm. A. (Sci. Ed.), *40*:509, 1951.
52. Kallings, L. O., Ernerfeldt, F., and Silverstolpe, L.: Acta path. microbiol. scand., *66*: 287, 1966.
53. Kallings, L. O., Ringertz, O., Silverstolpe, L., and Ernerfeldt, F.: Acta pharm. suecica, *3*:219, 1966.
54. Kariya, T., Marcus, A. D., and Benton, B. E.: J. Am. Pharm. A. (Pract. Ed.), *14*:297, 1953.
55. Katz, M., and Poulsen, B. J.: *In*: Part 1. Brodie, B. B., and Gillette, J. R. (eds.): Concepts in Biochemical Pharmacology. New York, Springer-Verlag, 1971. p. 103.
56. Katz, M., and Shaikh, Z. I.: J. Pharm. Sci., *54*:591, 1965.
57. Kligman, A. M.: JAMA, *193*:140, 151, 1965.
58. Lane, C. G., and Blank, I. H.: Arch. Derm., *54*:497, 1946.
59. Lantrol Brochure. Malstrom Chemical Corp., Newark, 1959.
60. Laug, E. P., Vos, E. A., Kunze, F. M., and Umberger, E. J.: J. Pharmacol. Exp. Ther., *89*:52, 1947.

61. Lehman, A. J., and Draize, J. H.: Quart. Bull. Ass. Food & Drug Off. U.S., *23*:150, 1959.

62. Lerner, M. R., and Lerner, A. B.: Dermatologic Medications. Chicago, Year Book Publishers, 1960.

63. LeVan, P., Sternberg, T. H., and Newcomer, V. D.: Calif. Med., *81*:210, 1954.

64. Lockie, L. D., and Sprowls, J. D.: J. Am. Pharm. A. (Sci. Ed.), *38*:222, 1949.

65. Lubowe, I.: J. Soc. Cosmet. Chem., *6*:19, 1955.

66. MacKenna, R. M. B., Wheatley, V. R., and Wormall, A.: J. Invest. Derm., *15*:33, 1950.

67. McKenzie, A. W.; Arch. Derm., *86*:611, 1962.

68. McKenzie, A. W., and Aitkinson, R. M.: Arch. Derm., *89*:741, 1964.

69. McKenzie, A. W., and Stoughton, R. B.: Arch. Derm., *86*:608, 1962.

70. "Malcaloid." The Inerto Co., San Francisco, 1957.

71. Mali, J. W. H.: J. Invest. Derm., *27*:451, 1956.

72. Marzulli, F. N.: J. Invest. Derm., *39*:387, 1962.

73. Marzulli, F. N., Callahan, J. F., and Brown, D. W. C.: J. Invest. Derm., *44*:339, 1965.

74. Mendes, R. W., Morris, R. M., and Brown, E. T.: Drug Cosmet. Ind., *95*:34, 1964.

75. Meyers, D. B., Nadkarni, M. V., and Zopf, L. C.: J. Am. Pharm. A. (Sci. Ed.), *38*:231, 1949.

76. Michelfelder, T. J., and Peck, S. M.: J. Invest. Derm., *19*:237, 1952.

77. Pail, D., and Todd, C. W.: American Perfumer, *77*:62, 1962.

78. Peck, S. M., and Glick, A. W.: J. Soc. Cosmet. Chem., *6*:330, 1956.

79. Plaxco, J. M., and Husa, W. J.: J. Am. Pharm. A. (Sci. Ed.), *45*:141, 1956.

80. Plein, E. M., and Plein, J. B.: J. Am. Pharm. A. (Sci. Ed.), *46*:705, 1957.

81. Plein, J. B., and Plein, E. M.: J. Am. Pharm. A. (Sci. Ed.), *42*:79, 1953.

82. Poulsen, B. J., Young, E., Coquilla, V., and Katz, M.: J. Pharm. Sci., *57*:928, 1968.

83. Powers, D. H., and Fox, C.: Proc. Scientific Section, Toilet Goods Assoc., *28*:21, 1957.

84. ———: J. Soc. Cosmet. Chem., *10*:109, 1959.

85. Price, J. C., and Osborne, G. E.: J. Am. Pharm. A. (Pract. Ed.), *19*:679, 1958.

86. Rosenthaler, L.: Pharm. act helv., *18*:262, 1943.

87. Rothman, S.: Physiology and Biochemistry of the Skin. p. 27. Chicago, University of Chicago Press, 1954.

88. Rowe, V. K., Spencer, H. C., and Bass, S. L.: J. Ind. Hyg. Toxicol., *30*:332, 1948.

89. Sagarin, E., Cosmetics Science and Technology. p. 105. New York, Interscience, 1957.

90. Salisbury, R., Leuallen, E. E., and Chavkin, L. T.: J. Am. Pharm. A. (Sci. Ed.), *43*:117, 1954.

91. Scheuplein, R. J.: J. Invest. Derm., *45*:334, 1965.

92. ———: J. Invest. Derm., *48*:79, 1967.

93. Scheuplein, R. J., Blank, I. H., Brauner, G. J., and Mac Farlane, D.: J. Invest. Derm., *52*:63, 1969.

94. Scheuplein, R. J., and Ross, L.: J. Soc. Cosmet. Chem., *21*:853, 1970.

95. Schneller, G. H., and Hutchinson, J. L.: Neomycin. 1. Pharmaceutical information. American Cyanamid Co., 1954.

96. Schorr, W. F.: Am. Perfumer Cosmet., *85*:39, 1970.

97. Schwarz, T. W.: Am. Perfumer Cosmet., *86*:39, 1971.

98. Shaw, J. M., and Growe, F. W.: Arch. Derm., *71*:379, 1955.

99. Shelmire, J. B.: Invest. Derm., *26*:105, 1956.

100. ———: Arch. Derm., *82*:24, 1960.

101. Smyth, H. F., Jr., Carpenter, C. P., and Weil, C. S.: J. Am. Pharm. A. (Sci. Ed.), *39*:349, 1950.

102. ———: J. Am. Pharm. A. (Sci. Ed.), *44*:27, 1955.

103. Sperandio, G. J.: Am. Perfumer Cosmet., *78*:99, 1963.

104. Steigleder, G. K., and Raab, W. P.: J. Invest. Derm., *38*:129, 1962.

105. Stoughton, R. B., and Fritsch, W.: Arch. Derm., *90*:512, 1964.

106. Strakosch, E. A., and Clark, W. G.: Am. J. Med. Sci., *205*:610, 1943.

107. Sulzberger, M. B., Cortese, T. A., Fishman, L., Wiley, H. S., and Peyakovich, P.: Ann. N.Y. Acad. Sci., *141*:437, 1967.

108. Sulzberger, M. B., and Witten, V. H.: Arch. Derm., *84*:189, 1961.

109. Talbot, J. R., MacGregor, J. K., and Crowe, F. W.: J. Invest. Derm., *17*:125, 1951.

110. Tiedt, J., and Truter, E. V.: Chem. and Ind., 403, 1952.

111. Tregear, R. T.: J. Soc. Cosmet. Chem., *13*:145, 1962.

112. ———: Physical Functions of Skin. New York, Academic Press, 1966. p. 21.

113. Treherne, J. E.: J. Physiol., *133*:171, 1956.

114. Veegum—Uses and Properties. Bull. No. 29. R. T. Vanderbilt Co., New York.

115. Wagner, H.: Am. Perfumer and Aromatics, *75*:23, 1960.

116. Wagner, J.: J. Pharm. Sci., *50*:379, 1961.

117. Warshaw, T. G.: J. Soc. Cosmet. Chem., *4*:290, 1953.

118. Wells, F. V., and Lubowe, I. I.: Cosmetics and the Skin. New York, Reinhold, 1964. p. 8.

119. Wolven, A., and Levenstein, I.: TGA Cosmetic Journal, *1*:34, 1969.

120. Wurster, D. E., and Kramer, S. F.: J. Pharm. Sci., *50*:288, 1961.

121. Zeutlin, H. E. C., and Fox, C. L.: Invest. Derm., *11*:161, 1948.

9

T. Werner Schwarz, Ph.D., *Associate Professor of Pharmacy and Pharmaceutical Chemistry, School of Pharmacy, University of California, San Francisco*

Molded Solid Dosage Forms: Suppositories

Suppositories are solid medications for insertion into body cavities. Currently, only rectal and vaginal suppositories are in use. They disintegrate in the body cavity either by melting or by dissolution. The term vaginal suppository is now used rather loosely and is often applied to vaginal tablets. (*Pessary* is an obsolete term for a vaginal suppository.) Rectal suppositories are an infrequently used but long known form of medication that is employed for both local and systemic distribution of a drug.

HISTORY

Suppositories were known to the Assyrians about 2600 B.C.,[28] to the Egyptians a thousand years later and to the ancient Greeks and Romans. While the Egyptians confined the use of suppositories to the treatment of local conditions, Hippocrates used them also to improve breathing in children and Dioscorides to produce sleep. Galen, in the second century, applied suppositories for their purgative effect only.

The vehicle was at first a shaped chip of wood or bone, which was dipped into a coating mixture of warm fat or honey and ground drug. The chips were retrieved, cleaned and used again. Other core materials, which were introduced later, were pieces of soap, raisins, vegetable or cabbage stock and pieces of cloth.[18] The suppository ranged in size from a small pellet to one weighing as much as 20 g.[15]

The lack of dosage uniformity in such diverse forms of rectal application is probably responsible for the neglect of the suppository in subsequent centuries. Paracelsus, like Galen, used suppositories, for a purgative effect only. With the discovery of cocoa butter in the 18th century and the intro-duction in the 19th century of molds, first of paper, then wood and, finally, metal, the use of suppositories became more widespread.

There is no consensus about the etymologic origin of the word suppository, which is the same in Romanic and Germanic languages. However, the most likely origin is from the Latin participle *suppositus,* which means placed underneath. Until the last century, the term was applied mostly to shaped medication inserted into any body cavity except the mouth; in the beginning of the 20th century urethral suppositories, called *bougies,* were not uncommon.*

As a useful form for drug administration, suppositories have been more popular in Europe than in the United States. In recent years about one percent of all prescriptions in the U.S. have been for rectal suppositories; a good many suppository preparations exist that do not require a prescription.

PURPOSE OF SUPPOSITORY MEDICATION

The suppository is a rational form of medication for the treatment in both the rectum and the vagina of local conditions, such as hemorrhoids and infections. Also, since drugs are absorbed from mucous membranes, suppositories have been used for systemic distribution when the oral administration of drugs was not suitable, as in infants or debilitated patients and in conditions in which nausea or gastrointestinal disturbances in general are present.

Suppositories have been used to obtain prolonged action of drugs. The introduction of sustained-action oral dosage forms has largely eliminated this particular applica-

---

* A urethral insert of nitrofurazone is still in use.

tion of suppositories. Absorption of drug from the rectal mucosa directly into the venous circulation may bring about a faster onset of action than is found after oral administration[22, 64] and avoids enzymatic decomposition of numerous drugs in the gastrointestinal tract.

ANATOMY OF RECTUM AND CONDITIONS FOR ABSORPTION OF DRUG INTO BLOOD CIRCULATION

The rectum, as the terminal portion of the intestine, begins at the rectosigmoid junction and ends in the anus. It has a length of about 15 cm., two thirds of which follows the curvature of the lower spine. At the height of the coccyx, the rectum of the erect human bends to a more horizontal position and turns downward just above the anal sphincter. Normally, the rectum is empty except for a small amount of mucus which in the adult averages 2 ml. and has a pH corresponding to that of blood.[32]

The absence of villi in the rectum is an indication that it has no primary absorptive function. However, diffusion through and between the epithelial cells of the mucosa takes place. The submucosal region is rich in lymphatic and blood vessels. The venous circulation in the vicinity of the rectum consists of three branches: the inferior hemorrhoidal vein near the anal sphincter, the middle hemorrhoidal vein, which receives blood from the capillaries of the middle region of the rectum, and the superior hemorrhoidal vein, which is near the upper section of the rectum. The paired inferior and middle hemorrhoidal veins drain into the inferior vena cava, while the superior hemorrhoidal vein joins the inferior mesenteric vein, which empties into the portal vein. Many of the small blood vessels drain into the inferior and the middle hemorrhoidal veins. This has given rise to the assumption that rectally administered drugs are carried directly into the vena cava, bypassing the liver, where most drugs undergo metabolic changes.

This assumption is, at best, only partially correct. There are extensive anastomoses between superior and middle hemorrhoidal veins and also between the latter and the inferior hemorrhoidal veins. According to the course of venous flow, a drug absorbed in the lower part of the rectum should enter the vena cava; a drug placed in the upper part of the rectum should diffuse into blood vessels which lead to the liver. To test this hypothesis, K. Bucher[3] administered ^{33}P as disodium phophate to rats. During a period of half an hour, blood was collected at the entry of the portal vein to the liver and from the vena cava at its junction with the thorax. From a suppository inserted into the lower part of the rectum, about one fourth of the radioactive sodium phosphate went to the liver, three fourths went directly to the vena cava. When four times as long a suppository was inserted (actually, a tampon was used), the same amount of ^{33}P was found in both places. It was shown subsequently by x-ray studies of barium sulfate suppositories that a suppository does not remain in the lower portion of the rectum but moves upward into the region where veins that lead to the liver predominate.[61] Hennig[32] also studied the migration of radiopaque suppositories in the rectum. He found that the suppository, regardless of its shape, came to rest between 4 and 6 cm. above the anal sphincter. There was no further ascent although different vehicles showed different distribution along the rectal walls after disintegration. In another study the suppository mass was found to spread up to 12 cm. from the sphincter.[27] While rapid disintegration of a suppository favors absorption of the drug by blood vessels connected mainly with the vena cava, variations in the spread of different vehicles along the mucosa, as well as the extensive anastomoses, preclude a conclusive statement in regard to the immediate course of a drug inserted into the rectum of man. For most drugs, however, it is immaterial whether or not they bypass the liver during their first circulation after absorption.

Lymphatic flow, which is exceedingly slow compared with blood flow, does not contribute to the transportation of the drug from the rectum, according to Bucher.[3] However, in an investigation of the rectal absorption of sulfanilamide in dogs, it was found that slightly more drug was transported via lymph than via blood and that the rate of transport was faster via lymphatic vessels.[24]

QUANTITATIVE STUDIES OF DRUG ABSORPTION FROM SUPPOSITORIES

The earliest chemical evidence of rectal absorption was recorded in 1874,[32] when iodide could be identified in the urine shortly after rectal administration of an aqueous solution of potassium iodide. There is, as expected, faster uptake from a solution than from a suppository, and Rapp[62] found, in the case of methylene blue, that the dye appeared in the urine twice as fast when given as an enema as when given as a cocoa butter suppository. These studies were followed by attempts to evaluate the effect of the vehicle and of the form of the drug used, i.e., whether salt, acid or base.[7, 70] However, these investigations were confined to the determination of the onset and the duration of drug action. Further knowledge was required in regard to the comparative amounts absorbed from orally and rectally administered drug and, as a corollary, the rectal dose relative to the oral dose. Such studies in man are beset with several difficulties. Many investigators have tried to solve attendant problems by animal experiments or in-vitro studies. In view of the large number and variety of available suppository vehicles, a screening method which is both simpler and more convenient than absorption studies in man or animals is highly desirable.

The systemic action of drugs inserted into the vagina was proved for cats and dogs[44] and for humans.[67] In the latter investigation, it was found that methylene blue was not absorbed from the vagina, while potassium iodide, and sodium salicylate were well absorbed. All three compounds are absorbed from the rectum. In medical practice, vaginal suppositories are limited to their local effect; whenever systemic action via suppositories is desired, the rectal route is chosen. Nevertheless, systemic action of a drug administered vaginally is a distinct possibility.

THE PATH OF DRUG FROM RECTAL SUPPOSITORY

In order to determine in vivo the uptake of drug from a rectal suppository, the concentration of drug in blood or urine or a pharmacologic response can be measured. It depends on the metabolic fate of the drug which of these three alternate methods is likely to give reliable data.

The absorption of drug from a suppository through the rectal mucosa into the circulation involves at least two steps, which are independent of each other: (1) release of drug from vehicle, and (2) diffusion of drug through mucosa. The drug is then transported via veins or lymph vessels into the blood circulation. There the drug is subject to several processes: (1) elimination as such; (2) detoxication or metabolism and subsequent elimination, and (3) distribution in tissue fluid. Thus the drug concentration in blood is subject to the above factors, to which should be added the possibility of protein-binding in both blood and tissue fluid. The resulting interrelations may be represented schematically:

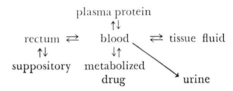

Several pathways are reversible. The release of drug from the suppository vehicle depends on the relative affinities of drug for the vehicle and rectal fluid. Low affinity between drug and vehicle and solubility of drug in the aqueous mucus favor release of drug and its availability for subsequent diffusion through mucous membrane. Conversely, high affinity between drug and vehicle and poor solubility in aqueous mucus retard the absorption rate and decrease amounts of drug available for absorption. This has been documented by the painstaking experiments of Eckert,[20] who compared the in-vitro release of the water-soluble procaine hydrochloride with that of the fat-soluble aminopyrine from various bases at different temperatures. Figure 9-1 shows the release of both drugs from cocoa butter suppositories at different temperatures. From 32.5°, the softening point of the mass, the amounts of both drugs released increased with temperature. At 34.3°, the melting point of the mass, six times as much of the suspended procaine hydrochloride was set free as at the softening point; there was only little more than twice as much aminopyrine

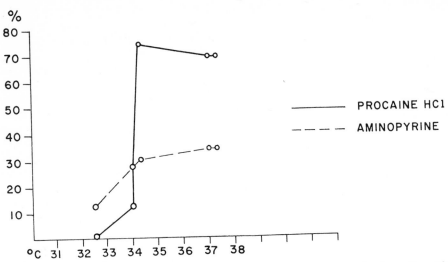

FIG. 9-1. Amount of drug released from cocoa butter suppositories after 90 minutes, as a function of temperature. (Eckert, V.: Ph.D. dissertation, Bern, Switzerland, 1958)

released during the change from softening to melting point. This behavior of the two drugs in cocoa butter is typical for most of the fatty vehicles examined in this study, which was summarized by Eckert and Mühlemann.[21] Drugs which were suspended in the suppository were effectively released only at the melting point. Up to 70 percent of drug was released after 90 minutes. Below the melting point but above the softening point, release of a suspended drug was less than 10 percent in the same interval.

Thus, rates of release from vehicle and transport of drug to the mucosa are essentially functions of the lipid/water distribution coefficient of the drug. A further factor is the physical state of the vehicle. Until it liquefies, reaction of drug with mucus is limited to the surface of the suppository. Drugs that are set free only after dissolution of the suppository in the small amount of mucus present in the rectum have a slow onset of action. Therefore, it is very likely that the transport from vehicle to mucus is the rate-determining step in the path of the drug to the site of action. The pharmacokinetics of rectal application were described by Diller and Bünger, who divided the process into three stages: (1) rate of drug release from suppository; (2) rate of uptake by body fluids; and (3) rate of urinary excretion.[19]

Since transport across the rectal mucosa is a passive diffusion process, it can go in either direction. However, the concentration gradient favors the direction from rectum to the submucosa and the vessels of the hemorrhoidal veins. The rectal epithelial membrane is lipoidal in character and appears to have a pH different from that of the rectal fluid. A slightly acidic zone has been postulated with a pH of about 5.3 along the lumen of the small intestine[34] and of about 6.5 for the colon.[69] The presence of such an acid membrane in the rectum has been proposed by Kakemi and coworkers.[35] In their rectal perfusion studies in rats, the ratios of distribution of several undissociated drugs in rectum and plasma pointed to a membrane pH of about 5.4. The character of this membrane adds to the complexity of the absorption process.

In Figure 9-2 change of absorption rate of sulfisoxazole with changing pH is illustrated. The absorption rate increases, passes through a maximum and then decreases with increasing pH. The peak is at the isoelectric point, while minimal absorption coincides with the pK's, thus indicating that the rectal absorption rate is a function of the drug's degree of ionization and is highest for

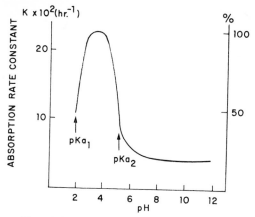

FIG. 9-2. Rectal absorption rate of sulfisoxazole vs. pH after 1 hour. (Modified from Kakemi, K., *et. al.*: Chem. Pharm. Bull., *13*:865 and 971, 1965)

the undissociated form. The authors, who used an experimental procedure similar to that of Riegelman and Crowell,[66] confirmed also the latter's tentative finding that rectal absorption is a first order process. Susceptibility to enzymatic interaction, affinity for protein, specific detoxication mechanisms and kidney clearance are some of the factors which determine the fate of the drug in the body.

DETERMINATION OF DRUG UPTAKE, IN VITRO

Any attempt to simulate biologic conditions in vitro must follow the qualitative and the quantitative factors as closely as possible. To simulate the rectum, e.g., by a tube through which water at 37° passes, totally disregards the volume, the viscosity and the chemical composition of the rectal mucus. It also disregards the pressure of the rectal walls against the suppository, which hastens its disintegration. Yet many conclusions in regard to action of drugs from suppository medication have been based on experimental procedures of this type. Hennig[32] described a melting-point tube for suppositories which approaches in-vivo conditions better than any other method reported. He compared the disintegration time of radiopaque suppositories in man with the time for complete melting of identical suppositories at 38° in his device. For cocoa butter suppositories,

the disintegration time in vivo was between 3 and 4 minutes, the melting time was 3 minutes 50 seconds; for the synthetic cocoa butter substitute (Witepsol), the times were almost twice as long: 5 to 7 minutes in vivo and 6 minutes 25 seconds in the melting tube. For suppositories made from polyethylene glycol, the disintegration times were between 40 and 60 minutes in vivo, 55 minutes in vitro. However, these similarities did not hold for another synthetic fat (since discontinued) and suppositories that had been prepared several days before the measurements. Similar results, based on a similar method, confirmed Hennig's report.[74]

DETERMINATION OF DRUG UPTAKE IN VIVO: IN ANIMALS

With his special method of determining melting points, Hennig was able to approximate the disintegration time of suppositories in vitro. However, this gave him no clue as to the diffusion of the drug through the mucosa and the pharmacologic efficacy of the rectal route.

While Hennig relied on urinary excretion data from human subjects, many investigators turned to animals to obtain comparable data on drug absorption from suppositories. With animals, it was feasible to conduct experiments utilizing radioactive tracers, which can be followed with relatively simple measurements and great accuracy. Bucher,[3] while at Berkeley, California, was the first to apply radioactive tracers to solve problems of rectal medication. Canals and coworkers[9] compared rectal and oral absorption of radioactive calcium salts. Peterson and coworkers[59] and Cemeli and Bardet[10] were the first to compare the effect of suppository vehicles on the absorption of drugs by means of radioactive tracers. The assumption in the radioactive studies was that the drug passes irreversibly through the mucosa into the blood circulation. Nevertheless, there is the possibility of the drug or its metabolite containing the tagged element diffusing back into the rectum. The radioactive count does not differentiate between the original drug and a therapeutically ineffective metabolite.

However, distribution of drug in animals can be measured in several other ways. In cases in which blood or urinary determination cannot be carried out because of drug accumulation in the body or difficulty of chemical or physico-chemical measurements, the physiologic response can be measured. For example, it was found that the methyl ester of nicotinic acid, after absorption, causes hyperemia and a rise in temperature in guinea pigs.[11] Experiments with different vehicles[11] bore out the previously stated principle that lack of affinity between drug and vehicle favors absorption. Best results were obtained with glycerinated gelatin as a vehicle; cocoa butter gave a delayed response and polyethylene glycol a poor response. Hassler and Sperandio[31] used the hypnotic effect of water-soluble barbiturates to evaluate the effectiveness of vehicles. Fatty vehicles gave quick onset and short duration of action; water-soluble vehicles caused delayed onset and prolongation of action. More recently, the hypoglycemic responses of rabbits to tolbutamide and tolbutamide sodium were measured.[40] In this study the glucose level could be correlated with the tolbutamide concentration in the blood. Again, the more water-soluble sodium salt gave a quicker response than the acid.

The drugs that were used more frequently in animals were acetylsalicylic acid and sodium salicylate, which are a related pair of compounds, one being almost nondissociated and relatively water-insoluble, the other being dissociated and very soluble in water. Pairs of sulfa drugs and barbiturates, their acids being relatively undissociated while their salts are not, were also used.

Results of studies relating in-vitro to in-vivo experiments were reported by Kuhne.[40] The author prepared suppositories of two pairs of drugs, phenobarbital and its sodium salt, and atropine and its sulfate, in several vehicles. These suppositories were administered to rabbits. To measure absorption of phenobarbital, its serum content was repeatedly determined by paper chromatography. In the case of atropine, the response was followed by measuring the diameter of the pupil. Both drug pairs in the same suppository bases were also subjected to diffusion through a semipermeable membrane; however, the alkaloid determination was not carried out quantitatively. Aside from melting characteristics of suppositories, the only drug pair evaluated comparatively was phenobarbital and its sodium salt. Nevertheless, the water-insoluble drugs, phenobarbital and atropine, did not pass from the suppository through the membrane in the in-vitro setup, while both passed through the rectal mucosa into the circulation of rabbits. Therefore, the author concluded from his experiments, which were patterned after those of Eckert and Mühlemann,[21] that in-vitro results cannot serve as a basis for the prediction of in-vivo effects.

All these reports do not result in a simple consensus. Often considerable differences in blood levels resulted from variations in the suppository vehicle. Yet the chemical differences between vehicles were so small that the significant differences in blood levels were surprising. If any one rule stands out so far, it is the one stated already that the drug which is more soluble in the mucus is likely to be absorbed faster and better from a fatty vehicle. Like most rules, it has its exceptions. Furthermore, the magnitude of solubility differences has no relation to quantitative differences in rates and amounts of drugs absorbed. No equivalent statements may be made for aqueous vehicles.

DETERMINATION OF DRUG UPTAKE, IN VIVO: IN MAN

Not only the variations in results with animals but also the uncertainty of applying conclusions from animal studies to man led investigators to turn to human subjects. Both blood level and urinary excretion data have been used to measure the uptake of drug after rectal administration.

The applicability of results of animal studies to man was experimentally examined by Schwarz and Bichsel,[71] who tested absorption from suppositories containing sulfisomidine and its sodium salt in man. Previously, the same drugs in the same vehicles were examined by Pennati and Steiger-Trippi in rabbits.[58] Maximum absorption in rabbits was obtained with the synthetic triglyceride Massupol. In man, maximum absorption was obtained with polyethylene glycol. In both series the superior vehicle caused significantly higher absorption of the drug than the other vehicles.

A comparison of in-vitro data with blood levels of drugs in man was carried out by Neuwald and Kunze.[54] They chose three salicylates for their tests: acetylsalicylic acid, calcium acetylsalicylate and sodium salicylate. The solubilities in water are respectively 1 in 300, 1 in 6, and 1 in 0.9.[46] They found that in the in-vitro diffusion, 75 percent of the amount of sodium salicylate present in the suppository passed through the membrane, 41 percent of calcium acetylsalicylate and only 3 percent of acetylsalicylic acid (Fig. 9-3). The in-vivo data were collected in five blood determinations within 4 hours; after that time blood concentration decreased. Surprisingly, the plasma concentration of all three compounds was about the same after 2 hours. While sodium salicylate reached the peak concentration within 30 minutes, the two other compounds required considerably more time. The maximum concentration for both aspirin and calcium aspirin was reached only after 3 hours, although after 2 hours both were nearly at peak concentration; the more water-soluble calcium salt was trailing slightly (Fig. 9-4). These

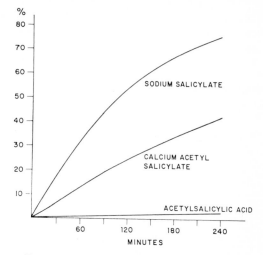

FIG. 9-3. Drug diffusion in vitro from Witepsol suppositories. (Adapted from Neuwald, F., and Kunze, F.: Arzneim. Forsch., *14*:1029 and 1162, 1964)

findings by Neuwald and Kunze not only refute their own in-vitro data but also are in disagreement with results of several animal experiments. However, their data matched

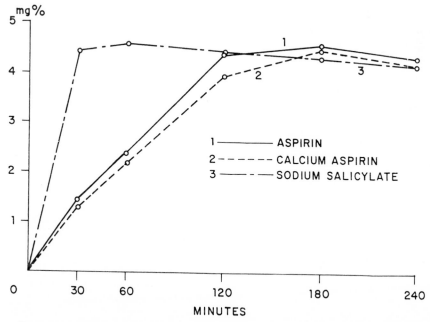

FIG. 9-4. Plasma concentration of salicylic acid after administration of equivalent doses of aspirin (1), calcium aspirin (2), and sodium salicylate (3), in Witepsol suppositories. (Neuwald, F., and Kunze, F.: Arzneim. Forsch., *14*:1029 and 1162, 1964)

fairly well those of two other teams who examined the absorption of acetylsalicylic acid from cocoa butter. Making adjustments for the different doses used, the plasma concentrations are compared in Table 9-1. Neuwald and Kunze drew the inescapable conclusion from their data that the evaluation of suppository medication for man cannot be based on animal experiments, much less on in-vitro diffusion studies.

SUPPOSITORY VEHICLES

In addition to the form in which the drug is used, the vehicle has great influence on the release of the drug and its subsequent transport through the wall of the rectum. A vast number of suppository bases exist; however, the following discussion will be confined to those bases that are readily available in the United States.

Suppositories disintegrate in the rectum by one of two processes. They either melt or dissolve. The various vehicles can be classified accordingly.

VEHICLES THAT MELT AT BODY TEMPERATURE

A suitable vehicle for suppositories must melt below body temperature, and it must be of firm consistency for easy insertion even in a warm climate. This narrows the temperature range between softening and melting to a few degrees. The vehicle must also be nonirritating, nonabsorbable, inert and compatible with drugs that are given rectally. It must be stable during storage. Most fats and waxes which melt near 37°, soften considerably below that temperature. An ex-

TABLE 9-1.   PLASMA CONCENTRATION OF ACETYLSALICYLIC ACID

	AFTER COCOA BUTTER SUPPOS. (mg%)	AFTER ORAL TABLETS (mg%)
Neuwald and Kunze[54] (after 2 hours)	3.35	
Cacchillo and Hassler[8] (after 2 hours)	3.5	5.4
Samelius and Åström[68] (after 90 minutes)	4.6	5.2

ception is cocoa butter, which melts just above 34°, softens at 32.5° and congeals at 27.5°.[21] Theobroma oil, as it is called in the *U.S.P.* (cocoa butter and cacao butter are common synonyms), has been in use as a suppository base for two centuries.[28] It is a mixture of triglycerides, in which oleic contributes about one third of the acid constituents of the esters.[65] Like many triglycerides, cocoa butter exhibits polymorphism. Its various configurations have different melting characteristics. The normal beta form is stable up to its melting point. When heated above this temperature, cocoa butter is transformed to a metastable form which congeals below 20° and melts around 24°. The return to the stable beta form may take several days. At 35°, less than 1 percent of the solid fat remains unmelted, at 36° virtually none. Without seed crystals present, cocoa butter solidifies very slowly. Solidification is more rapid at temperatures below 22°, even for the stable beta configuration; 16° appears to be the optimum temperature for solidification and contraction.[43] The presence of crystal seeding is essential to produce solidification within a reasonable period. Substances which dissolve in cocoa butter lower its melting point. For example, the presence of chloral hydrate in cocoa butter lengthens the solidification time and the period of transition from the metastable to the stable modification. During this period the softening point may be well within room temperature range. Addition of higher melting waxes produces no significant change.[4]

The incorporation of aqueous solutions into cocoa butter requires the addition of an emulsifier, which was first suggested in 1926.[14, 29, 83] A water number for cocoa butter of 20 to 30, cited in the literature, represents water occluded upon congealing; no true emulsion is formed.[6, 49] The effect of surface-active agents on the release and the absorption of drug from suppositories is not uniform. Both increase and decrease of release and absorption have been reported.[26, 29, 32, 37, 38, 60, 66, 78, 85] Furthermore, storage stability of cocoa butter suppositories that contain water is poor.[15, 53] Rancidification is accelerated and changes in consistency take place.

The importance of water absorption for cocoa butter has been overrated. It is true that water-soluble drugs can be dispersed more uniformly in emulsified fat and thus become available upon release, perhaps in molecular or colloidal dispersion. However, water-soluble components are released more slowly from a stable emulsion, particularly of the w/o type, than from a dispersion. Mühlemann and Neuenschwander clearly demonstrated this in their in-vitro studies.[48]

Because of the several drawbacks of cocoa butter, many combinations of fats and waxes were suggested for use as suppository vehicles, yet none of the vehicles approached the widespread use and popularity of cocoa butter.[29] Largely as a result of the shortage of cocoa butter during World War II, new fatty bases were developed in Europe. Several surveys of lipid and water-soluble suppository bases were published.[2, 57, 65] Some of the materials listed have been discontinued, others are not readily available, and some have been suggested for suppository manufacture although their chemical, physico-chemical and compatibility data are nowhere published.

The vehicles with a fatty composition, which are listed in Table 9-2, are available from suppliers in the United States.

Aside from cocoa butter, the largest number of studies published deal with the Witepsol bases. Witepsol H 15 disintegrates almost as fast in the rectum as cocoa butter, as was demonstrated with barium sulfate suppositories.[51] The melting times were 4 minutes for cocoa butter, 6 minutes for Witepsol. The higher melting Witepsol enables the suppository to ascend more in the rectum before disintegration, while a cocoa butter suppository, melting at a lower temperature and more rapidly, is more likely to cause leakage. Unlike cocoa butter, the Witepsols are not subject to structural

TABLE 9-2.   LIPID VEHICLES*

VEHICLE	COMPOSITION	MELT-ING RANGE (°C.)	CONGEAL-ING RANGE (°C.)	SPE-CIFIC GRAV-ITY	IODINE NUMBER	SAPONI-FICATION VALUE
Cocoa Butter	Mixed triglycerides of oleic, palmitic, stearic acids	30–35		0.86	35–43	188–195
Cotmar†	Partially hydrogenated cottonseed oil	35–89			70	
Dehydag Suppository‡						
Base I	Hydrogenated fatty	33–36	32–33	0.9	8	200
Base II	alcohols and esters	37½–39½	36–37½	0.88	12	140
Base IV	Glycerides of saturated fatty acids C_{12}–C_{18} 9 ranges	29–37	26½–34	0.97		215–240
Base G	Branched fatty alcohols	31–41 5 ranges			below 10	15–45
Paramount B§	Modified coconut oil	34½–35½	33		below 3	240
Wecobee R‖	Triglycerides derived	33½–35½	31–32		below 4	240
Wecobee SS	from coconut oil	40½–43	33–35		4	236
Witepsol #						
H 12	Triglycerides of satur.	32–33½	29–31	0.95	below	245
H 15	fatty acids C_{12}–C_{18}			to	7	240
E 85				0.98		230
S 55	Partial glycerides and triglycerides of satur. vegetable fatty acids C_{12}–C_{18}	33½–35½	29–32	0.95 to 0.98	below 7	220 to 230

* All vehicles except cocoa butter contain small amounts of emulsifiers.
† Procter and Gamble, Cincinnati, Ohio 45601.
‡ R. E. Flatow Co., 2344 Sixth St., Berkeley, Ca. 94710.
§ Durkee Famous Foods, Jamaica, N.Y.
‖ Drew Chemical Corp., 522 Fifth Avenue, New York, N.Y. Of the 7 WECOBEE suppository bases, a low and a high melting product were selected.
Riches-Nelson, Inc., Greenwich, Conn. 06838. Of the 12 WITEPSOL suppository bases, the lowest and the highest melting were selected in addition to the most widely used.

changes at temperatures above their melting points. They absorb water, due to the presence of glycerol mono- and diesters as emulsifiers. The fatty acids in the triglycerides, of which Witepsols are composed, are derived from natural saturated fats of acid chains between C_{12} and C_{18}, with lauric acid being predominant. The interval between softening and melting is small and the masses congeal just one or two degrees below their softening points. Witepsols solidify rapidly after being poured at their melting temperature into the mold, and chilling of the mold is unnecessary. Witepsols contract more upon solidification than cocoa butter, thus eliminating the need for lubricating the mold. Witepsol H 15 can be mixed with other Witepsols. As Figure 9-5 illustrates, combinations of Witepsol H 15 and E 85 cover a wide melting point range. Waxes, which are used to compensate for melting point lowering in cocoa butter, are not as suitable for Witepsols, nor are they necessary. Even 20 percent of chloral

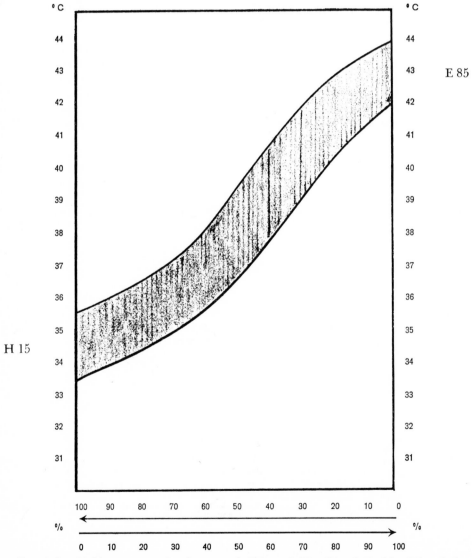

FIG. 9-5. Melting range of mixtures of Witepsol H 15 and E 85. (Chemische Werke, Witten)

hydrate when incorporated into Witepsol H 15 lowered the melting point to only 31° and the congealing point to 24°.[17] Witepsols are nearly white and practically odorless. They have a slightly greater density than cocoa butter.

The Dehydag Suppository Mass I is similar to Witepsol H 15 in appearance, melting and congealing ranges, while Suppository Mass II has slightly higher melting (37.5° to 37.5°) and congealing ranges (36° to 37.5°). Mass IV, also called Massa Estarinum, comes in a variety of melting ranges, each having a spread of no more than two degrees. The Dehydag Suppository Mass G represents a departure from glycerides. It consists of saturated fatty alcohols with chain lengths of C_{12} to C_{18}, which are combined to branched compounds up to 36 carbons in such a way that several distinct, narrow melting ranges are obtained. None of the Dehydag masses exhibits polymorphism. They may be heated above their melting points without lowering their congealing temperatures and, like Witepsol, contract upon congealing more than cocoa butter. Waxes or high-melting alcohols may be added to raise the melting points of these bases.

No in-vivo tests have been published for the other vehicles in Table 9-2. Wecobee bases[76] are derived from coconut oil by re-esterification of fractionated coconut fatty acids with glycerin and hydrogenation. The incorporation of glycerol monostearate and propylene glycol monostearate makes them emulsifiable (w/o type). The Wecobee bases, which are available in several melting ranges, appear to be similar to the Witepsols and Dehydag Suppository Masses I and II, which are also derived from coconut fatty acids.

WATER-SOLUBLE VEHICLES

Water-soluble vehicles represent a relatively new trend. The introduction of water-soluble vehicles was probably aided both by the observation that drugs from enemas were rapidly absorbed and by the emergence of new suitable materials. Rapp noticed in 1927 that methylene blue appeared in the urine sooner after it was administered in an enema than after it was given in a cocoa butter suppository.[62] Two decades later it was shown that penicillin sodium and also aminophylline were better absorbed from an enema than from cocoa butter suppositories.[45, 80]

A variety of products, all of which are wholly or partly polymers of ethylene oxide, have been suggested for suppository vehicles. It was assumed without question that the rectum, like the rest of the intestine, is perfused with fluids, in which water-soluble bases readily dissolve. However, the quantity of fluid in the rectum is very small and insufficient to effect ready dissolution of a suppository. There is no evidence that the presence of a hydrophilic mass forces water from surrounding tissue into the rectum. Of course, a strongly hygroscopic material will draw fluid from the mucous membranes with which it comes in contact while at the same time causing irritation. Suppositories formulated with water-soluble vehicles and a melting point considerably higher than body temperature take a relatively long time to

TABLE 9-3.   WATER-SOLUBLE VEHICLES

	MELTING RANGE (°C.)	CONCEALING RANGE (°C.)	SPECIFIC GRAVITY
Polyethylene Glycol* 1000		37–40	1.15
Polyethylene Glycol 1540		43–46	1.15
Polyethylene Glycol 4000		53–56	1.15
Polyethylene Glycol 6000		58–63	1.20
Polyoxyethylene (30) Stearate†	35–40		
Polyoxyethylene (40) Stearate†	38–43		
Polyoxyethylene Sorbitan Monostearate‡	35–39		
Glycerinated Gelatin			

* As Carbowax®, Union Carbide Corp., New York, N.Y. 10017. As Polyglycol®, Dow Chemical Co., Midland, Mich.
† As Myrj® 51 and Myrj® 52, Atlas Chem. Ind., Wilmington, Del.
‡ As Tween 61®, Atlas Chem. Ind., Wilmington, Del.

disintegrate in the rectum. During that time, the patient will have to suppress the normal defecation reflex which tends to expel the suppository.

The most popular water-soluble vehicles are the polyethylene glycols (abbreviated PEG), which were first suggested as suppository bases in 1939.[47] Commercially best known as Carbowaxes they exist in a molecular weight range from 200 to 20,000. At room temperature, the lower members of the series are liquid, PEG 1000 is a soft solid, and the higher members are waxlike. They melt between 37° and 63° and are easily shaped into suppositories. Even in an excess of water they dissolve slowly. PEG 1000 melts slightly above body temperature; however, it softens several degrees below that point, so that, alone, it is not a suitable suppository vehicle. By adding a small amount of PEG 4000 or 6000, a mass is obtained which is firm for insertion, yet softens afterward to spread in the rectum and thus dissolves faster than the higher melting compounds. For a comparison of various PEG suppository formulations and their disintegration times in man see Table 9-4.

A formula of 10 percent PEG 4000 and 90 percent PEG 1000[58] gave superior absorption of a sulfa drug, sulfisomidine, in man.[71] Cacchillo and Hassler[8] incorporated 10 gr. of aspirin in a PEG suppository, which consisted of 40 percent PEG 6000, 30 percent PEG 1540 and 30 percent PEG 400. Plasma levels 2 hours after rectal administration and after oral administration of 10-gr. tablets were compared. The plasma level after administration of the PEG suppository was 93 percent of the level after tablet ingestion, while aspirin in a cocoa butter suppository resulted in a plasma concentration of 65.5 percent of that obtained after the oral dose. Schwarz and Bichsel,[71] measuring urinary excretion of sulfisomidine, obtained barely half as much excretion after rectal administration of PEG suppositories as after oral administration. The amount of drug recovered from a cocoa butter suppository was only one fifth of that obtained after oral administration. In these experiments, the absorption of the dissociated salt, sulfisomidine sodium, from any of the vehicles averaged twice as much as the absorption of the undissociated acid.

In tests on rats with sodium salts of barbiturates Hassler and Sperandio[31] observed a quicker onset of action than with cocoa butter suppositories and twice as long a duration of action after PEG suppositories.

Its solubility in water makes PEG a suitable vehicle for vaginal suppositories. However, the slow dissolution of PEG in the rectum may make it difficult to suppress the defecation reflex. PEG suppositories, regardless of their composition, have the advantage of stability in warm weather. Incorporation of water decreases the stability of PEG suppositories and may lead to crystallization and change in consistency. Addition of hexanetriol helps to prevent this.

Kakemi and his group demonstrated in experiments with rats that, contrary to a number of reports in the literature, PEG depresses the absorption of unionized sulfonamides. The higher the molecular weight of the PEG, the greater was the inhibitory

TABLE 9-4.   DISINTEGRATION TIMES OF VARIOUS PEG SUPPOSITORIES IN MAN

PEG FORMULA	PER-CENT	BaSO$_4$ (g.)	DISINTE-GRATION TIME (min.)	REFERENCE
1. PEG 1000	96	0.5	15	Collins, *et al.*[13]
PEG 4000	4			
2. PEG 1540	94	0.5	40	Collins, *et al.*[13]
Hexanetriol (1, 2, 6)	6			
3. PEG 1540	33	0.8	20	Wellauer, *et al.*[84]
PEG 6000	47			
PEG 400	20			
4. PEG 1540	33	0.5	30–50	Setnikar and Fantelli[74]
PEG 6000	47			
PEG 400	20			

effect.[36] A number of drugs form complexes with PEG, which delay their release from the vehicle. PEG undergoes slight changes upon aging, which may be the cause of the occasional irritation by PEG suppositories.

In spite of these drawbacks, a good many proprietary suppositories are made with PEG as the vehicle.

Tween 61, which is composed partly of ethylene oxide units, was employed as the suppository vehicle for salicylic acid and sodium salicylate in dogs. Unexpectedly, the absorption of salicylic acid within 6 hours was several times faster and greater than that of the sodium salt.[42] Similarly, absorption of the acid was far greater from PEG, while absorption from cocoa butter was about the same for both acid and salt. With a synthetic triglyceride, Witepsol S-55, as the base, acid was again absorbed much faster than the salt. Yet when several sulfa drugs were administered in Witepsol S-55 to human subjects, only the salt form was absorbed in therapeutically significant amounts and the acid form hardly at all.[16]

Glycerinated gelatin as a suppository base was tested in mice with radioactive iodine. It resulted in higher blood levels than another water-soluble suppository base, Tween 61; lowest levels were produced by cocoa butter.[59] Charonnat and coworkers[11] observed in their tests with lipid-soluble methyl nicotinate in guinea pigs that glycerinated gelatin caused a stronger and longer response than cocoa butter which, in turn, was superior to PEG. (See Fig. 9-6.)

The glycerinated gelatin used by Charonnat was a mixture of 10 g. of gelatin, 60 g. of glycerin and 30 g. of water. This is slightly different from the formula in *U.S.P. XVIII,* originated by Tice and Abrams,[79] which consists of 20 g. of gelatin, 70 g. of glycerin and 100 g. of water. The absorption of sulfisomidine sodium in rabbits resulted in slightly higher blood levels from a modified glycerinated gelatin* than from either cocoa butter or PEG, but it was slower than from cocoa butter and faster than from PEG.[58]

Results of in-vitro tests only have been published for polyoxyethylene stearates, which were proposed as suppository bases by Gross and Becker.[30]

Glycerin suppositories, which are also recognized in the *N.F. XIII,* are made with 91 percent of glycerin, with 9 percent of sodium stearate as the gelling agent. They are used locally to induce and facilitate bowel movement.

Gelatin has found a new use in rectal administration with the introduction of rectal gelatin capsules.† These are soft gelatin capsules, filled with vegetable oil, surface-active agents and drug. The gelatin capsules represent a stable drug form with regard to shelf life and warm climate. They can hold a larger dose of drug than can suppositories of similar size and they disintegrate rapidly in the rectum. In studies with rectal barium sulfate capsules in man, disintegration and emptying of the capsules was complete within 10 minutes.[84] Rectal gelatin capsules for any drug have to be made to order. Several studies were conducted in Europe, where the capsules were first introduced. The results show that drug absorption varies with the drug used but is, by and large, similar to that from lipid vehicles.[1, 33, 52, 71]

A good many formulas for suppository vehicles have been published without, however, any indication of drug release or absorption. Some of these formulas, such as the cetyl ester of phthalic acid or a combination of cetyl and oleyl alcohols, are used by industry. It is not the intent in this chapter to list all vehicles or special formulations that have been reported or are in use.

The uncertainties in regard to the absorption of a drug, which are due partly to the vehicle, and the limit of the amount of drug that may be incorporated, which is due to the fixed size of the suppository, led to the development of a suppository which is mostly drug and very little vehicle. Such a suppository was prepared by lyophilization.[41] The authors envisioned such suppositories primarily for vaginal application. A similar idea was pursued some years earlier by administration of a drug rectally by insufflation. Although the method of insufflation was imprecise and the results uneven, absorption was prompt and in therapeuti-

---

* 25 g. of gelatin, 20 g. of glycerin, 18 g. of PEG 400, 37 g. of water.

† R. P. Scherer Corp., Detroit.

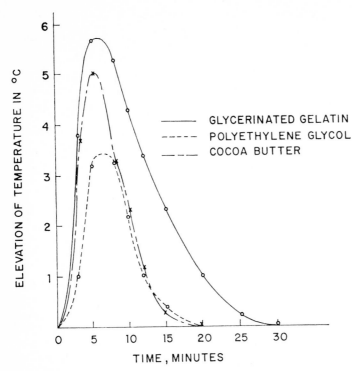

cally significant amounts.[45] In tests with lyophilized suppositories containing sulfisomidine sodium with only 9 percent of carrier material, absorption was greater than from suppositories made with either cocoa butter or a synthetic triglyceride and was surpassed only by suppositories made with PEG.[72] In other studies with lyophilized suppositories absorption was found to be poor and uncertain.[1] Figure 9-7 illustrates the results of absorption studies of sulfisomidine sodium from 5 different vehicles in male students. Even from the best vehicle, PEG, only half as much was absorbed as was absorbed from orally administered capsules. Urinary excretion data were used for comparison. The absorption of a corresponding amount of the acid sulfisomidine was less than that of the sodium salt for all vehicles tested.

In another experiment comparing oral and rectal administration, using 0.75 g. of aspirin as the drug, absorption from rectal suppositories made with Witepsol was equal to that from oral tablets, while both PEG and cocoa butter resulted in lower values (Fig. 9-8). Plasma levels in humans after 1 hour were used in the evaluation.[68] The similarity of blood levels after oral and rectal administration of aspirin is apparent also from Table 9-1 (p. 286). Recently Parrott substantiated the equivalence of the rectal and oral routes for aspirin as well as sodium salicylate, provided that suitable vehicles were used for the suppositories.[56] Indomethacin is another drug which was effectively administered by suppository although the rectal dose was higher than the oral.[39] In another experiment with aspirin in man, the drug was absorbed faster from a suppository than from a rectally administered suspension, but not as fast as after oral administration.[18] In comparing the oral and rectal routes of absorption in the case of Lincomycin® hydrochloride, highest blood levels were obtained after the oral dose, while a rectally administered solution gave lower blood levels and the suppository the lowest. A more suitable suppository base than PEG, which was employed as vehicle, would probably have resulted in levels closer to those obtained after the oral and rectal solutions.[82]

In comparing the various results of in vivo tests, one is struck with the lack of agreement in them. It is evident that no one

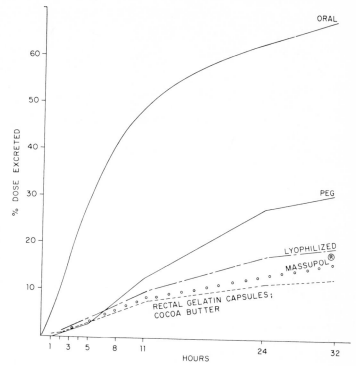

FIG. 9-7. Cumulative urinary excretion of sulfisomidine sodium after oral and suppository administration. The curves for rectal gelatin capsules and cocoa butter almost coincide. (After Schwarz, T. W., and Bichsel, K.: Pharm. Acta Helv., *38*: 861, 1963)

vehicle can be established unequivocally as superior to others; release of drug as a function of solubility in and disintegration of the vehicle appears as a paramount factor.[77] Exceptions exist, however, and they may well be due to differences among drugs tested and to variations in experimental setup and condition of test subjects or animals.

Neither the *U.S.P.* nor the *N.F.* specifies suppository vehicles in the monographs. The *U.S.P.* mentions several vehicles: theobroma oil, glycerinated gelatin, hydrogenated vegetable oils, mixtures of polyethylene glycols of various molecular weight and fatty acid esters of polyethylene glycol. Minor deviations in composition are allowed to maintain suitable consistency of the base under different climatic conditions.[81]

SIZE AND SHAPE OF SUPPOSITORIES

Rectal suppositories for adults weigh 2 or 3 g. and 1 g. for children. The *U.S.P.* designates 2 g. as the usual size. The

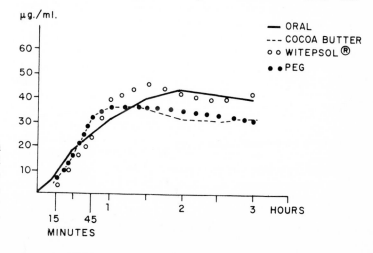

FIG. 9-8. Mean plasma concentration of salicylic acid after oral and rectal administration of 0.75 g. of aspirin. (After Samelius, Y., and Åström, A.: Acta pharmacol. tox., *14*:240, 1958)

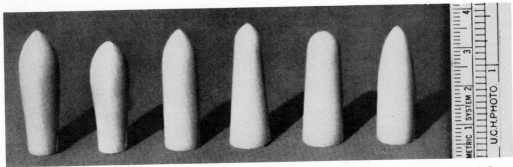

F<small>IG</small>. 9-9.   Shapes of 2-g. suppositories. (Actual size). (Chemical and Pharmaceutical Co., Inc., 260 West Broadway, New York, N. Y. 10013)

shape of rectal suppositories is tapered resembling a cone, torpedo or bullet; the bullet shape, tapered on both ends, is better retained in the rectum. Two-gram suppositories of several shapes are reproduced in actual size in Figure 9-9. Vaginal suppositories are usually globular or oviform and weigh about 5 g. each.[81]

DOSAGE

The preceding discussion of drug absorption from rectal suppositories makes it obvious that a definite rectal dosage cannot be derived from the oral or parenteral dose of a drug. The problem of proper dosage in suppositories was well summarized by Eiler:[22]

Many of the discrepancies concerning dosage and much of the uncertainty over the usefulness of suppositories may be attributed to a lack of appreciation of the influence of the base on the availability of the drug. The intensity of the pharmacologic response from a given drug is related to the concentration of that drug in the blood and the tissue fluids, and the time required for the onset of the response is related to the time required to attain the desired concentration. The actual concentration that is attained depends upon the magnitude of two opposing rates: the rate with which the drug is supplied to the blood and the rate with which it is removed from the blood by excretion and detoxication. The dose of the drug influences both the rate of supply and the duration of the response. Under favorable conditions (small dose, low availability, or poor absorption) the rate of supply may be so slow, in comparison to the rate of removal, as to give a greatly delayed response of a low intensity.

From the few studies comparing oral and

suppository administration, one may conclude that, with optimum absorption from a suppository, the dose should be at least of the same magnitude as the oral dose, and, more often, a multiple of it. Trimethobenzamide is an example of the former (oral dose: 250 mg., rectal dose 200 mg.), aminophylline an example of the latter (oral dose 200 mg., rectal dose 500 mg.). For topical effect, both rectally and vaginally, the dose depends on the clinical response; even then variations in dosage may be considerable, due to the influence of the vehicle on the release of drug.

PREPARATION OF SUPPOSITORIES

Two methods mainly are used; the compression or cold process and the fusion or hot process. In the compression method, the drug is mixed with the shredded vehicle, and the mixture then is forced into a mold and subsequently extruded. In industrial mass manufacture, a hydraulic press is used, while a simple press, such as the Whitall-Tatum machine,* is employed in small-scale production (Fig. 9-10). The Whitall-Tatum compression machine is applicable to few vehicles besides cocoa butter and altogether not very satisfactory. Its main drawback is the distortion of the suppository due to heat generated by the pressure applied to the mass. This can be partly remedied by chilling the mold and the cylinder with the suppository mass in it prior to expressing the suppositories. A water-cooled suppository press is therefore preferable.† Both machines

---

* Armstrong Cork Co., Lancaster, Pa.
† Available from Chemical and Pharmaceutical

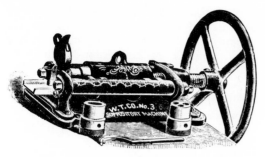

FIG. 9-10. Hand press for shaping suppositories.

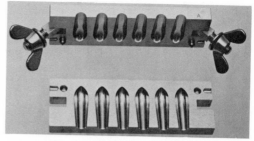

FIG. 9-11. Suppository mold. (Chemical and Pharmaceutical Co., Inc., New York)

have molds for 1-g. and 2-g. rectal suppositories and 5-g. vaginal suppositories. Another compression device is the Applebaum press, which has the advantage of compactness, but, unfortunately, the only samples known to this writer are made with such poor tolerances that they leak badly upon compression. Since they are made of nonanodyzed aluminum, cocoa butter is discolored during compression.

The fusion process is the principal method for the preparation of suppositories. All vehicles, whether fat-soluble or water-soluble, can be shaped into suppositories by first melting the mass and incorporating the drug and then pouring the mass into the mold just before it congeals. Molds for the fusion process come in sizes to accommodate from 6 to 500 suppositories (Fig. 9-11). They are made of aluminum or brass or nickel-copper alloy. The inner surface must be smooth to produce non-sticking suppositories. Molds of nickel-copper alloy produce better suppositories than aluminum molds.

When using cocoa butter as a vehicle, the molds should be lubricated to prevent sticking of the mass to the metal surface. Other suppository bases require no lubricant, since they contract more upon solidification than does cocoa butter. In the process of pouring the mass, it is important to keep a suspended drug evenly dispersed and to wait until just before congealing to avoid settling of drug in the tip of the suppository and thus assure uniform drug distribution.[23, 75] Some drugs markedly lower the congealing point of the

Industry Co., Inc., 260 West Broadway, New York, N.Y. 10013.

vehicle. To compensate for a lowered melting point, fats of higher melting point than the vehicle may be added. More recently lipophilic thickening agents were employed such as aluminum stearate or fumed silica.‡ These and other agents were found, however, to interfere with the release of drug in the few cases examined.[25, 63]

Uniform distribution of the drug in the suppository is essential for rapid absorption. Because of the contractibility of the mass on solidification, slightly more liquid mass must be poured than fits the mold cavity. Any excess is scraped off after congealing. Fusion molds should not be chilled (unless ambient temperature is above 25°) before the mass is poured because rapid solidification may lead to cracks in the center of the suppositories and breakage upon removal from the mold. To hasten solidification and to facilitate removal of the suppositories, the mold with the mass in it may be chilled in ice or in a refrigerator after the mass has congealed.

When using cocoa butter, one must be mindful of the configuration changes cocoa butter undergoes when heated above its melting point. As pointed out previously, cocoa butter will congeal to the stable beta configuration as long as seed crystals are present. Therefore, it is desirable to melt the cocoa butter to a creamy consistency only and not to a clear melt. Then the drug can be added and the mixture poured. When the mold temperature is kept several degrees below the solidification point of the mass, congealing without cracking will result promptly if the mass is poured at just above

‡ As Aerosil® or Cab-O-Sil®.

the congealing temperature. This applies equally to all suppository masses.

To find the correct quantity of vehicle for a suppository formula, one must know the volume of vehicle displaced by the drug. Lists of displacement factors for a number of drugs in cocoa butter can be found in the literature. Frequently, however, the displacement figures differ significantly.[4, 55] Differences are due to variations in particle size and melting temperature, i.e., whether the determinations were carried out with a creamy or a clear melt. An updated list was published by Münzel.[50] The factors can be used for any lipid vehicle which has the same specific gravity as cocoa butter. However, the experimental determination of the displacement factor for any drug and vehicle is quite simple. For example, using a 12-cavity mold, a quantity of vehicle known to be insufficient is added to the correct amount of drug for 12 suppositories. The mixture is poured into the mold, leaving one or two cavities unfilled; the excess is scraped off after congealing and returned to the pouring dish; a little more pure vehicle is added, melted together with the excess of drug-vehicle mixture, and poured into the unfilled cavities. More pure vehicle is added in the same way until all 12 holes are correctly filled. After removing the hardened suppositories from the molds, they are again melted, mixed and poured. Since actually a slight excess is poured into each cavity and some mass adheres to the pouring vessel, less than 12 suppositories are obtained on the final pouring. However, from the total weight of the 12 suppositories, the amount of vehicle per suppository is readily calculated, since the amount of drug added is known. This method circumvents the uncertainties inherent in the reported displacement factors. When using vehicles significantly different from cocoa butter in composition or specific gravity and in case of more than one drug being incorporated, the experimental determination is the only reliable one. It is not recommended to use the method described for just one cavity in the mold. The holes in a suppository mold are not always of identical size.

The removal of suppositories from the mold is occasionally difficult. Lack of lubricant, mistakes in cooling the mold or in pouring temperature may contribute to the sticking or cracking of suppositories. To avoid transfer of suppositories from the mold to the package, Schwarz and Nenneman in 1954 proposed shaped aluminum foil strips which would serve as both a mold and a package for suppositories. Transfer of the suppositories and the need for a lubricant would thus be eliminated.[73] Such strips, made of thin plastic, and also individual plastic cones for pouring suppositories are now commercially available.

Cocoa butter suppositories can be fashioned by hand also. The mass is rolled into a cylinder, divided and the individual pieces shaped by hand. Dusting powder such as starch is usually needed for the manual operation. It must be used sparingly, lest the mass lose its plasticity and crack.

Among the methods of preparation, the fusion process yields the best results. It permits better distribution of the drug and the final product is well shaped, uniform and smooth-surfaced in appearance. The method requires care and a little skill. A well machined mold also facilitates the release of the finished suppositories.

The number and the variety of suppositories containing prescription drugs have increased during the last years. The ready availability of new vehicles, their superior ability to release the drug, and their ease of handling should make the suppository a more frequently used form of medication. It has a definite place among drug forms, and the pharmacist with his knowledge of new vehicles and their drug release properties can assist the physician to achieve a better utilization of suppository medication.

STORAGE OF SUPPOSITORIES

Commercially manufactured suppositories are usually foil-wrapped. This protects them somewhat during storage, simplifies handling and hides blemishes but does not significantly affect their stability. Water-containing suppositories dry out on storage, foil-wrapping notwithstanding. Special wrappers exist which provide better storage stability for water-containing suppositories. They are discussed in the companion volume to this book, *Prescription Pharmacy* (2nd

TABLE 9-5. OFFICIAL SUPPOSITORIES

SUPPOSITORY	THERAPEUTIC USE	ROUTE OF ADMINIS- TRATION	DOSE
U.S.P. XVIII			
Aminophyllin	Smooth muscle relaxant	Rectal	500 mg.
Aspirin	Analgesic	Rectal	60 mg.–2 g.
Chlorpromazine	Tranquilizer	Rectal	100 mg.
Diethylstilbestrol	Estrogen	Vaginal	0.1–1 mg.
Iodochlorhydroxyquin	Local anti-infective	Vaginal	250 mg.
Metronidazole	Antitrichomonal	Vaginal	500 mg.
N.F. XIII			
Bisacodyl	Cathartic	Rectal	10 mg.
Candicidin	Local antifungal	Vaginal	3 mg.
Ergotamine Tartrate and Caffeine	Migraine analgesic	Rectal	2 mg. 100 mg.
Furazolidone and Nifuroxime	Local antibacterial and antiprotozoan	Vaginal	Furazolidone 0.25% Nifuroxime 0.4%
Glycerin*	Rectal evacuant	Rectal	Glycerin 91% Sodium Stearate 9%
Prochlorperazine	Antiemetic, tranquilizer	Rectal	2.5–25 mg.
Trimethobenzamide Hydro- chloride and Benzocaine	Antiemetic	Rectal	Trimethobenzamide HCl 200 mg. Benzocaine 2%

* Children's size: 1 g.

ed., p. 275, Philadelphia, Lippincott, 1970). Glycerin suppositories and the rarely encountered glycerinated gelatin suppositories are sufficiently hygroscopic to require storage in tight glass containers at temperatures below 25°. Suppositories made from low-melting vehicles obviously must be stored in a cool place. For suppositories made with cocoa butter, the *U.S.P.* requires storage in "well-closed containers preferably at a temperature below 30°."

Suppositories are dispensed customarily in compartmented containers to prevent deformation or adhesion during transport (see *Prescription Pharmacy,* Chap. 7).

The *U.S.P.* lists 6 and the *N.F.* 7 suppositories. Five of the 13 suppositories are for vaginal application. However, very many more drugs are used in suppository form. *U.S.P.* and *N.F.* monographs on suppositories do not specify a vehicle. Thus the choice of vehicle is left to the pharmacist or the manufacturer, who is expected to use the most effective. Unfortunately, data on comparative studies of vehicles for specific commercially produced suppositories are hardly ever found in the pharmaceutical literature. Without such documentation, knowledge of vehicles of commercially avail-

able suppositories, whether official or not, can serve at best as an introductory guide. Even then, the information provided by manufacturers about the suppository vehicle is spotty and incomplete and is of little usefulness to the pharmacist in the preparation of suppositories or in advising the physician in case of a sensitivity reaction. Neither the proportions of the ingredients nor their chemical designations are listed unambiguously on the labels or in the package inserts.

REFERENCES

1. Ackad, P.: Ph.D. Dissertation, Hamburg, Germany, 1964.
2. Anschel, J., and Lieberman, H. A.: Drug and Cosm. Ind., 97:507, 1965.
3. Bucher, K.: Helv. physiol. pharmacol. acta, 6:821, 1948.
4. Büchi, J.: Pharm. acta Helv., 20:407, 1945.
5. Büchi, J., and Oesch, P.: Pharm. acta Helv., 19:365, 1944.
6. ———: Pharm. acta Helv., 20:37, 1945.
7. ———: Pharm. acta Helv., 20:129, 1945.
8. Cacchillo, A. F., and Hassler, W. H.: J. Am. Pharm. A (Sci. Ed.), 43:683, 1954.
9. Canals, E., et al.: Ann. pharm. Franc., 9:318, 1951.
10. Cemeli, J., and Bardet, L.: Galenica acta (Spain), 9:235, 1956.
11. Charonnat, R., et al.: Ann. pharm. Franc., 7:627, 1949.

12. Coldwell, B. B., *et al.*: Clin. Toxicol., *2*:111, 1969.
13. Collins, A. P., *et al.*: Am. Prof. Pharm., *23*: 231, 1957.
14. Cooper, J.: Pharm. J., *117*:371, 1926.
15. Von Czetsch-Lindenwald, H.: Suppositorien. Editio Cantor, Aulendorf, Germany, 1958.
16. Delfs, F.-M., and Kuhne, J.: Arzneim. Forsch., *13*:304, 1963.
17. Del Pozo, A., and Cemeli, J.: Galenica acta (Spain), 7:137, 1954.
18. Deipgen, P.: Das Analzäpfchen in der Geschichte der Therapie. Thieme, Stuttgart, Germany, 1953.
19. Diller, W., and Bünger, P.: Arzneim. Forsch., *15*:1445, 1965.
20. Eckert, V.: Ph.D. Dissertation, Bern, Switzerland, 1958.
21. Eckert, V., and Mühlemann, H.: Pharm. acta Helv., *33*:649, 1958.
22. Eiler, J. J., *in* Lyman, R. A.: American Pharmacy. ed. 3, vol. I, chap. 21, p. 378. J. B. Lippincott, Philadelphia, 1951.
23. Elste, U., *et al.*: Dt. Apoth. Ztg., *106*:568, 1966.
24. Fabre, R., *et al.*: Ann. pharm. Franc., 5:585, 1947.
25. Falk, G., and Voigt, R.: Pharmaz. Zentralhalle, *105*:573, 1966.
26. Fincher, J. H., *et al.*: J. Pharm. Sci., *55*:23, 1966.
27. Geissberger, W., *et al.*: Helv. med. acta, 17: 465, 1950.
28. Griffenhagen, G.: Am. J. Pharm., *125*:135, 1953.
29. Gross, H. M., and Becker, C. H.: J. Am. Pharm. A. (Sci. Ed.), *42*:90, 1953.
30. ———: J. Am. Pharm. A. (Sci. Ed.), *42*: 498, 1953.
31. Hassler, W. H., and Sperandio, G. J.: J. Am. Pharm. A. (Pract. Ed.), *1*:26, 1953.
32. Hennig, W.: Ueber die rektale Resorption von Medikamenten. Juris, Zürich, Switzerland, 1959.
33. Höbel, M., and Talebian, M.: Arzneim. Forsch., *10*:653, 1960.
34. Hogben, A. M., *et al.*: J. Pharmacol. Exp. Ther., *125*:275, 1959.
35. Kakemi, K., *et al.*: Chem. Pharm. Bull., *13*: 861, 1965.
36. ———: Chem. Pharm. Bull., *13*:969, 1965.
37. ———: Chem. Pharm. Bull., *13*:976, 1965.
38. Kata, M.: Die Pharmazie, *24*:395, 1969.
39. Kerckhoffs, H. P. M., and Huizinga, T.: Pharm. Weekblad, *102*:1255, 1967; through Internat. Pharm. Abstracts, 5:548, 1968.
40. Kuhne, J.: Ph.D. Dissertation, Braunschweig, Germany, 1960.
41. Lang, E., and Speiser, P.: Schweiz. Apoth. Z., *96*:506, 1958.
42. Loewenthal, W., and Borzelleca, J. F.: J. Pharm. Sci., *54*:1790, 1965.
43. Lovegren, N. V., and Feuge, R. O.: J. Am. Oil Chem. Soc., *42*:308, 1965.
44. Macht, D. I.: J. Pharmacol. Exp. Ther., *10*: 509, 1918.
45. Mandel, E. E., and Thayer, F. D.: J. Lab. Clin. Med., *33*:135, 1948.
46. Merck Index. ed. 7. Rahway, N.J., 1960.
47. Middendorf, L.: Münch. med. Wschr., *86*: 95, 1939.
48. Mühlemann, H., and Neuenschwander, R. H.: Pharm. acta Helv., *31*:305, 1956.
49. Münzel, K.: Schweiz, Apoth. Z., *90*:132, 1952.
50. Münzel, K., Büchi, J., and Schultz, O.-E.: Galenisches Praktikum. p. 668. Wissenschaftliche Verlagsgesellschaft, Stuttgart, Germany, 1959.
51. Neuwald, F.: Pharm. Z., *104*:670, 1959.
52. Neuwald, F., and Ackad, P.: Deutsche Apoth. Z., *105*:1245, 1965.
53. Neuwald, F., and Bohlmann, W.: Pharm. Z., *103*:666, 1958.
54. Neuwald, F., and Kunze, F.: Arzneim. Forsch., *14*:1029, 1162, 1964.
55. Oesch, P.: Ph.D. Dissertation. Zürich, Switzerland, 1944.
56. Parrott, E. L.: J. Pharm. Sci., *60*:867, 1971.
57. Pennati, L., and Steiger-Trippi, K.: Schweiz. Apoth. Z., *96*:205, 1958.
58. ———: Pharm. acta Helv., *33*:663, 1958.
59. Peterson, C. F., *et al.*: J. Am. Pharm. A. (Sci. Ed.), *42*:731, 1953.
60. Plaxco, M., *et al.*: J. Pharm. Sci., *56*:809, 1967.
61. Quevauviller, A., and Jund, Y.: Ann. pharm. Franc., 9:593, 1951.
62. Rapp, R.: Pharm. Z., *72*:312, 1927.
63. Regdon, G., and Kedvessy, G.: Pharm. Zentralhalle, *107*:507, 1968.
64. Ridolfi, N. S., and Kohlstaedt, K. G.: Am. J. Med. Sci., *237*:585, 1939.
65. Riegelman, S. *in* Sprowls, J.: American Pharmacy. ed. 5, vol. I, chap. 19. J. B. Lippincott, Philadelphia, 1960.
66. Riegelman, S., and Crowell, W. J.: J. Am. Pharm. A. (Sci. Ed.), *47*:115, 1958.
67. Robinson, G. D.: J. Obstet. Gyn. (Brit.), *32*: 496, 1928.
68. Samelius, Y., and Åström, A.: Acta pharmacol. tox., *14*:240, 1958.
69. Schanker, L. S.: J. Pharmacol. Exp. Ther., *126*:283, 1959.
70. Schroff, E.: Pharm. Z., *76*:1239, 1931.
71. Schwarz, T. W., and Bichsel, K.: Proc. 21st Intern. Congress Pharm. Sci., Pisa, Italy, 1961, p. 809.
72. ———: Pharm. acta Helv., *38*:861, 1963.
73. Schwarz, T. W., and Nenneman, M.: Report, A.Ph.A. Convention, Boston, 1954; Pacific Drug Rev., 66 (No. 10):26, 1954.
74. Setnikar, I., and Fantelli, S.: J. Pharm. Sci., *51*:566, 1962.
75. Setnikar, I. and Fontani, F.: J. Pharm. Sci., *59*:1319, 1970.
76. Silverman, H. I.: J. Am. Pharm. A. (Sci. Ed.), *49*:716, 1960.

77. Steinke, G., *et al.*: Arznei. Forsch., *16*:1576, 1966.
78. Tardos, L., *et al.*: Die Pharmazie, *14*:526, 1960.
79. Tice, L. F., and Abrams, R. E.: J. Am. Pharm. A. (Pract. Ed.), *14*:24, 1953.
80. Truitt, E. B., *et al.*: J. Pharmacol. Exp. Ther., *100*:309, 1950.
81. United States Pharmacopeia, 18th Revision, Bethesda, Md. 1970. pp. 4, 813.

82. Wagner, J. G., *et al.*: J. Clin. Pharmacol., *8*:154, 1968.
83. Waxman, P., and Eiler, J. J.: J. Am. Pharm. A. (Pract. Ed.), *6*:232, 1945.
84. Wellauer, J., *et al.*: Pharm. acta Helv., *35*: 619, 1960.
85. Whitworth, C. W., and LaRocca, J. P.: J. Am. Pharm. A. (Sci. Ed.), *48*:353, 1959.
86. Widmann, A.: Pharm. & Ind., *22*:348, 1960.

10

L. L. Augsburger, Ph.D., *Assistant Professor of Pharmacy, University of Maryland School of Pharmacy*

Powdered Dosage Forms

GENERAL CONSIDERATIONS

Powders may be defined as dry mixtures of pulverized drugs and/or chemicals which are used internally or externally. Although the use of "powders" as a dosage form has declined in recent years, powders as starting points in the manufacture of other dosage forms have become increasingly important, and along with this has come the recognition of the importance of *particle size*.[25] Particle size can have a significant effect on the physical, chemical, and therapeutic properties of a drug.[50, 53] For example, the particle size of a drug can influence its availability for absorption from dosage forms. Drugs may be inhaled from aerosols or insufflations for local or systemic effects. The particle size of the inhaled drug determines where it is deposited in the respiratory tract and, hence, its therapeutic effectiveness.

For reasons related to stability, certain drugs are formulated as powders intended to be reconstituted as solutions or suspensions by the pharmacist at the time of dispensing. In these, as well as in the preparation of any solutions or suspensions, particle size is of particular practical importance because it affects dissolution time in preparing solutions and settling time in suspensions.

Particle size is also an important consideration in the blending and handling of powders. Variation in particle size can cause separation of chemicals during mixing operations or during shipping. The control of particle size is an important aspect of obtaining proper powder flow properties. Poorly flowing powders are difficult to blend. High-speed capsule filling machines and tablet presses require freely and uniformly flowing powders or granules in order to obtain uniform capsule or tablet weights. It is apparent that any discussion of powdered dosage forms must begin with a discussion of the reduction and classification of particle size, powder flow properties, and blending.

PARTICLE SIZE REDUCTION

Comminution, or *grinding,* may be defined as the process of particle size reduction. Particle size reduction is carried out by the community pharmacist on a small scale by manual methods such as trituration and levigation. Industrially, comminution is carried out on a large scale in mills of various types.

Large-Scale Comminution. Mills, in general, are the most inefficient pharmaceutical machinery in use. Most of the energy expended in reducing particle size is wasted. Many particles receive impacts lacking sufficient force to fracture them and are eventually fractured by some needlessly forceful blow.[75] To break a particle, the force applied must exceed the elastic limit of the material; when this is not exceeded, the particle deforms elastically. In elastic deformation the applied energy is stored as the particle deforms. Upon removal of the force, the applied energy is given off as heat as the particle returns to its original state. In general, energy is wasted not only in elastic deformation of particles but also in particle-particle friction, friction between particles and the mill surfaces, elastic deformation of mill components, noise, vibration, heat, and frictional losses in the machinery.[75] The reduction of particle size in mills is usually the result of crushing, impact, cutting, grinding or wearing down by friction (attrition), or a combination of these. Mills employed in the pharmaceutical industry typically include hammer, roller, rotary cutter, ball, and fluid energy mills.[75]

Typical of the *hammer mill* is the Fitzpatrick comminuting machine (Fig. 10-1). Hammer mills are primarily impact mills. Either swinging or stationary hammers or blades are affixed to a high-speed rotor mounted in a chamber. The chamber is bounded on the bottom by an interchangeable grid or screen through which the milled material must pass. The rapidly rotating hammers strike against the feed material, breaking it into smaller fragments which are swept against the grid. Rotor speed, type of hammer, and size of the grid openings are important factors governing the particle size of the product.[19] Flat-edge (blunt) hammers are generally used for pulverizing and tend to create a large number of *fines*. Knife-edge hammers are generally used for chopping, sizing, etc., when fines are undesirable or when fibers and tissues must be severed.

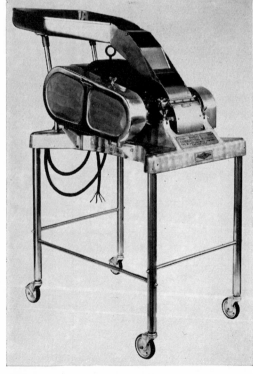

FIG. 10-1.   Fitzpatrick Model D comminuting machine. Machine is assembled ready for use.

Although the size of the grid openings has a limiting effect on the particle size of the discharged product, product particle size varies for a given grid or screen according to the rotor speed. The discharged product is actually smaller than the nominal dimensions of the grid opening because the particles exit at an angle, rather than radially, and "see" the openings as narrowed slits. The effect is exaggerated at high rotor speeds, at which this angle approaches a tangent. Thus, finer particles are produced with a given grid at higher speeds. Speeds that are too low result in a mixing action rather than comminution. Rotor speeds that are too high may not allow sufficient time for the material to fall between blades for hammering. This may be resolved without a reduction in speed by using hammers with smaller top dimensions.

In addition to comminuting vegetable and chemical materials, hammer mills can be used to process wet or dry granulations, disperse powder mixtures, and mill ointments. Because of the heat generated in milling, some models are equipped with jackets through which coolant circulates. This permits the milling of materials with low melting points and materials containing volatile constituents.

The *roller mill* reduces particle size through crushing, or crushing and shearing. In its simplest form, the roller mill consists of two rollers revolving at different speeds in opposite directions. The distance between the rollers is variable, and the surfaces may be either smooth or corrugated. There are many variations of roller mills available, some employing as many as five rollers. These mills are generally not suitable for fine grinding and are used extensively for milling ointments.

The comminution of animal or vegetable drugs presents special problems because of the tough, fibrous nature of the material. These drugs are often processed in *rotary cutter mills* such as the Wiley Mill (Fig. 10-2). This mill provides a continuous cutting or shearing action through blades attached to a horizontal rotor which come into close proximity to similar blades mounted around the housing as the rotor rotates. The relatively coarse product is dis-

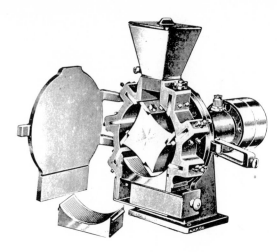

FIG. 10-2. Wiley mill.

charged through a screen mounted at the bottom of the mill housing.

Versatile and simple to operate, *ball mills*[46] are among the most commonly used of mills. A ball mill consists of a cylindrical container that lies on its side and is rotated

about its longer axis. The mill that appears in Figure 10-3 is typical. The material to be milled and the grinding medium balls or other shapes are sealed within. Although often used synonymously, the terms "ball mill" and "pebble mill" should be differentiated. *Ball mill* usually refers to a mill that uses steel balls as the grinding medium, whereas *pebble mill* usually refers to a mill employing flint pebbles or manufactured ceramic shapes. The grinding action is the result of impact of the grinding medium and attrition by the medium and against the mill lining as the mill rotates.

One of the most important factors determining grinding action is mill speed. The most desirable speed is one that induces a cascading action of the medium (Fig. 10-4). When cascading occurs, the balls or pebbles break away from the mill wall at an angle of about 45° to 60° from the horizontal and fall and roll over one another in a coherent, mobile mass. As can be seen in Figure 10-4, impact is achieved as the balls or pebbles

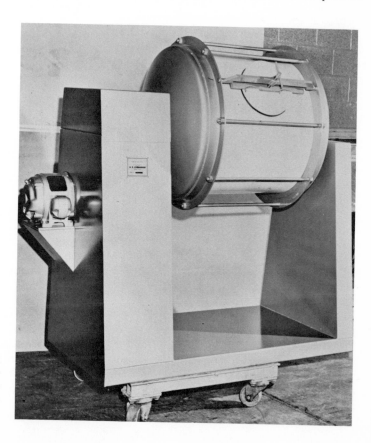

FIG. 10-3. Modern ball mill. (Norton Chemical Process Products Division, formerly U. S. Stoneware, Akron, Ohio)

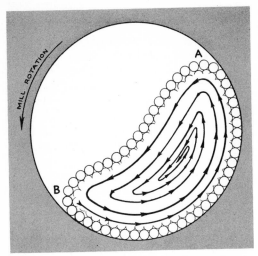

FIG. 10-4. Diagram of cascading action in a ball mill during grinding. (Norton Chemical Process Products Division, formerly U. S. Stoneware, Akron, Ohio)

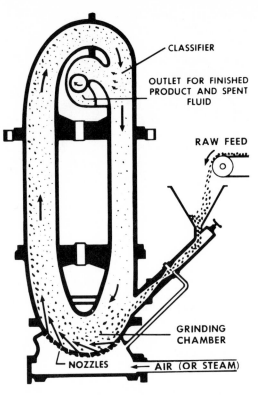

FIG. 10-5. Diagram illustrating the principles of operation of the Jet-O-Mizer® fluid energy mill. (Fluid Energy Processing & Equipment Co., Hatfield, Pa.)

fall from point A to point B, the potential energy at point A being converted to kinetic energy on falling. Loss of milling efficiency occurs at speeds high enough to throw the grinding elements clear of the contents (cataracting) or at speeds too low, so that slippage occurs. Slippage may lead to scoring of the mill lining and flattening of the grinding elements.

Mills are commonly filled from 45 to 55 percent of their internal volumes with the medium and, for dry grinding, usually enough of the material to be ground is added to fill the voids up to the level of the medium. The greater force of impact of larger grinding elements is desirable for grinding tough, large materials. Small grinding elements, however, produce finer particles because a fill of a given volume requires more of the medium, and a greater number of contacts are produced with each revolution of the mill. Generally, a medium made from high density materials provides greater impact and grinding effectiveness than a medium of the same size composed of low density materials. Ball mills are useful for the wet milling of slurries as well as for dry milling and are capable of fine grinding to submicron sizes. Blending and dispersing of dry powders may also be carried out in ball mills.

Fluid energy mills permit the continuous grinding of nearly any solid to a particle size in the micron or submicron range, a range that is well beyond the capacity of mills of many other types. The Jet-O-Mizer® is typical (Fig. 10-5). Basically, the mill consists of a hollow, vertical, elongated torus. At the bottom of the mill, fluids such as air or steam are introduced at high pressures through specially designed nozzles. Typically, air pressures of from 45 to 115 psig.* or steam at pressures between 100 and 250 psig. may be used. In pharmacy, compressed air is generally used, because many drugs have low melting points or are thermolabile.[75] As the fluid expands, gas streams

* Psig. is pounds per square inch gage. This is the pressure as read on a pressure gage. Pressure gages are commonly set to read zero at sea level where the air pressure is 14.7 pounds per square inch. Thus, in order to convert gage pressure (psig.) to absolute pressure (psia., or pounds per square inch absolute), it is necessary to add 14.7.

usually at velocities of from 200 to 500 m.p.h. are created. The material to be ground is continuously introduced into the region where the fluid is introduced, referred to as the grinding chamber, where the particles are trapped in the turbulent high-velocity gas streams and rapidly pulverized through particle-particle impact and attrition. As the gas circulates, the processed material is carried up and around the mill, and centrifugal force stratifies the entrained particles according to their size, so that the larger, heavier particles are pulled toward the periphery. On passing the reverse outlet, a portion of the circulating gas is diverted out of the mill, carrying with it only those smaller particles capable of being diverted from their path. The larger particles, with their greater centrifugal force, are carried past the reverse outlet and back to the grinding chamber for further milling. The selectivity of this built-in classification feature results in products with narrow particle size distributions.

As a further advantage, the expansion of the compressed air provides an inherent cooling effect which tends to counteract heat generated by the milling operation itself. Since particle size reduction is primarily a result of particle-particle interaction, there is minimal contamination of the product from the mill. Small percentages of additives may be blended with other materials as they are being processed, and, in other applications, materials may be ground and coated simultaneously by introducing a spray of the coating solution. Wet slurries may be dried almost instantaneously, and chemical reactions may be carried out in the fluid energy mill.

Manual Methods. *Trituration* is the principal method of comminution in the community pharmacy. It is the process of reduction of particle size by rubbing in a mortar and pestle. Particle size reduction is the result of both pressure and attrition as the pestle is firmly pressed down and given a circular motion over the inner surface of the mortar. Trituration also results in blending when two or more substances are processed in the mortar. Care must be taken to scrape the sides down with a spatula frequently. The mortars most frequently found in the pharmacy are Wedgwood, porcelain, or glass. Of the three, Wedgwood and porcelain mortars are preferred for particle size reduction because their roughened surfaces provide greater attrition than is possible with the smooth surface of a glass mortar. Their surfaces are also more porous than glass which makes them more susceptible to staining and more difficult to clean than glass mortars. Generally, glass mortars are preferred for dissolving substances or for mixing substances such as dyes and iodine which would stain Wedgwood or porcelain.

Levigation is the process of reducing particle size by first forming a paste of the solid with a minimum amount of a levigating agent and then triturating the paste in a mortar or on a slab with a spatula or a muller. A muller is a round, flat-surfaced glass instrument. When levigating on a slab, a circular or figure-8 path is often traced. Frequently the slab is a pill tile. The levigating agent may be water or other liquid in which the material is insoluble. Levigation is most commonly used in the extemporaneous preparation of ointments, in which case the levigating agent is frequently a small portion of the ointment base. The efficiency of particle size reduction by levigation depends in large measure on the viscosity of the paste which tends to hold the particles in place so that they can be pulverized by the rubbing process.

Pulverization by intervention is reduction of particle size with the aid of a second agent which can be readily removed from the pulverized product. Although the process varies according to the material to be pulverized, the term in pharmacy today usually applies to particle size reduction of camphor. Camphor, which otherwise is difficult to triturate, may be readily triturated when a few drops of alcohol or other volatile solvent are added. The pulverized camphor is readily recovered as the solvent evaporates.

Special Processes. Particle size reduction may be accomplished by processes designed primarily for other purposes, such as purification, preservation, etc. For example, fine particles may be produced by controlled precipitation from solution through change of solvents or temperature, or by application of ultrasonic vibration. Other processes which may be used to prepare powders for dosage forms include sublimation, freeze drying, and spray drying. The latter two processes, which are of particular importance in pharmaceutical technology, are discussed below.

Freeze Drying[30, 54, 79, 96] is also known as gelsiccation, drying by sublimation, lyophilization, and cryodesiccation. Freeze drying refers to the removal of water by sublimation from frozen products at low temperatures. The process is used to dry biological products such as blood serum, plasma, certain antibiotics such as penicillin, and other substances that are heat-labile and cannot be dried by the usual application of heat. In ordinary drying, the phase change is from liquid to vapor. However, if conditions are reduced to below the *triple point* temperature and pressure, e.g., of water (0.0099° C., 4.57 mm. Hg), the water sublimes, i.e., the phase change is directly from the frozen solid to vapor. The process may be visualized by referring to Figure 10-6. Along curve AO, water is in equilibrium with its vapor. Ice and vapor are in equilibrium along the sublimation curve, CO. Curve BO is the

melting curve where ice and water are in equilibrium. Only the labeled phase can exist in each region and the three phases are in equilibrium at point O, the triple point. Below this point, where freeze drying takes place, only ice and vapor phases exist. In general, the process of freeze drying involves (1) freezing the material, (2) reducing the pressure over the frozen sample, under which conditions the ice vaporizes without conversion to a liquid, (3) careful introduction of heat to maintain sublimation, and (4) continual removal of the vapor.

Freeze drying is usually carried out in the temperature range of −10 to −40° C.[54] The material should be frozen in thin layers, because sublimation takes place slowly (about 1 mm. thickness per hour).[30] Thin layers are created in bottles, vials, and ampuls by rotation or spinning during the freezing process. In small-scale production, the bottles, vials, etc., may be frozen in a cold bath such as a mixture of dry-ice and acetone. Standard refrigeration units are preferred for large-scale production. In bulk processing, the material is frozen in flat, shallow trays. In this case, the product may be frozen in freeze dryers equipped with

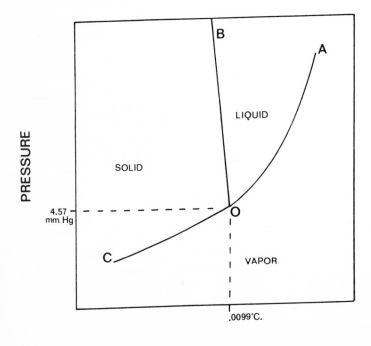

Fig. 10-6. Schematic representation of the triple point of water.

hollow shelves through which a coolant circulates or in deep freezing chambers.

It is important that the freezing process be as rapid as possible. Rapid freezing gives rise to small ice crystals. If freezing takes place too slowly, large crystals are formed which could damage cellular tissues. Rapid freezing also minimizes the concentration of solutes. Slow freezing causes solutes to concentrate near the top of a tray or toward the inside of a bottle as pure water crystallizes out. High local concentrations of salts could form which tend to denature protein. Heat-labile materials which separate in this fashion would be more vulnerable to the application of heat during the actual drying process.

Freeze drying is slow and the equipment is expensive relative to its drying capacity.[30] However, for certain heat-labile materials, it may well be the only possible means of drying. When properly packaged and stored, freeze-dried products exhibit extended shelf-lives. Chemical changes, enzymatic activity, and microbial growth are inhibited at low moisture levels. Certain drugs which are unstable in the presence of a solvent or vehicle may be dispensed as freeze-dried powders which are intended to be reconstituted as solutions or suspensions by the pharmacist at the time of dispensing. With these powders, which may contain all necessary adjuvants, such as flavors, buffers, suspending agents, etc., the solutions or suspensions are easily reconstituted, since freeze-dried solids are highly porous and expose a large surface to the solvent or vehicle. Since product sterility can be retained in freeze drying, parenteral solutions or suspensions may be similarly freeze dried in ampuls or vials for reconstitution by the clinician or pharmacist at the time of usage.

Spray drying[9, 54, 55] is a process for converting solutions or suspensions into dry, free-flowing powders in a single drying step. The solution or suspension is atomized or "sprayed" into an enclosed chamber into which heated air is also introduced. The atomization process produces very fine, generally spherical droplets with large surface areas that dry almost instantaneously. Rapid evaporation from this large surface and concomitant uptake of latent heat of vaporization keep the product temperature

below that of the hot air, thus making the process a suitable one for many heat-sensitive materials. The finer particles produced are capable of being carried out of the chamber with the effluent exhaust air and are collected in cyclone collectors. The coarser particles which fall out in the chamber may be collected through appropriate discharge ports.

A case-hardened outer shell of dried solids may form around droplets at the beginning of drying. The subsequent vaporization of moisture trapped within case-hardened particles causes them to balloon, and, if the pressure of the trapped vapor is great enough, holes may be blown through the shells. This exposure of internal surface adds to the total particle surface. Since dissolution occurs at surfaces, product dissolution would be rapid.

There are three basic schemes for mixing the spray and hot air: cocurrent, countercurrent, or a combination of the two (mixed flow). Maximum protection against overheating is afforded by the cocurrent design where the spray and hot air are introduced together from the same direction, and the wettest particles first encounter the hottest air. This also results in rapid initial drying which encourages case-hardening and ballooning. Agglomeration is less common in cocurrent dryers because the particles dry rapidly. Generally, cocurrent dryers are the most prevalent types in commercial use because designs are simpler and a wide range of products can be handled.[9]

The utility of spray drying in the pharmaceutical industry has been summarized by Lieberman and Rankell.[54] Materials sensitive to heat and/or oxidation can be spray dried without degradation. These include heat-sensitive materials such as pepsin and vitamins A and D, and easily oxidized materials such as epinephrine and ascorbic acid. Because the particles are spherical, spray-dried powders are free flowing and, therefore, suitable for use in formulations intended to be tableted or filled into capsules.[54]

Spray drying also provides a means of microencapsulation or coating of small solid particles or liquid droplets.[54] The coating may serve to mask taste and odor, improve stability, impart enteric properties, or provide sustained release. Small solid particles may be coated by spray drying a suspension of the powder in a solution of the coating material. As the solvent evaporates, a film of the coating material is deposited onto the particles. Oily liquids may be encapsulated by spray drying an emulsion of the oil in water. Gums such as acacia or starch are used as stabilizers. As the water evaporates, a dry shell of the gum forms around the oil droplets. "Dry" flavor oils are produced in this manner.[54]

Solid particles may also be encapsulated by spray congealing or spray chilling.[54] In this process, a suspension of the powder in molten waxy, fatty material is sprayed into the chamber. Cold air, rather than hot air, is introduced which causes the spray droplets to congeal. Spray congealing is primarily used to prepare sustained-release formulations and for masking taste.[54]

PARTICLE SIZE ANALYSIS AND CLASSIFICATION

The various methods of comminution can produce appropriate degrees of fineness in powders intended for various purposes. Regardless of the process, powders cannot be produced with perfectly uniform particle size. There is always a distribution of sizes. Because of the important relationship of particle size to drug properties and pharmaceutical processes, it is essential that particle size be measured and controlled.

One of the difficulties inherent in the measurement of particle size is that particles are usually irregular in shape. As such, irregular particles have no single unique dimension with which to define their size. However, since the size of a sphere is uniquely determined by its diameter, resort is made to expressing the particle size of irregular particles in terms of the diameter of a sphere equivalent to the particle in some property, i.e., an equivalent spherical diameter.[24] For example, d_s, the *surface diameter,* is the diameter of a sphere having the same surface area as the irregular particle. The *volume diameter,* d_v, is the diameter of a sphere having the same volume as the particle. The diameter of a sphere with the same projected area as the particle in its most stable position when viewed from above is the *projected area diameter,* d_p. The *Stokes' diameter,* d_{st}, is the diameter of a sphere with the same density and sedimentation rate in a given fluid as the particle in question. The diameter of a sphere that is just able to pass through the same square aperture as the irregular particle is the *sieve diameter,* d_{sieve}.

The equivalent spherical diameter measured relates to the method of particle size analysis. For instance, the *projected area diameter* is measured by observing the particles under a microscope. A graticule is used to superimpose a series of standard circles of known area and diameter over the field. The circles are visually compared against the cross sectional area of each particle. The *Stokes' diameter* is measured by sedimentation methods which depend on the fact that larger particles settle faster than smaller particles through a suspending medium. The Coulter Counter is an instrument which gives the *volume diameter.* In the Coulter Counter, a suspension of the particles in a conducting medium is pumped through an orifice. An electrode is positioned on either side of the orifice. As each particle passes through the orifice, it displaces its own volume of electrolyte which results in an increased resistance between the electrodes which produces a voltage pulse proportional to the particle volume (see Chap. 6).

Since a powder is a collection of various particle sizes, average particle size is not sufficient information in itself to characterize the sample. An infinite number of collections of particles may have the same average diameter. The *frequency of occurrence* of particles in various size groups must be determined. A plot of frequency of occurrence against the means of the size groups forms a particle size distribution curve that adequately describes the sample.

In order to standardize particle size, the *U.S.P.* and *N.F.* have adopted such descriptive terms as "Very Coarse," "Coarse," "Moderately Coarse," "Fine," and "Very Fine" to distinguish the various degrees of subdivision of vegetable and animal drugs and of chemical substances. These terms relate to the proportion of powder capable of passing through the openings of certain standard sieves in a specified period of time when subjected to standard agitation usually in a mechanical sieve shaker. The specific definitions of these terms are given in Table 10-1. Standard sieves are of wire mesh and are identified by a *sieve number* or *mesh number* which refers to the number of openings per linear inch. Hence, sieve number is inversely related to the aperture or opening size. Although several sieve series are in use, the most commonly used series in pharmacy is the U.S. Sieve Series which is also the series adopted by the *U.S.P.* and *N.F.* Some of the standard sieves in this series are listed in Table 10-2. The dimensions of the square apertures in successive sieves progress in the ratio of $\sqrt{2}$. Specifications for type of wire, wire diameter, and permissible variations in openings and wire diameter are given in the official compendia.

TABLE 10-1. OFFICIAL DEFINITIONS OF TERMS DESCRIBING THE DEGREE OF FINENESS OF VEGETABLE AND ANIMAL DRUGS AND CHEMICAL SUBSTANCES

Powders of Vegetable and Animal Drugs

Very Coarse (No. 8 powder)
100% pass through No. 8 sieve; not more than 20% may pass through a No. 60 sieve

Coarse (No. 20 powder)
100% pass through a No. 20 sieve; not more than 40% may pass through a No. 60 sieve

Moderately Coarse (No. 40 powder)
100% pass through a No. 40 sieve; not more than 40% may pass through a No. 80 sieve

Fine (No. 60 powder)
100% pass through a No. 60 sieve; not more than 40% may pass through a No. 100 sieve

Very Fine (No. 80 powder)
100% pass through a No. 80 sieve

Chemical Substances

Coarse (No. 20 powder)
100% pass through a No. 20 sieve; not more than 60% may pass through a No. 40 sieve

Moderately Coarse (No. 40 powder)
100% pass through a No. 40 sieve; not more than 60% may pass through a No. 60 sieve

Fine (No. 80 powder)
100% pass through a No. 80 sieve

Very Fine (No. 120 powder)
100% pass through a No. 120 sieve

TABLE 10-2. NOMINAL DIMENSIONS OF SELECTED STANDARD SIEVES

SIEVE NO.	APERTURE SIZE	
	MM.	MICRONS
8	2.38	2380
10	2.00	2000
20	0.840	840
40	0.420	420
60	0.250	250
80	0.177	177
100	0.149	149
200	0.074	74
325	0.044	44

The official fineness definitions are at best only an approximate indication of particle size and particle size distribution. The "Very Fine" designation for vegetable and animal drugs and the "Fine" and "Very Fine" designations for chemical substances only define the upper size limit of the powders. There is no limit to how fine these powders may be. Furthermore, while particle size standards based on sieve aperture sizes are often suitable controls for many pharmaceutical processes, it is in the subsieve range where the effect of particle size on the properties of drugs usually becomes significant.[24] The subsieve range, which has been defined to include particle size from one micron to a somewhat arbitrary 50 microns or more, requires more sophisticated means of particle size analysis. Some of these methods include microscopy, sedimentation, and the Coulter Counter. The student is referred to the excellent review by Edmundson[24] for a discussion of methods of particle size analysis and the means by which size frequency distributions are determined and utilized.

POWDER FLOW PROPERTIES

One of the properties of powders which is of great concern to pharmacists is the extent to which free flow will occur. Many pharmaceutical processes require freely flowing powders. The control of weight variation of both capsules and tablets is dependent upon the reproducibility of powder flow into fixed volume receptacles. Powders that do not flow readily cannot be successfully metered into empty capsule shells by high speed automatic filling equipment. In tablet production, the powder or granulation must flow readily and uniformly from the hopper into the die cavities of the tablet press in order to obtain uniform tablet weights (see Chap. 14). Dusting powders must be free-flowing to facilitate delivery through sifter caps and spreading when applied to the body. Poorly flowing, cohesive powders are also difficult to blend uniformly because the particles resist differential movement. The dispensing pharmacist, on the other hand, may find that powders that are too fluid are difficult to hand-pack into capsules.

The flow properties of powders vary considerably, ranging from those that flow readily and uniformly through small orifices to those that will not maintain uniform flow under any circumstances.[21] Particulate solids resist flow because of "classical" solid-to-solid *friction,* and because of *cohesion* or cohesionlike forces acting between the particles.[11] Cohesion between particles is normally attributed to nonspecific van der Waals forces. However, a structural cohesion is possible, owing to the mechanical interlocking of certain irregularly shaped particles, and a layer of adsorbed moisture can produce cohesiveness through the effect of surface tension at points of contact. In addition, the frictional movement of particles may lead to the build-up of electrostatic charges which can cause particles to attract each other.

Frictional and cohesive resistance to flow become more significant as particle size is reduced because there are more points of contact per unit weight of powder. Van der Waals forces often predominate over gravitational forces at particle sizes of about 10 microns and less.[67] Such particles are said to be "sticky" and are too cohesive to flow readily through orifices. Gravitational forces predominate with larger particles because these forces increase in relation to the cube of the diameter, and the particles would not be cohesive unless other forces were involved.[67] Gravitational effects are also greater with denser particles; hence, high particle density encourages powder fluidity.

Particle shape and surface texture have an important influence on flow properties. Rough irregular particles present more points of contact than smooth spherical particles and are less free-flowing.[74]

Particle size distribution is also important. Large proportions of fines can inhibit flow because the fine particles themselves are inherently poor flowing and because fines can fit into the voids between larger particles and encourage packing and powder densification.

The frictional and cohesive forces in a powder are reflected in the *angle of repose.*[67] The angle of repose is the maximum angle possible between the free surface of a loosely piled conical heap of powder and the horizontal plane. Since frictional and cohesive forces oppose the gravitational forces acting on particles, the greater these forces are in relation to gravitational forces, the greater will be the angle of repose. For most pharmaceutical powders, this angle is in the range of 20 to 40°.[74] Actually, the exact angle depends somewhat on the conditions of measurement and the method used. Four main methods of measuring angles of repose were critically evaluated by Train,[97] who concluded that most methods are satisfactory for comparing samples during routine quality control tests. Although the tangent of the repose angle has often been equated with the coefficient of interparticulate friction, the indiscriminate use of this relationship may result in error, since it assumes that there is no cohesion between particles.[35]

Flow properties are often inferred from angle of repose measurements. A higher angle of repose implies a greater *resistance to flow* than a lower angle of repose. However, several recent studies have demonstrated little or no correlation between the angle of repose and powder *flow rates,*[23, 32, 93] and it has been suggested that the movement of a powder may be more appropriately evaluated by a *dynamic* measurement, such as through a *flow meter,* than by a *static* method, such as the angle of repose.

Danish and Parrott[23] described a *flow meter* consisting of a vertically mounted cylinder bounded on the bottom by various circular plates. A different circular orifice was drilled through each plate so that orifice size could be varied by interchanging the plates. Flow rate was determined by collecting and weighing the material discharged through a given orifice in a given time. One of the difficulties of using flow through tubes or orifices as a means of evaluating fluidity is that some powders flow so poorly that flow cannot be initiated. Gold et al.[31] described a flow meter that helps alleviate this problem. In their apparatus, a vibrator could be attached to hoppers with orifices of various diameters, and the weight of powder discharged could be recorded continuously as a function of time. Not only could overall flow rates be determined, but the uniformity or lack of uniformity in flow could be inferred from the fluctuations in the continuous tracings.

Poorly flowing powders present many problems in the pharmaceutical industry, and considerable effort has been expended in finding ways to overcome poor fluidity. One method, previously described, is through spray drying which results in generally spherical free-flowing particles. In tableting, it is common practice to improve flow properties by forming larger particles through a granulation procedure. Compressibility is also improved by granulation. Other possible methods include controlled crystallization in chemical production to produce the most symmetrical particles, the careful control of humidity in production areas along with the use of antistatic agents to reduce static charges, the use of vibrators and positive feed devices to promote continuous flow, and the use of glidants.[57] The term *glidant* was first used by Munzel to define agents that enhance the flow properties of granulations when added in small quantities.[90] The term is presently understood to apply to dry agents that enhance the flow properties of powders as well as granular solids. The use of glidants in powder formulations intended for encapsulation is a widely accepted procedure. Examples of substances employed as glidants include talc, starch, and certain synthetic colloidal silicas, such as Cab-O-Sil® (Cabot Corp., Boston, Mass.). In general, the colloidal silicas consist principally of siilcon dioxide and are characterized by ultrafine particle size and low bulk density.[7] Glidants are fine particles which appear to coat the particles of the bulk powder and enhance flow properties by

acting through one or more possible mechanisms which include:[47]

1. Filling in irregularities and reducing surface roughness;
2. Physically separating the bulk particles, thereby reducing attractive forces;
3. Reducing electrostatic charges;
4. "Scavenging" moisture; and
5. Acting as "ball bearings" between the bulk particles.

There is usually an optimum concentration of glidant, often 1 percent or less, beyond which there is no further improvement in flow properties and possibly a deterioration of flow properties. This appears to depend largely on the nature of the bulk powder and its particle size.

Glidants must be differentiated from *lubricants*. Lubricants are agents which reduce friction between adjacent surfaces in relative motion to one another.[74, 90] Lubricants may be added to powders which are to be encapsulated or to granulations or powders intended to be compressed into tablets. Their principal role in tableting is to prevent the sticking of tablets to the die wall and facilitate ejection of the tablet from the die (see Chap. 11). In capsule formulations, they serve a similar role in certain automated capsule-filling operations. Certain lubricants, such as magnesium stearate, also appear to possess glidant properties.[32, 47]

BLENDING

Blending and the prevention of unblending are of fundamental importance to pharmacy. A powder blend should be as uniform as possible to assure the proper amount of medication in each dosage unit. Once thorough blending is achieved, it is essential that the powder remain blended during any subsequent operations and handling.

General Considerations.[27, 98] The blending of solid particles is affected by shape, density, size and size range of the particles, and surface effects such as adsorbed liquid films, electrostatic charges, and van der Waals forces. Small particles are difficult to blend because they exhibit poor fluidity. However, more important than actual particle size is *particle size range.* All drugs and chemicals should be reduced to approximately the same size prior to weighing and mixing, since the large and the small particles tend to become segregated. Under agitation, as in a blender, the fines tend to "dust out" at the top, and the larger particles tend to settle, under the influence of gravity, to the bottom of the vessel. Under conditions of flow, larger particles roll farther and faster than smaller particles. In certain mixtures of fines with larger irregular particles, the smaller particles may become segregated at the bottom of a vessel during agitation by falling through the voids between larger particles. Even if a good mixture of dissimilar particle sizes could be achieved, the condition must be regarded as unstable because subsequent agitation or vibration encountered during storage or processing could result in segregation.

Another factor related to particle size which can adversely affect the randomness of a blend is the tendency of very small particles to coat larger particles. A uniform blend could be achieved only if the coated ingredient were uniform in size. Otherwise, fractions of the coated ingredient that were of smaller particle size, and thus possess more surface area per unit weight, would be coated with a disproportionately large amount of the coating ingredient.

Even with particles of the same size, large *differences in density* can promote segregation, because the heavier particles tend to settle. However, since the densities of most drugs and adjuvants are not greatly different, this effect may be generally regarded as being of little significance.[74]

The effect of *particle shape* on blending is attributable largely to its effect on powder flow properties. All other things being equal, regular shapes are easier to mix than irregular shapes. Irregular shapes are generally less mobile, and, at the extreme, complex shapes may interlock, or flat needle-shaped particles may bundle, to impede powder flow in the blender.

Forces acting at surfaces can cause groups of particles to hold together as aggregates and resist uniform dispersion in the powder bed. These forces include weak van der Waals forces, electrostatic charges, and the surface-tension effects of adsorbed liquid films at points of contact between particles. Because they act at surfaces, their influence is greatest on finer particles which have a larger surface area per unit weight. Probably the most important of these three forces is *electrostatic charge* which is considered the principal cause of unblending in the blender. Under the motion of blending, electrostatic charges may be induced as surface electron states become unbalanced through particle-particle friction. As a result, one species of particles may preferentially attract each other and repel other particles. In other instances, one species may be preferentially attracted to the walls of the blender. Although electrostatic repulsive or attractive forces themselves may not be great enough to induce very much particle movement, the motion of the blender provides sufficient mobility for segregation to occur. To prevent unblending, the simplest approach is to avoid overworking the powders by stopping the blender when maximum blending has occurred. In addition, segregation may usually be prevented if the ingredients are introduced into the blender in alternate layers. This reduces blending time and reduces build-up of charges. The addition of a small amount of moisture may help, since this increases particle surface conductivity and reduces the tendency for charges to build-up. Other possible approaches include the addition of small quantities of surfactants or glidants.

No blend of solid particles can be truly homogenous.[27, 56] Even if perfect blending could be achieved, there is a statistical chance that a given random sample of this blend will not contain the same amount of active ingredient as another random sample of the same size. This is referred to as *sampling error.* How great this probable error is depends on the number of particles of active ingredient in the blend. The smallest sample of a blend in which accuracy of blending affects its use is the *critical quantity.* From a pharmaceutical point of view, the critical quantity is the smallest unit of dosage, e.g., the amount to be filled into a capsule or compressed into a tablet. The fewer the number of particles of the active ingredient in the blend, the greater the probable error in content of active particles in each critical quantity. From the desired percentage concentration of active ingredient in the blend and the size of the critical quantity, the weight of active ingredient required in each critical quantity may be determined. The corresponding number of particles of active ingredient required in each critical quantity may then be determined from a knowledge of the particle size of the active ingredient. Generally, any blend that would require fewer than 100 particles of active ingredient per critical quantity is questionable and should be investigated.[27] In order to minimize sampling error, the active ingredient should be reduced to the smallest practical size.

The problem of sampling error is especially acute for low-dose drugs, for which the active ingredient represents only a minute fraction of the over-all blend. In such cases, it may be necessary to abandon the blending approach and introduce the active ingredient in another fashion, e.g., a particle-counting or particle injection scheme. It may also be feasible to introduce the drug as a solution (see section on *Liquid-Solids Blending,* below), or to adsorb the drug uniformly on a bulk filler which is then used in forming the blend.

Blenders and Methods. Blending requires the differential movement of particles. In order to attain this movement, the blending operation must cause the powder bed to expand, allowing space between particles for movement, and must apply suitable force to move the particles.[98] Thus, all processes for the mixing of powders are based on agitation produced by some method or device. Generally, two types of large-scale blenders are employed in the pharmaceutical industry: mechanical mixers and tumbling mixers.[27, 29] In *mechanical mixers,* agitation is produced through the action of moving screws, blades, or paddles. In *tumbling mixers,* motion is imparted to the powders by rotating the vessel containing the powder about an axis. The Patterson-Kelly twin shell tumbler blender is illustrated in Figure 10-7. With each rotation, the powder mass is alternately divided and recombined, thereby providing an efficient intermeshing effect. These blenders are available in small sizes suitable for laboratory use as well as in production

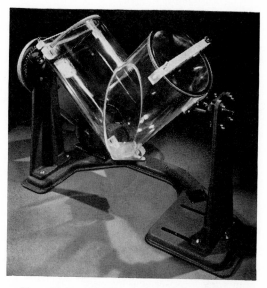

Fig. 10-7. Standard plastic laboratory twin shell blender. The dust-tight shell is made of heavy, transparent Lucite. (Patterson-Kelley Co., East Stroudsburg, Pa.)

sizes. Where precision blending is involved, tumbler types are better than the mechanical mixers, since blending action can be sustained more thoroughly throughout all parts of the powder bed.

The dispensing pharmacist usually accomplishes blending by *spatulation, trituration,* or *sifting.* As a general rule, each ingredient should be pulverized separately before weighing and blending. The general principle to be followed in all cases is to begin with the ingredient present in the smallest quantity (or the most potent) and add an approximately equal volume of the diluent or other drug. The two powders are mixed thoroughly. Then a quantity of additional diluent or other drug equal in volme to the bulk already mixed is added and the powders are mixed again. This process, which is repeated until all the powders have been mixed, is called *geometric dilution.*

When powders of the same color are mixed, it is impossible to determine visually when a uniform blend has been produced. While the use of geometric dilution usually ensures a uniform blend, some pharmacists prefer to add a small quantity (e.g., about 0.1%) of a dry certified dye, such as amaranth, as a tracer.[4] When the dye is uniformly dispersed, the blend is presumed thoroughly mixed.

Blending is most frequently accomplished by the dispensing pharmacist with the mortar and pestle. This method, called *trituration,* has the principal advantage of accomplishing both comminution and blending in one operation. If particle reduction is required, the rough interior surfaces of Wedgwood or porcelain mortars are preferred over the smooth surface of the glass mortar. Heavy trituration results in a fine, dense powder. Gentle trituration may be employed if it is desired that the finished product have the properties of lightness and diffusibility in liquids. The mortar and pestle should be occasionally scraped with a spatula, particularly during heavy trituration which sometimes causes caking and sticking to the sides of the mortar and the end of the pestle. When the powders to be mixed are already in a state of fine subdivision, simple blending may be carried out in the glass mortar and pestle. In other instances, the glass mortar may be preferred for drugs that might stain porcelain or Wedgwood mortars.

The properties of lightness and bulkiness in powder blends can be obtained by *spatulation* or *sifting,* although neither of these methods is considered suitable for the blending of potent substances. Mixing by spatulation is accomplished by running a spatula through powders on a pill tile or sheet of paper. Mixing by sifting is usually accomplished by passing the powders several times through a kitchen-type flour sifter. In either case, particle sizes and densities should be approximately the same for all ingredients.

Liquid-Solids Blending.[26] The term liquid-solids blending is generally applied to blends in which the liquid is a relatively minor constituent, and the blends usually retain the appearance and behavior of "dry" powders. The process may be used to add granulating solutions to precision powder blends or for the addition of active ingredients as solutions to filler powders or granulations. Other applications include the addition of flavor oils to powdered dentifrices or perfume oils to cosmetic powders. The particles retain their individual identities. The liquid may be bound to the solid particles through adsorp-

tion, absorption, entrapment within fissures or pores, or chemical reaction. At times it is difficult to determine which of these is occurring, and often two or more processes are occurring simultaneously. The liquid added may be totally or partially removed after processing.

Generally, solids pick up liquids in relationship to their specific surface area (surface area per unit weight), the affinity of the surface for the liquid, and the surface tension of the liquid. The uniform distribution of liquid on the solid particles on a weight-to-weight basis requires uniform particle size. The reason for this is that a given weight of smaller particles has a larger surface area for holding liquids than the same weight of larger particles.

In the foregoing, it is assumed that all particles in the blend have the same ability to attract and hold moisture on their surfaces. Although the particles may initially appear dry, actual moisture content may vary, especially if there are hygroscopic materials present. Since the capacity to attract and hold liquids depends largely on how much moisture is already present, the moisture content of some materials may require adjustment. Thus, an initial drying step may be required to enhance the moisture-holding capacity of particles. When dry, certain materials may have so great an affinity for moisture that it would be difficult or impossible to distribute a liquid uniformly in the bulk powder blend. In such cases, the powder may be "prepped" with water prior to adding the principal liquid ingredient.

Liquids with low surface tensions make liquid-solids blending easier because they tend to wet and spread easily over solid surfaces.

Precision in liquid-solids blending requires (1) that both liquid and solid be finely divided, (2) that both be suspended in space, and (3) that fresh material be continuously exposed by keeping both liquid and solid in motion.[26] In practice, a mist of the liquid may be sprayed into the moving powders in a blender. A special feature available with Patterson-Kelly twin shell blenders allows the mist to be sprayed within the mobilized powders as the blender rotates. This is accomplished with a high-speed whirling agitator bar which enters through the walls and extends across the axis of rotation of the blender. The bar is driven by a separate drive mechanism. Liquid passes into the hollow bar and is sprayed as fine droplets through annular orifices by centrifugal force as the bar rotates at high speeds. Knifelike blades extending from the orifices create a small void about the whirling bar which is bounded by highly mobilized particles into which the mist is sprayed.

When the powder consists of more than one component, the materials must first be dry-blended to the desired degree of precision before adding any liquid. The addition of a substantial quantity of liquid inhibits any further solid-solid blending.

POWDERS AS A DOSAGE FORM

Powders (Latin, *pulvis*; plural, *pulveres*) may be defined as dry mixtures of pulverized drugs and/or chemicals which are used externally or internally. Although originally intended as a convenient means of administering dried vegetable drugs, the use of powders has been extended over the years to include mixtures of two or more powdered pure chemicals present in definite proportions. Powders are compounded in bulk or in divided doses (*chartulae*).

As a dosage form, powders offer several advantages. For example, quantities of drugs too large to be practical as tablets or capsules may be conveniently administered as powders. Children and certain adults who have difficulty swallowing tablets or capsules may often be able to take powders. The small particle size of powders provides more rapid dispersion of ingredients than tablets which must first disintegrate. The last-mentioned factor may allow for a better coating of mucosal surfaces as compared with compacted dosage forms in the treatment of gastrointestinal disorders. Capsules and tablets of very soluble drugs (e.g., chloral hydrate, iodides, bromides) may produce local irritation of the gastrointestinal tract and consequent nausea and vomiting, owing to the formation of localized high concentrations of drug. The rapid dispersion of powders reduces this local irritation. Because

they may be readily compounded by the pharmacist, powders offer the physician greater flexibility in dosage and in drug combinations than is possible with prefabricated dosage forms.

On the other hand, a powder is not an ideal dosage form for unpleasant tasting medication. Because of the large surface area exposed, powders make poor dosage forms for drugs that are subject to deterioration on exposure to atmospheric oxygen and moisture.

Powders to be taken orally may be placed on the tongue and washed down with a drink of water or other liquid. Alternatively, the powder may be mixed in water or other liquid and immediately swallowed. The latter procedure is particularly desirable if the powder is large in volume. Unpleasant tasting drugs may often be rendered more palatable if mixed with jam, honey, or fruit juice.

Bulk Powders. When accuracy of dosage is not critical, powders may be dispensed in bulk. Bulk powders for oral administration are limited to those which the patient can safely measure with a spoon or by the "capful." These generally include laxatives, antacids, dietary supplements, and analgesics. Other bulk powders include dusting powders, douche powders, dentifrice powders, and insufflations.

Bulk powders may be dispensed in pasteboard boxes or widemouth screw-cap glass jars. Glass jars are preferred if the powder is hygroscopic or deliquescent, or if it contains volatile ingredients.

Dusting powders are dispensed in sifter-top cans. All dusting powders should be impalpable and grit free, particularly if they are to be applied to traumatized areas. Generally, extemporaneously prepared dusting powders should be passed through a 100-mesh sieve.

Insufflations are powders usually intended to be blown into body cavities such as the ear, nose, throat, or tooth sockets. Administration requires, as an accessory, an *insufflator*. The Abbott Aerohaler® is a unique insufflator used for the administration by inhalation of isopropylarterenol sulfate. In general, insufflators suffer from the inability to control dosage and the tendency for the powders to cake or agglomerate. With the application of pressurized packaging technology to pharmacy, medicinal and pharmaceutical aerosols have been developed which largely overcome these problems (see Chap. 13).

Bulk powders intended to be used externally or locally should always bear *External Use* or *Local Use* auxilliary labels.

Divided Powders. Powders may be prescribed in divided doses. Once the ingredients have been triturated, weighed, and blended by geometric dilution according to the principles and considerations previously described, the blend must be subdivided into the required number of doses. The individual doses may be weighed or the powder may be subdivided into doses by the *block and divide* method. Each dose is placed on a small sheet of paper which is neatly folded around the powder to form a packet.

Weighing. Dividing the powder by weighing each dose is by far the more nearly accurate of the two methods and is really the only safe method for potent drugs. Because there are significant differences in weight between weighing papers, the same pair of balanced weighing papers are used for each weighing, and each weighed dose is transferred to the paper in which it is to be wrapped. Loss of powder during compounding is unavoidable. In order to be certain that there will be sufficient powder for the last dose, enough powders may be compounded for one or two extra doses and the excess discarded. This procedure may not be used for divided powders containing narcotics or other similarly controlled substances where only the amount prescribed may be used. Working carefully, however, it is possible to prepare the prescribed number of divided powders containing a controlled substance within the usually accepted limits of ±5 percent compounding error.[76]

Block and Divide Method. This method should not be used for potent drugs. Since this method is not as accurate as weighing, several powders should be weighed as a check of accuracy.

The powder is generally placed on a pill tile and formed into a rectangular pile of uniform depth and packing. With the edge of a spatula, the entire rectangular bed is marked off by sight into small, uniform, rectangular portions equal in number to the number of prescribed doses. The scale on the pill tile may be used as an aid in dividing. The smaller blocks of powder are then separated with the spatula and transferred to powder papers. Powders that are too fluid are difficult to block and are best divided by weighing.

Powder Papers. The papers in which divided powders are traditionally folded are called powder papers. Commonly used papers include white, lightweight bond, vegetable parchment, glassine, and waxed paper. The paper of choice for hygroscopic or deliquescent powders is wax paper because of its waterproof qualities. If only limited moisture resistance is required, glassine or parchment may be satisfactory. Bond paper, which has no moisture-resistant capabilities, is commonly preferred for its neat, aesthetic appearance. Thus, it is common practice to double-wrap hygroscopic powders, using glassine, parchment, or wax paper as the inner paper and bond as the outer paper. Powders containing volatile ingredients should be similarly double wrapped.

The size powder paper required depends on the amount of the dose and the size of the powder box in which the folded powders are dispensed. Powder papers are available commercially which have been precut to the most popular sizes. These include 2¾ × 3¾ inches, 3 × 4½ inches, 3¾ × 5 inches, and 4½ × 6 inches.

Folding. With practice a neat, uniform appearance can be obtained by following the steps below which outline the traditional folding of powder papers (see Fig. 10-8):

1. The long edge of the paper is folded down about ½ inch. Several papers may be folded at one time to save time and promote uniformity (Fig. 10-8, A).
2. The papers are then placed on the counter in a convenient arrangement, with the folded tops away from the pharmacist.
3. The individual doses are placed on the center of each paper (Fig. 10-8, A).
4. The lower edge of the paper is brought up and inserted completely into the top fold (Fig. 10-8, B).
5. The top fold is folded down toward

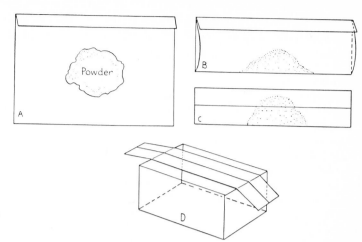

Fig. 10-8. Steps in the folding of powders in papers.

the pharmacist until the remainder of the paper is divided approximately in half (Fig. 10-8, C).

6. The folded paper is then centered lengthwise over an open powder box of the size intended to be used. The equal overhanging ends are folded down while pressing in on the sides of the box (Fig. 10-8, D). The ends are then folded back completely and the end folds creased sharply by pressing with a spatula.

The powders are usually placed in the box with the folds away from the pharmacist. Usually, all top folds are up, but occasionally they may be alternately up and down. The appearance is not as neat with the latter procedure, but it allows more folded papers to be placed in the box and minimizes the tendency for several to "pop-out" when a single powder is removed.

Envelopes. The use of powder papers as a dosage form is declining. The lack of interest in divided powders is reflected in the lack of advances made in developing new ways of packaging divided powders. However, the problems of folding powder papers and of protecting ingredients from the atmosphere may be avoided by using small cellophane or polyethylene envelopes. After the weighed dose is placed within, the open end may be folded over and heat sealed to provide an airtight enclosure. Other specially designed polyethylene envelopes are available which may be sealed simply by pressing the open end together between the fingers.

Powder Boxes. Divided powders may be dispensed in the older, slide-type boxes or in the newer, more attractive shouldered boxes with hinged or removable lids. Since the label with directions to the patient is placed either on or, preferably, inside the lid, hinged boxes are preferred because they prevent accidental exchange with the lids from other boxes.

Granules. Granules may be defined as generally irregular agglomerates of small particles which behave as single larger particles.[26] Typically, they are in the 4- to 12-mesh size range. Although granules may be prepared by several wet or dry methods, they are often prepared by blending powders with a liquid that serves as an adhesive. The wet, cohesive mass formed may then be passed through a screen, and the wet granules are then dried and classified.

Granulation offers a number of advantages. Granules generally flow well and powders are often granulated prior to tableting to improve flow properties as well as compressibility (see Chap. 14).* Also, granulation may prevent segregation in powder mixtures since each granule, would contain the correct proportions of ingredients. Hence, any segregation of the granules would not adversely affect the homogeneity of the overall mixture. Dust problems associated with the handling and processing of fine powders may be minimized by granulation, and granules are less likely to cake than fine powders.

---

* These are finer granulations. Granulations in the 12- to 20-mesh range are not uncommon in tableting.

They are generally more stable than powders when exposed to the atmosphere because less surface is exposed. Granules, rather than very fine powders, may be preferred for making solutions because powders are often difficult to wet and tend to float on the solvent surface.

Drugs that are unstable in aqueous solution or suspension are often prepared in the form of granules; the solution or suspension is "reconstituted" by the pharmacist by adding a specified amount of water to the granules just prior to dispensing. Even under refrigeration, these "reconstituted" preparations exhibit limited stability, and the pharmacist should advise the patient about proper storage conditions and the product expiration date. An example is Abbott's Erythrocin® Ethyl Succinate Granules. When reconstituted, an oral suspension is formed containing activity equivalent to 200 mg. of erythromycin base in each 5 ml. (teaspoonful). The manufacturer recommends that the suspension be refrigerated after reconstitution and used within 10 days. Similarly, Upjohn's Sugracillin® Flavored Granules yield oral solutions containing either 125,000 or 250,000 units of penicillin G per 5 ml., depending on the formulation. These solutions should be refrigerated after reconstitution and used within two weeks.

Bulk granular products are not intended for potent medication since, as in the case of other bulk powders, the patient measures doses by the teaspoonful. These products may be either effervescent or noneffervescent. Examples of *noneffervescent* bulk granules are Senokot® Granules (Purdue Frederick), Serutan® Toasted Granules (J. B. Williams), and Somagen® (Upjohn). Bromo Seltzer® (Warner Lambert) and Sal Hepatica® (Bristol Myers) are examples of effervescent granulations. Alka Seltzer® (Miles) is an effervescent granulation compressed into a tablet.

Effervescent granulations (effervescent salts) are granulated mixtures of a soluble medicinal agent, and citric acid or tartaric acid (or both), and a bicarbonate, usually sodium bicarbonate. These mixtures are intended to be dissolved in water and taken either during or immediately after effervescence. The carbonated solution provides a vehicle that masks the taste of saline or otherwise unpleasant tasting medication. Effervescent powder mixtures are purposely formed into relatively coarse granules to reduce the rate of dissolution in water and thereby provide a more controlled reaction. The violent, uncontrolled effervescence of the reacting mixture in powder form would cause spillage from the container.

The proportions of acids required is determined from the stoichiometry of the reactions between them and the bicarbonate. A mixture of the two acids is preferred because the use of tartaric acid alone produces granules that are too friable and imparts a salty taste, and the use of uneffloresced citric acid alone yields sticky mixtures which are difficult to handle. A good working formula has been found to be:[28]

	Percent
citric acid	19
tartaric acid	28
sodium bicarbonate	53

The reacting mixture may be regarded as a basic formulation to which the active ingredients are added. Typically, the patient takes a heaping teaspoonful. This is generally assumed to be 5 grams, although this weight may vary somewhat according to the bulk density of the product. On this basis, the finished product is designed so that each 5 grams contains the prescribed dose of medication, the balance being the basic effervescent formulation. The total amount of preparation is based on the total number of doses required.

Granules should be packaged in tight, dry, widemouth glass jars. Storage is best in a cool place.

CAPSULES

Capsules (Latin, *capsulae*) are solid dosage forms in which the medication is contained within hard or soft gelatin shells. The medication may be a powder, a liquid, or a semisolid mass. The French pharmacist, Mothes, is credited with inventing the soft gelatin capsule, for which he was granted a French patent in 1834. A two-piece hard gelatin capsule was patented by the Englishman James Murdock, in 1848.

Capsules are usually intended to be administered orally by swallowing them whole. In certain instances, the capsules may be emptied and the contents used as a divided powder. Occasionally, capsules may be administered rectally or vaginally, in which cases moistening with warm water often assists insertion. AVC Suppositories® (National Drug) are soft gelatin capsules intended for vaginal insertion; Emesert Inserts® (Arnar-Stone) are soft gelatin capsules intended for rectal administration.

Capsules are neat and elegant in appearance. Enclosing the medication within capsule shells provides a tasteless, odorless means of administering medication, and the ready solubility of gelatin at gastric pH's provides for rapid release of medication in the stomach. Since hard gelatin capsule products may be extemporaneously compounded by the pharmacist, this dosage form offers physicians greater flexibility in dosages and drug combinations than is available with prefabricated medication.

On the other hand, capsules are not suitable containers for liquids that dissolve gelatin, such as aqueous or hydroalcoholic solutions. Very soluble salts, such as bromides or iodides, should not be dispensed in capsules. The rapid release of such materials may cause gastric irritation, owing to the formation of localized areas of high drug concentration.

Hard Gelatin Capsules. The two-piece, telescoping hard gelatin capsule is used by the pharmacist in prescription compounding and by pharmaceutical manufacturers for most prefabricated capsule products. Hard gelatin capsules consist largely of gelatin, sugar, and water. Attractive and distinctive colors are achieved through the addition of certified dyes, and titanium dioxide is often added as an opaquing agent. An opaque color may be specifically desired to conceal capsule contents or to provide protection against light.

Manufacture.[52] According to the United States Pharmacopeia, *gelatin* is prepared by the partial hydrolysis of collagen obtained from skin, bones, and white connective tissues of animals. Its physical and chemical properties vary somewhat, according to its source and the method of extraction. Accordingly, to produce capsules with high clarity and the desired firmness and plasticity and to assure batch-to-batch uniformity, manufacturers usually establish specifications to control properties such as Bloom strength (gel strength), color, pH, viscosity, and the presence of inorganic materials, as well as particle size and bacterial content.

Mixtures of gelatins derived from pork skin and bone are used in capsule manufacture: bone gelatin contributes firmness and pork gelatin contributes plasticity, flexibility, and clarity. The most objectionable inorganic material appears to be calcium phosphate which is chiefly found in bone gelatin and which may impart a haze to finished capsules if present in too large quantities.

Particle size is important because it affects the preparation of the gelatin solution from which the capsules are cast: High proportions of coarse particles prolong the hydration time; too many fines results in excessively rapid hydration, with the formation of incompletely wetted gelatin masses which are difficult to dissolve.

The capsule shells are cast by dipping cold metallic molds, or pins, into carefully heated gelatin solutions (Fig. 10-9); 150 pairs of pins, representing cap and body portions, are dipped simultaneously. As the cap and body pins are dipped into different solutions, different colored caps and bodies may be produced. The time required to cast the film varies according to the size of the capsule, with larger capsules requiring longer dipping times. After dipping, the pins are withdrawn and rotated 2½ times to distribute the gelatin uniformly over the pins. During spinning, the gel may be firmed with a blast of cooled air. The coated pins are then passed through a series of 4 drying kilns where the degree and rate of drying are carefully controlled. After drying, the body and cap portions are stripped individually from the pins with bronze jaws and delivered into collets. The collets are rotated, and a blade is brought to bear against the cap and bodies to trim them to the appropriate lengths. Finally, the finished caps and bodies are aligned, joined, and ejected.

Storage. Capsules should be stored in tightly closed glass containers, protected from dust and extremes of humidity and

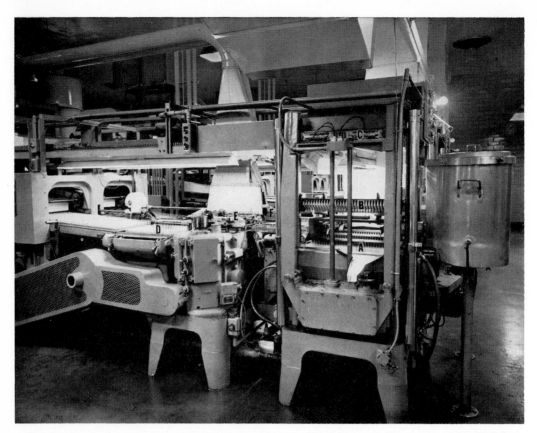

Fig. 10-9. Automatic capsule-making machine at Eli Lilly and Company. (A) Stainless-steel body molds are dipped in gelatin solution; molds for caps are treated similarly on the opposite side of the machine; (B) molds are rotated as they are raised to the top of the machine to ensure uniform distribution of gelatin; (C) molds are conveyed to the drying kiln; (D) molds are conveyed from the drying kiln; (E) dried gelatin is stripped from the molds and trimmed and bodies and caps joined; (F) finished capsules are delivered on other side.

temperature. Capsules normally contain from 10 to 15 percent of moisture. However, when stored under conditions of high humidity, sufficient moisture may be absorbed to soften the gelatin and make it tacky. On the other hand, when stored under conditions of low humidity, the capsules may dehydrate and become brittle.

Sizes. Empty gelatin capsules for human use are available from manufacturers in 8 sizes, ranging from 000 (the largest) to 5 (the smallest). These are illustrated in Figure 10-10. The exact capacity by weight of any given capsule size obviously varies according to the density and compressibility of the formulation. As a guide, manufacturers list the approximate capacities of each size capsule for 5 commonly used drugs on the

capsule box. The weights of aspirin and volumes in ml. of water are listed in Table 10-3.

For veterinary use, empty gelatin capsules

TABLE 10-3.   CAPSULE CAPACITIES*

CAPSULE SIZE	WATER VOLUME IN ML.	ASPIRIN APPROXIMATE WEIGHT (GRAMS)
000	1.37	1.00
00	0.95	0.65
0	0.68	0.50
1	0.50	0.32
2	0.37	0.25
3	0.30	0.20
4	0.21	0.15
5	0.13	0.10

* Data from Parke, Davis & Co.[71]

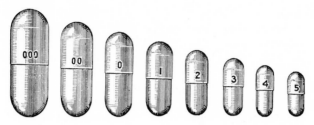

Fig. 10-10. Actual sizes of empty gelatin capsules.

are available in three large sizes: Nos. 10, 11, and 12 (Fig. 10-11). Their approximate capacities are, respectively, 30, 15, and 7.5 grams.

Extemporaneous Filling. All powders should be triturated and blended by geometric dilution, exercising all previously described considerations and precautions. For ease of swallowing and greater patient acceptance, a pharmacist generally chooses the smallest capsule that will contain the prescribed dose. The dose of medication may often conveniently be of sufficient bulk to fill a capsule. In other instances, each required dose may lack sufficient bulk to fill even the smallest available capsule, thus requiring the addition of an appropriate amount of inert diluent such as lactose. Occasionally, other inert materials must be added to the formulation to separate physically or chemically incompatible substances or to act as sorbents to prevent the sorption of moisture by deliquescent or hygroscopic substances. In general, the quantity of drug(s) required in each capsule is first determined and any inert diluents, protectives or sorbents are added as required. At times, the total bulk per dose may exceed the capacity of the largest available capsule, or youngsters and elderly persons may have difficulty swallowing anything but the smallest capsules. In these cases, the pharmacist may halve the dosage per capsule and dispense twice the originally prescribed

number of capsules with directions for the patient to take 2 capsules per dose, rather than one.

As in the case of compounding of divided powders, some loss of powder during manipulation and filling is unavoidable, and there is likely to be insufficient powder to adequately fill the last capsule. To avoid this problem, the pharmacist may usually prepare enough powder to fill one or two more capsules than required. However, as has been previously mentioned, this procedure may not be used if the prescription contains narcotics or other similarly controlled substances.

The choice of capsule size ultimately must be determined by making trial weighings of filled capsules. As previously noted, guidance may be had by referring to the table of approximate capsule capacities for common substances which is usually provided on the box of empty capsules. Capsules ordinarily available for prescription use are either clear-colorless or clear-pink. Although colorless capsules are routinely used, pink capsules may be used to distinguish two similar appearing capsule preparations for the same patient or to help disguise the appearance of unsightly contents. Colors other than pink may be achieved extemporaneously by dipping empty capsules into solutions of FD&C dyes in 70 percent alcohol (see reference 99 for further details). The pharmacist should be careful to note the size and color of the capsule selected on the prescription to assist in the compounding of refills.

When the proper size capsule has been determined, the required number of empty capsules are selected and set aside for filling. This procedure helps to prevent the inadvertent filling of the wrong number of capsules and avoids the possibility of contami-

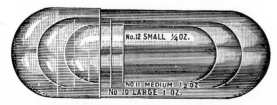

Fig. 10-11. Veterinary capsules.

nating the stock capsules with powder, as might occur if the capsules were removed singly during the filling operation.

The usual procedure is to fill the capsules by the *punch method*. The powder formulation is formed with a spatula on a pill tile or sheet of paper into a pile with a uniform depth of about ⅓ to ½ the length of the capsule body. The cap is removed and the empty capsule body is held between thumb and forefinger and repeatedly pressed downward into the pile until it is full. The cap is replaced and the filled capsule is weighed using an empty capsule of the same size as a tare. The same empty capsule may be used as a tare for each capsule to be filled in a prescription, because any differences in weight between empty capsules of the same size would be insignificant compared to the weight of the filled capsule. The weight of the filled capsule may be adjusted to the proper weight by pressing more powder into the body, or by tapping a little out. When potent drugs are involved, each capsule should be weighed. If nonpotent drugs are to be encapsulated, an experienced pharmacist may weigh the first two or three capsules to get a "feel" for the degree of compression that corresponds to the proper weight and thereafter only weigh occasional capsules as a check of uniformity. To give a full appearance, the capsule may be tapped gently on the cap end to distribute the powder uniformly. Alternatively, the capsule may be squeezed gently or rolled between the fingers.

After filling, some traces of powder inevitably remain on the outside of the capsules. Not only may this present an unsightly appearance, but the drug may be bitter tasting or have an unpleasant odor. Powder traces may be removed by wiping each capsule with gauze or cloth. The capsules may be placed within the fold of a clean towel and rolled back and forth, or shaken in the towel by gathering it into a bag around the capsules.

Obviously, cleanliness is of utmost importance in handling capsules. Hands should be clean and dry. Any traces of moisture can make capsules sticky, cause dry powders to adhere, and leave fingerprints. One method of keeping hands dry is to rub them thoroughly with a towel before the filling of each cap-

sule. Another approach is to use the cap of another capsule as a holder for the bodies during filling. Probably the best way to avoid the problem of moist fingers and assure sanitary filling is to wear finger cots or rubber gloves.

Granular substances and other free-flowing powders that lack sufficient cohesiveness to pack well by "punching" may be pushed into capsules with a spatula, or individually weighed doses may be carefully poured into capsules from weighing papers.

When small quantities of a potent drug are involved, a pharmacist may often place a small tablet containing the appropriate dose of the drug in each capsule along with any diluents or other less potent medication. Manufacturers have used such a technique to separate two incompatible substances by inserting a coated tablet of the offending substance into the capsule. A similar procedure that may be readily employed by the pharmacist is to pack one of the offending substances into a small capsule which may then be inserted in larger capsules along with the other ingredient(s) and any diluents.

Fixed oils and other liquids that do not dissolve gelatin may be filled into hard gelatin capsules with a pipet or calibrated dropper. Care should be taken to avoid getting any of the liquid on the outside of the capsules. The capsules are sealed by moistening the lower part of the inner surface of the caps with water. This may be conveniently accomplished with a camel's hair brush or by pressing the cap down into a pledget of cotton which has been moistened with water. The moistened cap is best put on with a slight twisting motion; this promotes a complete seal by spreading the moisture. Prior to dispensing, the integrity of the seal should be checked by allowing the capsules to rest on a blotter or filter paper for a while.

Liquids may often be sorbed onto inert carrier powders to form "dry" powders suitable for capsule filling. If this is not possible without unduly increasing the bulk or if the liquid is viscous, a plastic, doughlike "mass" can be formed which may be filled into the capsules. Such a mass could also contain any powders that may have been prescribed with the liquid. The general procedure is to roll the mass into a uniform pipe on a tile. The pipe is then completely subdivided into uniform pieces equal in number to the number of prescribed doses. As these pieces are each put into an empty capsule, they should be slightly longer than the capsules to ensure complete fill.

To facilitate the small-scale filling of capsules, hand-operated devices such as the Universal Model illustrated in Figure 10-12 are available. This model has a capacity of 24 capsules at a time; capacities of up to 144 capsules at a time are possible with other models. Although the capsules must be placed in the device manually, the caps are removed and replaced mechanically. The powder is distributed uniformly into the capsules by spreading it over a perforated tray which holds the powder over the empty bodies. A tamper is used to pack the capsules.

Industrial Filling. [18, 39, 43, 89] The industry uses semi-automatic and fully automatic

equipment for the large-scale filling of capsules. Regardless of the process, all have in common the basic operations of (a) removal of caps, (b) filling of the bodies, (c) replacement of caps, and (d) ejection of filled capsules.[18]

The classical semi-automatic Elanco No. 8 Capsule Filling Machine* is illustrated in Figure 10-13. This machine is capable of filling all capsule sizes from 000 through 5 and attains its maximum rated capacity (with skilled operators) of 15,000 to 20,000 capsules per hour with capsule sizes 1 to 4. Capsules are aligned in the rectifier (5) and delivered into the perforated capsule filling ring. The ring is rotated on a turntable, and a vacuum pulls the bodies into the lower half of the ring, leaving the caps in the upper half of the ring. The top and bottom halves

* Elanco Products Co., division of Eli Lilly and Co., Indianapolis, Indiana.

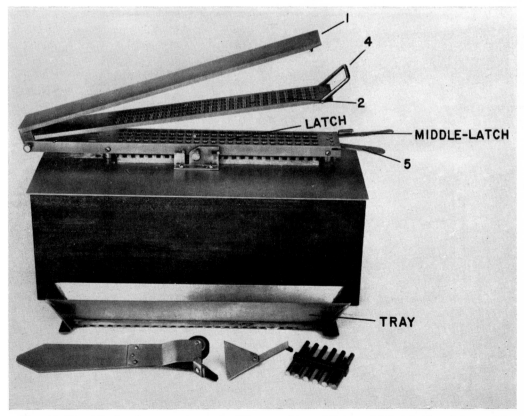

FIG. 10-12.   The hand-operated capsule-filling machine. (Universal Model. Chemipharm, New York 7, N. Y.)

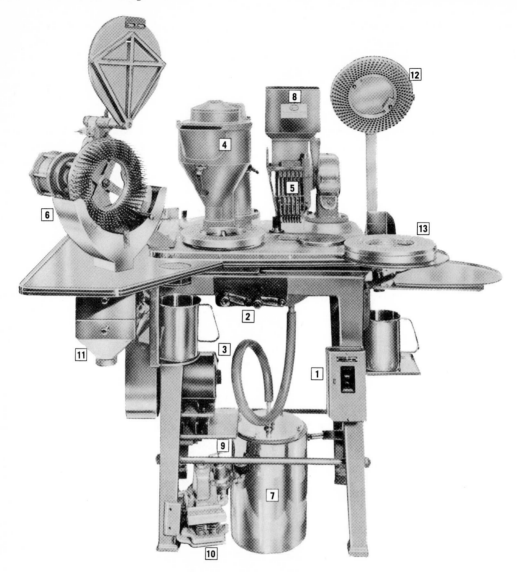

PARTS IDENTIFICATION

1. Motor Switch
2. Weight Control Levers
3. Drive Motor
4. Powder Hopper
5. Rectifier Head
6. Capsule Closing Assembly
7. Filter Can

8. Capsule Hopper
9. Air Line Regulator and Pressure Gauge
10. Foot Control Valve for Closing
11. Receptacle Box
12. Filling Ring (Cap Section)
13. Filling Ring (Body Section)

FIG. 10-13. Semi-automatic machine for filling hard gelatin capsules. (Eli Lilly & Company, Indianapolis, Indiana)

of the filling ring are separated manually, and the cap half of the ring (12) is set aside. The body half of the ring (13) is then moved to another turntable where it is rotated mechanically under a powder hopper (4). The hopper contains an auger which feeds the powder into the bodies. When the capsule bodies are filled, the cap and body rings are rejoined and the unit is placed against a peg ring (6). A retaining plate is placed against the other side of the capsule ring, and the peg ring, driven by air pressure, pushes the caps and bodies together. The retaining plate is removed and the capsules are ejected. Similar equipment is available from Parke, Davis.*

A major factor affecting fill weight is the rate of rotation of the body ring under the hopper. All other things being equal, slower rotation speeds generally produce fill weights higher than those produced by more rapid rates of rotation, because at slower speeds each empty capsule body spends more time under the hopper. Because capsule weights tend to increase with higher powder levels in the hopper, the maintenance of a relatively constant powder level helps to control weight variation. Also, powder formulations should flow freely and uniformly if constant weights are to be maintained, and in this regard glidants appear to be useful. For example, working with the Parke-Davis machine, Ito *et al.*[45] found meaningful reductions in capsule weight variation in test runs with lactose and with cornstarch when a silica type glidant was used. Also, in an evaluation of several factors affecting encapsulation using the Lilly machine, Reier *et al.*[78] showed that the use of talc as a glidant seemed to reduce weight variation in the several formulations studied.

Recent years have seen the development of several fully automatic capsule filling machines. One of these, the Zanasi model RV-59/R,† is unique in that the powder is first formed into slugs which are then delivered into the capsules. The operational features of the Zanasi machine were described by Stoyle.[89] Forty-eight stationary

dies are arranged around a turntable. Above the table are twelve groups of 4 movable dies. The capsules are rectified and fed into 4 movable dies at a time. The movable dies bearing capsules are then pushed down onto the stationary dies. Vacuum holds the bodies in the stationary dies and the caps are then retained in the movable dies which retract toward the center of the turntable where they remain until the bodies are filled. Capsule fill is accomplished by means of two sets of four specially designed tubes. The tubes are open at one end, and each contains a movable piston. The tubes dip into powder hoppers to pick up the desired dose which is compressed into slugs by the pistons. Carrying the slugs, the tubes are then positioned over the open bodies where the pistons eject the slugs into the capsules. As two tubes of each group are discharging slugs, the other four are picking up powder and forming new slugs. Weight can be adjusted by varying the height of the piston and, to some extent, by varying the level of the powder in the hopper. Powder formulations should possess good flow properties and be sufficiently compressible to form good slugs. Adequate lubrication (e.g., magnesium stearate) is required to facilitate ejection of the slugs from the tubes. After filling, the caps are re-positioned over the bodies, and the two portions are joined by means of pins. Ejection pins from below then push the capsules into cleaning dies where they are held by a pair of rubber rings. A vacuum in the chamber formed by the rubber rings assures closure and cleans the capsules, and the finished capsules are finally ejected. This machine is capable of filling as many as 17,300 capsules per hour.

Automatic filling equipment based on two different dosing principles is available from Hofliger and Karg.‡ The DOS Mikro machine accomplishes dosing through an auger fill and is available in models rated at capacities of up to 400 capsules per minute. In the ST models, which are rated at capacities of up to 600 capsules per minute, rapidly reciprocating plungers compress the powders into capsule bodies. The plungers

---

* Parke-Davis Type #8 Capsule Filling Machine, Parke, Davis & Co., Detroit, Michigan.

† Fratelli Zanasi S. p. A., Bologna, Italy.

‡ Hofliger and Karg, Waiklingen (near Stuttgart), Germany.

act through a shoe which supports a bed of powder over the empty capsule bodies.

Locking and Sealing of Capsules. Methods of locking or sealing caps and bodies together have been developed by several manufacturers. For example, Parke-Davis' Kapseals® are hard gelatin capsules the cap and body portions of which are sealed together by a narrow band of colored gelatin. More recently, unique cap and body configurations have been developed that permit the mechanical locking of the two halves when joined. For example, Elanco's Lok-Cap® (Fig. 10-14) utilizes a 3-segment raised collar around the inner cap shoulder which provides a positive friction lock when the body is inserted. Locking action with Parke-Davis' Snap-Fit® capsules is due to matching interlocking rings formed in the cap and body portions which engage when the caps and bodies are joined. Another method of locking capsules is offered by Hofliger-Karg in which a small hot probe is momentarily brought to bear against the cap where it overlaps the body to form a spot weld. Also noteworthy is a capsule-banding machine available from Zanasi which can be used independently or in conjunction with their automatic capsule filling machine.

These techniques serve to prevent the accidental separation of capsules during handling and shipping. Safeguards such as these have become particularly important with the development of high-speed automatic filling and packaging equipment and with the advent of beadlike sustained-release capsule products which would otherwise tend to separate on handling because the fills are not compacted and offer little frictional resistance to separation. In addition, both the banded and the mechanically locked capsules provide a deterrent to tampering.

Soft Gelatin (Elastic) Capsules.[38, 44, 59, 86] The composition of soft gelatin differs from that of hard gelatin in that the sugar is replaced by a plasticizer which imparts elastic properties to the gelatin. However, up to 5 percent of sugar may be added to the formulation to give "chewable" properties to the shell.[86] Commonly used plasticizers include glycerin and sorbitol, or mixtures of these. Other polyhydric alcohols may be used.

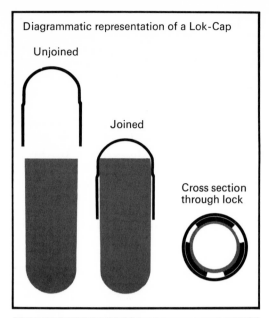

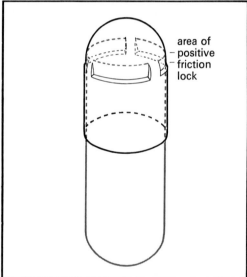

Fig. 10-14. Sketch illustrating the locking principle of the Lok-Cap® (Eli Lilly & Company, Indianapolis, Indiana)

Soft gelatin capsules may be formed in many shapes—oblong, spherical, or elliptical, among others. Capacities may range from 1 to 480 minims. Spherical or oval capsules have been called pearls or globules.

Soft gelatin capsules provide an attractive, odorless, and tasteless form of medication. In addition, they are hermetically sealed, making them uniquely suitable for liquids, volatile drugs, and drugs subject to atmospheric oxidation. Compared with hard gelatin capsules as a dosage form, they suffer the disadvantage of not being easily and readily prepared on a small scale. Although once a part of extemporaneous compounding, filled soft gelatin capsules are now exclusively mass produced, usually with equipment that automatically forms and fills the capsules at the same time. The usefulness of soft gelatin capsules is not limited to oral medication or as a form of rectal or vaginal suppositories. Topical, eye, ear, and nose preparations as well as a variety of cosmetics and foodstuffs may be dispensed in soft gelatin capsules.

The fill may be single liquids, blends of miscible liquids, solutions, suspensions, semisolids, dry powders, or slugs. Only liquids that do not dissolve the shell may be used. Examples include animal, vegetable, or mineral oils and the polyethylene glycols.

Originally, Mothes made soft gelatin capsules by dipping small leather molds into a hot gelatin solution. After cooling, the shell was stripped off, filled with medication, and sealed with several drops of the gelatin solution. Technological advances have brought about many changes in the manufacture of soft gelatin capsules, and Mothe's method contrasts sharply with modern methods of mass production.

Plate Process. This semi-automatic batch process was the earliest commercial means for the manufacture of soft gelatin capsules. The process involves placing an oversize sheet of still soft gelatin on a die plate. The sheet is drawn by vacuum into the die cavities to form pockets which are filled with a liquid or semisolid medicament. The unused half of the sheet is folded back over this and the plate is put under a die press which simultaneously seals and stamps out the capsules.

Rotary Die Process. The first continuous process for the manufacture of soft gelatin capsules was the rotary die process which was invented by R. P. Scherer in 1933. Contemporary rotary die machinery is shown in Figure 10-15, and the essential features of the process are diagrammed in Figure 10-16. In this process, the gelatin solution is spread onto two rotating drums to form a pair of continuous sheets of gelatin which are fed between two matched rotary dies. The injection wedge guides the gelatin sheets between the rotary dies, and as the sheets are brought together between the matching die cavities, the fill is simultaneously injected under pressure by means of a metering pump, causing the gelatin to swell into the cavities to form the capsules. At the same time, the pressure of the converging dies seals the capsules and also serves to cut the capsules from the gelatin sheets. The injection wedge heats the gelatin to the proper temperature for sealing. The filled capsules are then deposited on a conveyor which first carries them through a naphtha wash to remove the mineral oil used to lubricate the gelatin strips, and then to an infrared rapid drying stage where most of the water is removed from the shells. Final drying to a moisture content of from 6 to 10 percent is accomplished in forced-air drying tunnels where the moisture content of the shells is allowed to come to equilibrium with relatively dry air (20 to 30% relative humidity at 70 to 75° F.).[86]

This machine is capable of encapsulating anything pumpable that will not adversely affect the gelatin shell. The precision positive displacement pump provides a remarkable fill volume accuracy of ±1 to 3 percent.[86]

Reciprocating Die Process. Developed in 1949 by the Norton Company, this process resembles the Scherer process except that the capsules are formed, sealed, and cut out by the action of vertically positioned reciprocating dies. The action of the dies first forms the capsules as open sacks in the gelatin ribbons which are automatically filled with the drug material. As they pass through the dies, the further reciprocating action of the dies seals and cuts out the capsules. Although the original process requires a pumpable fill, a newer development allows dry beadlike or pelleted substances to be filled in soft gelatin capsules.

Accogel Process. Developed in 1948 by the Lederle Laboratories Division of the American Cyanamid Company, the Accogel, or Stern, machine is another rotary-die type machine for the continuous processing of soft gelatin capsules. This machine is unique in that it is the only one capable of accurately filling dry powders into soft gelatin capsules. Not limited to dry powders, the Accogel machine may be used to encapsulate pumpable fills as well as slugs and pelletized materials.

Official Tests for Capsules

Weight Variation Test. Permissible variations in the weights of individual capsules are provided by the *U.S.P.* and *N.F.* for

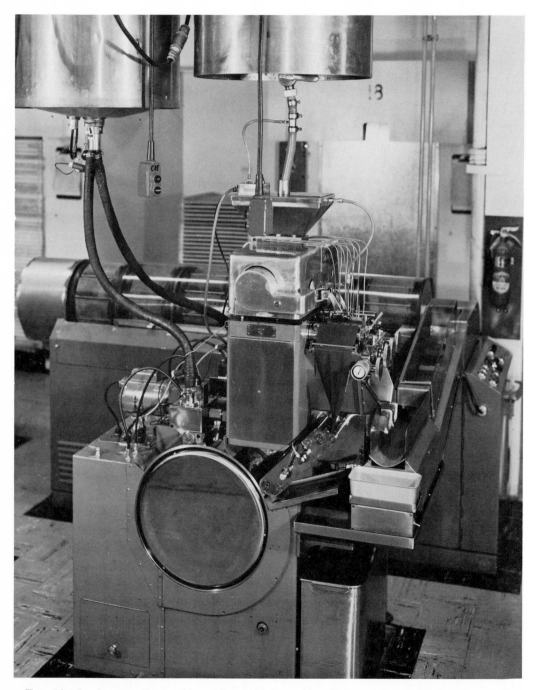

Fig. 10-15.   Rotary die machine for producing soft gelatin capsules. (R. P. Scherer Corporation, Detroit, Michigan)

official capsules which are not required to meet the content uniformity test. In general, the procedure is to weigh 20 intact capsules and determine the average weight. Official requirements are said to be met if the weight of each capsule falls between 90 and 110 percent of the average weight of the sample.

If any of the capsules should fail this requirement, the official compendia provide that the net weight of each capsule be compared to the average net weight of the sample. This removes the possibility that the variability in capsule shell weight may be causing the capsules to fail the first part of

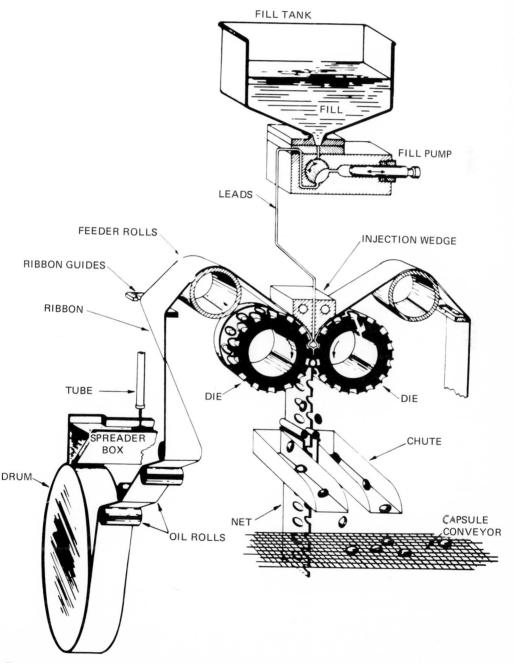

FIG. 10-16.   Diagram of rotary die process. (R. P. Scherer Corporation, Detroit, Michigan)

the test. No more than two of the net weights may deviate from the average net weight by more than 10 percent, and none may deviate by more than 25 percent. If from 2 to 6 of the net weights deviate from the average by 10 to 25 percent, the net weights of an additional 40 capsules are determined, and the net capsule weight of each of the now sixty capsules is compared against the average net capsule weight of all sixty. Official requirements are said to be met if no more than 6 of the net capsule weights deviate from the sixty-capsule mean by 10 percent, provided that none of the deviations exceeds 25 percent.

Hard gelatin capsules must be emptied with the aid of a small brush or cotton pledget and the weight of each empty shell subtracted from its respective filled gross weight to determine the net weight. In the case of soft gelatin capsules, individual shell weights are determined by cutting the capsules open with a suitable clean, dry instrument, removing the contents with a suitable solvent, and allowing the shells to dry for a prescribed period of time prior to weighing.

This test was designed primarily for evaluating commercial capsules. The student should note that the test measures precision rather than accuracy, since each capsule net or gross weight is compared against the sample mean rather than the true or correct value.

Content Uniformity. The control of weight variation may be generally presumed to be a sufficient control over the uniformity of actual drug content in individual capsules if the unit dose of the drug is large and there is relatively little diluent or excipient present. In the case of more potent, low-dose drugs that constitute a relatively small portion of the encapsulated mass, the control of weight variation does not offer sufficient assurance of the uniformity of drug content, since adequate blending may not have been achieved. As had been noted in a former section (see p. 312), even with perfect blending, uniformity of content cannot be reasonably assured if there are too few active drug particles in a critical quantity. Thus, with the increasing use of potent low-dose drugs, content uniformity in solid dosage forms has become an increasingly

important consideration, and the development of analytical procedures that make feasible single capsule or tablet assays has made possible the control of individual dosage unit variation of many drugs. Accordingly, the official compendia have established a content uniformity test for tablets and capsules containing 50 mg. or less of drug (so long as unit dose assays are feasible). The *N.F.* extends the concept to sterile solids as well.

In the official test, 30 capsules are selected and 10 of these are assayed individually. At least 9 of these must fall within 85 to 115 percent of the average of the tolerances specified in the monograph potency definition, and none may fall below 75 percent or above 125 percent of that average. If 1 to 3 of them fall outside of the 85 and 115 percent limits, the remaining 20 capsules are individually assayed, and the requirements are said to be met if no fewer than 27 fall within the 85 percent and 115 percent limits and none fall outside the 75 percent and 125 percent limits.

Disintegration. Although the official compendia have traditionally required tablets to pass a disintegration test, capsules have not been required to meet a disintegration time limit because of the rapidity with which the gelatin shell dissolves in the stomach. However, the compendia state that enteric capsules, i.e., capsules treated to resist gastric fluid (see p. 338), shall meet the requirements for the disintegration of enteric-coated tablets, and the student is referred to the official compendia for a discussion of this test.

Dissolution. Disintegration of a tablet or dissolution of a capsule shell does not imply complete dissolution of the active ingredient. Since the dissolution of a drug is considered to be an essential step in the absorption process, the availability of a drug for absorption from a dosage form largely depends on the drugs dissolving in gastrointestinal fluids. Often dissolution is the rate-limiting step (i.e., the slowest step) in the over-all absorption process. As will be discussed in a later section (p. 335), various factors, including the physicochemical properties of the drug, how it is formulated, and how it is processed can significantly affect drug availability. As an alternative to disintegration, the official dissolution test sets standards for the amount of drug that dissolves in a specified period of time under certain specific conditions.

No relationship should be assumed between any in-vitro dissolution test and availability in vivo unless a correlation has first been established between the dissolution data and the clinical tests. Presently, the official compendia have established a dissolution requirement for thirteen capsule and tablet dosage forms for which such a correlation has been made with specific formulations, and it may be anticipated that more tablets and capsules will be required to meet a dissolution requirement as the individual standards are developed. However, it is unlikely that such a requirement will be established for drugs that are sufficiently soluble or drugs that are in solution at the time of administration.[12]

A rotating basket dissolution apparatus is official in both the *U.S.P.* and *N.F.* In general, the capsule or tablet sample is placed in a basket formed from 40-mesh stainless steel fabric. A stirrer shaft is attached to the basket, and the basket is immersed in the dissolution medium and caused to rotate at a specified speed. The dissolution medium (900 ml., unless otherwise specified in the individual monograph) is held in a covered 1000-ml. vessel (such as a resin flask) made of glass or other inert transparent material. The lid has four holes: two to accommodate the stirrer shaft and a thermometer, two for sampling and fluids exchange. The dissolution medium is maintained at $37° \pm 0.5°$ by means of a suitable constant-temperature water bath. The stirrer speed and type of dissolution medium are specified in the individual monograph. Samples are withdrawn at specified intervals and assayed to determine the extent of dissolution. Six capsules or tablets are individually tested, and if one or two fail to meet the monograph requirements, 6 more are tested, and 10 of the 12 must meet the requirement.

Only the rotating basket assembly is specified in the *U.S.P.* However, the *N.F.* also specifies an oscillating basket assembly which is essentially the traditional tablet disintegration apparatus. Each *N.F.* monograph specifies which test apparatus to use. For complete details of both dissolution apparatus and test procedures, the student is referred to the official compendia.

SPECIAL PROBLEMS IN POWDERED DOSAGE FORMS

Hygroscopicity and Deliquescence

The sorption of water can have a profound effect on the physical and chemical stability of pharmaceutical powders. The presence of moisture encourages chemical reactions that may lead to loss of potency or to the formation of an insoluble reaction product on the drug surface which may inhibit drug availability.[76] If not kept dry, an effervescent salt may react slowly on storage, resulting in a mixture no longer capable of effervescence. At the very least, sorbed moisture can result in poor powder flow properties.

Moisture usually condenses on the surface of a substance exposed to the atmosphere. At a given temperature, condensation increases with increases in the partial pressure of water vapor in the atmosphere to which the substance is exposed. *Hygroscopicity* is the ability of a substance to attract and retain moisture, a characteristic that varies widely with the nature of the substance.[15, 73, 91] In general, water molecules are strongly attracted by surface ions and dipoles. Because it is a surface phenomenon, the amount of water adsorbed by a given weight of powder at a given temperature and water vapor pressure increases as the specific surface area of the powder increases. The term *adsorption* strictly applies to the uptake of material at surfaces and should be differentiated from *absorption* wherein the material penetrates into the bulk of the absorbing substance; the more general term *sorption* is applicable to either phenomenon.[15]

Some of the compound may dissolve in the sorbed water to form a saturated solution on the surface of the solid. Since the vapor pressure over a solution of a nonvolatile solute is less than that of the pure solvent, the vapor pressure of water over the saturated solution must be depressed. The lowering of the vapor pressure of the solvent depends on the relative number of solute particles in solution.* Thus, if the solubility of the compound is high, the water vapor pressure over the saturated solution may be depressed to below that of the partial pressure of water vapor in the atmosphere. If such is the case, more water will be sorbed, and more of the compound will dissolve, the cycle leading ultimately to complete dissolution of the compound. This phenomenon in which a compound sorbs water and dissolves on standing when exposed to the atmosphere is called *deliquescence*.[15, 16] A compound will deliquesce only if the water vapor pressure over a saturated solution of the compound is less than the partial pressure of water vapor in the atmosphere to which it is exposed. Examples of compounds that are known to deliquesce when exposed to usual ambient humidities are calcium chloride, choline chloride, methacholine bromide, and potassium acetate.

Generally, a divided powder is not an ideal dosage form for hygroscopic materials. Divided powders containing such substances should be double wrapped, as previously described, to exclude moisture. However, better protection from atmospheric moisture is possible with sealed polyethylene envelopes.

In the case of gelatin capsules, the shell itself does not provide hygroscopic contents adequate protection from atmospheric moisture;[92] therefore, capsules containing such materials should be packaged in tight moistureproof containers. Inclusion of a tube or packet of desiccant helps to maintain dryness on repeated opening of the container during use.

Depending on the relative hygroscopicity of the gelatin shell and its contents, a capsule shell may gain moisture from, or lose moisture to, its contents.[44, 92] Thus, deliquescent materials may dehydrate capsule shells sufficiently to cause splitting or

cracking. This has been observed, for example, with potassium acetate.[41]

The physical stability of divided powders and capsules containing hygroscopic materials may be improved by adding to the powder inert finely divided substances which preferentially sorb moisture. The colloidal silica type glidants, for example, have the ability to sorb large quantities of moisture. Traditionally, pharmacists have used materials such as magnesium oxide, magnesium carbonate, talc, and starch. Husa and Becker[41] made a study of several sorbents in various deliquescent capsule formulations. In most cases, they found that inert sorbents were not helpful when the capsules were stored in an open container. When the capsules were stored in airtight glass containers, it was found that inert sorbents were not usually needed. However, in some instances physical stability was improved by the addition of a sorbent. Most effective in this regard were magnesium carbonate and light magnesium oxide, followed by heavy magnesium oxide and talc. Starch and lactose were least effective. Magnesium oxide should be used with caution because its alkalinity in the presence of moisture causes ester hydrolysis.

Efflorescence

The water of crystallization in crystal hydrates is bound reversibly within the crystal lattice, and the hydrate exerts a definite vapor pressure. When exposed to an atmosphere in which the partial pressure of water vapor is less than the vapor pressure of the hydrate, the hydrate will spontaneously give up some or all of its water of crystallization, i.e., it will *effloresce,* to form a lower hydrate or the anhydrous form.[15, 16] Examples of drugs that effloresce in low humidity include citric acid monohydrate, sodium borate, terpin hydrate, and zinc sulfate.

On a weight basis, a hydrated drug is less potent than its corresponding lower hydrate or anhydrous form, and the difference may be significant. Thus, if a hydrated drug effloresces in a dry atmosphere, an overdose may result if the loss of water of crystallization is ignored during weighing.[76]

---

* This is a *colligative* property, i.e., a property that depends on the relative number of solute particles in solution, rather than their nature. Other colligative properties of solutions are osmotic pressure, boiling point elevation, and freezing point depression.

The heat and pressure of trituration promote the release of water of crystallization. Damp masses may result when such hydrates as sodium sulfate, ferrous sulfate, alum, and sodium phosphate are triturated. In such cases, light mixing or the addition of inert sorbents is helpful; however, it is preferable to use the anhydrous form of the salts. When these forms are not available, the hydrates may be dried prior to mixing.

Eutectics

An interesting phenomenon which occasionally occurs when two chemicals of relatively low melting points are mixed together is the formation of a liquid or a pasty mass. It is commonly known that impurities lower melting points. When two chemicals are mixed together—for example, in the compounding of solid dosage forms—each may act as an impurity in respect to the other and cause a mutual lowering of melting points. If the original melting points are low, the intimate mixture of the two may lower the melting point to below room temperature and a liquid will be formed.

The pharmacist can generally expect liquefaction from the intimate mixing of substances having low intermolecular attractive forces, such as the phenolic, aldehydic, or ketonic compounds.[77] Pharmaceutical examples, include acetophenetidin, acetylsalicylic acid, antipyrine, camphor, chloral hydrate, menthol, phenol, phenylsalicylate, and salicylic acid. How much liquefaction occurs depends on (a) the room temperature, (b) the original melting points of the substances involved, (c) the proportions in which the two substances are mixed, and (d) the presence of any additional substances which may delay liquefaction or sorb the liquid upon formation.

The influence of temperature and composition on the amount of liquefaction can be best illustrated by means of a phase diagram.[22] The familiar binary phase diagram for a simple eutectic is illustrated in Figure 10-17. The melting point (or freezing point) of each of the two compounds is lowered by the other compound. The lowest melting blend of A and B occurs at point E, the *eutectic point,* and the composition of this mixture is the *eutectic mixture* in a physicochemical sense. The latter should be differentiated from a *pharmaceutical eutectic mixture,* which may be defined as two or more

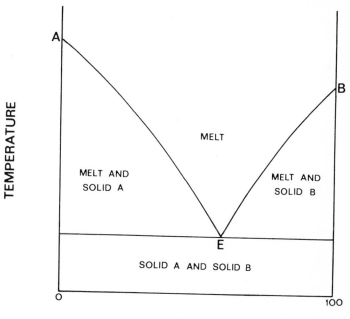

FIG. 10-17. Diagram of a simple binary eutectic system in which the two components are perfectly miscible in the liquid state and perfectly insoluble in the solid state. A, melting point of pure compound "A"; B, melting point of pure compound "B"; E, the eutectic point.

substances which liquefy to any extent when intimately mixed at room temperature.[77] Along AE, pure compound A separates from the melt; long BE, pure compound B separates. The temperature at the eutectic point is the *eutectic temperature,* and this is the lowest temperature at which a liquid phase can exist in the system. The solid which forms below the eutectic temperature consists of a fine-grained physical mixture of compounds A and B.

As can be seen, there will always be some liquid at temperatures above the eutectic temperature, regardless of the composition. However, under curve AE, the relative proportion (mass) of solid A to liquid increases at a given temperature in mixtures richer in compound A. Similarly, under curve BE, the relative proportion of solid B to liquid increases at a given temperature in mixtures richer in component B. For any given mixture of A and B under curves AE and BE, the relative proportion of solid to liquid decreases with increases in temperature.

In the foregoing discussion is has been assumed that the crystals which separate out are the pure components. In certain systems, the components which crystallize out under curves AE and BE may precipitate out with some of the other component in the form of mixed crystals or solid solutions. Some degree of solid solution formation may be anticipated in all binary systems; however, the degree of solubility is usually not sufficient to be considered significant.[33, 58] Goldberg et al.[33] indicated that, for practical purposes, solid solution formation may be considered significant if one component is soluble (in the solid state) in the other to the extent of 5 percent or more; more recently, others have suggested that this limit may be somewhat high.[17] Solid solutions are homogeneous single phases, and may be interstitial (the molecules of one component occupying the interstitial spaces of the other's crystal lattice) or substitutional (the molecules of one component replacing molecules of the other in the crystal lattice).[58] As will be discussed in a later section (p. 336), solid solution formation has important implications for drug availability from solid dosage forms.

It is clear that any mixture that has a eutectic temperature below room temperature will exhibit some degree of liquefaction.

There are two approaches to the dispensing of pharmaceutical eutectic mixtures. Both involve the addition of inert, high-melting, finely divided substances. In one case, the two solids with low melting points may be mixed separately with the inert powder and the two triturations lightly blended together; or alternatively, one of the troublesome ingredients may be mixed with the inert powder before mixing with the other ingredients by light trituration.[40] This technique is intended to separate the troublesome ingredients, but may serve to only delay liquefaction. However, sufficient inert powder may have been used to sorb any liquid that might eventually form. Husa and Becker[40] evaluated several such protectives and found magnesium carbonate and light magnesium oxide to be the most effective of those tested, followed by heavy magnesium oxide. Talc, lactose, and various starches appeared to be the least effective. Magnesium carbonate appears to be the agent of choice because, in certain instances, magnesium oxide (light or heavy) caused cementlike masses to form which did not disintegrate in a 0.5 percent solution of hydrochloric acid.

In the second approach, the liquid is allowed—and even encouraged—to form, and enough of an inert sorbent such as magnesium carbonate or kaolin is added to cause dryness.[10] Since, in the former approach, it is difficult to predict whether or not the amount of protective that had been added would be enough to sorb any liquid that might eventually form, the latter method of preforming the eutectic may be the more practical one.

Addition of Liquids

Pharmacists are occasionally required to incorporate small quantities of liquids in powders. As was previously pointed out in the section on *Blending,* care should be taken to achieve as good a blend as possible of the dry powders before adding the liquid. The liquid may be added, small portions at a time, to a portion of the powder, with trituration, and the remainder of the powder added in portions while triturating.

Fluidextracts and tinctures may be concentrated over a water bath or the pharmacist may replace the alcoholic preparation with an equivalent amount of the corresponding powdered extract. When an alcoholic preparation is concentrated, the resulting small volume of liquid should be sorbed with an inert powder such as lactose, which may then be incorporated into the powder blend.

Small quantities of volatile oils are often incorporated into powders as flavors. When volatile oils or any other volatile ingredients such as camphor or menthol are incorporated into powders, care should be taken to prevent their loss by evaporation. Divided powders should be double wrapped or sealed in individual polyethylene envelopes. Bulk powders and capsules should be packaged in tight glass containers.

Mixtures That Explode

Mixtures of strong oxidizing agents, such as potassium chlorate or potassium permanganate, with organic materials, such as sugar, starch, sulfur, and tannic acid, are potentially explosive and should not be triturated. Although the ingredients may be individually triturated and then lightly mixed by spatulation or tumbling, such mixtures should never be dispensed.

FACTORS AFFECTING DRUG AVAILABILITY FROM POWDERED DOSAGE FORMS

Drug availability refers to delivery of the drug to the site of absorption in a form in which it will be absorbed. Generally, the availability of a drug for absorption is affected by the physicochemical properties of the drug itself, and by the type of dosage form and how it is formulated.

Some Physicochemical Properties of the Drug Affecting Availability

Particle Size and Surface Area. When drugs are administered orally in solid dosage forms, certain events must take place before absorption can occur. Tablets disintegrate to produce fragments, granules, and aggregates of primary particles. Capsule shells dissolve

to release aggregates of powdered drug and any excipients present. Primary drug particles are produced following a deaggregation process. In all cases, however, dissolution of the drug must occur in gastrointestinal fluids before absorption can occur. For drugs that are inherently slowly dissolving, the dissolution step may well be the slowest step in the over-all absorption process. In such cases, the absorption process is said to be dissolution rate limited. Some drugs may dissolve so slowly that absorption is never complete.

The factors governing dissolution rate were described by Noyes and Whitney[70]:

$$\frac{dw}{dt} = KS(C_s - C)$$

where $\frac{dw}{dt}$ is the dissolution rate, K is the dissolution rate constant, C_s is the solubility of the material in the dissolution medium, C is the concentration of the material in the dissolution medium at any given time, t, and S is the surface area of the dissolving substance. According to the model, a diffusion layer consisting of a saturated solution (concentration $= C_s$) surrounds the dissolving particle, and the rate of dissolution depends on the rate of diffusion of solute molecules through the diffusion layer to the body of the solution (concentration $= C$) down the concentration gradient $(C_s - C)$. The constant K incorporates the diffusion layer thickness and diffusion coefficient. It is apparent that anything that increases the solubility of the drug also increases the dissolution rate. The Noyes-Whitney relationship also points up the direct relationship between dissolution rate and surface area. The greater the surface area, the greater the rate of dissolution. In the case of dissolution rate limited absorption, anything that would increase the rate of dissolution would also increase the rate of absorption. When a drug is so slowly soluble that normally absorption is not complete, an increase in dissolution rate results in an increase in not only the rate of absorption but also in the total amount of drug absorbed.

For a given weight of drug, particle size is inversely related to surface area. Thus, a given weight of micronized drug would be expected to exhibit a faster rate of dissolution than the same weight of larger particles. Although more efficient absorption resulting from the administration of drugs in smaller particle size has been reported in several instances, the classic example is griseofulvin.[6] It was found that 0.5 g. of griseofulvin micronized to a particle size of 2.6 μ produced blood levels in man similar to 1 g. of the drug at a particle size of 10 μ.

Particle size reduction does not necessarily result in a faster rate of absorption. An increase in specific surface area has no influence on readily soluble drugs, i.e., when dissolution rate is not the rate determining step in absorption. For example, no effect of particle size on absorption rate was observed with soluble tetracycline hydrochloride.[64]

Crystal Form. Drug availability may also be significantly influenced by crystal form. Many drugs are known to exhibit *polymorphism*—that is, they are capable of existing in more than one crystal form. The solubility of a *metastable* (less stable) form of a compound is greater than its corresponding *stable* form and may well be preferred in the development of a dosage form. In one example, polymorphic form II of methylprednisolone was found to have 1.2 times the water solubility of the stable form (I).[8] The absorption rate of form II was found to be 1.7 times that of form I from pellets implanted subcutaneously in rats. The in-vitro dissolution rate of form II was shown to be about 1.4 times that of form I.[34]

The *amorphous* or *noncrystalline* form of a drug is more soluble than its crystalline form, and this may significantly affect blood levels. For instance, crystalline novobiocin produced no detectable blood levels on oral administration, whereas the amorphous form produced significant blood levels and therapeutic activity.[60]

Salt Form. The salt form of a compound can influence the rate of absorption of a drug through its effect on dissolution rate.[63, 65] For instance, the water-soluble salts of most weak acids are intrinsically more rapidly soluble than the weak acids themselves. Surprisingly, this is also true in acidic media, such as would be encountered in the stomach. This is so because the salt

acts as a buffer to raise the pH in the diffusion layer around the particles, thus increasing C_s in the Noyes-Whitney equation (p. 335). Precipitation of the free acid may occur in the bulk of the acidic solution; however, this also encourages absorption because the drug usually precipitates as ultrafine particles. The significance of salt form was demonstrated, for example, with tolbutamide where the sodium salt resulted in greater blood sugar lowering than the free acid after one hour in man.[66]

Hydrates. The anhydrous form of a drug may be more desirable than the corresponding hydrate from the point of view of dissolution rate. The anhydrous forms of caffeine, theophylline, and glutethimide have been reported to exhibit higher dissolution rates than their corresponding hydrates.[85]

Formulation Factors Affecting Drug Availability

In addition to particle size and the other physicochemical properties of the drug, factors that may affect the availability of drugs from powders include the nature of the diluents or other formulation components and their possible interaction with the active ingredient. Other factors are introduced when powders are encapsulated. Since the economic importance of capsules as a dosage form far overshadows that of powders in contemporary pharmacy, this section will be devoted primarily to capsules.

Drug Particle Size. The importance of particle size in drug availability has already been discussed. The usual approach with poorly soluble drugs is to subject the drug to an appropriate mechanical comminution process. A unique approach to particle size reduction was reported by Sekiguchi and Obi.[83] These investigators formed a *eutectic mixture* of a poorly soluble drug, sulfathiazole, with a water-soluble carrier, urea. The eutectic temperature of this mixture is well above room temperature so that the mixture was solid. To form the mixture, the two components were blended and melted. The melt was then solidified by chilling and pulverized. According to the principles discussed on page 333, the solid eutectic mixture consists of a fine-grained physical mixture of the two substances.

Thus, when such a mixture is exposed to aqueous fluids, the water-soluble carrier is rapidly washed away, leaving a dispersion of ultrafine crystals—in this case, of sulfathiazole. These investigators confirmed that the eutectic mixture did, indeed, yield both a faster dissolution rate in vitro and a faster absorption rate in vivo than the pure crystals.

As an extension of this concept, Goldberg et al.[33] described what they considered the "ultimate achievement of this approach," i.e., *solid solution* formation. A solid solution formed between a poorly soluble drug and a water-soluble carrier would leave the drug molecularly dispersed in gastrointestinal fluids when the carrier washes away. Goldberg et al.[33] noted from Sekiguchi and Obi's phase diagram that the sulfathiazole-urea system actually exhibits a significant degree of solid-solid solubility. They further noted that the enhanced rates of dissolution and absorption reported by those investigators were likely due at least as much to solid solution formation as to eutectic mixture formation alone. An extensive review of the current status of this technology and the pharmaceutic utility of solid dispersion systems has been presented by Chiou and Riegelman.[17]

Hard Gelatin Capsules. The over-all dissolution rate of a drug from capsules may be regarded as a function of several variables[69]: (1) the dissolution rate of the shell, (2) the rate of penetration of the dissolution medium into the powder, (3) the rate at which the powder mass deaggregates, and (4) the nature of the primary particles. The formulation factors influencing the in-vitro and the in-vivo dissolution rates of drugs from capsules have been listed by Wagner.[101] These include the amount and nature of adjuvants, including diluents, lubricants, surfactants (if used), and others. Also noted were steps taken to reduce bulk (such as granulation), particle size and size distribution, the degree of powder compaction during filling, and the composition and characteristics of the capsule shell.

As was pointed out in previous sections, the dissolution of the capsule shell is generally considered to take place rapidly and to be a negligible factor in drug availability. However, the shell may influence the very early stages of drug release. Whitley and Mainville[103] found that the in-vitro dissolution of some formulations did not begin until a "minute or so" after the test began, and attributed this to the "gelatin capsule effect."

Newton et al.[68, 69] conducted statistically designed experiments to evaluate the effect of various formulation variables on the in-vitro availability of a hydrophobic drug, ethinamate, from capsules. Three levels of diluent (lactose at 0, 10, and 50%), lubricant (magnesium stearate at 0, 1, and 5%), and surfactant (sodium lauryl sulfate at 0, 1, and 10%) were evaluated. In general, their results may be summarized as follows:

1. Increasing the concentration of the water-soluble diluent lactose to 50 percent produced an increase in drug release, apparently by making the powder matrix more hydrophilic.

2. The presence of the hydrophobic lubricant magnesium stearate had the general effect of making the powder bed less easily wetted by the dissolution medium, thus reducing drug release.

3. The general effect of the surfactant is to make the powder bed more easily wetted by the dissolution medium and hence, enhance drug release. The effect of the lubricant may be offset by the presence of a surfactant.

An interesting case illustrating the influence of formulation on drug availability involved *diphenylhydantoin*.[3] Australian physicians had observed in the course of their practice that an unusual number of patients using a particular product were exhibiting symptoms of diphenylhydantoin toxicity. When the manufacturer was consulted, it was found that the filler had been changed from calcium sulfate to lactose. The increased incidence of toxic reactions appeared to be due to an increase in the physiological availability of the drug when lactose is the filler.

Aguiar et al.[1, 2] found that the differences in drug availability among four different lots of *chloramphenicol* capsules could be related to their rates of *deaggregation* in vitro. The capsules, which contained equivalent amounts of the drug, were produced by different manufacturers. The product exhibiting the highest blood levels and fastest rate of absorption in man also showed the fastest rate of deaggregation; the product yielding the lowest mean blood levels showed the slowest deaggregation rate. The two products giving intermediate blood levels showed intermediate deaggregation rates.

Poor deaggregation may be due to the presence of a hydrophobic lubricant. Samyn and Jung[82] found that the in-vitro release of a water-soluble dye from experimental capsule formulations was severely retarded by the presence of 5 percent magnesium stearate. After dissolution of the capsule shell, a wet powder mass of high consistency formed which only slowly eroded and dissolved. Data were presented which suggested that this high consistency mass was the result of limited penetration of the powder mass by the dissolution medium.

Seemingly inert fillers may complex with the active ingredient. A classical example is the *tetracyclines,* which were originally formulated using dicalcium phosphate as the filler. It was found that the calcium formed a poorly soluble complex with the drug, making some of the drug unavailable for absorption.[14]

Soft Gelatin Capsules. Recent studies have suggested that, with proper formulation, liquid-filled soft gelatin capsules may be more desirable than tablets for low dose drugs, poorly soluble drugs, or drugs for which rapidly attained high blood levels are desired.[36, 37] Soft gelatin capsules appear to sorb water on contact and split at the seams to release their liquid fill. The proper choice of vehicle may promote rapid dispersion of the drug content. In two similar studies, a combined total of 20 different drugs were formulated in soft gelatin capsules using a rotary die process, and their in-vitro release characteristics were compared with those of commercial tablets of the same drugs purchased on the open market (except chloramphenicol, which the investigators tableted themselves). In preparing the liquid fill for the soft gelatin capsules, the drugs were dissolved in polyethylene glycol 400, or suspended in various polyols with 1 to 3 percent of a nonionic surface-active agent. In other instances, the vehicle was the surfactant itself or a mixture of nonionic surfactants. In all cases, the dissolution rate from soft gelatin capsules was faster than from the corresponding tablets.

It was concluded that, with the proper choice of vehicle, it is possible to solubilize many low-dose, poorly soluble drugs, but high-dose and very insoluble drugs are better encapsulated as suspensions. The use of solubilizers and/or surface-active agents appears to enhance drug solubility and/or dispersibility in the dissolution medium, and this offers promise for improved absorption rates. However, no comparative in-vivo studies were reported.

Enteric Coated Capsules. Capsules that have been coated or otherwise treated to resist dissolution in gastric fluids but release their contents in the intestine are said to be *enteric.* Such delayed release of medication may be desired if the drug is inactivated in gastric fluids or if the drug is irritating to the gastric mucosa. In other instances, a high local concentration of the drug may be especially desirable in the intestine, as in the case of anthelmenthics.

Depending on the nature of the enteric coating material, breakdown in the intestine may depend on one or more of several factors. The coating may be insoluble at gastric pH's but dissolve in the less acidic, but not necessarily alkaline, environment of the intestine. Other materials may be digested by intestinal enzymes or emulsified by bile salts. Still other coatings may gradually break down with time, owing to moisture penetration and erosion, and ultimately release their contents in the intestine. Typical of materials used for enteric coating are shellac, cellulose acetate phthalate, and fatty, waxy materials such as beeswax, carnauba wax, and stearic acid. One approach for rendering gelatin capsules enteric that has met with only limited success is treatment with formaldehyde. The gelatin is hardened as the formaldehyde reacts with the gelatin to form methylene bridges and cross links.

Although he is seldom called upon to do so, the pharmacist has several approaches at his disposal for the *extemporaneous enteric coating* of hard gelatin capsules. In the older method, the filled capsules are carefully dipped in melted salol (phenyl salicylate).

In more recent years, the use of salol has largely given way to a mixture consisting of 45 parts of n-butyl stearate, 30 parts of carnauba wax, and 25 parts of stearic acid.[88] In practice this mixture is heated to about 70°C. to form a melt. Half of the capsule is first coated by dipping one end into the melt with tweezers. The capsule is removed, the coat is allowed to harden, and then the other end is dipped to form a coat that slightly overlaps the first coat.

An alternative procedure for the extemporaneous enteric coating of capsules that avoids heat and adds less bulk to the capsules is to dip them into a 10 percent solution of cellulose acetate phthalate in acetone.[72] After immersing the capsule in the solution, it is removed with tweezers, held for a minute, and then placed on gauze to finish drying. Three coats are usually applied. Disintegration in the intestine is due to hydrolysis by intestinal enzymes and ionization of the phthalate carboxyl groups in the less acidic conditions found in the intestine. More recently, two polylvinyl acetate resins were recommended for coating solutions, consisting of 12 percent of the resin, 10 percent of castor oil (as a plasticizer), and 78 percent acetone.[20]

Sustained Release.[84, 87, 94] When medication is administered, a peak blood level is reached which immediately begins to fall as the drug is detoxified or eliminated. Ordinarily, enough drug must be administered in a capsule or tablet to produce a blood level somewhat in excess of the minimum therapeutic concentration so that a therapeutic level can be maintained for several hours. Frequently, after 3 or 4 hours, the blood level will have fallen to well below the minimum effective level, and another dose must be administered. A larger single dose may be given which will take longer to be detoxified or eliminated and thus sustain the blood level above the minimum effective level for a longer period of time, but the initial peak concentration may well be capable of producing toxic reactions.

As an alternative to this, a *sustained release* dosage form may be designed to provide a therapeutic blood level of a drug which is reached relatively rapidly and is maintained within relatively narrow limits

for extended periods of time, usually 10 to 12 hours.[84] Accordingly, blood levels are more uniform and there is a minimum of the highs and lows associated with divided dosage therapy; the drug is more efficiently utilized, and total drug intake is reduced. From the patient's point of view, as well as that of the nursing staff, administration is more convenient, since a single dose provides all-day or all-night medication. In general, a sustained release dosage form may be regarded as consisting of two parts: (1) an immediate release portion, and (2) a sustained release portion which, ideally, gradually releases medication at a rate equal to the rate at which the drug is eliminated or detoxified.

Certain drugs are more suitable for sustained release formulation than others.[84] Drugs such as antibiotics or muscle relaxants may have large doses, possibly making sustained release dosage forms inappropriately large. Others, such as the digitalis glycosides or reserpine, would not be suitable because they are inherently long acting. Sustained release dosage forms do not lend themselves to adjustment or manipulation of dosage; therefore such dosage forms are more suitable for drugs used in the management of chronic conditions, rather than acute illnesses. After release of the initial portion of the medication, a sustained release dosage form is designed to release medication gradually as it passes through the gastrointestinal tract; therefore the drug should, ideally, be uniformly absorbed throughout the gastrointestinal tract.

Numerous approaches to the designing of sustained release dosage forms are possible; several involve capsules. The Spansule* is a hard gelatin capsule containing many specially coated beads.[84] The medication is usually pan-coated onto the surface of sugar-starch beads using a nonaqueous solution of the drug. A portion of these drug-coated beads is intended to provide the initial release of medication, and these receive no further treatment. The remainder (approximately ⅔ to ¾ of the beads) are then pan-coated with a fatty, waxy material such as

---

* Registered Trademark, SmithKline Corporation.

beeswax or glyceryl monostearate or a cellulosic material such as ethyl cellulose. Different portions of the beads receive different thicknesses of coating. Usually three or more such batches are blended to provide the desired sustained release pattern. Release is primarily dependent on moisture penetration of the fatty material which, in turn, depends on the composition and thickness of the coat. If the dose of the drug is large, granules of the drug itself replace the beads in the process (e.g., Fortespan*).

Medules† are also an encapsulated coated bead product.[84] The granules of the sustained release portion are coated with styrene-maleic acid copolymer. The coat is pH sensitive and disintegrates at intestinal pH's. Release is also dependent on the stomach emptying rate.

Strasionic‡ resins represent a completely different concept in sustained release capsules.[84] Here, for example, in Biphetamine‡ capsules, a cationic drug is sorbed onto a cationic exchange resin. The resin consists of a polystyrene cross linked with divinyl benzene and sulfonated to render it cationic. Drug release depends on both pH and electrolyte concentration in gastrointestinal fluids.

Another approach is to form an insoluble complex by reacting a drug possessing an amine group with tannic acid in an alcoholic solution.[84] After precipitation, washing, and drying, the complex may be either encapsulated or tableted. The solubility of the complex is greatest at gastric pH's and diminishes at intestinal pH's. Too rapid dissolution in the stomach is avoided by adding pectic or galacturonic acids for their buffering effect.

Although no sustained release capsules or tablets are currently official, an in-vitro release test for such preparations was first adopted in the Second Supplement to N.F. XII, and formally incorporated in N.F. XIII. This test procedure is presented in the interest of (1) providing a useful means of setting appropriate test criteria for assuring product uniformity of the majority of sustained release products, (2) promoting interlaboratory uniformity in such testing, and (3) providing guidelines and direction in the development of acceptable testing procedures. The procedure is not intended to establish official specifications for any preparations official in the *N.F.* Naturally, as with any such in-vitro test procedures, suitable in-vitro release limits can be established only when the data have been correlated with in-vivo studies and clinical evaluation.

In general, the test apparatus consists of 5 round screw capped bottles clamped to a shaft which rotates at 40 r.p.m. in a constant temperature water bath (37 $\pm$0.5°C.). The device has a rotational capability of from 6 to 50 r.p.m. An appropriate number of sustained release capsules or tablets are placed in each of the bottles along with 60 ml. of an extraction fluid. There are five extraction fluids representing pH's of 1.2, 2.5, 4.5, 7.0, and 7.5. These are comprised of simulated gastric fluid, T.S. (pH 1.2), simulated intestinal fluid, T.S. (pH 7.5), or stated mixtures of these two fluids. Beginning with the pH 1.2 fluid, each extraction fluid is replaced with the next higher pH fluid after 1, 2, 3.5, 5, and 7 hours of rotation. To determine the drug release rate, one bottle is removed from the test at each time interval, and the sample residue is assayed for drug content.

REFERENCES AND BIBLIOGRAPHY

1. Aguiar, A. J.: Physical properties and pharmaceutical factors influencing absorption of chloramphenicol and chloramphenicol palmitate. Drug Inf. Bull., 3(1):17, (1969.
2. Aguiar, A. J., Wheeler, L. M., Fusari, S., and Zelmar, J. E.: Evaluation of physical and pharmaceutical factors involved in drug release and availability from chloramphenicol capsules. J. Pharm. Sci., 57:1844, 1968.
3. Anon.: Diphenylhydantoin. Clin-Alert, No. 299, Dec. 8, 1970.
4. Ansell, H. C.: Introduction to Pharmaceutical Dosage Forms. pp. 265–286. Philadelphia, Lea and Febiger, 1969.
5. Arnold, K., Gerber, N., and Levy, G.: Absorption and dissolution studies on sodium diphenylhydantoin capsules. Canad. J. Pharm. Sci., 5(4):89, 1970.
6. Atkinson, R. M., Bedford, C. B., Child, K. J., and Tomlik, E. G.: Effect of particle size on blood griseofulvin levels in man. Nature, 193:588, 1962.

---

* Registered Trademark, SmithKline Corporation.
† Registered Trademark, The Upjohn Company.
‡ Registered Trademark, Strasenburgh Labs.

7. Augsburger, L. L., and Shangraw, R. F.: Effect of glidants in tableting. J. Pharm. Sci., 55:418, 1966.

8. Ballard, B. E., and Nelson, E.: Physicochemical properties of drugs that control absorption. J. Pharmacol. Exp. Ther., 135:120, 1962.

9. Belcher, D. W., Smith, D. A., and Cook, E. M.: Design and use of spray driers. I. Principles and applications. II. Design and costs. Chem. Eng., 70(20):83, 1963; 70(21):201, 1963.

10. Bellafiori, I. J.: Stabilization of capsules and eutectic mixtures against liquefaction. J. Am. Pharm. A. (Pract. Ed.), 14:580, 1953.

11. Benarie, M. M.: Rheology of granular material. II. A method for the determination of the intergranular cohesion. Brit. J. Appl. Physics, 12:514, 1961.

12. Blake, M. I.: Role of the compendia in controlling factors affecting bioavailability of drug products. J. Am. Pharm. A., NS11:603, 1971.

13. Blubaugh, F. C.: Mixing Methods, Equipment and Control. Paper presented before the Industrial Pharmaceutical Technology Division, A.Ph.A. 114th Annual Meeting, Las Vegas, April 9–14, 1967.

14. Boger, W. P., and Gavin, J. J.: An evaluation of tetracycline preparations. New Eng. J. Med., 261:827, 1959.

15. Bowden, S. T.: The Phase Rule and Phase Reactions. pp. 74–76. New York, Macmillan, 1960.

16. Campbell, A. N., and Smith, N. O.: The Phase Rule and Its Applications. pp. 224–227, 235–238. New York, Dover, 1951.

17. Chiou, W. L., and Riegelman, S.: Pharmaceutical applications of solid dispersion systems. J. Pharm. Sci., 60:1281, 1971.

18. Clement, H., and Marquardt, H. G.: The Mechanical Processing of Hard Gelatin Capsules. News Sheet 3/70. Capsulgel A. G., CH-4000 Basel, Switzerland.

19. Comminution. Bulletin INF-61. The Fitzpatrick Company, Chicago, Illinois.

20. Cook, C. H., Jr., and Webber, M. G.: An extemporaneous method of preparing enteric-coated capsules. Am. J. Hosp. Pharm., 22:95, 1965.

21. Craik, D. J.: The flow properties of starch powders and mixtures. J. Pharm. Pharmacol., 10:73, 1958.

22. Daniels, F., and Alberty, R. A.: Physical Chemistry. Ed. 2, pp. 244–246. New York, John Wiley & Sons, 1961.

23. Danish, F. Q., and Parrott, E. L.: Flow rates of solid particulate pharmaceuticals. J. Pharm. Sci., 60:548, 1961.

24. Edmundson, I. C.: Particle Size Analysis. In Bean, H. S., Beckett, A. H., and Carless, J. E. (eds.): Advances in Pharmaceutical Sciences. Vol. 2, pp. 95–177. New York, Academic Press, 1967.

25. Felmeister, A.: Powders. In Remington's Pharmaceutical Sciences. Ed. 14, p. 1626–1648. Easton, Pa., Mack Publishing Co., 1970.

26. Fischer, J. J.: Liquid-solids blending. Chem. Eng., 69(3):83, 1962.

27. ———: Solid-solid blending. Chem. Eng., 67(16):107, 1960.

28. Foote, A. P.: Powdered Dosage Forms. In Sprowls, J. B. (ed.): American Pharmacy. 6 Ed., pp. 331–366. Philadelphia, J. B. Lippincott, 1966.

29. Fowler, H. W.: Mixers. 2. Powder mixers. Manuf. Chem., 33:5, 1962.

30. ———: Dryers. 2. Conduction and radiation dryers. Manuf. Chem., 32:301, 314, 1961.

31. Gold, G., Duvall, R. N., and Palermo, B. T.: Powder flow studies. I. Instrumentation and applications. J. Pharm. Sci., 55:1133, 1966.

32. Gold, G., Duvall, R. N., Palermo, B. T., and Slater, J. G.: Powder flow studies. II. Effect of glidants on flow rate and angle of repose. J. Pharm. Sci., 55:1291, 1966.

33. Goldberg, A. H., Gibaldi, M., and Kanig, J. L.: Increasing dissolution rates and gastrointestinal absorption of drugs via solid solutions and eutectic mixtures. I. Theoretical considerations and discussion of the literature. J. Pharm. Sci., 54:1145, 1965.

34. Hamlin, W. E., Nelson, E., Ballard, B. E., and Wagner, J. G.: Loss of sensitivity in distinguishing real differences in dissolution rates due to increasing intensities of agitation. J. Pharm. Sci., 51:432, 1962.

35. Hiestand, E. N.: Powders: Particle-particle interations. J. Pharm. Sci., 55:1325, 1966.

36. Hom, F. S., and Miskel, J. J.: Enhanced dissolution rates for a series of drugs as a function of dosage form design. Lex et Scientia, 8(1):18, 1971.

37. ———: Oral dosage form design and its influence on dissolution rates for a series of drugs. J. Pharm. Sci., 59:827, 1970.

38. Hosman, P. S.: One million air-conditioned capsules per day. Drug & Cosmetic Ind., 73:768, 1953.

39. Hostetler, V. B., and Bellard, J. Q.: Capsules. I. Hard Capsules. In Lachman, L., Lieberman, H. A., and Kanig, J. L. (eds.): Theory and Practice of Industrial Pharmacy. pp. 346–359. Philadelphia, Lea and Febiger, 1970.

40. Husa, W. J., and Becker, C. H.: Incompatibilities and prescriptions. III. The use of inert powders in capsules to prevent liquefaction due to formation of a eutectic mixture. J. Am. Pharm. A. (Sci. Ed.), 29:78, 1940.

41. ———: Incompatibilities in prescriptions. IV. The use of inert powders in capsules to prevent liquefaction due to deliquescence. J. Am. Pharm. A. (Sci. Ed.), 29:136, 1940.

42. Husa, W. J., and Macek, T. J.: Incompatibilities in prescriptions. V. The use of calcium phosphate and silica gel in capsules

to prevent liquefaction. J. Am. Pharm. A. (Sci. Ed.), *31*:213, 1942.

43. Irwin, G. M., Dodson, G. J., and Ravin, L. J.: Encapsulation of Clomacran Phosphate, 2-Chloro-9-[3-(dimethylamino)propyl] acridan phosphate. I. Effect of flowability of powder blends, lot-to-lot variability, and concentration of active ingredients on weight variation in capsules filled on an automatic capsule-filling machine. J. Pharm. Sci., *59*:547, 1970.

44. Ito, K., Kaga, S-I., and Takeya, Y.: Studies on hard gelatin capsules. I. Water vapor transfer between capsules and powders. Chem. Pharm. Bull., *17*:1134, 1969.

45. ———: Studies on hard gelatin capsules. II. The capsule filling of powders and effects of glidant by ring filling method-machine. Chem. Pharm. Bull., *17*:1138, 1969.

46. Jar, Ball and Pebble Milling, Theory and Practice. Bulletin P-291. Norton Chemical Process Products Division (Formerly U.S. Stoneware, Inc.), Akron, Ohio 44309.

47. Jones, T. M.: The effect of glidant addition on the flowability of bulk particulate solids. J. Soc. Cosmetic Chem., *21*:483, 1970.

48. Jones, T. M., and Pilpel, N.: Some angular properties of magnesia and their relevance to material handling. J. Pharm. Pharmacol., *18*:1825, 1966.

49. King, R. E.: Tablets, Capsules, and Pills. *In* Remington's Pharmaceutical Sciences. Ed. 14, pp. 1649–1680. Easton, Pa., Mack Publishing Co., 1970.

50. Lamy, P. P.: Importance of particle size in pharmaceutical practice. Hosp. Pharm., *1* (11):29, 1966.

51. ———: Factors affecting absorption and availability of drugs. Pharm. Times, *35*(12): 32, 1969.

52. Lappas, L. C.: The Manufacture of Hard Gelatin Capsules. Paper presented at meeting of the Research and Development Section of the American Drug Manufacturers Association, Atlantic City, N.J., October 8, 1954.

53. Lees, K. A.: Fine particles in pharmaceutical practice—chemical and pharmaceutical aspects. J. Pharm. Pharmacol., *15*:43T, 1963.

54. Lieberman, H. A., and Rankell, A.: Drying. *In* Lachman, L., Lieberman, H. A., and Kanig, J. L. (eds.): Theory and Practice of Industrial Pharmacy. pp. 22–48. Philadelphia, Lea and Febiger, 1970.

55. Marshall, W. R., Jr.: Principles of spray drying. I. Fundamentals of Spray-Dryer Operations. II. Elements of Spray-Dryer Design. Chem. Eng. Prog., *46*:501, 1950; *46*:575, 1950.

56. Mattocks, A. M.: Qualities of compressed tablets: potency variation. Am. J. Pharm. Ed., *30*:110, 1966.

57. Milosovich, G.: Direct compression of tablets. Drug & Cosmetic Ind., *92*:557, 656, 662, 667, 1963.

58. Moore, W. J.: Physical Chemistry. Ed. 3.,

pp. 133, 151. Englewood Cliffs, N.J., Prentice Hall, 1964.

59. Muller, G.: Methods and machines for making gelatin capsules. Manuf. Chemist, *32*:63, 1961.

60. Mullins, J. D., and Macek, T. J.: Some pharmaceutical properties of novobiocin. J. Am. Pharm. A. (Sci. Ed.), *49*:245, 1960.

61. Munzel, K.: The influence of formulation on drug action. Pharm. acta helv., *46*:513, 1971.

62. Nelson, E.: Measurement of the repose angle of a tablet granulation. J. Am. Pharm. A. (Sci. Ed.), *44*:435, 1955.

63. ———: Comparative dissolution rates of weak acids and their sodium salts. J. Am. Pharm. A. (Sci. Ed.), *47*:297, 1958.

64. ———: Influence and dissolution rate and surface area on tetracycline absorption. J. Am. Pharm. A. (Sci. Ed.), *48*:96, 1959.

65. ———: Symposium: Clinical drug evaluation. XVII. Physicochemical and pharmaceutic properties of a drug that influence the results of clinical trials. Clin. Pharmacol. Ther., *3*:673, 1962.

66. Nelson, E., Knoeckel, E. L., Hamlin, W. E., and Wagner, J. G.: Influence of absorption rate of tolbutamide on the rate of decline of blood sugar levels in normal humans. J. Pharm. Sci., *51*:509, 1962.

67. Neumann, B. S.: The Flow Properties of Powders. *In* Bean, H. S., Beckett, A. H., and Carless, J. E. (eds.): Advances in Pharmaceutical Sciences. Vol. 2, pp. 181–221. New York, Academic Press, 1967.

68. Newton, J. M., Rowley, G., and Tornblom, J. F. V.: The effect of additives on the release of drug from hard gelatin capsules. J. Pharm. Pharmacol., *23*:452, 1971.

69. ———: Further studies on the effect of additives on the release of drug from hard gelatin capsules. J. Pharm. Pharmacol., *23*: 156S, 1971.

70. Noyes, A. A., and Whitney, W. R.: The rate of solution of solid substances in their own solutions. J. Am. Chem. Soc., *19*:930, 1897.

71. Parke-Davis Empty Gelatin Capsules. Bulletin PD-R-0491-1a-1P (6-71), Parke, Davis & Co., Detroit, Mich.

72. Parrott, E. L.: An extemporaneous enteric coating. J. Am. Pharm. A., *NS1*:158, 1961.

73. ———: Student experiments in pharmaceutical technology. III. Humidity. Am. J. Pharm. Ed., *30*:470, 1966.

74. ———: Student experiments in pharmaceutical technology. II. Flowability of powders. Am. J. Pharm. Ed., *30*:205, 1966.

75. ———: Milling. *In* Lachman, L., Lieberman, H. A., and Kanig, J. L. (eds.): Theory and Practice of Industrial Pharmacy. pp. 100–119. Philadelphia, Lea and Febiger, 1970.

76. ———: Solid Dosage Forms. *In* Sprowls, J. B., Jr., (ed.): Prescription Pharmacy. Ed.

2, pp. 103–162. Philadelphia, J. B. Lippincott, 1963.

77. Patel, N. K.: Experiments in physical pharmacy. IV. Pharmaceutical eutectic mixtures. Am. J. Pharm. Ed., *34*:47, 1970.

78. Reier, G., Cohn, R., Rock, S., and Wagenblast, F.: Evaluation of factors affecting the encapsulation of powders in hard gelatin capsules. I. Semi-automatic capsule machines. J. Pharm. Sci., *57*:660, 1968.

79. Remington's Practice of Pharmacy. Ed. 12. Martin, E. W. and Cook, E. F. (eds.) pp. 155–157. Easton, Pa., Mack Publishing Co., 1961.

80. Rosenstein, S., and Lamy, P. P.: Some Aspects of Polymorphism. Am. J. Hosp. Pharm., *36*:598, 1969.

81. Rowe, E. J.: Capsules. *In* Martin, E. W. (ed.): Husa's Pharmaceutical Dispensing. Ed. 6, pp. 76–95. Easton, Pa., Mack Publishing Co., 1966.

82. Samyn, J. C., and Jung, W. Y.: *In* Vitro dissolution from several experimental capsules. J. Pharm. Sci., *59*:169, 1970.

83. Sekiguchi, K., and Obi, N.: Studies on absorption of eutectic mixture. I. A comparison of the behavior of eutectic mixture of sulfathiazole and that of ordinary sulfathiazole in man. Chem. Pharm. Bull., *9*: 866, 1961.

84. Shangraw, R. F.: Timed Release Pharmaceuticals. I. and II. The Maryland Pharmacist, *39*:218, 1963; *39*:280, 1963.

85. Shefter, E., and Higuchi, T.: Dissolution behavior of crystalline solvated and nonsolvated forms of some pharmaceuticals. J. Pharm. Sci., *52*:781, 1963.

86. Stanley, J. J.: Capsules. II. Soft Gelatin Capsules. *In* Lachman, L., Lieberman, H. A., and Kanig, J. L. (eds.): Theory and Practice of Industrial Pharmacy. pp. 359–384. Philadelphia, Lea and Febiger, 1970.

87. Stempel, E.: Patents for prolonged action dosage forms. Drug & Cosmetic Ind., *98*(1): 44, 118; *98*(2):36, 139, 145, 146, 148, 1966.

88. Stoklosa, M. J., and Ohmart, L. M.: A practical method of extemporaneous enteric coating. J. Am. Pharm. A. (Pract. Ed.), *14*: 507, 514, 515, 1953.

89. Stoyle, L. E., Jr.: Evaluation of the Zanasi Automatic Capsule Filler. Paper presented to Industrial Pharmacy Section, A.Ph.A.,

113th Annual Meeting, Dallas, Texas, April 25–29, 1966.

90. Strickland, W. A., Jr.: A new look at tablet lubricants. Drug & Cosmetic Ind., *85*:318, 1959.

91. ———: Study of water vapor sorption by pharmaceutical powders. J. Pharm. Sci., *51*: 310, 1962.

92. Strickland, W. A., Jr., and Moss, M.: Water vapor sorption and diffusion through hard gelatin capsules. J. Pharm. Sci., *51*:1002, 1962.

93. Sumner, E. D., Thompson, H. O., Poole, W. K., and Grizzle, J. E.: Particle size distribution and hopper flow rates. J. Pharm. Sci., *55*:1441, 1966.

94. Swintosky, J. V.: Design of oral sustained-action dosage forms. Drug & Cosmetic Ind., *87*:464, 465, 548, 549, 551, 1960.

95. Tawashi, R.: Particulate solids. flow properties and mixing. Drug & Cosmetic Ind., *106*(2):46, 50, 52, 148, 1970.

96. Thompson, T. N.: Freeze Drying. Med. Electronics and Data, *2*(5):56, 1971.

97. Train, D.: Some aspects of the property of angle of repose of powders. J. Pharm. Pharmacol., *10*:127T, 1958.

98. ———: Mixing of pharmaceutical solids: the general approach. J. Am. Pharm. A. (Sci. Ed.), *59*:265, 1960.

99. Tuckerman, M. M., and Martin, A. N.: Coloring and flavoring empty gelatin capsules in the prescription laboratory. J. Nat. Pharm. A., *2*(3):60, 1955.

100. Wagner, J. G.: Biopharmaceutics. 19. Rate of dissolution. IV. Measuring *in vivo* rates of dissolution from capsules and tablets. Drug Intelligence and Clin. Pharm., *4*:92, 1970.

101. ———: Biopharmaceutics. 20. Rate of dissolution *in vitro* and *in vivo*. V. Factors affecting rate of dissolution of drugs from tablets and capsules and interpretation of dissolution rate data from *in vitro* testing of tablets and capsules. Drug Intelligence and Clin. Pharm., *4*:132, 1970.

102. White, R. C.: The manufacture of efferverscent salts. J. Am. Pharm. A., *10*:609, 1921.

103. Whithey, R. J., and Mainville, C. A.: A critical analysis of a capsule dissolution test. J. Pharm. Sci., *58*:1120, 1969.

11

Gilbert S. Banker, PH.D., *Professor of Industrial Pharmacy and Head, Industrial and Physical Pharmacy Department, School of Pharmacy and Pharmacal Sciences, Purdue University*

Tablets and Tablet Product Design

INTRODUCTION

Solid oral dosage forms are the most important and the most widely used class of drug delivery systems designed to produce systemic drug effects. With the exception of insulin therapy, parenteral routes of drug administration are not employed for self-administration of drugs. It can safely be estimated that well over 90 percent of all self-administered drugs employed for a systemic effect are administered by the oral route. Solid oral dosage forms represent the preferred drug delivery system for the oral route because they are unit dosage forms in which one tablet or capsule represents one dosage unit of the drug; therefore, they deliver the dose accurately. Oral liquid dosage forms, such as solutions, elixirs, syrups, suspensions, and emulsions, are commonly designed to contain one dose of drug in 5 to 15 ml. Dosage measurement is imprecise, by a factor of at least 20 to as much as 50 percent, when liquid products are self-administered by the patient.

Pharmaceutical manufacturers are always hopeful that new systemically active drugs will be effective in oral dosage forms because a drug that is effective only on parenteral administration will usually be restricted to use in physicians' offices or hospitals. Unless such a drug has unique advantages, it is not likely to have wide or extensive use. Manufacturers like the conventional compressed tablet because it best lends itself to rapid mass production and is the least expensive of the solid dosage forms to produce. Capsules, whether hard gelatin or soft elastic capsules, require a capsule shell enclosure to contain the drug. The cost of the filled capsule thus begins with this shell, which may cost from one-tenth to one-

half cent or more per unit. The cost of the shell enclosure is omitted entirely in the standard uncoated compressed tablet. Additionally, the cost of filling the capsule shell may be greater than that of fabricating the entire compressed tablet, particularly if a simple tablet granulation process is employed. Until recently (about the last decade), all hard gelatin capsules were filled on manually operated machines. Automatic capsule machines now exist and are finding increasingly wide usage, but they are much slower (less than 1,000 capsules per minute) than modern high speed tablet machines (up to 12,000 tablets per minute).

Compressed tablets are easy to carry (a capsule may come open) and are compact and easy for the pharmacist to store. They are the lightest in weight per dosage unit and, hence, the cheapest to package and ship. Consider, for example, that one dose of drug in a liquid product with the typical 5 ml. dose weighs about 5 g. By comparison, one dose of a drug in tablet form typically weighs from about 200 to 600 mg. These weight differences may be of no great significance to the pharmacist, but they are significant to the pharmaceutical manufacturer who must ship millions of dosage units per year from one end of the country to the other, and abroad. Higher manufacturer's shipping costs are of course passed along to the pharmacist and the consumer. Liquid dosage forms are not convenient for the ambulatory patient to use in going about everyday activities since few of us carry teaspoons in our pockets. Also, dose administration may be limited to meal times.

Another major advantage of tablets and capsules is that every single dosage unit can be identified as to manufacturer and

345

absolute product identity. Coated tablets may be imprinted with an edible ink for identification; uncoated tablets may be embossed with their identification code using engraved tablet punches. Thus, the identity of such coded products is never lost, regardless of separation from the original or prescription container. Rapid product identification, at best, can be a life and death matter in cases of accidental or purposeful overdosing or of therapeutic incompatibility or drug reaction. At least, absolute product identity is helpful to the pharmacist and physician in verifying the identity of products about which patients may have questions. Presently, most drug manufacturers are identifying individual drug doses of solid dosage forms only, and even that identification is not complete at the time of this writing. Individual dose identification of liquid products requires individual dose packaging, an expensive practice, but one resorted to in some hospitals.

Another advantage of solid dosage forms is their inherently greater chemical stability, compared to liquid dosage forms. Drugs in solution are most prone to chemical decomposition. At any given temperature, drugs in the dry state may be expected to be in their most stable form and have the greatest shelf life. Likewise, chemical incompatibilities between drugs or between drugs and excipients are diminished in the dry state. In tablet systems, compression of the tablet components into a dense, compact mass can bring reactants into such intimate contact that physical incompatibilities, such as eutectic formation, become a problem, whereas no such problem occurs in a loose powder-filled capsule. Often, such reactions in tablets can be circumvented by employing layered tablets.

Lastly, solid dosage forms can readily be designed to provide controlled drug dissolution so that the rate of drug release, and not the inherent absorbability of the drug, determines the rate of drug absorption. Thus, dosage form release may influence the blood level patterns generated and, consequently, the safety of the drug product. Most drug products provide for immediate and uncontrolled drug absorption, with resultant sharp, high-peak blood levels which,

on overdosing, may cause toxic reactions or death. For some classes of drugs, including most if not all depressant drugs, such uncontrolled drug release cannot be considered to be optimized drug delivery from a safety standpoint. Similarly, control of drug absorption rate and duration along the gastrointestinal tract can influence drug effectiveness and reliability. Such control of absorption following oral administration is best achieved with solid dosage forms.

Occasionally, it may be desirable to prevent drug dissolution in the stomach for drugs that are nauseating (diethylstilbestrol, emetine, atabrine) or irritating (potassium chloride) if released there. Other drugs are chemically degraded in the stomach if allowed to dissolve there (erythromycin) and must be protected against dissolution in the stomach. *Enteric coating* of tablets is commonly employed to prevent gastric drug dissolution. Continuous *sustained drug release* over an 8- to 12-hour period following oral administration of a dosage unit can be achieved with solid dosage forms; it is simplest to fabricate for tablets and is much more difficult to produce with liquid products. Such continuous drug release may be desirable to reduce the frequency of dosing (sustained release), or to produce a more uniform therapeutic response.

In summary, solid oral dosage forms, most notably tablets, provide advantages—to the pharmacist, in storage, dispensing, and control; to the patient, in convenience of use; and, to the physician, of product identification, dosage accuracy and precision, improved control, and more reliable therapy. Accordingly, prescriptions for drugs in tablet dosage form outnumber the sum total of prescriptions for all other dosage forms filled in the community pharmacy.

TYPES AND CLASSES OF TABLETS

Tablets may be classified according to the type of drug delivery system they represent as well as according to their method of manufacture. Tablets may be manufactured by compression in a die between two punches or by molding. A summary of the various types of tablets classified according to method of manufacture and type of drug delivery system is given in Table 11-1. Most tablets are manufactured by compression and are intended to be swallowed intact. In the following section, tablets will be classified according to type of drug delivery system.

Oral Tablets for Ingestion

Oral tablets for ingestion are designed either to be swallowed intact, usually aided by a swallow of liquid, or to be chewed prior to swallowing. The latter tablets are termed *chewable tablets* or simply *chewables*. Chewable tablets are designed primarily for administration to children, vitamin products being the biggest area of application. A third type of tablet for oral ingestion is first placed in a half-glass of water in which it is dissolved or dispersed, after which the user drinks the solution or suspension mixture. The most important tablet in this third class is the *effervescent tablet* in which an acid-base reaction involving citric and/or tartaric acid plus sodium bicarbonate

generates carbon dioxide in water, providing very rapid tablet dispersion and dissolution as well as a pleasant tasting carbonated drink.

Classes 1 through 8 under "oral tablets for ingestion" in Table 11-1 represent tablets intended to be swallowed intact. Tablets in the class of *compressed tablets* or *standard compressed tablets* are uncoated and are usually intended to provide rapid drug release on oral administration. However, some uncoated tablets are comprised of drug compressed in a polymer or plastic matrix and provide prolonged drug release. Some *coated tablets,* notably sugar-coated and film-coated tablets, are designed to provide rapid drug release while the coating serves to mask the taste or odor or to provide improved chemical stability. *Sugar-coated tablets* are especially hazardous in the hands of young children who mistake them for candy. *Chocolate-coated tablets* are only of historical interest. Both *layered tablets* and *compression coated tablets* may represent either two compressions (two layers or a tablet within a tablet) or three compressions (three layers or a tablet within a tablet within a tablet). Layered tablets and compression coated tablets are typically employed either to separate two or more reactive substances in a single tablet or to provide repeat drug action from a rapid and a slow release component. Two layer tablets do not provide complete separation of reactive components but greatly reduce the surface area for reaction compared to mixed ingredients in the standard compressed tablet. Three layered tablets can provide complete separation of reactive components by interposing an inert middle layer. It should be noted that the classification in Table 11-1 is not absolute and a tablet in one class can also belong to a second class. For example, a compression coated tablet may be designed to provide enteric protection or a layered tablet, repeat action.

Frequently, a pharmaceutical manufacturer can achieve a particular objective in the *design* of an oral tablet for ingestion by any of several approaches. As described previously, reactive ingredients may be separated in one of the forms of multiple compressed tablets. Reactive ingredients may also be separately granulated, one or both of the granule fractions coated, and the mixed granulations compressed. Reactive materials such as vitamins may be embedded in wax or other carriers to permit compression in standard tablets with other normally reactive components. In vitamin-mineral combinations reactive vitamins and minerals frequently have been separated between the tablet core and the sugar coating layer, some of the active materials being added in the sugar coating proper. Likewise, a variety of techniques may be used to provide an enteric coating or repeat drug action or sustained drug release. The specific approach used by a given drug company for a particular drug product design objective depends on many factors including past company experience and expertise with various tableting techniques, tableting equipment currently "in-house," cost factors, ability to reproduce the desired product precisely (i.e., safety and reliability considerations), and the efficacy of the various products as manufactured by the various techniques or in the various tablet forms.

Broadly speaking, there are two classes of drugs administered orally in tablet form: *insoluble drugs intended to exert a local effect,* such as antacids and adsorbents, and *soluble drugs intended to exert a systemic effect* following absorption. With both classes of drugs, careful attention to product design and manufacture is essential to produce efficacious and reliable products. The effectiveness of antacids and adsorbents is typically related to particle size, surface area, and the effect of granulation and tableting on surface properties. Before a drug in tablet form can exert a systemic effect, it must be absorbed, and dissolution must precede absorption. Unfortunately, both *agglomeration* (the *granulation* step) and *compaction* (tablet *compression*), which are involved in tablet making, may be expected to retard the drug dissolution process. This may not affect drug availability for amine basic drug moieties with a high equilibrium solubility, rapid dissolution rate, and good absorbability along the intestinal tract. However, the availability of acidic drug moieties, which are best absorbed in the upper gastrointestinal tract, and drugs that are slowly

soluble or have a low equilibrium solubility can be greatly influenced by tablet design and manufacturing methods.[109] Dramatic differences in bioavailability for a sparingly soluble drug from two types of tablets are shown in Figure 11-1. Phenylindanedione is an oral anticoagulant drug whose bioavailability is greatly influenced by relatively minor changes in tablet formulation. The physician typically establishes an individualized dosage regimen for each patient on anticoagulant therapy based on measured blood clotting or prothrombin times. The area under the blood level curve in Figure 11-1 indicates relative availability of each phenylindanedione product; in this case one product is at least twice as available as the other. Figure 11-1 illustrates the hazard of product substitution with such drugs. If the pharmacist substitutes the more bioavailable for the less available product the patient would be overdosed and internal bleeding could ensue. If the pharmacist substituted the less bioavailable for the more available product the patient would be underdosed and may have a coronary or other type of cardiovascular crisis owing to clot formation.

The steps that may be involved in drug release and dissolution from tablets (Fig. 11-2) are related to processing factors that affect availability. Drug dissolution from the deaggregated particles typically exceeds dissolution from all the other steps in tablet disintegration and dissolution, owing to the much greater surface area of the deaggregated particles. The lengths of the arrows in Figure 11-2 for the three possible dissolution steps reflect the contribution typical of each dissolution step to the drug in solution in the G.I. contents for a standard uncoated tablet. When a very slowly releasing sustained action tablet is desired, the disintegration step is usually minimized so that a slow release from the tablet provides the protracted dissolution needed. The general order of availability which may be expected from various types of oral dosage forms is shown in Figures 11-3 and 11-4. As these figures suggest, very careful consideration of product design and manufacture is essential to obtain the best availability and reliability of drug action for many drugs administered in tablet form. Numerous ex-

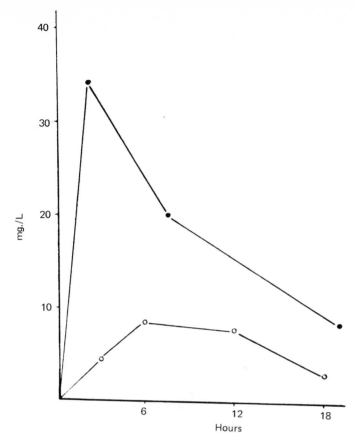

FIG. 11-1. Plasma levels of phenylindanedione following administration of 0.4 g in two types of tablets. (Schulert, A. R., and Weiner, M.: J. Pharmacol. Exp. Ther., *110*:451, 1954. Copyright © The Williams & Wilkins Co., Baltimore)

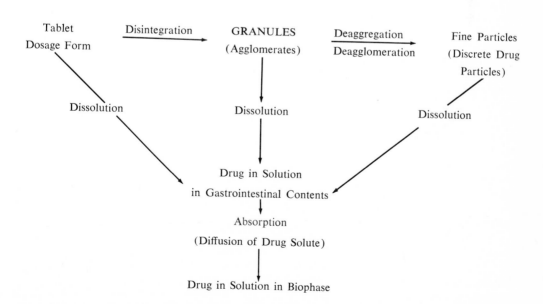

FIG. 11-2. Schematic representation of disintegration, deagglomeration, and dissolution of a tablet dosage form which must precede drug absorption.

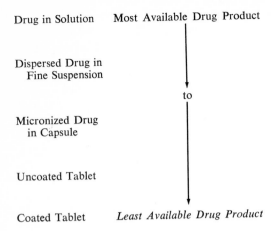

Drug in Solution   Most Available Drug Product

Dispersed Drug in
Fine Suspension

to

Micronized Drug
in Capsule

Uncoated Tablet

Coated Tablet   *Least Available Drug Product*

Fig. 11-3. The general order of bioavailability, which may be expected for drugs with "limited" solubility or absorption limited to a site high in the G.I. tract, according to dosage form type.

amples may be found in the literature illustrating a lower order of availability for tablet forms of drug delivery, as exemplified in

Figures 11-5 and 11-6. But, if a tablet product is properly designed, it should produce equivalent availability to any other oral dosage form.

Tablets Used in the Oral Cavity

Tablets used in the oral cavity (see Table 11-1) are placed in the mouth but not swallowed.

Buccal and sublingual tablets, though not swallowed, are intended to provide systemic drug action. These tablets are small, flat, usually oval dosage forms to be inserted in the buccal, or cheek, pouch (*buccal tablets*) or beneath the tongue (*sublingual tablets*). The drug is absorbed directly through the oral mucosa, thereby avoiding the acid and enzymatic environment of the stomach and the drug-metabolizing enzymes of the liver. Only a few drugs are commonly administered by the oral mucosal route: the vasodilator glyceryl trinitrate; steroids, such as methyltestosterone, testosterone propionate, and estradiol; and, possibly, some miscellaneous hormones and drugs, such as pancreatic

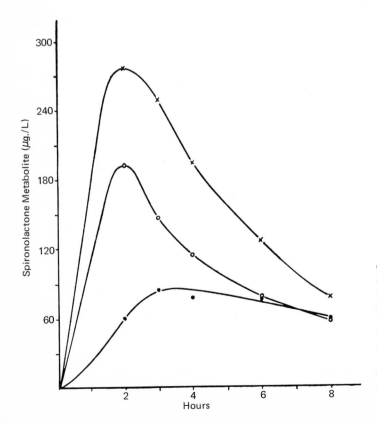

Fig. 11-4. Plasma levels of spironolactone metabolite after administration of 400 mg. of spironolactone in commercially available tablets (●); 100 mg. of powdered drug in gelatin capsules (○); and 100 mg. of micronized drug in gelatin capsules (×). (After Bauer, G., *et al.*: Arzneim-Forsch., *12*:487, 1962)

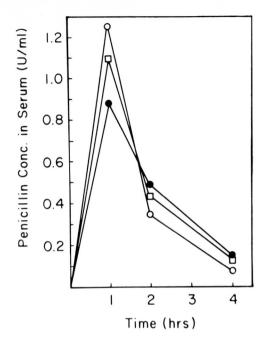

Fig. 11-5. Descending order of availability of 200,000 U of penicillin V in man, from an aqueous suspension (most available), a capsule form, and a tablet form (least available). (Putnam, L. E., *et al.*: Antibiot. Ann., 1955-56, p. 483. With permission of the Society for Industrial Microbiology)

lipotropic hormone factors, hesperidin, and nicotinic acid. Drugs that may be absorbed via the oral mucosa have several possible advantages: (1) Avoidance of the gastric environment and the decomposition it may produce with some steroids and hormones; (2) a more rapid onset of drug action than occurs with tablets which are swallowed; (3) reduction of nausea, with drugs that produce this effect when swallowed (methyltestosterone), and (4) more efficient drug utilization (lower dose), owing to avoidance of inactivation by liver drug-metabolizing enzymes. Drugs absorbed from the gastrointestinal tract enter the mesenteric circulation which feeds directly into the liver via the portal vein. Drug absorption from the oral cavity involves drug diffusion into the blood and lymph canals through the sublingual or oral mucosa. Blood is supplied to this region via the external carotid artery and is returned via the jugular veins into the general circulation rather than going directly to the portal vein. Many steroids in practical doses are either relatively or totally inert if ingested, owing to inactivation by liver enzymes. This loss of potency can be circumvented by other modes of administration such as intramuscular injection, implantation of tablets, use of vaginal suppositories, or absorption through the oral mucosa. The latter method, in many instances, is preferable.

Since most drugs, including weakly acidic drug moieties, are probably absorbed primarily in the upper small intestine,[11, 25, 116] the tablet must disintegrate, the drug dissolve, and the stomach empty at least partially

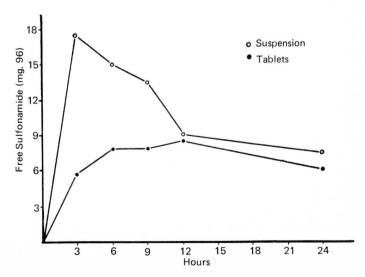

Fig. 11-6. Average blood levels of free sulfonamide in children following oral administration of sulfadimethoxine (1 g/M²) in tablets and in suspension. (Sakuma, T., *et al.*: Am. J. Med. Sci., *239*: 142, 1960)

before drug absorption can begin. Therefore, a time lag of 30 minutes or more (corresponding to the time required for the drug to be dissolved and leave the stomach) is typical before a drug effect is exerted after swallowing a tablet. On the other hand, total drug absorption typically occurs within 30 minutes after buccal or sublingual tablets have been administered, and an onset of action of 5 to 10 minutes or less is common with vasodilator drugs. Buccal and sublingual tablets are designed not to disintegrate but to dissolve slowly over a 15- to 30-minute period. The tablets are usually composed of drug plus a bland base. The tablet composition should not promote salivation, which would result in swallowing dissolved drug, thereby circumventing the purpose of the buccal or sublingual routes. On filling a prescription for buccal or sublingual tablets, the pharmacist should always counsel the patient to ensure that the patient knows how to use the tablets properly.

Troches or lozenges and dental cones— the other two classes of tablets used in the oral cavity—are intended primarily to exert a local effect in the mouth or throat. The terms lozenge and troche are used synonymously today for any form of tablet intended to be held in the mouth for slow dissolution and release of drug to provide prolonged (up to 30 minutes) contact of drug with the mouth and throat. The drugs used in this form today are primarily local anesthetics, antiseptics, astringents, or antitussives. Lozenges may also contain antihistaminics, analgetics, and decongestants; however, such drugs must be absorbed to exert their effect. Lozenges were historically known as pastilles, and are commonly called cough-drops when discoid shaped and formulated for antitussive action with the drug in a flavored hard sugar candy, glycerinated gelatin, or sugar-gum base. Lozenges may be made by a fusion or a candy molding process or by compression. Most troches are manufactured by compression as are other tablets. Dental cones are a tablet form intended to be placed in the empty socket following a tooth extraction, usually for the purpose of preventing local multiplication of pathogenic and saprophytic bacteria associated with tooth extractions.

The cones may contain an antibiotic or antiseptic, typically in a filler of sodium bicarbonate, sodium chloride, amino acid, or lactose. The cones are formulated and compressed so that a small volume of serum or fluid will cause disintegration and dissolution in 20 to 40 minutes with the cone loosely packed in the extraction site.

Tablets Administered by Other Routes

Implantation tablets, also known as *pellets,* are small sterile tablets, cylindrical or rosette-shaped and usually not over 8 mm. in length, for subcutaneous implantation in man or animals to provide very prolonged drug effects—for 3 to 6 months or longer. In man, use of this dosage form is limited to very potent drugs which are not orally absorbed, notably steroids such as desoxycorticosterone, testosterone, or estradiol. The major advantage of the dosage form is to provide continuous therapy over many months without the need for repeated parenteral dosing. Over long periods of time this form of therapy can be most economical. Also, it may provide the most even and uniform hormone therapy.

The immediate and potential disadvantages of *implantation therapy* are: the surgical technique which may be required for implantation, the difficulty of maintaining a constant drug release rate as the pellet changes geometry with dissolution, the possibility of a histopathological (tissue toxicity) reaction against the implanted "foreign body," and the need to employ a surgical technique to terminate the therapy should such termination become necessary.

Implantation tablets are usually comprised of pure drug, compressed from a crystalline form and individually sterile-packed. Any additives must be completely soluble in physiological fluids to avoid a granuloma type tissue reaction. Pellets may be implanted by surgical incision or by a special injector comprised of a hollow needle and plunger (Kearn injector). Possibly because of these disadvantages and unresolved safety questions, implantation therapy in man has not received wide use. In veterinary practice, however, it is very common, and a number of antibiotics, steroids, and antiparasitics are frequently administered in this form. Here, the cost and convenience of a single administration for prolonged effect are major factors.

Vaginal tablets, also termed *inserts,* are generally ovoid or pear-shaped tablets made by compression and intended to undergo dissolution and drug release in the vaginal cavity. The tablets are usually used in the treatment of trichomonas vaginitis and contain organic iodine (iodochlor or iodohydroxyquinoline compounds) or other antiseptics, astringents, or steroids in a soluble base of lactose or sodium bicarbonate. The tablets may be buffered to provide a pH favoring the action of a particular antiseptic agent. A plastic tube inserter with a plunger for tablet insertion is usually supplied to enable the patient to place the tablet in the upper region of the vaginal tract. Some vaginal tablets are dispensing type tablets to be dissolved in a given volume of water to prepare a proper strength vaginal douche. The pharmacist has an obligation to be sure the patient understands the proper use of whichever type of vaginal tablet is being dispensed, to ensure proper, safe, and effective use and to prevent injury to the patient through misuse of the tablets or the applicator.

Tablets Used to Prepare Solutions

Hypodermic tablets were once fairly widely used in medicine because the physician could carry vials of hypodermic tablets of many different kinds in his bag and required only one bottle of sterile water for injection to prepare extemporaneously any injection solution he chose. Hypodermic tablets are little used today because their use increases the chance of injection of a nonsterile solution and stable, safe, and reliable solutions for injection are now commercially available for most drugs. Since the physician practices most of his medicine in his office or a hospital today, the advantage of portability of the tablet for injection is far outweighed by the disadvantages of the dosage form in most medical situations.

Dispensing tablets are intended to be added to a given volume of water by the pharmacist or consumer to produce a solution of fixed concentration. Antiseptic materials, such as quaternary ammonium com-

pounds, merbromin, mild silver proteinate, or bichloride of mercury, were most commonly prepared as dispensing tablets. Most dispensing tablets contain toxic and very hazardous (often lethal) drug doses if swallowed. Such tablets should always be dispensed with a poison label. Bichloride of mercury was prepared in coffin-shaped dispensing tablets with an embossed skull and crossbones to emphasize their toxicity. Nevertheless, many cases of poisoning have resulted from misuse of dispensing tablets which accounts in part for their decreasing use.

Tablet triturates were originally an extemporaneous tablet form of potent drugs that the pharmacist could prepare. The drug was usually mixed with lactose and possibly some binder, such as powdered acacia. The powder mixture was moistened to produce a moldable, compactable mass and was then forced with a spatula into the holes drilled through a plastic or wooden mold. The moist tablets were forced out of the mold with a peg board, whose pegs matched the holes in the mold, and allowed to dry. Tablet triturates (lactose-based dispensing tablets) are now made primarily by compression with a tablet machine.

TABLET DESIGN AND MANUFACTURE

Granulation

Compressed tablets are manufactured by compressing crystalline or granular solids in a die between two punches (Fig. 11-7) under loads of a thousand pounds or more. Tableting pressures are typically in the thousands of pounds per square inch range. Powders resist compression into tablets, owing to two factors: entrapped air and poor particle-particle adhesion on compression. The result is that tablets prepared from powders tend to be soft and of poor appearance regardless of the compression pressure. In addition, powders generally have poor flow properties. Materials to be compressed into tablets at production speed should flow readily from feed hoppers and into the die cavities. Materials with poor flow properties will not fill the dies uniformly, and a high intertablet weight variation re-

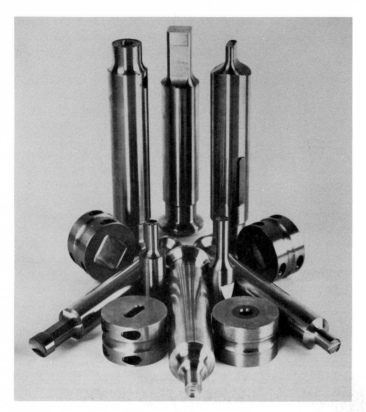

FIG. 11-7. One of the most critical factors in tablet making is the tooling (punches and dies) with which the tablets are made. The tooling utilizes hard steel alloys and the parts are machined precisely to close tolerances. (Thomas Engineering Co., Hoffman Estates, Ill.)

sults. To overcome the compression and flow problems of powders, *granulations* are prepared. Granulations are agglomerated powders in which the powder particles are bonded together by adhesive materials, pressure, or both, into occluded particles as large as 6 to 8 mesh and as small as 40 to 80 mesh. Satisfactory granulations are the key to effective tablet making.

Tablet granulations have a number of physical properties that can affect the tableting operation and resulting tablet properties. A knowledge of these granule properties, their method of determination, and their probable effect on the compression process and the resulting product is fundamental to tablet product design. *Granule true density* (the density of the individual granule) for a particular drug product is usually directly related to final tablet density. *Granule bulk density* (density of the granulation per se) is directly related to the weight of material that will fill a given die cavity. Achieving a high granulation bulk density may be a critical consideration with

flocculant, low density materials, such as aluminum and magnesium antacid compounds, in order to achieve the desired dose of material in a single tablet. *Granule shape* may affect both bulk density and flow. Spherical particles produce the highest possible bulk density. Irregular particles produce a low bulk density. Spherical particles have the lowest interparticle friction as they roll over one another; hence, they have the best flow properties. The micromeritics or particle characteristics of granulations prepared by five different granulation methods and a detailed discussion of relationships between these characteristics has been reported by Fonner *et al.*[33]

Components

In addition to the drug(s), nearly all tablets contain one or more binders, disintegrants, and lubricants. Unless the drug has a dose of several hundred milligrams or more, the tablet must also contain a diluent (Fig. 11-8). Optional components of tablets are colorants, flavors, and sweeteners.

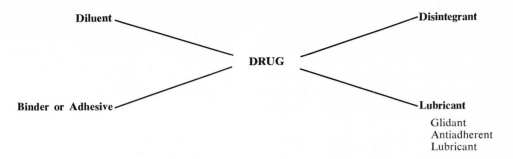

Fig. 11-8.   The basic components of a compressed tablet.

Diluents. The purpose of the diluent is to provide tablet bulk. Tablets that are to be swallowed intact generally are about ¼ inch in diameter or larger and weigh 250 mg. or more. Smaller tablets are not appreciably easier to swallow but become more difficult to handle. Consequently, if the amount of drug is inadequate to produce the tablet bulk, a filler or diluent is used. The diluent must meet several basic criteria, notably compatibility and nonreactivity with the drug, chemical stability, physical stability, and physiological inertness. Preferably, the diluent should be acceptable as a food additive, making it acceptable to the FDA for all drug product use. It should have no adverse effect on drug bioavailability.

A classic case of the effect of a diluent on *bioavailability* is the effect of calcium salts on the availability of tetracycline antibiotics (Fig. 11-9). Divalent and trivalent cations form insoluble complexes and salts with these antibiotics which strongly interfere with the drugs' absorptions following oral administration.[8] An example of a drug-excipient *chemical incompatibility* is the reaction of amine drug bases with the common excipient, lactose, in the presence of an alkaline lubricant, such as a metal stearate, which results in a tablet that discolors with age.[21, 27]

A further consideration in diluent selection is whether the diluent is contraindicated for some segment of the population. If the drug is one that is taken chronically, several grams of a given tablet diluent might be taken daily. Sodium chloride is strongly crystalline, compresses very well, and is an

FIG. 11-9. The effect of various excipients (one a calcium salt) on the absorption of tetracycline in man: Solid line, citric acid filler; dashed line, sodium hexametaphosphate filler; dotted line, dicalcium phosphate filler. (Boger, W. P., and Gavin, J. J.: New Eng. J. Med., *261*:827, 1959. Reprinted by permission of the New England Journal of Medicine)

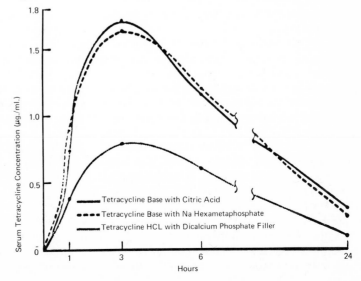

Tetracycline Base with Citric Acid
Tetracycline Base with Na Hexametaphosphate
Tetracycline HCL with Dicalcium Phosphate Filler

excellent low-cost tablet diluent. However, since many "many persons such as those with hypertension or various heart or kidney conditions" are on low salt diets, the use of sodium chloride as a diluent is avoided. Likewise, sucrose is avoided as a diluent, since sugar consumption also is limited in some conditions.

When acceptable to the drug system, insoluble calcium salts, such as dibasic calcium phosphate or calcium sulfate, are good low-cost diluents. Both of these diluents in their usual forms exist as dihydrates. The fact that a diluent exists as a hydrate does not preclude the use of such material, even with hydrolyzable drugs, provided that the hydrate does not release its water under any projected storage temperature for the product. Hydrates contain their water in bound form, not available for chemical reaction. The two named hydrates may be dried to contain little free (unbound) moisture from the atmosphere. Consequently, such materials are widely used as diluents for vitamins, steroids, and other water-sensitive drugs.

A number of *granular* or *coarse crystalline diluents* are employed in tablet making, some having been specially prepared for that purpose. These include spray-dried lactose, anhydrous lactose, calcium sulfate, microcrystalline cellulose (available in several colors), some specialty grades and forms of starch, and others. These materials are directly compressible with drug substances, usually after the addition of a lubricant.

Chewable tablets were made possible through the application and use of several hexahydric alcohol sugars.[24] Mannitol, though more costly, is less hygroscopic than sorbitol and is usually preferred in chewable tablets. These materials have a pleasing sweet taste, chemical stability, and a cooling sensation on chewing and dissolution in the mouth due to their negative heat of solution.

Binders and Adhesives. *Adhesives* are materials used in solution to wet-granulate powders and facilitate powder agglomeration. Most granulating agents have adhesive properties and include materials such as gelatin and acacia solution, liquid glucose, sucrose syrups, starch paste, and lactose[26, 83] as well as aqueous solutions of cellulosic

polymers such as sodium carboxymethylcellulose (CMC), methylcellulose (MC), hydroxypropylmethylcellulose (HPMC), and others. Mucilages of colloidal clays, sodium alginate, and other natural gums[44, 51, 65, 82] are also used.

Alcoholic or organic solvent solutions of HPMC, ethylcellulose (EC), polyvinylpyrrolidone (PVP), or hydroxypropylcellulose (HPC) may be used for water-sensitive drugs. Fortunately, these are FDA acceptable polymers which are soluble in alcohols or alcohol-chlorinated hydrocarbon mixtures. However, care must be exercised since EC is not water soluble and will retard drug release. Also, PVP has been reported to complex and bind drugs, and even though this polymer is completely water soluble, evidence should be obtained to assure that the polymer is not reducing drug availability.[49, 50]

Starch paste is typically used as a partially hydrolyzed 10 percent dispersion containing dextrins and dextrose to achieve the binding effect of sugar while retaining starch's disintegration properties. One reason for the popularity of starch paste as a binder is the fact that while functioning as an adhesive, it has less retardant effect on tablet disintegration and drug dissolution than most other binders. Some pharmaceutical manufacturers process their starch paste through a heat exchanger to bring the paste to a particular elevated temperature and cool it at a precise rate, thereby achieving the same degree of hydrolysis from one batch to another. A partially hydrolyzed starch paste is a dispersion with a translucent-white appearance. On complete hydrolysis a clear dextrose solution is obtained.

Binders are materials added as dry powders to powdered or granular materials which are to be tableted to provide bonding and cohesion of the components in slugging or tableting operations. Materials used as binders include microcrystalline cellulose, powdered or spray-dried acacia, colloidal clays, amylose, and polyvinylpyrrolidone.[59, 87]

Tablet cohesion is best achieved when the binding component is used in solution as an adhesive. A more cohesive tablet is produced with a lower concentration of adhesive in solution than with the adhesive used in dry form. Additionally, some poorly compressible materials can be successfully tableted only when a liquid adhesive and wet-granulation procedure are employed.

Most binders and adhesives, by the very nature of their mechanism of action, have a retardant effect on drug dissolution and release from tablets. Whether or not this retardation of drug release together with that imposed by compaction into the tablet form will be reflected in a reduction in drug availability depends on drug dose, solubility in gastrointestinal contents and rate of drug dissolution, extent of retardation of dissolution, and region of drug absorption along the gastrointestinal tract. The retardation effect of the binder/adhesive may be ameliorated, wholly or in part, by the proper use of tablet disintegrating agents.

Disintegrants. Compression of even very soluble drugs under the loads employed in the tableting operation can result in a dense compact tablet which requires hours to disintegrate and dissolve. Indeed, such compacts may often be observed to be eliminated in the feces nearly intact, having traveled through the entire gastrointestinal tract without substantial dissolution. To ensure that a compressed tablet will break up into small particles in the gastrointestinal tract to produce complete drug dissolution and full bioavailability, it is essential that the tablet be properly designed. *Disintegrants* are materials added to tablets to cause them to break up and fragment after ingestion, usually in the stomach.

Disintegrant materials used in tableting are typically materials that sorb water and swell on hydration. The best and fastest acting disintegrants are those that hydrate and swell in the acid environment of the stomach (pH 1 to 3). The ability of a material to sorb water, to increase tablet porosity, to promote capillary action, and/or to function as a *wick* to draw water into the tablet substrate to effect disintegration have been proposed as the mechanism(s) of disintegration.[23]

The most commonly used tablet disintegrant is *cornstarch,* although potato, wheat, and other starches have been used. The wide acceptance of starch is based on its status as a food material, its very low cost, and its efficiency as a disintegrant in tablets at 5 to 20 percent concentrations. Figure 11-10 illustrates the effect of starch concentration on drug dissolution rate. Powdered starch suffers at least three disadvantages as a tablet disintegrant: the material alone or in high concentration has poor compression properties (i.e., it does not form a cohesive compact), it has poor flow properties, and it is hygroscopic, sorbing up to 20 percent w/w of water in humid atmospheres. Some new forms of starch have been developed specifically for use in tablets, which have improved flow and compression properties. Examples of such specialty starches are the "Sta-Rx"* starches.

In addition to the starches, a great many materials have been used as disintegrants. *Microcrystalline cellulose* is an excellent disintegrant. It may be compressed directly into tablets. It flows well and does not readily sorb moisture; however, it is costly in comparison to starch. Various mineral clay powders are used, including *bentonite* and the lighter colored *Veegum*† products. Natural and modified natural products used as disintegrants include cellulose wood materials such as Solka-Floc,‡ [5, 32] as well as alginic acid,[37] natural sponge,[22] bentonite,[43] and Veegum† clays,[37, 45, 96] pulp,[54] carboxymethylcellulose,[55] guar gum,[28] and others.[85, 114, 119]

A very effective means of achieving rapid tablet disintegration is to employ a chemical *effervescent reaction* generated by citric acid and/or tartaric acid plus sodium bicarbonate. This approach, though effective, has two shortcomings: the resultant tablets are unstable if subjected even briefly to a humid atmosphere, and the carbon dioxide if generated in an appreciable amount may produce some discomfort and belching. An effervescent reaction is often employed to provide rapid dissolution of many brands of a common dispensing tablet, e.g., saccharin tablets.

Disintegrating agents often may be thought to function as drug dissolution

---

* A. E. Staley Mfg. Co., Decatur, Ill.
† R. T. Vanderbilt Co., New York, N.Y.
‡ Brown Co., Milton Village, Mass.

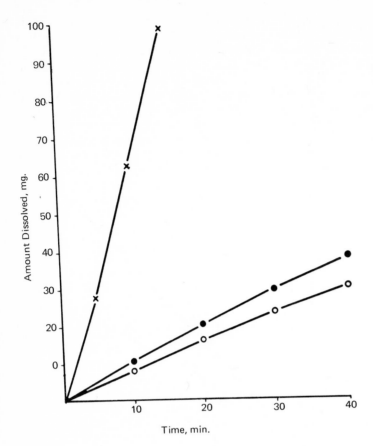

Fɪɢ. 11-10. Effect of starch content on the dissolution rate of salicylic acid contained in tablets: ○, 5%; ●, 10%; x, 20% starch. (Levy, G., *et al.*: J. Pharm. Sci., *52*:1047, 1963)

promoting agents, because of their ability to cause tablet break-up and particle deaggregation and deagglomeration (see Fig. 11-1). In addition, *wetting agents* or *surfactants,* such as dioctyl sodium sulfosuccinate[19] and sodium lauryl sulfate,[117] are occasionally added to tablets and other solid oral dosage forms to promote drug dissolution. It has been suggested that surfactants promote wetting of the tablet matrix and the deagglomerated particles to improve tablet disintegration and drug dissolution.[52] Fig. 11-11 shows the effect of sodium lauryl sulfate on the dissolution of salicylic acid from compressed tablets. Experimentally, large amounts of surfactants have been added to solid dosage forms to improve drug bioavailability by partially removing the mucin layer of the gastrointestinal mucosa and by the resultant irritant effect on the mucosa. To date, the small improvement in drug absorption resulting from such techniques has been more than offset by the accompanying diarrhea and other side effects.

The method by which disintegrants are incorporated into a tablet product during manufacture can have a pronounced effect on disintegrant effectiveness. The major portion of the disintegrant is usually mixed with the drug-excipient powdered materials prior to granulation. The remaining portion of disintegrant is added with the finely powdered lubricant to the granulation just prior to compression. Adding the disintegrant in this divided manner is often more effective from two standpoints: (1) The most effective lubricants are water repellent. Coating the granules with such water-repellent materials has the effect of retarding tablet disintegration. By combining a powdered disintegrant material with the lubricant, the continuous water-repellent coating of the granules is broken, and the retardant effect of the lubricant is diminished. (2) The mixed lubricant and disintegrant powder,

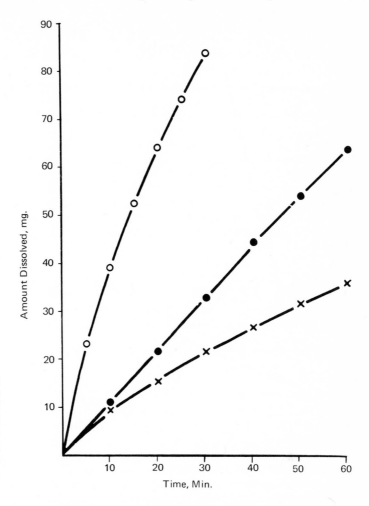

FIG. 11-11. Effect of a lubricant and a surfactant on the dissolution rate of salicylic acid contained in compressed tablets: x, 3% magnesium stearate; ●, no additive (control); ○, 3% sodium lauryl sulfate. (Levy, G., and Gumtow, R. H.: J. Pharm. Sci., *52*:1140, 1963)

which is added to the granulation just prior to the compression step, is termed the *running powder*. Adding disintegrant in the running powder may also provide a cushion between the granules, reducing granule cohesion, and facilitating tablet disintegration.

There are many variables influencing the rate of tablet disintegration or the time required for total disintegration and subsequent drug dissolution. Wagner[115] has enumerated some of these variables, which include:

1. the diluent used, its concentration relative to the drug, and its method of incorporation;

2. the method of tablet granulation and tablet manufacture employed;

3. the type and concentration of binder used;

4. granule size and size distribution;

5. the lubricant used and its concentration and method of incorporation;

6. the presence of a surfactant and its nature and method of incorporation;

7. compression pressure and speed of compression;

8. the drug itself and its properties, i.e., solubility, particle size, and surface characteristics;

9. age of the finished tablets and their method of storage, and

10. at least six additional factors for coated tablets.

Lubricants. With the exception of a few crystalline materials which themselves possess some lubricant action, such as sodium chloride, tableting on production equipment is not possible without proper granulation lubrication. Tablet lubricants serve two immediate purposes: to reduce adhesion or sticking of powdered materials to the punch faces, which would produce a rough or pitted tablet surface, and to reduce the ejection force needed to expel the compressed tablets from the dies of the tablet machine. Unlubricated granulations produce tablets which after tight compaction in the die have high die wall friction on ejection. This friction may cause the tablets to fracture and split, may score the die walls, producing excessive wear and a rapid increase in die bore diameter, and may produce other machine damage including wear of the lower punch heads and damage to the ejection cam. It is not difficult to identify an inadequately lubricated granulation: A rotary tablet machine will produce a distinctive cyclic grating sound as each lower punch works against its cam track as it attempts to drive the tablet from its die. The tablets themselves will bear vertical striations along their edges, reflecting the high frictional force of ejection along the die wall.

Tablet lubricants may serve a third role. Just as the finely powdered lubricant coating the granulation particles reduces friction between the compacted granulation and the die wall, it also reduces friction between the coated particles as they tumble over each other in flowing from the hopper and into the die cavities. This reduced interparticle friction in the granulation bed is reflected by improved granulation flow and frequently a reduction in tablet weight variation.

According to the primary function of lubricant materials in the three roles just discussed, lubricants have been classified as follows[81]:

1. *Lubricants*: Materials that reduce friction between surfaces, in this case the tablet cylindrical surface (edge) and the die wall. Metallic stearates such as magnesium or calcium stearate, mineral oil (usually applied as a spray from an organic solvent solution), and high melting point waxes, such as the high molecular weight polyethylene glycols, are the best lubricating materials.

2. *Anti-Adherents*: Materials that reduce adhesion and sticking of the granulation components to the punch faces. Punch faces should retain their highly polished appearance throughout a tableting run. When punch face sticking becomes appreciable, "pocked" tablets result which are underweight. Two good anti-adherents are talc and cornstarch, both of which, however, are poor lubricating materials.

3. *Glidants*: Materials that reduce interparticle friction and promote granulation flow. Cornstarch and colloidal silicas are good glidants.

No known material is highly efficient in all three categories. Accordingly, combinations of lubricants are often selected to provide the necessary total lubrication effect.

Unfortunately, many materials that are good tablet lubricants are also hydrophobic and may have an undesirable effect on drug bioavailability from tablets. Figure 11-11 shows the effect of magnesium stearate, a widely used lubricant, on the dissolution of salicylic acid from compressed tablets. Thus, lubricants may inhibit wetting of tablet, granule, or primary particle surfaces through a "raincoat" effect if enough is added to coat the particles in the tablet granulation.

A need has long existed for a good water-soluble lubricant for those tablets intended to produce clear solutions; i.e., hypodermic tablets, certain dispensing tablets, and effervescent tablets. Unfortunately, the best lubricants are water repellent and quite hydrophobic. Materials that have been used as soluble tablet lubricants include polyethylene glycol (PEG) 4,000, higher molecular weight PEGs, surfactants,[19, 28, 52, 55, 73, 79, 81, 85, 114, 115, 117, 119] sodium chloride, sodium benzoate,[67, 100, 104, 109] sodium oleate,[100, 122] sodium stearate,[84, 100] and others.[80, 86, 98] Boric acid[16] was one of the best water-soluble lubricants but is now known to pose a toxicity hazard.[12, 16, 91] No highly effective and safe water-soluble tablet lubricant is known.

Other techniques have been employed to reduce the need for tablet lubricants, especially where soluble lubricants are concerned, including chrome plating of punch faces and die walls or Teflon coating of punch faces. The problem has been to find a coating for punches and dies that possesses adequate durability under the thousands of pounds of pressure and abrasive abuse incurred in tableting.

Other Tablet Components. Other components may be incorporated into tablet formations but are less essential to tablet manufacture and product quality than those already mentioned; these are *coloring agents, flavors, sweeteners,* and *adsorbents.*

Tablets are colored for esthetic reasons and for elegance, and to hide differences in color or speckling when either the drug or an additive is off-white. Pastel shades are most often used for coloring uncoated tablets because it is easier to achieve uniform colors with such shades. The color is added to uncoated tablets in either of two ways: (1) the dye is dissolved in water, a suitable solvent, or the granulating agent and the powder mixture is wet massed to a uniform color, or (2) lake dye is added to the tablet powder mixture, blended well, and granulated by whatever procedure is desired. The wet granulation procedure employing dissolved dye produces the most uniformly colored tablets provided that no color migration occurs during drying (the dye often moves with the solvent to the top of the granulation on drying). When wet granulation is not to be employed, *lake dyes* are indicated. Lake dyes are dyes that have been strongly adsorbed on alumina and aluminum hydroxide.

Two classes of dyes are permitted in oral drug products, *F.D. and C. dyes* (foods, drugs, and cosmetics) and *D. and C. dyes* (drugs and cosmetics). The F.D. and C. dyes have generally been established as the safest, since they are permitted in foods and have higher permissible ingestion limits. They are the only class of dyes used by many companies in oral products. Furthermore, for those drug products that are classified as foods, such as vitamin products, F.D. and C. dyes must be used. The third class of dyes, *External D. and C. dyes,* are permitted only in topical products.

The use of dyes in tablet products causes several problems. First, most dyes tend to fade or lose color on aging, especially on exposure to light,[30, 62–64, 106, 107] the rate of fading depending upon the composition of the tablet and the protection from light afforded by the container. High intensity light sources, light cabinets, and accelerated stability testing methods are required to evaluate color stability in tablets.[40, 88] Second, over the last decade the Food and Drug Administration has decertified many dyes, some because they were carcinogenic when fed in very high doses to animals. When a dye is decertified, the manufacturer must either seek a blend of the remaining dyes to match the lost color, which may be impossible, or change the appearance of the product, which creates marketing problems.

Flavors and sweeteners are indispensable in the formulation of chewable tablets or effervescent tablets. The drug industry is presently faced with the loss of all effective synthetic non-sugar sweeteners. Cyclamates were lost as synthetic sweeteners because they were carcinogenic in massive doses in animals. The safety of saccharin is currently under study. Its permitted uses as a synthetic sweetener are limited, and its future as a sweetening agent is presently uncertain. Other synthetic sweeteners, such as ammoniated glycyrrhizin, are much less efficient. Hundreds of oils, oil extracts, and flavor principles are used to flavor drug products. These materials are only now coming under the full scrutiny of the FDA as food and drug additives. Many will undoubtedly be decertified in the years ahead.

Adsorbents are occasionally used in tablet formulations to sorb small quantities of a liquid, such as the oily free-base form of a drug or an organic solvent solution of the drug or a fluidextract, into the tablet excipients. Light magnesium oxide, magnesium carbonate, kaolin, bentonite, and other materials have been used for this purpose.

Methods of Tablet Manufacture

There are three basic methods of preparation of compressed tablets. Each method has its own advantages, disadvantages, and limitations.

The Wet Granulation Method. This is the oldest method of tablet preparation and probably continues to be the most widely used, although many manufacturers strive to use more streamlined manufacturing methods for new tablet products. The wet granulation method involves dampening or wet massing the tablet powder mixture with a liquid-adhesive granulating agent, followed by wet screening or granulation to agglomerate the powder. The disadvantage of the wet granulation process is that it involves many separate manufacturing steps, numerous handling operations, and a drying step, all of which are time consuming and costly. The process does not lend itself to automation.

The greatest disadvantage of this process is the problem of reproducing a granulation from one lot to the next. Factors such as the chemical variation between lots of polymeric binding agents; differences in solvation of the polymers or gums in the granulating agent; moisture content, particle size, and other variables in the powders being granulated; amount of granulating agent added and rate of addition; wet-massing mixing time; rate of feeding the wetted powder to the granulating machine; and other variables can influence a range of properties of the resultant granulation. These granulation properties include particle size and particle size distribution, granule density and hardness, granule shape, granulation bulk density, compressibility, and even drug content uniformity and bioavailability. Figure

11-12 illustrates the effect of granule size on in-vitro drug dissolution release.

The individual steps in the wet granulation process of tablet preparation include the following:

1. Weighing
2. Milling
3. Sieving
4. Dry Powder Mixing
5. Wet Massing
6. Granulation
7. Drying
8. Sizing
9. Lubrication
10. Compression

WEIGHING. A typical weighing operation is shown in Figure 11-13. The figure illustrates several of the precautions taken by manufacturers in weighing components of a product. Two men are involved in the operation to double check both the identity and the quantity of each component according to the product work sheet which is a photocopy of the master formula for the product. The work sheet accompanies the product throughout all steps in manufacture. In Figure 11-13, the man on the left is touching a dust-exhaust duct which is exhausting air from the weighing site to keep the area dust

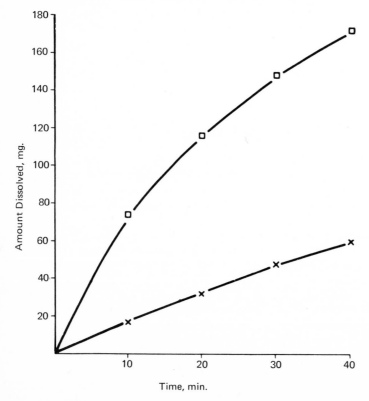

FIG. 11-12. Effect of granule size on the dissolution rate of salicylic acid in compressed tablets; x, 40 to 60 mesh; □, 60 to 80 mesh granules. (Levy, G., *et al.*: J. Pharm. Sci., *52*:1047, 1963)

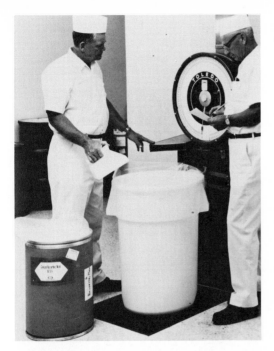

FIG. 11-13. The weighing step in a tablet production operation. (Rowell Laboratories, Baudette, Minnesota)

to a very fine particle size such that 100 particles are required to produce the same dose, an error of one or two particles per tablet is now only an error of ±1 to 2 percent. Therefore, as the number of particles making up the dose increases, the statistical probability of producing an accurate dose also increases.

The greatest possible number of drug particles will exist (6×10^{23} particles/mole) when the drug is in solution, and, accordingly, potent drugs are sometimes added in solution in the granulating agent. This may or may not provide a better *uniformity of distribution* of the drug than dry mixing of micronized powder. Drugs that are highly soluble in the wetting or granulating agent tend to migrate to the surface of a slab of drying granulation as the massing solvent evaporates. Such migration leads to a reduction in the mixing uniformity of the drug in the granulation and a greater variation in intertablet drug content.

SIEVING. The initial sieving operation may be undertaken for two reasons: (1) to remove foreign materials which may be present in common bulk diluents such as sugar or starch, and (2) to control particle size by removal of lumps of loosely agglomerated powder from drug or excipient materials. The sieving operation is often accomplished by charging the powder blender through a vibrating power-driven sieve.

MIXING. A variety of equipment reflecting a number of mechanical approaches is employed to achieve powder mixing. The twin-shell or V blender (Fig. 11-14) is an efficient powder mixer, often producing optimum mixing in as little as five minutes. A version of the twin-shell blender, known as a liquids-solids blender, contains a high speed rotating bar running horizontally through the unit which has the ability to feed liquid products into the blender during operation. This blender has the capability of mixing, wet massing and even agglomerating (granulating) the powder in one piece or equipment and in one continuous operation.

A number of *trough type mixers* with horizontal mixing devices are used in mixing and massing. The ribbon blender (Fig. 11-15), which contains a series of spiral steel ribbons to move the powder back and forth

free and to minimize the chances of contamination of one drug product by another. Note too the cleanliness of the entire work area and the fact that only one chemical container is permitted at the weighing station at a time. A record is made on the work sheet of the lot number of every drug or excipient material going into the product, and each weighing is initialed by the individual responsible for the verification of the identity and quantity of that component.

MILLING. A milling step to produce a fine particle size of the drug may be required prior to sieving and mixing. A micronized or finely milled powder dispersion is of particular importance with potent drugs administered in doses in the fractional milligram to several milligram range. The larger the number of particles to a given dose of drug, the less significant is the presence of a few drug particles more or less in one tablet or another. For example, if only 10 particles or crystals of drug comprise a single dose, tablets that happen to contain one particle too many or too few will have a dose error of ±10 percent. If the same drug is milled

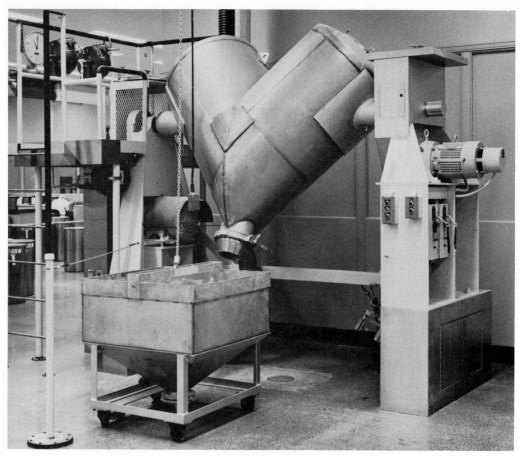

FIG. 11-14. A twin-shell or V-blender powder mixer. (The Upjohn Co., Kalamazoo, Michigan)

in the trough, can function as a good powder blender but does not function well for wet massing. Conversely, the so-called *dough mixer* or mass mixer, with its heavy S-shaped blade, is effective for wet massing but is a poor powder mixer. One trough mixer combines a high shear rate with sufficient power to be used for wet massing and is reportedly effective for both mixing and massing (Fig. 11-16). If effective powder mixing followed by wet massing of the powder can be accomplished in the same piece of equipment, at least one product transfer and handling step can be eliminated. There are also a number of *planetary mixers* used in tablet making. In these, the mixing blade enters a cylindrical mixing container vertically from the top, similar to the common kitchen mixer but on

a much larger scale. Such mixers are good massing mixers for incorporating liquids into powders, but they are typically poor powder mixers.

Other mixers are used to extinguish a potent drug throughout a diluent forming a drug-concentrate. The *pot mill,* in which from one to three balls as large as bowling balls roll in a rotating mushroom-shaped pan, is a classical drug-triturate mixer. The *muller* or *chaser mill,* in which a vertical wheel held by pressure against the base of a cylindrical drum, rotates about its axis (Fig. 11-17), also provides the drug extinguishing effect, combining drug particle size reduction with dispersion throughout a diluent. If the diluent is a reasonably hard crystal of an inorganic substance, such as sodium bicar-

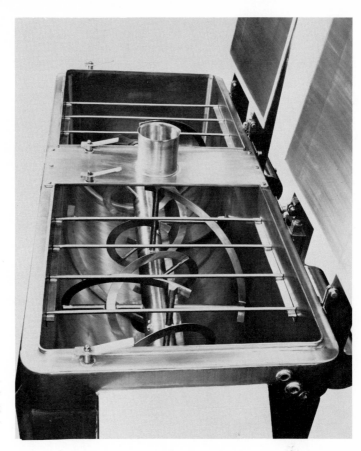

Fig. 11-15. Ribbon blender powder mixer in cut-away view showing spiral mixing ribbons. (J. H. Day Co., Cincinnati, Ohio)

bonate, the extinguishing effect on a softer organic material, such as a potent steroid, is accentuated.

The *massing operation* in which the granulating agent is added to powder mixture requires 10 to 20 minutes of mixing-kneading action in the typical mass mixer. The end point of the massing operation must be determined by the operator and is indicated when the damp powder will pack to the consistency of a dry snowball, and crumble into fragments, not powder, under finger pressure.

The *granulation step* is accomplished by forcing the moistened powder through a screen in an oscillating granulator (Fig. 11-18) or in a hammer mill. The resulting granular material is dried on trays in a *hot air circulation oven* or in a *fluid bed drier* (Fig. 11-19). If an organic solvent is used in wet granulation, particularly a potentially inflammable or explosive solvent such as one containing an alcohol or acetone, care must be taken in drying. If an oven is used, preliminary solvent evaporation in air may be advisable, and the oven must be the air circulation type which is set to operate at a high air flow rate so that an explosive solvent vapor concentration is never reached in the oven. The explosive limits of various solvents in air, expressed as vapor concentrations, are reported in the *Merck Index*[103] and various chemical handbooks, and air flow rates through an oven for a given solvent and given evaporation rate may be calculated to determine the relative hazard under any set of operating conditions.

A great disadvantage of the wet granulation process has been the oven drying time of 12 hours or longer, which made tablet making at least a two day process. In a *fluid bed drier* (Fig. 11-19), warm air is forced upward through a porous grid, fluidizing and partially suspending the gran-

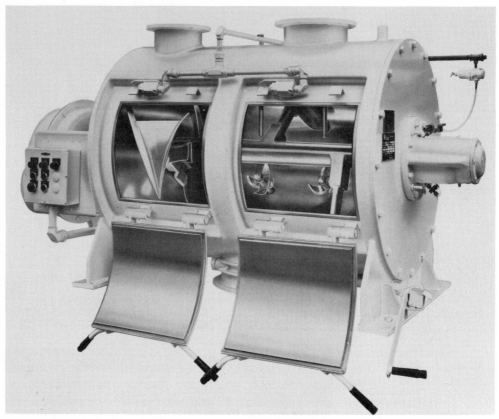

Fig. 11-16.   Lodige high shear trough mixer for powder mixing and wet massing. (Little-ford Bros., Inc., Cincinnati, Ohio)

ules in the warm air steam and reducing drying times to an hour or less. Fluid bed drying now permits tablets to be made by wet granulation in a single day.[70, 93] The fluid bed drier also produces a granulation in which all portions of the granulation are equally dried, a situation which may not exist for oven-dried materials. Furthermore, in the fluid bed drier drug migration during drying is usually not a problem, owing to the continuous agitation of the granulation. Equipment is available to convert fluid bed driers to continuous granulators and driers.[89, 92] A spray-head is mounted in the fluid bed drier, and the drier is loaded with dry powder which is fluidized and sprayed with granulating agent to produce particle-particle agglomeration, after which the agglomerates are dried by the conventional fluid bed techniques.

SIZING.   Particles may agglomerate and lump during drying, particularly in an oven, and a *sizing* or *dry screening operation* is usually required after drying. An *oscillating granulator* is often used for this sizing step. The screen used for sizing should have slightly larger openings than that used to prepare the original granules if excessive powder is not to be formed and granulation lost during sizing. If, for example, a 20-mesh screen is used for granulation, a 16-mesh screen would be a good selection for sizing.

LUBRICATION.   The lubrication step is the point at which the lubricant or running powder is added to the granulation. Some pharmacy students, in first making tablets, make the error of mixing the lubricant with the other tablet ingredients prior to wet granulation. The lubricant must, however, be on the granule surface to be effective. Since lubrication is a surface phenomenon, the finer the lubricant particle size the better the

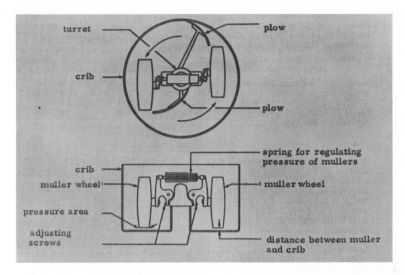

FIG. 11-17. A muller or chaser mill for extinguishing (mixing and grinding) potent drugs. (Blubaugh, F. C.: Mixing Methods Equipment and Control, presented at Industrial Pharmaceutical Technology Symposium, APhA Academy, Las Vegas, Nev., April 10, 1967)

surface coverage of the granulation and the more effective the lubricant.

Although the wet granulation process can suffer from numerous disadvantages, the process may be the best approach to tablet-making for very potent drugs given in minute doses. It also provides a method of producing very uniformly colored tablets when a soluble dye is incorporated in the granulating agent.

The Dry Granulation Method. The original dry granulation method is also known as *double compression* or *slugging*. Typically, the process involves compressing a powder mixture into a rough tablet or "slug" on a heavy-duty rotary tablet press. The slugged

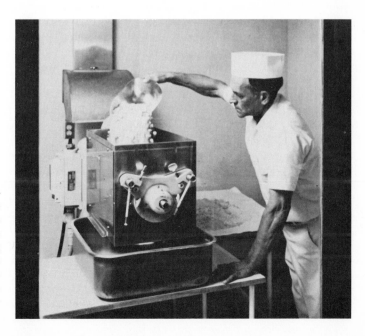

FIG. 11-18. The oscillating granulator employs two oscillating metal members to force the wet powder mass through a screen, producing the granulation. Note the operation is being conducted in an isolated room. (Rowell Laboratories, Baudette, Minn.)

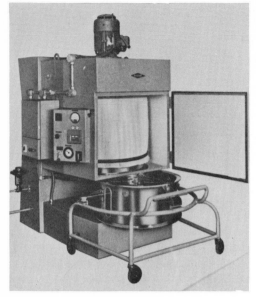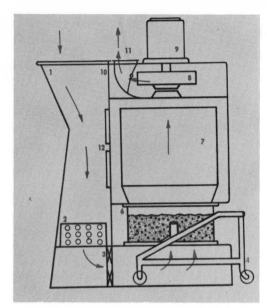

Fig. 11-19.   Fluid-bed drier (*Right*) schematic view: 1, Air inlet duct; 2, air heater; 3, air pre-filter; 4, product portable carrier; 5, fluidized product; 6, product container; 7, exhaust air filter; 8, exhauster fan; 9, fan motor; 10, control damper; 11, outlet air duct; 12, pressure "blow-out" panels. (The Fitzpatrick Co., Elmhurst, Ill.)

tablet is crude because of the poor compression properties of most powders. The slugs are then broken up into granular particles by a grinding operation, usually by passage through an oscillating granulator, and the resultant granules are lubricated and recompressed. The steps in the operation are basically the following, after the weighing of the ingredients:

1. Mixing
2. Compression (Slugging)
3. Grinding (Slug Reduction or Granulation)
4. Mixing (Relubrication)
5. Recompression

No wet binder or moisture is involved in any of the steps. The primary area of application of the method is accordingly the tableting of hydrolyzable or water-sensitive drugs. A less frequent application is the densification of a flocculant, low-density powder to permit compaction of a dose into a single tablet of reasonable size. The slugging or double compression method requires fewer steps than wet granulation and avoids the time and handling required for a drying step.

In the slugging operation, dry binders such as spray dried or powdered acacia or microcrystalline cellulose may be added to the drug powder to permit formation of a cohesive slug. It is usually necessary to add one or more lubricant materials to the powder to be slugged to reduce powder adhesion to the punches and to facilitate ejection of intact slugs from the dies. The result is that a typical tablet prepared by double compression contains lubricant throughout the tablet matrix and not simply at granule boundaries as in a wet granulated tablet. Because the double compression tableting process usually requires two lubrication steps (with most lubricants being water repellent) and tends to produce high density, hard tablets, drug dissolution and release are frequently retarded and drug bioavailability may be reduced.[56]

The double compression method also has the disadvantage of being a slow production operation. The rate limiting factor in double compression is the formation of the slugs themselves. Very large heavy duty rotary machines are used for slugging, to prepare slugs 1 to 2 inches in diameter and to produce the heavy compressive punch loads required. Even though the slugs are made very large, the slugging process, in terms of pounds of material processed per hour, tends to be slow. Additionally the excessive powder produced on granulation may need to be screened out, reslugged, and reground before the final tablets are made. After the slugs are ground to granular size, the pressure used for recompression to produce the final tablets usually has to be greater than that used to produce the slugs. Thus, the harder the slugs, the harder the finished tablet may have to be and the poorer the drug dissolution and release and bioavailability may become.

To overcome some of the shortcomings of double compression, notably the low production rate, the need for two lubrication steps, and the variability in slug density, several other devices for dry powder compaction have been developed and investigated.[46] One such device is the Chilsonator,* which utilizes paired, grooved cylindrical rolls which are held at a fixed clearance, regardless of powder fill between them, by hydraulic rams. Powder is augered into the nip of the paired rolls and is compressed into a serrated sheet of compacted powder at a reported rate of up to 400 kg. per hour. The sheet may then be ground to granular proportions, lubricated, and tableted. Other powder compactors, such as the Hutt Compactor† and pelletizing machines, such as are used to prepare charcoal briquettes, have been employed for powder compaction in dry granulation processes.

The Direct Compression Method. Direct compression is a method of tablet making in which (1) crystalline drugs with intermediate to large doses are directly compressed without a prior granulation step, or (2) powdered drug is combined with a pregranulated or coarse particulate diluent and the mixture is directly compressed. The great advantages of direct compression are the simplicity of the process, avoidance of a granulation step, avoidance of moisture and drying steps, minimal materials handling,

rapidity of the total process, and optimum possible bioavailability of drug(s) from the resulting tablets. The process has no major disadvantages, but it has distinct limitations. Only a few crystalline drugs lend themselves to direct compression—e.g., sodium chloride, aspirin, or methenamine. When powdered drug is combined with pregranulated diluent, the drug content of the finished tablet often cannot exceed 20 to 25 percent of total weight without losing compressibility and tablet cohesion. At the other extreme, potent drugs with doses below 10 to 25 mg. may separate from the coarser diluent granulation in the hopper or feed frame, producing a nonuniform mixture and lack of uniformity of content in the resultant tablets. When the drug has a low dose, a small particle size must be used to achieve uniformity of tablet content. The differences in particle size and density between the drug and the diluent may lead to stratification and separation of drug and diluent.

Direct compression of the few crystalline drugs that lend themselves to this process is a relatively old and long-employed process. With the development and application to tableting of *spray-dried lactose* as a diluent, the approach was extended to many drugs which were not directly compressible themselves. Spray drying is accomplished by atomizing droplets of concentrated solutions or suspensions in a tower of hot air. Drying occurs as the product drops to the bottom of the tower. The resultant product is spherical, it is frequently of very uniform particle size, and has superior flow properties.

Newer *direct compression diluents* include special coarse crystalline grades or pregranulated forms of anhydrous crystalline lactose, calcium phosphate, calcium sulfate dihydrate, granular mannitol, crystalline sorbitol, and microcrystalline cellulose.[17, 40, 47, 57, 78] *Microcrystalline cellulose* is particularly interesting because it satisfies several criteria of an ideal direct compression diluent: it compresses directly without added binders or gums which could retard drug dissolution, has good flow properties, produces rapid tablet disintegration, is chemically compatible with a wide range of drugs, has low moisture content, and is physically, chemi-

---

* The Fitzpatrick Co., Chicago, Ill.

† Hutt, Inc., Schluchtern-Heilbronn, West Germany.

cally, and physiologically inert. The drawback of microcrystalline cellulose is its relatively high cost. The material, in addition to being a good dry binder, also acts as a disintegrant and is often contained in direct compression formulations in 5 to 15 percent concentration when another material is the primary diluent.

Many drug companies would like to convert to the direct compression method of tablet manufacture for established products, in order to streamline tablet production procedures, and they have the technology to do so. However, a change in tablet formulation is usually required to convert from wet granulation or slugging to direct compression, necessitating the filing of an amended new drug application and costly reverification of product safety and efficacy. Consequently, such changes in manufacturing approach for existing products have occurred slowly. Direct compression is, however, carefully considered for most new products as potentially the manufacturing method of choice.

For drugs with potential problem in regard to bioavailability on oral administration, tablets may be more difficult to design and manufacture than capsules or a liquid oral form. It is often found that direct compression interferes less with drug availability than either wet granulation or slugging, because the latter methods require double compaction or the use of liquid adhesives which may (and frequently do) inhibit drug release.

Tablet Compression

Tablets are manufactured by compression in a *die* between two *punches*. The tablet machine is a device which holds the punches and dies, feeds granulation into the die cavity, provides pressure, and ejects the formed tablet from the die. The bottom punch moves up and down in the die but never leaves it. The distance the bottom punch is set to drop in the die determines the size of the die cavity, the amount of granulation that will be fed into the die cavity from a *feeding device* and consequently, the tablet weight. With the bottom punch in its lowest position and the die cavity filled, the *compression step* is accomplished by the top punch which descends into the die and compacts the granulation.

Basically, there are two types of tablet machines—single punch machines and rotary machines. The *single punch machine* (Fig. 11-20) is a stamping press containing one die and one top and one bottom punch. All of the compression is applied by the top punch which descends to "stamp out" a tablet. A feeding shoe, fed from a hopper above, contains the granulation and moves back and forth over the die to fill it when the bottom punch is down. The shoe then moves out of the way so that the top punch can descend for compression. After compression, the top punch lifts and the bottom punch carries the completed tablet to the level of the top of the die. The feed-shoe then sweeps across the die to kick the tablet down a discharge shoot. The bottom punch drops and the feeding shoe refills the die. The single punch tablet machine is limited in output to from 60 to 150 tablets per minute, which is too slow for commercial production. It does not typically contain an overload device to prevent jamming if excessive pressure is applied, and, being a stamping press, it tends to compress air in the die during tablet compression. One of the few remaining uses of the single punch machine is preparation of very large tablets for veterinary use, and even this is being taken over by special rotary machines.

In the *rotary tablet machine* (Fig. 11-21) from 4 to 69 sets of punches and dies are used. A heavy metal table containing the dies rotates, as does the "head" of the machine containing the top punches and the "foot" containing the bottom punches. These three rotating members are all driven by a central shaft or "post" of the machine and are thus synchronized. A hopper feeds granulation into an elongated feed frame which may cover 8 to 12 inches or more of the track the dies move under when the bottom punches are in the down position. In Figure 11-21, the feed frame is enclosed and is to the left-front, below the stainless steel hopper. The feed frame may contain revolving motor-driven spindles or other devices to introduce or force granulation into the dies. The compression

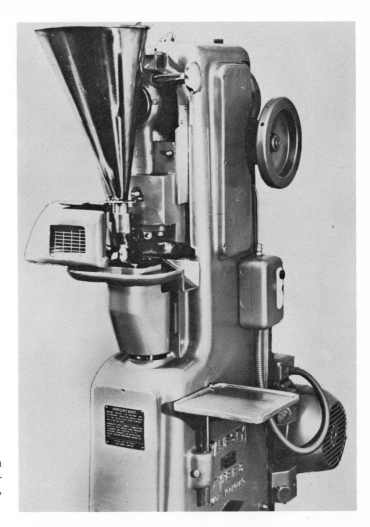

Fig. 11-20. A single punch tablet machine. (Thomas Engineering, Hoffman Estates, Ill.)

cycle begins when both the upper and the lower punches, moving together on a cam track, move between two pressure wheels. The upper pressure roll or wheel (top left of Fig. 11-21) is shown at the point at which the top punches are in their lowest position. An identical roll is out of sight for application of pressure to the lower punches. The heads of the tablet punches are flanged, as shown, to ride in the slotted grooves of the cam track which guides the punches up and down in their circuit around the machine. The pressure rolls are connected to a lever-arm or other pressure release device to permit them to lift if a double tablet or other overload is generated. Thus, a properly set-up rotary tablet machine should not jam or break punches as a result of compression overload. If square tablets or tablets of any shape other than round are being made, the cylindrical holes through the head of the machine into which the top punches are dropped must be slotted or have a groove to match a ridge running along the punch barrel which keeps the punches from turning in the head of the machine. This is essential if the punch with noncircular shape is to drop into the die and perfectly match a similarly shaped die cavity.

Rotary machines can produce as many as 12,000 tablets per minute in the largest and most sophisticated models—a clear advantage over single punch machines. A single machine operating at 12,000 tablets per minute has a production capacity of over 5 million tablets in a single 8-hour day. In

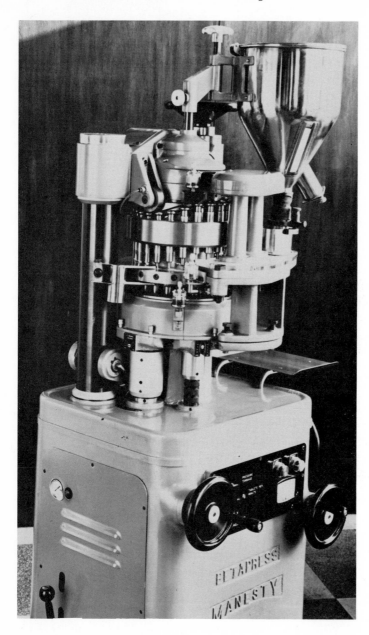

FIG. 11-21. A rotary tablet machine. Refer to text for operating description. (Thomas Engineering, Hoffman Estates, Ill.)

addition, the compression cycle in a rotary machine is a squeezing action which is much less likely to entrap air and create tableting problems. Formulations and granulations are frequently encountered that cannot be successfully compressed on a single punch machine but run quite well on a rotary tablet machine.

Three major advances have been made recently in *rotary tablet machine design and control,* and these advances are having an effect on tablet product quality. They are:

(1) Very high speed machines;

(2) Instrumented tablet machines, and

(3) Automated tablet machines.

Figure 11-22 shows the latest of *very high speed tablet machines* capable of producing up to 12,000 tablets per minute. Figure 11-23 shows the control panel for this sophisticated machine which includes a tachom-

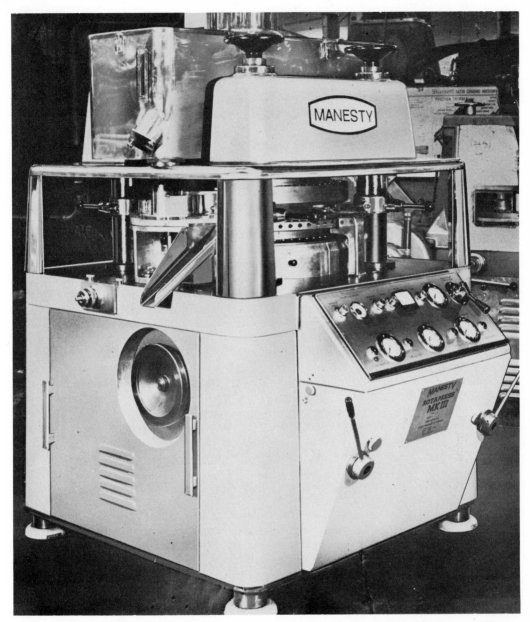

Fig. 11-22.   A modern high speed tablet press, the Manesty Rotapress Mark III. (Thomas Engineering, Hoffman Estates, Ill.)

eter, precompression (tamping to partially exclude air) and final compression gauges, overload warning lights, lubricating oil pressure gauge (at these speeds moving parts of the machine must be kept lubricated), speed control buttons which if held down either speed or slow the machine, a clutch lever, air pressure gauge, an ammeter to indicate electrical demand, and the start-stop button. For maximum high speed operation, granulation flow must be good, even with induced die feeding, and tablet weight variation may be the limiting factor.

Instrumented tablet machines are equipped with electronic devices to monitor machine performance. The most common monitoring

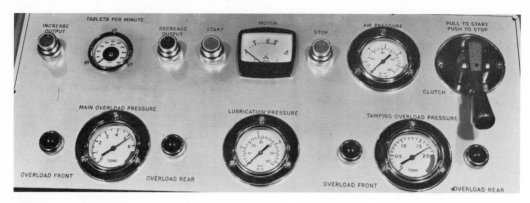

Fig. 11-23. The control panel of the Manesty Rotapress Mark III. (Thomas Engineering, Hoffman Estates, Ill.)

device is the *strain gauge,* which is a sensing unit capable of measuring deformation, strain, and load in and applied to a metal structural unit. Strain gauges, if applied to the beam of the pressure roll, can measure the compressive force applied to each tablet. If applied to the lower punch ejection cam, the strain gauge can monitor the forces required to eject the completed tablets. If all the punches in a rotary machine are carefully gauged to be the same length and if the granulation is reasonably standardized as to particle size distribution, the tablet compression force and variations in that force will reflect tablet weight and weight variation, respectively. In Figure 11-24, a strain-gauge instrumented machine is shown connected to an oscilloscope for strain gauge read-out. Strain gauge outputs monitoring several different machine functions may be switched into a single oscilloscope through a control box. Print-out from the strain gauges may also be put on tape for a permanent record. Strain gauge monitoring data not only provide information on tablet weight and ejection forces but can provide information on machine malfunctioning or punch wear. Other machine monitoring involves measurement of electrical power demand. A jump in power demand may indicate pressure overload or machine malfunction.

The most recent and exciting tableting advance is *automated tablet production.* The tablet weight is sensed by a monitoring device, for example a strain gauge on the pressure roll beam, and the data are fed to a computer. The computer is programmed with the optimum tablet weight and its acceptable upper and lower limits of tolerance. If the measured tablet weight approaches or exceeds the limits, the computer resets tablet weight through a synchronous motor connected to the machine's weight adjustment. In other, less automated systems, the machine is not connected to a computer and does not have the ability to reset itself, but it constantly monitors its own performance and automatically shuts itself off when the strain gauge read-out indicates that tablet weights are approaching either of the limits of tolerance. The operator then must make the necessary adjustments before restarting the machine.

The significance of the automated tablet machine is that the weight of every single tablet can be monitored, and the control of tablet weight and weight variation is absolute. Tableting pressure and resultant tablet hardness, porosity, and probable rate of dissolution and release are thus also monitored and controlled.

EVALUATION OF TABLETS

Tablets are evaluated according to their chemical and physical characteristics.

Chemical Characteristics

The chemical characteristics of tablets involve their (1) *potency,* (2) *content uniformity,* and (3) *purity.*

The **potency** of official tablets is usually given in terms of milligrams of drug per tablet and is determined by means of an

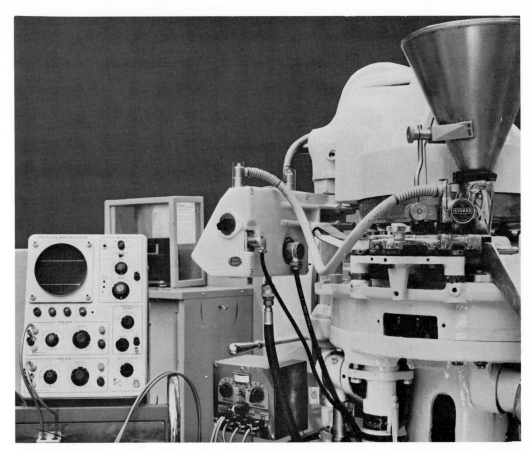

Fig. 11-24.   An instrumented tablet machine with oscilloscope read-out. (The Upjohn Company, Kalamazoo, Mich.)

official analytical method which involves grinding several tablets in a mortar and analyzing a portion of the resulting powder. For example, if twenty 300-mg. Aspirin Tablets U.S.P. were subjected to the official assay, they might be found to contain a total of 6.2 g. of aspirin. Thus, the average potency would be 310 mg. per tablet. Since the *U.S.P.* states that the actual potency must fall between 95 and 105 percent of the labeled potency (i.e., between 285 and 315 mg. per tablet for tablets labeled 300 mg.) the assayed tablets meet the *U.S.P.* specifications for potency.

Of the twenty tablets, however, 10 tablets may have contained 250 mg. of aspirin and 10 may have contained 370 mg. of aspirin. Such a variation in potency could lead to ineffectiveness or overdosing or, at least,

marked variation in therapeutic response. It is for this reason that tablets are subjected to additional tests which preclude great tablet-to-tablet variations in potency. One such test is the *Weight Variation Test.** In this test, individual tablets are weighed to assure that the tablet-to-tablet variation in weight is not excessive. This test is prescribed by the *U.S.P.* as a means of assuring uniform potency for Aspirin Tablets, U.S.P., and it is effective for aspirin and other high-dose drugs where the tablets are essentially all (90 to 95%) active ingredient.

The weight variation test is not sufficient to assure uniform potency for tablets of low-dose drugs, in which excipients make up the

* United States Pharmacopeia, 18th Revision, p. 950.

bulk of the tablet weight.[9, 10, 35, 36, 53] In this case, a *Content Uniformity Test** is applied in which 30 tablets are selected and at least 10 are individually assayed. Nine of the 10 tablets must contain not less than 85 percent nor more than 115 percent of labeled potency and the tenth tablet may contain not less than 75 percent nor more than 125 percent of labeled potency. If these conditions are not met, the remaining 20 tablets must be individually assayed, and none may fall outside the 85 to 115 percent range. In evaluating a particular lot of tablets, the content uniformity test should be applied to several samples taken from various parts of the production run according to accepted statistical sampling procedures.

What appears to be a relatively wide content uniformity range (i.e., 85 to 115%) may be difficult to achieve in practice with potent low-dose drugs. There are three factors inherent in the tablet manufacturing process which may cause difficulties in achieving narrow ranges of content uniformity: (1) *nonuniform distribution* of drug throughout the powder mixture or granulation, (2) *Segregation* of the powder mixture or granulation during the manufacturing process, and (3) *Tablet weight variation.*

Figure 11-25 illustrates the problem of *nonuniform distribution* of irregularly shaped

* United States Pharmacopeia, 18th Revision, p. 930.

drug particles of various sizes throughout a mixture of irregularly shaped diluent particles of various sizes. It is not difficult to comprehend why a perfect physical mixture never occurs geometrically (uniform physical placement of the drug particles in space) or statistically (equal probability that all portions of the mixture will contain a given number of drug particles). Reduction in drug particle size may help distribution, but it also may promote segregation.

The greatest potential for *segregation* or drug-excipient separation occurs with powder mixtures intended for direct compression and with wet granulations in which drug migration is likely. In the former case, separation is promoted by vibration in the machinery and by differences in the particle sizes and densities of the drug and excipients. In the latter case, separation is more likely when the drug is very soluble in the granulating fluid. Since the uniformity of the tablets cannot be better than that of the granulation, it may be advisable to determine the drug content uniformity of the granulation before compression. Corrective steps taken before compression are simpler, less expensive, and less likely to have a deleterious effect on tablet properties, such as dissolution rate or in-vivo availability, than grinding and recompressing the tablets after they have once been made.

Although a small *variation in tablet weight* does not guarantee a similarly small

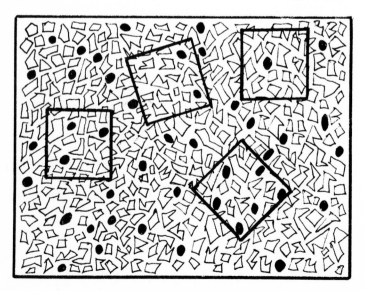

FIG. 11-25. Illustration of a powder mixture; angular open particles represent excipient, dark circles represent drug. The one square inch squares represent identical size powder samples, which contain as few as one to as many as six drug particles. Solid dosage forms represent similar powder or granule "samples." The presence of a large number of drug particles per dose is critical to low dose variation between tablets.

variation in content uniformity, a large variation in tablet weight precludes good content uniformity. The influence of various factors on tablet weight variation are discussed in the next section.

In considering the total concept of potency and uniformity of solid dosage forms, pharmaceutical scientists are more and more concerned with evaluating and controlling the *effective drug content* of the product. This is the amount of drug in the product that is present in an absorbable or bioavailable form. Evidence based on controlled studies in man[13, 14, 15, 29, 39, 68, 69, 76, 94] indicates that the effective drug content of solid dosage forms is frequently not 100 percent of the assayable drug content of the product. For some classes of drugs, such as the anticoagulants, as little as 50 percent or less of the labeled and assayed drug content in each dosage unit may be bioavailable. Likewise, if manufacturing parameters, such as compression load, influence bioavailability, the *effective content uniformity* of a batch of tablets will be dependent upon both the actual drug content per tablet and the bioavailability of that particular batch of the drug product. The variation in effective drug content uniformity is undoubtedly much greater in many cases than chemical content uniformity indicates. At some future date, for at least some classes of drugs such as the anticoagulants, the potency of various products may be expressed as an *effective bioavailable content* rather than a chemical content as at present. Such expressions would help physicians and pharmacists establish dosage regimens and could improve the safety of such drugs.

The **purity** of U.S.P. tablets is usually assured by utilizing raw materials (both active drug and excipients) which meet U.S.P. specifications. Any extraneous substance present in a raw material which is not specifically allowed in compendial specifications, or in well-defined manufacturer's specifications, renders the material unacceptable for pharmaceutical product use. Such extraneous substances may have unpredictable effects on product stability, safety, or efficacy. Occasionally, a well-defined impurity may appear in a tablet either from a raw material or from unavoidable decomposition of the drug. In these cases, a specification is set for the maximum permissible amount of the impurity. For example, Aspirin Tablets, U.S.P., may contain no more than 0.15 percent of free salicylic acid relative to the amount of aspirin present.

Physical Characteristics

It was earlier stated that in regard to quality, the physical properties of tablets and the proper control of these properties are as important to this dosage form as they are to any dispersed system. It is also now recognized that some of the fundamental physical characteristics of tablets, such as porosity, hardness, disintegration, drug dissolution and release, and friability, are subject to change on aging and according to storage conditions. When pharmaceutical formulators design a solid dosage form, particularly a tablet, attention must be paid not only to maintenance of chemical potency on aging (chemical stability) but also to maintenance of drug bioavailability on aging (physical stability). In establishing expiration dates for drug products, drug companies and the Food and Drug Administration should give the matter of maintenance of bioavailability on aging due consideration, since myriad changes in the physical properties of the drug, the excipients, or the tablet-matrix itself could retard bioavailability.

Weight and Weight Variation. The relationship, or lack of relationship, which may exist between weight variation and content uniformity of solid dosage forms was mentioned earlier. A small weight variation does not ensure good content uniformity between dosage units; a large weight variation precludes good content uniformity. Any of the following factors, alone or in concert, can produce excessive tablet weight variations: (1) poor granulation flow properties, resulting in uneven die fill; (2) a wide variation in granulation particle size, which results in a variation in die fill density as a function of particle size and particle size distribution at different points in the production run; (3) differences in lower punch length, which result in different size die cavities; (4) improper incorporation of glidant granulation flow promotors, and (5) tablet machines in mechanically poor condition or dirty, which prevents free punch movement.

Official weight variation tests for tablets and capsules are given in the *U.S.P.* They range from ±10 percent for tablets weighing 130 mg. or less to ±5 percent for tablets weighing over 324 mg.[110]

Thickness. At constant compressive load, tablet thickness varies with changes in die fill and tablet weight; with constant die fill, thickness varies with variations in compressive load. Some variation in tablet thickness in a particular lot of tablets or between different lots of the product is inevitable. Variation in tablet thickness should not be immediately apparent to the unaided eye under normal conditions, for obvious reasons of product acceptance by the consumer. A second practical aspect in control of tablet thickness relates to packaging. Both the effective and repeated use of packaging equipment and the consistent fill of the same product container for a given number of dosage units may be affected if tablet thickness varies.

In practice, the crown thickness of individual tablets may be measured with a micrometer, or five or ten tablets may be simultaneously measured in a holding tray with a sliding caliper scale. The micrometer method is the more precise but the more time consuming.

In general, tablet thickness is controlled within 5 percent of a standard value. Tablet thickness control may be impossible unless (1) the physical properties of raw materials are closely controlled, (2) the upper and lower punch lengths are accurately and continuously standardized,[105] and (3) the granulation properties, including density, particle size, and particle size distribution, are also carefully controlled. Tablet thickness cannot be controlled independently, since it is related to tablet weight, compaction, density, friability and, possibly, drug release and bioavailability. At present, the interrelationships of all these variables have not been precisely elucidated. Doubtless, pharmaceutical science will advance to the point where tablet granulations will be sufficiently standardized to permit optimization of all tablet characteristics.

Hardness. *Tablet hardness* is usually expressed as the load required to crush a tablet placed on its edge. Hardness is thus sometimes termed the *tablet crushing strength*. A number of testing machines have been developed to measure tablet hardness. One of the earliest testers, developed nearly 40 years ago, was the *Monsanto hardness tester*.[99] It was a threaded device with a knurled knob which was turned to drive a plunger against the tablet. The plunger also operated against a spring such that the fracture point of the tablet could be read against the spring load in kilograms. The *Strong-Cobb tester*,[1] introduced about 20 years ago, is still in use. With this device, a plunger, activated by pumping a lever arm, is forced by hydraulic pressure against the tablet which is held in an anvil. The force in kilograms required for tablet fracture is read on a hydraulic gauge.

The *Pfizer tester*[77] (Fig. 11-26), developed about 10 years ago, is a plier type device utilizing hand-gripping action to produce the force to fracture the tablet. The fracture force is read on a direct force gauge. This is probably the most popular hardness tester currently in use, but it suffers from the disadvantage that the force with which the tester is gripped, i.e., the rate

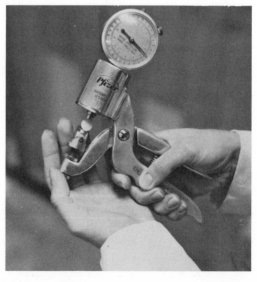

Fig. 11-26. The Pfizer tablet hardness tester. (School of Pharmacy, Purdue University)

at which the force is applied, affects the results. To overcome this disadvantage, an *electrically driven pneumatic tester* has been developed which is the most reproducible (and most expensive) of all the hardness testers developed to date. Although all the aforenamed testers read in kg. load or crushing strength, no two testers give identical readings for essentially identical tablets. Values obtained with the Strong-Cobb tester are reportedly 1.7 times those obtained with the Monsanto tester[71] and 1.4 to 1.7 times those obtained with the direct force loaded testers.[31]

Tablet hardness is frequently a useful method of controlling a tablet production operation, particularly when it is combined with measurements of tablet thickness. The suitability of a tablet in regard to mechanical stability during packaging and shipment can usually be predicted on the basis of hardness. Most manufacturers consider a tablet hardness of about 5 kg. to be minimal for uncoated tablets, though some chewable tablets may be somewhat softer. Tablet hardness is not an absolute indicator of friability (weight loss on attrition). Some very hard tablets tend to "cap" on attrition, losing their crown portions.

The hardness of a tablet is a function of the compressive force, the granule or crystal hardness and ability to deform under load, the binders used and their concentration, the granulation method, and other factors. Tablet hardness, in turn, influences tablet density and porosity. It may affect tablet friability and disintegration time (Table 11-2). It usually affects drug dissolution and release, and it may affect bioavailability (Fig. 11-27).

Friability. *Tablet friability* results in weight loss of tablets in the package container, owing to partial powdering, chipping, or fragmentation of the tablets on attrition or wear. Cotton or other cellulose materials are commonly placed in containers of tablets to keep them tightly packed to reduce "rattling" and frictional contact on shipping or other handling and agitation. The pharmacist may occasionally observe evidence of excessive tablet friability in the form of powder or tablet fragments in the bottom of a container. Excessive friability has the effect

TABLE 11-2. COMPRESSIONAL FORCE AND DISINTEGRATION TIMES FOR ASPIRIN, PHENACETIN AND CAFFEINE TABLETS PREPARED ON AN INSTRUMENTED ROTARY TABLET PRESS*

FORCE (LBS.)	DISINTEGRATION TIME (MINS.) w/o DISCS†	WITH DISCS‡
2170	15	4.7
2845	19	13.7
3650	27	20.7
4275	31	23.8
4715	33	24.8
5500	37.7	27.8
6080	42.5	27.2
6735	46.5	33.2
7225	52	32.5
7975	54	33.8

* Knoechel *et al.*: J. Pharm. Sci., *56*:116, 1967.
† Average time for 2 tablets tested individually.
‡ Average time for 6 tablets tested at same time; fluid was pH 1.3 in both cases.

of decreasing tablet weight and the drug dose remaining in the tablet. Tablets that are chipped or mechanically eroded and no longer have sharp edges are of reduced pharmaceutical elegance and reduced quality. They may also lack consumer acceptance. Tablet friability often reflects lack of cohesiveness on compression of the dry granulation from which the tablets are made.

Friability may be measured either by field trials (involving shipping tablets in their usual containers and shipping cartons back and forth across the country) or by use of a laboratory apparatus. The former method suffers from the fact that it is not a controlled procedure. It is accordingly difficult to interpret and is costly and time consuming. As a result, a laboratory tester[95] has been developed to quantify tablet friability (Fig. 11-28). This apparatus, *The Friabilator,* has a plastic chamber that is revolved at 25 r.p.m., dropping the tablets a distance of 6 inches with each revolution. Normally, the preweighed tablet sample is placed in the Friabilator which is operated for 100 revolutions, after which the tablets are reweighed. Conventional compressed tablets that lose less than 0.5 to 1.0 percent in weight on Friabilator testing are usually considered acceptable.

Some chewable tablets and most effervescent tablets have higher friability weight

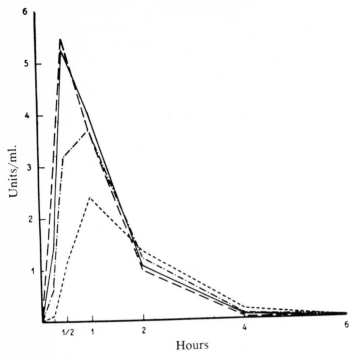

Fig. 11-27. Effect of tablet hardness and resultant disintegration time on the bioavailability of penicillin V, based on units of activity/ml. in the plasma of 10 fasting human subjects. Solid line, 1 minute disintegration; long-dashed line, 10 minute disintegration; dot-dash line, 30 minute disintegration; short dashed line, 75 minute disintegration. (Juncher, H., and Raaschou, F.: Antibiot. Med. Clin. Ther., *4*:497, 1957)

loss, which accounts for the stack packaging of effervescent tablets in a single column in special tablet vials. Hydrophobic drug substances which have weak crystalline structure, are difficult to wet and bind together by the usual granulation methods, and have poor cohesion on compression pose the greatest friability problem. Increasing compression pressure and tablet hardness may not reduce friability if the tablets tend to cap

(i.e., lose their crowns). When capping does occur, increasing compression pressure often makes the problem worse. When capping is observed on Friabilator testing, the tablets are considered to be unacceptable for commercial use regardless of the friability percentage loss value.

When concave punches are used in tableting, punches that are in poor condition and are worn at their surface edges produce

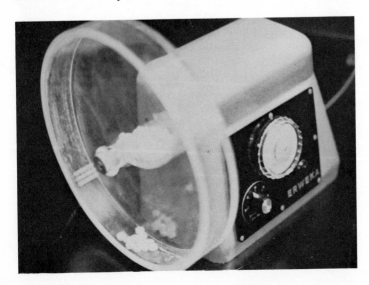

Fig. 11-28. The Roche Friabilator, illustrating the dropping of tablets during test. (School of Pharmacy, Purdue University)

tablets with "whiskers" at the tablet edge. Even though the resultant tablets may be well within weight variation limits, such tablets may produce high friability values because the "whiskers" will probably be removed in testing. Tablet friability may be profoundly affected by the moisture content of the tablet granulation and the finished tablets. Very dry granulations and tablets containing less than 0.5 to 1.0 percent of moisture may be much more friable than tablets containing 2 to 4 percent of moisture. For this reason, the manufacture of mechanically sound and maximally chemically stable tablets of some hydrolyzable drugs is very difficult.

Disintegration. The United States Pharmacopeia[110] has long had a disintegration test for tablets. The U.S.P. apparatus (Fig. 11-29) employs 6 glass tubes, 3 inches long open at the top end and held against a 10-mesh (10 wires per linear inch) screen at the bottom end of the basket rack assembly. In practice, one tablet is placed in each tube, and the basket rack is positioned in a 1-liter beaker of water, simulated gastric fluid, or simulated intestinal fluid at 37° ±2° such that the tablets remain at least 2.5 cm. below the liquid surface on their upward movement and descend to not closer than 2.5 cm. from the bottom of the beaker. A standard motor-driven device is used to move the basket rack assembly containing the tablets up and down through a distance of 5 to 6 cm. at a frequency of 28 to 32 cycles per minute. Perforated plastic discs (Fig. 11-29) may also be employed in the test, being placed on top of the tablets. The discs are mildly abrasive to the tablets and may or may not produce a more sensitive or meaningful test. The discs are useful for tablets that float.

To comply with U.S.P. standards, the tablets must disintegrate and all particles fall through the 10-mesh screen in the time specified. If any residue remains, it must have a soft mass with no palpably firm core. Specifications for disintegration time exist for all coated and uncoated tablets except very large tablets (such as effervescent tablets), tablets used to make hypodermic solutions, and troches or tablets to be chewed. Uncoated U.S.P. tablets have disintegration times as low as 5 minutes (aspirin tablets), but the majority of uncoated tablets have a maximum disintegration time of 30 minutes to one hour. Enteric-coated tablets should show no distinct evidence of dissolution or disintegration after 1 hour in simulated gastric fluid, and the same tablets run thereafter in the apparatus containing simulated intestinal fluid must disintegrate within 4 additional hours.

In regard to compressed tablets, the U.S.P. disintegration test tells the pharmacist one thing only—how long it takes for a tablet to break up and for all the particles to fall through the 10-mesh screen under the conditions of the test. The test may or may not correlate with tablet dissolution in vitro or with drug absorption in vivo. Some tablets readily disintegrate to regenerate the original granules from which the tablets were made; however, if these granules are slow to dissolve, the disintegration time may be completely unrelated to drug dissolution or bioavailability. The work of Levy[66] on the disintegration, dissolution, and absorption of commercial aspirin tablets (Table 11-3) not only indicates the lack of correlation which may exist between the U.S.P. disintegration test results and the performance of the products in vivo but also suggests the manner in which a development pharmacist could be misled by relying on disintegration data. Product A in Table 11-3 had by far the longest disintegration time, yet was the most nearly completely dissolved at 10 minutes

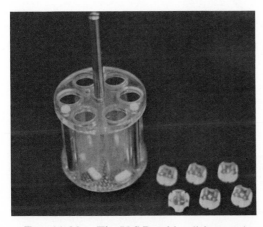

Fig. 11-29. The U.S.P. tablet disintegration basket with plastic discs.

TABLE 11-3.   DISINTEGRATION, DISSOLUTION AND GASTROINTESTINAL ABSORPTION VALUES FOR A SERIES OF COMMERCIAL ASPIRIN TABLETS*

PRODUCT	AVERAGE U.S.P. DISINTEGRATION TIME (SECONDS)	AVERAGE AMOUNT DISSOLVED IN 10 MINUTES (MG.)	AMOUNT EXCRETED IN URINE† (MG.)	
A	256	242	24.3	
C	< 10	165	18.1	Study I‡
E	< 10	127	15.9	
B	35	205	18.5	
D	13	158	13.6	Study II‡
E	< 10	127	12.1	

* Levy, G.: J. Pharm. Sci., *50*:388, 1961.
† In terms of apparent salicylic acid, 1 hour postadministration of two 0.3-g. tablets.
‡ Studies I and II were carried out with different test subjects and under somewhat different conditions.

and was the most rapidly absorbed based on 1-hour urinary elimination. The disintegration data in no way correlated with or predicted bioavailability in this study.

Dissolution. Drugs administered orally in solid dosage forms, such as tablets or cap-

sules, must dissolve in the contents of the gastrointestinal tract before drug absorption can occur. Often the rate of drug absorption is determined by the rate of drug dissolution from the dosage form. Therefore, if it is important to achieve high peak blood levels for a drug, it will usually be important to obtain rapid drug dissolution from the dosage form. For drugs absorbed high in the gastrointestinal tract (e.g., acidic drugs) which have a large dose and a low equilibrium solubility, rapid dissolution may be equally important. The design of the dosage form and the dissolution profile for such drugs may determine the total amount of drug absorbed as well as its rate of absorption. Thus, the rate of dissolution may be directly related to the efficacy of the product. Controlled drug dissolution is the basis of all sustained-release and controlled-release solid dosage forms, and factors such as physiological site of drug release, onset of drug action, and duration of drug effect may be intentionally modified by modifying drug dissolution rate.

Table 11-3 and Figure 11-30 show good correlation between in-vitro dissolution data and in-vivo bioavailability of aspirin prod-

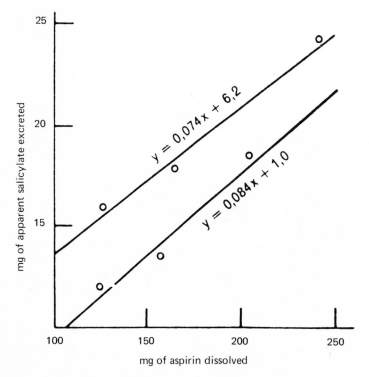

FIG. 11-30.   Correlation between in-vitro and in-vivo drug release for a series of commercial aspirin tablets. See Table 11-3 for raw data. (Levy, G.: J. Pharm. Sci., *50*:385, 1961)

ucts. Similar correlations have been observed with many drugs. Since in-vitro dissolution rate measurements can often be correlated with drug bioavailability or other in-vivo characteristics, the importance of dissolution testing as the major in-vitro test of tablet characteristics is obvious.

In the design of any *dissolution test* several operating variables must be considered: (1) the nature of the dissolution medium used, (2) the volume of the medium, (3) the method of mounting the dosage form in the apparatus, (4) the geometry of the apparatus, (5) the intensity of agitation, and, in some cases, (6) the presence of a dialysis membrane. Other variables include temperature, which is usually maintained at 37° or body temperature. If the dissolution test procedure is to correlate with drug product performance in vivo, the operating variables of the test should be relevant to the properties of the drug such as site of absorption from the gastrointestinal tract and solubility. In addition, a dissolution test should be capable of discriminating small differences in the dissolution and release behavior of a variety of drug products or of slight modifications in the design of a single product. A dissolution test may overdiscriminate or indicate release differences that are of no consequence in vivo. Still, such a test is much more desirable than one that underdiscriminates and does not reflect dissolution differences which are in fact significant in vivo.

The *dissolution medium* should reflect the medium at the site of absorption or above it in the gastrointestinal tract. For example, acidic drugs should be tested in simulated gastric fluid or in an acidic medium, since, for best absorption, they must dissolve in the stomach or upper small intestine. Dissolution testing of such drugs in simulated intestinal fluid at pH 7.4 would serve little purpose, since moderately acidic drugs would be nearly completely ionized and absorption would be inhibited at that pH. The volume of the dissolution medium should be adequate to dissolve all the drug in the dosage form, even if several liters of fluid are required. If drug solubility is so low that this is impracticable, a miscible organic solvent (e.g., alcohol) may be added to the

medium, or an elaborate dissolution cell employing a membrane system or a water-immiscible organic solvent layer may be used to provide a reservoir. It should be emphasized, however, that complex dissolution cells which attempt to simulate human physiology by means of elaborate glassware or animal membranes do not give any better correlations with in-vivo release than are obtained with simpler well-designed systems.

The method of mounting the dosage form in the dissolution apparatus should be precisely reproducible for all solid dosage forms, including coated and uncoated tablets as well as capsules. The dissolution apparatus should have a widely variable but highly controllable range of agitation intensities.

The *U.S.P. dissolution test apparatus* (Fig. 11-31) consists of a cylindrical vessel with a rounded bottom capable of holding 1,000 ml. of dissolution medium. The top of

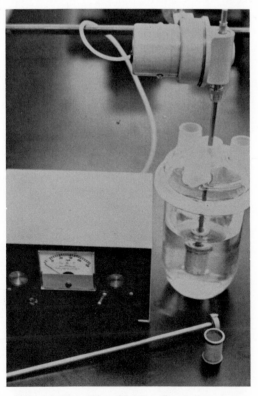

Fig. 11-31. The *U.S.P.* dissolution apparatus, showing the rotating basket in the dissolution flask plus the speed control box with tachometer. The dissolution flask is ordinarily mounted in a water bath and operated at 37°.

the vessel is flanged to accept a fitted cover with 4 ports. The shaft from the variable speed (25 to 150 r.p.m.) motor goes through the center port and is connected to the cylindrical stainless steel 40-mesh wire basket which holds the dosage form. The other ports are for a thermometer and for fluid withdrawal and return.

A dissolution test may employ intermittent sampling or continuous analysis of the dissolution medium. Figure 11-32 shows a U.S.P. dissolution apparatus (A) set up for continuous analysis. A pump (B) is used to draw fluid from the dissolution vessel and pass it into the flow cell of a UV spectrophotometer (C). The absorbance value read by the spectrophotometer is fed to a recorder (D) which plots drug concentration in the dissolution vessel versus time. *E* is the power supply for the spectrophotometer, and *F* is the speed control and tachometer which controls the stirring motor. The dissolution vessel is mounted in a water bath to provide temperature control.

When intermittent sampling is employed, corrections may be necessary to account for the volume and drug content of the samples removed for analysis or for dilution resulting from the addition of fresh medium

to maintain volume. When the dissolution medium is continuously analyzed using an arrangement such as that shown in Figure 11-32, these corrections are usually unnecessary, since the medium is returned to the apparatus after it is analyzed. Additional advantages of a continuously recording dissolution apparatus are convenience and operator efficiency and a continuous record of drug release which may reveal subtle differences in the release patterns of the tablets studied.

It is important to conduct a dissolution test properly and equally important to interpret the data properly. Dissolution results may be expressed in terms of the concentration of drug in the dissolution medium versus time, the amount of drug released from the dosage form versus time, or the amount of drug remaining unreleased from the dosage form versus time. Most commonly, the results are expressed in terms of the time required to release some predetermined fraction of the labeled amount of drug from the dosage form. For example, the *U.S.P.* specifies that 60 percent of the labeled amount of hydrochlorothiazide shall dissolve from Hydrochlorothiazide Tablets, U.S.P., in not more than 30 minutes. Such ex-

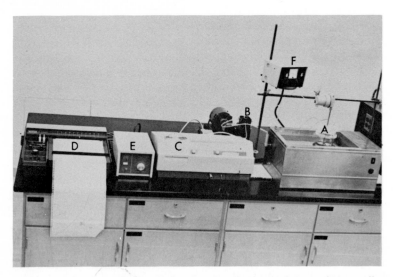

Fig. 11-32.   U.S.P. dissolution apparatus set-up for continuous dissolution monitoring and recording. (A) Dissolution apparatus; (B) pump; (C) UV spectrophotometer; (D) recorder; (E) power supply for spectrophotometer; (F) speed control and tachometer. (School of Pharmacy, Purdue University)

pressions of dissolution and release characteristics obviously suffer from the disadvantage that they do not account for the portion of the drug remaining unreleased. For example, it is entirely possible that 60 percent of the labeled amount of hydrochlorothiazide could be released from a given tablet in 5 minutes and also that 10 percent, or more, would never be released from the *same tablet*. Alternatively, it is possible for 60 percent to be released rapidly and for the remaining 40 percent to be released very slowly. Thus, the description of a dissolution process in terms of a single point in time is inherently risky. Such expressions are useful for quality control purposes once the dissolution characteristics of the drug and dosage form are well understood. For tablet product design purposes and for critical product comparisons, the time required for substantially complete (80 to 90%) release or amount released versus time profiles are most desirable.

TABLET COATING

The coating of solid dosage forms (pills) is a historical pharmaceutical process that can be traced back over 1,000 years. Coating of pills with vegetable gum mucilages was reported in the 9th century, with coatings of silver and gold leaf being reported a century later.[113] Still later, a "pearl coating" technique was developed, employing a talc composition which produced coated pills resembling pearls.[120] While these "pearls" and the gold and silver coated products were undoubtedly very elegant, talc is not only water insoluble but also water repellent, and gold and silver resist dissolution even in aqua regia. Consequently, most such products must have been eliminated in the same form in which they were given, i.e. intact. In light of the crude drug combinations of the day, such coatings may at least have served the purpose of "consumer protection."

Coating technology advanced in the middle and late 1800's, with all of the following pill coating techniques being reported; first gelatin coating;[58] first sugar coated pills made in Europe and used in the U.S.;[121] first sugar-coated pills manufactured in the U.S. by a Philadelphia pharmacist;[118] first enteric coated pills.[111] After tablets were introduced in the United States and manufactured here in the late 1800's, many of the same coating techniques were also applied to tablets.

Early coating was undertaken primarily for the purpose of improving product elegance, notably appearance. Much of the early coating of pills was done by the pharmacist, who coated his pills singly by such crude methods as dipping a pill on the point of a needle or held with forceps. A physician by the name of Upjohn recognized that many coated and uncoated pills did not break up in the body, and he developed a method of coating sugar beads with drug plus excipient to produce the so-called friable pill. The Upjohn Company began with this development, and early Upjohn labels depicted a thumb (presumably Dr. Upjohn's) crushing a friable pill.

In the first forty years of the 20th century, production techniques were developed for sugar- and enteric-coating of tablets. The most rapid development in both coating technology (compression coating, film coating, air suspension coating, and automated coating) and coating compositions (controlled release coatings for sustained release products and synthetic polymers for film coating) have occurred since about 1940. We have not seen the end of coating developments. When optimized drug products become a reality through scientific dosage form design to precisely control drug release, new and improved coating will be part of the picture. Some of these coatings will function as semipermeable membranes or as molecular sieves to exactly control drug release. Other coatings will control not only the rate of release of drugs in the body but the duration of residence of the dosage form at a particular body site. Some coated solid forms will be used in implant therapy to provide controlled drug release for months at a time. Even though it is more difficult than ever to meet all FDA requirements in bringing a new dosage form to the market place, a number of very exciting new advances in dosage form design are being developed which could revolutionize drug delivery.

Modern Justification for the Coating of Solid Dosage Forms

There are numerous valid reasons for coating solid dosage forms, and most of these reasons can be related to the concept of *the dosage form as a delivery system for drugs.* The dosage form is intended to deliver the drug chemically intact, to the absorption site, in an absorbable form. This means that dissolution must proceed at an optimum rate for maximum reliable therapeutic effect with the maximum possible safety margin.

Many drug products today are not delivery systems, but "dump systems," that is, they dump drug rapidly into the gastrointestinal tract. As a result, the rate of absorption depends upon the inherent absorption rate of the drug, not the delivery rate from the dosage form. For such dump systems, the therapeutic index (ratio of lethal dose in 50% of the subjects to effective dose in 50% of the subjects) would be the same for the drug product as for the drug administered in solution. In the controlled release system, where the absorption rate is dependent upon the drug delivery rate from the dosage form, it is possible for the drug product to have a higher therapeutic index (hence a greater safety margin) than the drug in solution or in a dump system.

For example, in one study with the antihistamine methapyrilene, an L.D.$_{83}$ (lethal dose in 83% of the animals dosed) was established in rats when the methapyrilene was administered in a dump system. The same dose in a controlled release system had an L.D.$_{.0}$.[41] The controlled release form, at the same time, produced *continuous* therapy in test animals (protection against allergic response to histamine vapor) over an 8-hour period, compared to only four hours protection with the dump system. Dump systems are rational for acidic drug substances, for which rapid dissolution is desirable to achieve complete or near complete availability; in therapeutic situations in which high peak blood levels are sought (perhaps some antibiotic therapy), or in situations in which rapid drug absorption reduces gastrointestinal irritation or other side effects.

For dangerous drugs (low therapeutic index), depressant drugs, or abused drugs, *controlled drug release* for the purpose of *improved safety* could well be more fundamental to optimum drug product design than longer duration of therapeutic effect. If depressant and dangerous drugs were designed as delivery systems rather than as dump systems, in many cases greater safety could be achieved along with equivalent therapeutic action, even if a somewhat longer time for onset of action might result. In the case of accidental or intentional overdose, for example, a significant fraction of a controlled release dosage form of a potent drug might be recovered with a stomach pump, whereas use of a stomach pump might be too late in the case of a dump system dosage form of the same drug.

Thus, if the dosage form is conceived as a true delivery system, the following are valid reasons for coating solid dosage forms:

1. *To control the site of release of the drug.* This is best illustrated in terms of enteric coating:

    A. Protection of the drug against gastric fluids which would destroy it by enzymic attack or acid catalyzed decomposition (Examples: a glandular product or proteinaceous drug in the former case; erythromycin in the latter case)

    B. Protection of the stomach against drugs that would be irritating or dangerous if released in the stomach (Examples: strong electrolytes, such as potassium chloride, or aspirin in ulcer patients)

    C. Retarded release of drugs that may exert an emetic effect if released in the stomach (Examples: emetine, atabrine, diethylstilbestrol, iron salts, and many anthelmintics)

    D. Delivery of the drug into the intestinal tract in the highest possible concentration without dilution by mixing with gastric contents (Examples: intestinal antiseptics and anthelmintics)

2. *To provide a controlled, continuous drug release rate.* This may be done for any of the following purposes:

    A. To produce a sustained or prolonged drug effect, with resultant diminished frequency in the drug dosing schedule

B. To improve the safety of drug products by reducing high peaks in the blood level–time profile, particularly in those cases where high peaks do not contribute to the therapeutic effect

C. To improve drug reliability either by delivering the drug to the duodenum and jejunum for optimum absorption[42, 48, 74] or by reducing the periods during which serum concentrations fall below the minimum effective concentration

3. *To maintain physical or chemical drug integrity.* This may be done for the following purposes:

A. To protect the ingredients against the atmosphere, notably water vapor and oxygen, and light. Hydrolyzable drugs and hygroscopic inorganic salts frequently require protection from water vapor in the air if adequate stability and shelf life are to be achieved. However, coatings that provide an effect barrier against water vapor are hydrophobic and generally retard drug dissolution. Coatings are less effective as oxygen barriers. Perfectly opaque coatings can be designed for light-sensitive drugs.

B. To separate reactive or incompatible ingredients. Certain combinations of active ingredients and/or excipients may undergo a detrimental chemical or physical reaction in the tablet. In the sugar coating process, the core or uncoated tablet may be sealed with a barrier coating and a second drug separated from the core by adding it with the sugar coating or as a separate coat. In many vitamin-mineral tablets, selected minerals, especially iron salts, are placed in the coating to provide chemical separation from the vitamins. Compression coated tablets can provide partial separation of reactants in the two-component product or complete separation in the three-component system. Occasionally, reactant materials are prepared as separate granulations, and

one or both granulations are coated to reduce reactant contact in the tablet. Ascorbic acid is commercially available with an ethylcellulose coating for such applications.

4. To produce a pharmaceutically better product. This is less related to the drug delivery concept but is perhaps equally as important. Some drugs have an unpleasant odor, or a decomposition product may have an odor, which can be contained by coating. Other drugs are off-white or darkly colored or may change color on aging without significant reduction in potency. Drugs that stain the skin and clothing are also candidates for coating. Additionally, certain drugs are among the most bitter substances known to man, e.g., quinine and its salts and derivatives and many antibiotics in the form of soluble salts. In uncoated form, unless they are quickly swallowed, tablets of such drugs may dissolve sufficiently to produce bitterness and make swallowing unpleasant if not impossible. Although these factors are not as dramatic as altering the toxicity or therapeutic effectiveness of a drug by changing the properties of the dosage form, they are nonetheless important in the clinical situation where the patient's psychological response to the product and its acceptance may be as important as his physiological response to the drug.

Theory and Design of Enteric and Controlled Release Coatings

Enteric coatings are designed to remain intact in the stomach but to quickly fail and release drug on entering the small intestine. *Controlled release coatings,* on the other hand, are designed to release drug at various rates on exposure to gastric or intestinal contents. They provide continuous controlled release as opposed to the delayed release of the enteric coated product.

A successful *enteric coating* must withstand the gastric environment for at least an hour but release the drug *very quickly* after it leaves the stomach. An enteric coating that requires one or two hours to fail and begin releasing drug after leaving the stomach will have already passed the upper small intestine where the absorption of most drugs is best and may be so far down the tract that complete drug release will not occur before the colon is reached. To rapidly trigger failure of an enteric coating high in the small intestine, advantage is taken of the differences in the lumen environment of the stomach and small intestine. The two major differences are *pH* and *enzyme content*.

The *gastric pH* in man is usually between 1 and 2.5, whereas the pH of the duodenum just outside the stomach is between 4.5 and 6.5. Effective enteric coating materials are often weak polymer acids which are insoluble at low pH's, at which they are predominantly unionized, but dissolve readily at higher pH's at which they are ionized to a significant degree. The degree of ionization of a weak acid as a function of its pKa and its pH environment is given by the Henderson-Hasselbalch equation.[75] The question is, "What is the ideal pKa for an effective enteric coating material?" Considering the upper and lower limits of the normal pH's in the stomach and duodenum, it can be estimated that an ideal enteric coating material should have a pKa of about 6, and the most widely used enteric coating material, cellulose acetate hydrogen phthalate, has a pKa exactly in this region.

Gastric enzymes—e.g., pepsin—do not attack fats, but pancreatin and lipase, which are secreted via the common bile duct into the duodenum very near the pylorus, have the ability to emulsify and digest many fats and waxes. Since the change in enzyme content between the stomach and the duodenum is more dramatic than the shift in pH, attempts have been made to utilize the fat emulsifying and digesting actions of bile and pancreatic fluid to trigger drug release from enteric-coated dosage forms. However, no fats or waxes, alone or in combination, have as yet been found that are sufficiently impervious to gastric fluid and are, also, rapidly attacked by duodenal enzymes to serve as effective enteric coatings.

On the other hand, fats and waxes have found wide application as *controlled release coatings* because they allow a gradual penetration of water which is almost completely independent of the pH of the environment. The rate of water penetration is dependent upon the thickness of the coating, and many substances have been employed as coatings.

Beeswax, carnauba wax, glyceryl monostearate, stearic acid, palmitic acid, and cetyl alcohol have been employed as coating materials for Spansule* products.† [6, 7] In a Spansule, the dose of the drug is distributed among a large number of pellets about 1 mm. in diameter. The pellets are coated with varying thicknesses of waxy or fatty materials. When they are exposed to gastrointestinal fluids, water penetrates the pellets at varying rates depending upon the thicknesses of their coats. Drug release is the result of sequential bursting of the pellets as the water reaches the cores. Each pellet releases a tiny dose of the drug.

There are a multitude of *release mechanisms* responsible for the action of both enteric and controlled release coatings. Most of the mechanisms that have been postulated are summarized in Table 11-4. Under actual experimental or clinical conditions, the most common is probably mechanism 5, i.e., some combination of any or all of the postulated mechanisms. Because of unavoidable biological variation in gastrointestinal pH and/or enzyme content, the most reliable release mechanisms are those which are solely dependent upon exposure to water. Two of the most promising sustained release techniques based on this type of mechanism are *diffusion of soluble drugs through membrane coatings* and *leach-out of soluble drugs from insoluble matrices*.

With modern polymer technology, it is possible to produce a polymer with almost any properties one wishes. If a polymer film with just the right size pores is coated onto beads containing the drug, drug release can be made to occur by *diffusion of the dissolved drug through the coating*. The rate of such diffusion is controlled by the thickness of the coating and the concentration of drug in solution inside the bead. Since modern coating technology allows very precise control of coating thickness and uniformity, such a system could be designed to give any release rate desired. In addition, the fluid inside the bead will be saturated with respect to the drug during most of the process, and

---

* Registered trademark, SmithKline Corporation.

† Developed by SmithKline Corporation.

TABLE 11-4. RELEASE MECHANISMS FOR ENTERIC AND CONTROLLED
RELEASE COATINGS

1. pH Triggered Release	Carboxylic acid polymers and copolymers
2. Enzyme Triggered Release	Fats, waxes, and their derivatives
3. Contact with Gastrointestinal Water and Fluids	Leach-out of soluble drugs from insoluble matrices Erosion and slow dissolution of soluble matrices Diffusion of soluble drugs through membrane coatings Slow hydration of pH and enzyme-insensitive coatings Desorption of sorbed and ion-exchanged drugs
4. Metered Stomach-Emptying of Drug-Containing Particles	Slow-releasing particulate drug matrices Slow-release coated beads
5. Combinations of Mechanisms 1–4	

the release of nearly the entire dose will occur at a constant rate (i.e., zero-order release), which is the most desirable sustained release pattern.

Sustained release tablets made by compressing mixtures of soluble drugs with insoluble materials, such as high melting waxes, release drug primarily by *leach-out of the soluble drug from the insoluble wax matrix*. Release rates of such systems are not as constant as those of membrane coated bead systems, owing to the changing geometry of the tablet as it wears away or to the lengthening of the diffusional pathway as drug must diffuse from deeper and deeper within the tablet core. But the release patterns are good enough, considering all the other clinical variables, and the system has a great advantage in terms of its simplicity and low cost of production. Modern techniques of assuring the reproducibility of raw materials and of controlling the parameters of the tableting process make it possible to mass produce such products very reliably.

Types and Forms of Tablet Coatings

The four basic types of tablet coatings in use today are sugar coatings, modified sugar coatings, film coatings, and compression coatings. The equipment and techniques, as well as the materials used, vary for the different types of coatings and will be discussed with each coating method.

Sugar Coating. Sugar coating is the oldest method for the coating of tablets and is still in common use, even though it has few

advantages and many disadvantages. An up-to-date pharmaceutical manufacturer who is looking for a method of coating a new drug product will probably carefully consider all the alternatives before accepting the sugar coating approach.

Disadvantages of sugar coating include the following:

1. Sugar coated tablets taste like, look like, and are mistaken for candy by children, resulting in accidental poisonings which might, in most cases, be avoided.

2. Sugar coating is an art requiring a highly skilled technician.

3. It is very time consuming, typically requiring 3 to 5 days to complete one lot of tablets.

4. The process is costly and utilizes a great deal of plant floor space compared with other methods.

5. The components of sugar coatings (sugar and gelatin solutions held at warm temperatures) can provide media for microbial growth, leading to microbiological contamination of the product at an unacceptable level.

6. Sugar coatings must be applied from an aqueous solution. This usually requires first sealing the tablet against water, which may affect drug availability adversely.

7. Sugar coatings are prone to crack on exposure to temperature cycling or rough handling.

8. Sugar is hygroscopic, and sugar coatings will pick up atmospheric moisture unless the final coated product is sealed.

9. Sugar coatings typically increase tablet weight 50 to 100 percent over the weight of the uncoated tablet.

The primary *advantage of sugar coating* is its outstanding high-gloss, pharmaceutically elegant appearance which may be difficult to match by other methods.

The *steps in sugar coating* are as follows:

Tablet Preparation. Tablets must be compressed hard enough to withstand the attrition of 80 to 120 pounds or more of tablets tumbling in a coating pan. They should be nonporous so as not to sorb water from the coating solution, which would produce very long drying times. The tablets must be assayed to ensure proper potency and uniformity of dose, and other specifications, such as dimensions, moisture content, and hardness or friability should be determined. Tablets prepared for sugar coating are often prepared with deep concave punches to produce a more nearly spherical or ovoid product than is produced by standard concave punches. A spherical tablet can be rounded with less coating than is possible with a standard shaped tablet.

Tablet Dusting and Sealing. The tablets are placed in a coating pan and rotated while an air exhaust is used to remove dust. In some cases, the tablets may be first placed on a screen and blown off with compressed air. Removal of excess dust is critical in smooth film coating and can be critical in effective tablet sealing. If a tablet contains a hydrolyzable drug or tends to be penetrated by water, the tablet core must be sealed against water penetration. The sealing coat may be food grade or "arsenic-free" shellac, or cellulose acetate phthalate. The sealing coat is applied as a thin continuous film which must cover the entire tablet to be effective. Since the sealing materials are water repellent and tend to delay drug release, *annealing agents,* such as polyethylene glycols or calcium carbonate, which do not substantially reduce the effectiveness of the water barrier during sugar coating but will dissolve in gastric fluid may be added to the sealer coat.

Tablet Rounding. In this step, the tablet is rapidly built up and rounded to produce a spherical or edge-free form. The process is also termed *subcoating.* A warm aqueous solution of sucrose, of sucrose, corn syrup, and acacia, or of acacia and tragacanth is applied to the tablets. This *smoothing syrup* may also contain dispersed starch, calcium carbonate, or dye. Enough solution is added to make the tumbling tablets begin to stick together. At this point, a *coating powder* is dusted into the pan. The powder adheres to the tacky tablet surface and builds up the tablet dimensions. Coating powders are mixtures typically containing precipitated chalk or finely powdered calcium carbonate, acacia, starch, powdered sugar, and/or talc. After each subcoating step, the tablets are allowed to dry for 15 to 20 minutes while tumbling in the revolving pan under a directed flow of warm air. A day or longer may be required to complete the subcoating and tablet-rounding steps. In a cross section of a sugar-coated tablet, the subcoat layer appears opaque and constitutes the bulk of the coating.

Sugar Coating. At the end of the subcoating step, the tablets are rounded or ovoid (if capsule shaped), are white or light buff colored, and have a very rough surface appearance. The sugar coating operation is now undertaken to smooth and color the tablets. The sugar solutions used for this step are less concentrated (about 60% w/v) than in the smoothing step. When water-soluble dyes are being used, the first applications of colored syrup are very dilute with respect to dye concentration. In subsequent applications, the dye concentration is increased. This provides for an even build-up of color and avoids mottling. Insoluble or lake dyes are often used in colored sugar coatings; since they are opaque, mottling is less of a problem. In a tablet cross section, the sugar coating layer is translucent and usually colored. The tablets are smooth and evenly colored but have a dull surface appearance at the end of this step.

Polishing. For the polishing operation, the tablets are usually transferred to a canvas-lined coating pan. The canvas lining buffs the tablets during polishing. Natural waxes, such as beeswax or carnauba wax, or synthetic waxes, such as chlorinated waxes, are applied from an organic solvent solution to produce the familiar high luster of an elegant sugar-coated tablet.

The five steps discussed above are the basic steps in sugar coating. Other steps may be added for special purposes. An enteric coating step may be added after, or in lieu of, the sealing step, if an enteric release profile is sought. Drugs may be incorporated in the coating (usually in the rounding or sugar coatings) to separate an incompatible ingredient from the core tablet or to provide repeat drug action (first drug release in the stomach, second drug release in the intestinal tract from an enteric coated core).

Certain control procedures may be desirable during the sugar coating operation—after the sealing or enteric coating steps, for example, to verify that the tablets are adequately sealed against water or gastric juice. If enteric coated tablets have not been adequately coated to meet the U.S.P. test, it would be desirable to know this before proceeding with a half-week's work completing the coating.

The numerous handling operations required tend to slow the sugar coating process and increase the cost. For example, the tablets may need to be removed from the pan and the pan washed at the end of the sealing step if there is any danger of the sealing coat (which will now also be coated on the interior of the pan) flaking off later in the operation. The pan will almost certainly have to be washed at the end of the rounding or subcoating step and again after the sugar-coating step. Finally, the tablets must be transferred, usually to a special pan, for polishing. In addition, it may be necessary to remove the tablets from the coating pan for oven or room temperature drying at one or more points in the operation. Since it may take a tablet coater a week or more to sugar coat one batch of tablets, each operator will frequently be working with four or five coating pans of tablets simultaneously (see Fig. 11-33).

Modified Sugar Coating. Modifications in the sugar coating operation were undertaken for two basic reasons: (1) to expedite the process, and (2) to improve the mechanical properties of the coating. Modifications have been made in both coating materials and coating methods.

Modified sugar coating materials usually incorporate into the normal sugar coating composition water-soluble polymers, such as sodium carboxymethylcellulose,[101] hydroxyethylcellulose,[102] polyvinylpyrrolidone,[30] and hydroxypropylmethylcellulose. These polymers are true film formers which add strength and flexibility, thereby reducing sugar coating thickness by 50 percent or more and

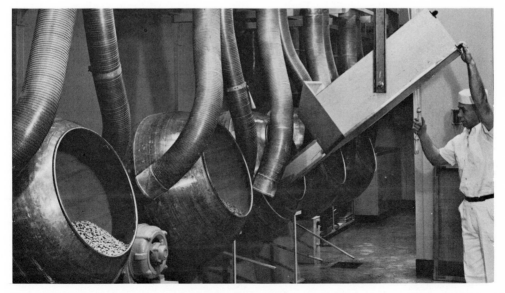

FIG. 11-33. A battery of conventional tablet coating pans, with one pan being loaded with uncoated tablets. (The Upjohn Co., Kalamazoo, Mich.)

greatly reducing coating times. Addition of a film former to the sugar coating allows it to be applied from a spray gun, which provides for more even coating and permits automation. These modifications reduce the operation to a 2- to 3-day process, at least doubling the capacity of a given coating facility.

EQUIPMENT REQUIREMENTS FOR SUGAR COATING. Sugar coating and modified sugar coating procedures require pans of various types and sizes and controllable hot air and exhaust systems for each pan. (Note the two large flexible pipes which are outside each pan in Figure 11-33. These are positioned in the pans during operation.) The hot air system usually consists of a steam or electric heat source and a fan and should be capable of producing dry air at temperatures between room temperature and 180°F., with an adjustable flow rate to accommodate the pan load. The exhaust system removes powder or organic solvent or water vapor from the pan. The exhaust system should have a greater volume capacity than the hot air system, to prevent dust from blowing out of the coating pan and contaminating other products and to prevent contamination of the room air with solvent vapor.

In addition, mixers, mixing tanks, and steam-jacketed kettles are necessary to prepare the coating solutions and hold them at appropriate temperatures. Drying ovens and drying trucks with trays as well as work bench space and storage space for raw materials and tablets in various process stages are required. Air conditioning of the coating facility to provide controlled temperature and low humidity, if not an absolute must, is highly desirable.

Film Coating. In this process, polymeric films are applied to tablets, usually by spraying an organic solvent solution of the polymer. The coatings are typically no thicker than the page of paper you are reading and are usually in the range of 0.002 to 0.010 inch in thickness. There is currently no tablet coating methodology that can match film coating for production capacity and economy. Today, most drug companies regard film coating as the preferred method for coating new products.

Advantages of film coating over other tablet coating methods are as follows:

1. The coating adds only 10 to 20 mg. to tablet weight.

2. The coating can be applied from an anhydrous solvent, so that tablet sealing is unnecessary.

3. The process readily lends itself to automation and is rapid (several hours versus several days for sugar coatings).

4. The coating is noncaloric and virtually flavorless, and is less likely to be mistaken for candy by children.

5. The identity of embossed tablets may be maintained, or the films may readily be imprinted for product identity.

6. The coating is flexible, elastic, and extremely resistant to chipping.

7. Film coating is basically a science, compared with sugar coating which is an art (thus, technician training is easier).

8. Film coated tablets can be prepared with little or no increase in disintegration time or rate of dissolution and release, compared with uncoated tablets.

9. Film-coating solutions in organic solvents are stable and are not growth media for microorganisms.

10. Systems can be readily designed to provide either enteric or rapid drug release.

The major *limitation of film coating* is organic solvent protection and pollution control. An important consideration is the explosive hazard of the organic solvent system used to prepare the polymer coating solution. Ideally, a nonflammable solvent system is used. If this is not possible, adequate air flow through the coating equipment together with restricted spray times must be adopted to preclude reaching an explosive air-solvent mixture in the coating pan. A second factor which may or may not be a limitation, is that film coated tablets will have no better appearance than the core tablets being coated, since the thin film has little "hiding power." Chipped, rough surfaced, or otherwise defective tablets will produce defective appearing film-coated tablets. Core tablets for film coating should be hard and smooth surfaced. Good quality, well polished punches should be used to prepare such tablets.

A film coating formulation consists of polymer, plasticizer, and solvent, all of which must be compatible. The polymer and the plasticizer should be soluble in a common solvent, and they should desolvate at about the same rate so as not to separate as the film forms. A film is a dried gel or network structure made up of crisscrossed, interspersed polymer chains. The plasticizer interposes itself between the high molecular weight polymer chains, reducing brittleness and increasing flexibility of the film. Plasticizers are usually low molecular weight, low melting, nonvolatile compounds which have functional groups similar to or identical to those on the polymer. Derivatives of cellulose are the most common of tablet film coatings. Cellulose is a polymer containing many hydroxyl groups, and a good plasticizer for cellulose would be a nonvolatile material with many hydroxyl groups. Thus, it is no surprise that glycerin and propylene glycol are good plasticizers for cellulosic polymers. Phthalic acid and phthalate esters are good plasticizers for polymers containing carboxyl groups. These are enteric and controlled release polymers.

Selection of Film Coating Materials. Since vitamins are classified as foods by the FDA, the polymer, plasticizer, and solvent (if any trace solvent residues remain in the film) used in film coating vitamins must be materials that are acceptable as food additives. Food additive approved materials are not required for coating materials used for drugs, but proof of safety and freedom from toxicity must be demonstrated for all such additives to drug products. Polymers that are not intended to retard drug release should have some solubility in water. To facilitate film coating they should also be soluble in an organic solvent system. Polymers that meet these criteria and also have food additive status are: hydroxypropylcellulose, hydroxypropylmethylcellulose, ethylcellulose (not water soluble by itself), and ethyl-methylcellulose mixed ethers. The polymers are often used in combination to obtain the best film properties. Solvents are selected for film coating on the basis of their chemical properties. Cellulose polymers, with their hydroxyl groups, tend to be soluble in hydroxyl-containing polar solvents (i.e., the lower alkyl alcohols). Film coating theory and practice and the design and evaluation of film coatings are more thoroughly discussed elsewhere.[2]

Film Coating Equipment. Two basic methods are used for film coating: spray coating in one of several types of coating pans, and air suspension coating.

The spray pan-coating process involves either spraying the polymer solution into a conventional solid-wall mushroom-shaped pan (Fig. 11-33) or into a "side-vented" coating pan (Fig. 11-34). The side-vented pan has thousands of holes in its periphery, and an exhaust plenum is located near that portion of the pan where the tablets tumble. The plenum draws air through the cascading tablet bed to accelerate the drying process. The preferred spray system is the airless type in which the coating solution is atomized at the nozzle by fluid pressure alone. Several programmed automated coating systems have been described[60, 61] in which solenoids and timers are used to operate the spray-gun valves. With these systems, the process proceeds automatically, with no more than a periodic check by the operator.

Air suspension coating is used for film coating and also lends itself to some sugar coating. In this process, the tablets are suspended in a stream of air in a cylindrical tower which is usually narrower at the bottom. (The device is similar to the fluid bed drier described and depicted in the tablet-making portion of this chapter.) The most widely used air-suspension coating device is the Wurster apparatus[18, 97, 123] named after its inventor. The coating solution is usually introduced at the bottom of the tower as a spray with the incoming high velocity air. The air suspension process is the most rapid coating method known because the very large volumes of heated air employed make drying extremely rapid. A batch of tablets can be film coated in the Wurster apparatus in as little as 10 or 20 minutes. One major difficulty exists with air suspension coating. The tablets are subjected to a great deal of attrition, and it is difficult or impossible to formulate some tablet systems into tablets hard enough to be coated by this technique. For some drugs, bioavailability may be adversely affected when tablets are made hard enough for air suspension coating.

Compression Coating. Compression coating is the process of making a tablet and compressing a second tablet around it. Figure 11-35 illustrates one type of compression

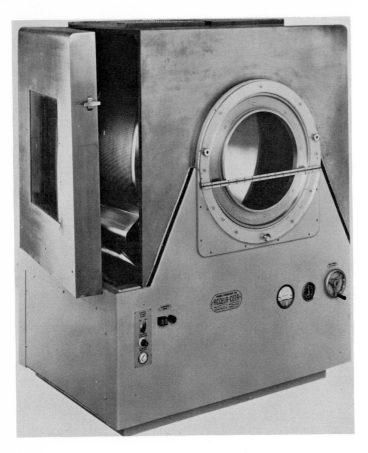

FIG. 11-34.   Accela-Cota side-vented coating pan. The perforated wall of the cylindrical revolving drum can be seen through the open door, with the fixed positioned exhaust plenum shown at the lower quadrant of the drum. (Thomas Engineering, Hoffman Estates, Ill.)

coating machine. It is actually two rotary tablet machines side by side, with a synchronized transfer mechanism that slides the core tablet from one machine to the other where it is deposited in the center of a die cavity half-filled with granulation. Additional granulation is then added and compressed around the first tablet. (Another type of "press coater" utilizes three rotary machines and produces a tablet within a tablet within a tablet.)

The major difficulty with compression coating lies in achieving a strong physical bond between the inner and the outer tablets. If the bond is weak, the tablets will cap, split, or otherwise come apart. Bonding is promoted by making the core porous and soft by compressing it with a low compression load. At the second compression step, such a core tablet is able to undergo additional compression and forms a "compact joint" at the boundary layer with the coating

tablet. A second method of promoting bonding is to incorporate waxy materials in the two granulations which tend to fuse together under compression.

Another major limitation of the compression coating process is that it is slow compared with other tableting processes. High speed operation may not produce sufficient bonding between the core and coat tablets and may cause the core tablets to be off-center in the coat tablet. Finally, the core and coat granulations must be made with accurately reproducible hardness and particle size or the end product may vary in quality.

In the past, many advantages were attributed to compression coating,[90] among them that the process can be made entirely anhydrous. Today, most manufacturers look to compression coating only when they have problems that cannot be solved by other means.

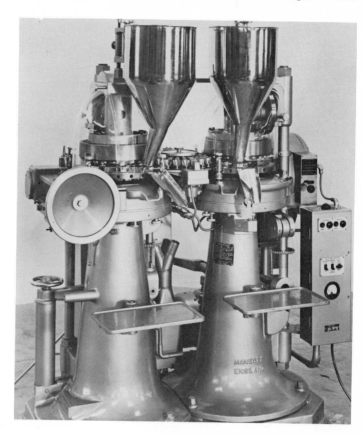

Fig. 11-35. Manesty Bicota compression coating tablet machine. (School of Pharmacy, Purdue University)

TABLET PRODUCT DESIGN

Factors that influence the bioavailability of drugs from tablet dosage forms have been discussed throughout this chapter. These factors may be summarized as in Table 11-5. The effects of various drug characteristics on bioavailability have been reviewed.[20, 72, 115]

In the design of a tablet dosage form for a new drug substance, the pharmaceutical scientist must keep in mind the *criteria for a drug product of high quality*. In addition to assuring *drug potency* and *purity* in the product, and maintenance of reasonable *chemical stability* for a minimum shelf life of one to two years, the scientist must consider three other criteria which may be difficult to achieve in the tablet dosage form. These criteria are full or substantially full *drug bioavailability,* a high order of *drug content uniformity,* and *physical stability* on aging. The physical stability of a tablet is related to changes with time in tablet hardness, density, porosity, friability, rate of drug dissolution and release, and bioavailability. These changes in properties with time should be determined, not only in the unopened container, but also while the drug product is subjected to conditions of temperature and humidity that simulate the real stress conditions the product might encounter under conditions of use. It is increasingly recognized today that the physical stability is fundamental to the quality of compressed tablets as well as to any other class of drug delivery system and can profoundly influence bioavailability and product effectiveness. In establishing expiration dates for tableted products, the maintenance of bioavailability is equally important to the maintenance of drug potency.

Preformulation research is undertaken on a new drug substance to characterize the substance physicochemically and pharmacologically and to provide an objective and rational basis for the subsequent design of a drug product with maximum safety, effectiveness, and reliability. Preformulation research is intended to remove the trial and

TABLE 11-5. FACTORS INFLUENCING THE
BIOAVAILABILITY OF DRUGS FROM ORAL
TABLET DOSAGE FORMS

Drug Characteristics

   Polymorphism
   Amorphous state
   Solvation
   Free acid, base, or salt form
   Particle size and distribution

Additives

   Disintegrants
   Lubricants
   Surfactants
   Complexing agents
   Solid solutions
   Binders

Processing Variables

   Method of disintegrant incorporation
   Granulation and compression method (wet, dry,
     or direct)
   Binder used and granule hardness
   Granule size and size distribution
   Composition and concentration of disinte-
     grant(s), lubricant(s), and other excipients,
     and ratio to drug dose
   Presence of a surfactant and method of its in-
     corporation
   Compressional pressure and compression dwell
     time
   Coating method employed (if any)

**Product Age and History of Environmental
Exposure During Aging**

error element and place product development on a firm scientific basis. It is doubly
critical in tablet drug product design. If a
drug poses a bioavailability problem, the
nature of the problem should be identified
before a particular approach to tablet design
is attempted. For example, a bioavailability
problem might be associated with destruction of the drug in the stomach (such as
erythromycin), and the solution to the problem is to get the drug into the intestinal tract
intact. On the other hand, a bioavailability
problem could be caused by the low equilibrium solubility of the drug, or poor dispersion, lack of wettability, and slow solubility rate of particles of the drug. The
solution in this case is exactly the opposite
of the erythromycin example and involves
achieving rapid tablet disintegration and as
complete drug dispersion in the stomach as
possible. By examining the characteristics of
the drug and analyzing potential problems,

rational drug product design becomes possible. Secondly, preformulation research is
important in tablet design because the tablet
dosage form can produce a great variety of
controlled drug delivery release patterns.
For example, release may be delayed to provide no release in the stomach followed by
rapid or slow continuous release in the intestinal tract. Or, very rapid release in the
stomach may be desired. Controlled prolonged zero-order or first-order release along
the entire gastrointestinal (G.I.) tract, with
or without an initial rapid fractional dose
release, is also possible.

The elements that should comprise a preformulation study are those which might
have bearing on the rational scientific design
of a tablet product with complete bioavailability and maximum safety, efficacy, and
reliability. The basic types of physical-
chemical and biological information which
make up a preformulation study, and the input of such information in product design
are depicted in Table 11-6.

The *chemical characterization* of a new
drug substance is relatively straightforward
today, using sophisticated techniques such as
mass spectroscopy and NMR. The development pharmacist thus usually knows the
molecular weight and exact chemical structure of the new drug when he receives it.
Alone or in cooperation with a physical
chemistry group, he will establish physical
characterization of the new drug substance,
including such points as the following:

Crystallography: Is the drug crystalline or
amorphous? If crystalline, does the drug
have more than one crystal form (polymorphs)? If polymorphs exist, are they bio-
logically active or inactive? In what crystal
form is the drug produced by the anticipated
method of manufacture? Particle size distribution of the powdered drug is determined, as are the true and bulk densities,
which may relate to encapsulation and tableting.

Solubility Characteristics: The equilibrium
solubility and dissolution rate of the drug in
water at several pH's are determined, including a low pH of about 2 (corresponding
to gastric pH), pH 3 to 4 (corresponding to
the upper intestinal tract), and perhaps pH
7. The fact that a drug has a high equi-

TABLE 11-6. THE COMPONENTS OF A PREFORMULATION STUDY AND THE
RELATIONSHIP OF PREFORMULATION TO PRODUCT DESIGN

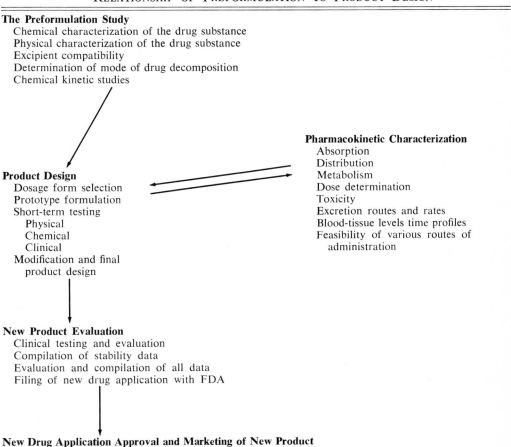

The Preformulation Study
    Chemical characterization of the drug substance
    Physical characterization of the drug substance
    Excipient compatibility
    Determination of mode of drug decomposition
    Chemical kinetic studies

Pharmacokinetic Characterization
    Absorption
    Distribution
    Metabolism
    Dose determination
    Toxicity
    Excretion routes and rates
    Blood-tissue levels time profiles
    Feasibility of various routes of
        administration

Product Design
    Dosage form selection
    Prototype formulation
    Short-term testing
        Physical
        Chemical
        Clinical
    Modification and final
        product design

New Product Evaluation
    Clinical testing and evaluation
    Compilation of stability data
    Evaluation and compilation of all data
    Filing of new drug application with FDA

New Drug Application Approval and Marketing of New Product

librium solubility does not ensure that it will dissolve rapidly, and indeed many very soluble antibiotics in compacted forms, even loose compacted forms, dissolve slowly. Solubility in solvents other than water will be determined if liquid dosage forms are planned for the drug. Stability at gastric pH should be determined if any oral form is anticipated.

Temperature and Humidity Sensitivity: Sensitivity of the drug to decomposition at elevated temperatures is normally a part of the chemical characterization in preformulation research. The physical characterization includes sensitivity to humidity, or heat and humidity (measured gravimetrically as moisture pick-up), physical change with moisture pick-up (such as liquefaction), and chemical decomposition (a problem if hy-

drolytic decomposition occurs). Whether or not the drug is sensitive to moisture or must be protected from moisture dictates the types of excipients which may be used with the drug as well as other product protection procedures which may be required such as coating or special packaging.

Excipient Compatibility: Since drugs may physically and chemically interact with excipients, an excipient compatibility screen is a very important part of preformulation research as far as solid dosage forms are concerned. The drug is typically combined with oxidizing and reducing agents plus several common excipients such as lactose, starch, microcrystalline cellulose, a calcium salt, etc. These screens for potential drug-excipient interaction can take several forms. Fortunately, some predictive screening tests, such as the use of *differential thermal analysis,* may be run in a matter of hours. DTA scans (thermograms) are run on the drug alone and in combination with various excipients. Drug-excipient interactions are often disclosed by comparing the thermograms of the mixture to the thermograms of the components. For example, decomposition is typically an exothermic process, and appearance of an exothermic thermogram peak in the mixture may predict an incompatibility problem. Other accelerated tests involve heating samples together at 40° to 60° for 10 to 30 days and reexamining the products for residual drug potency as well as for dissolution properties.

Mode of Drug Decomposition, Energy of Activation for the Drug, and Chemical Kinetic Studies: The activation energy associated with decomposition of a drug is a thermodynamic constant for the drug which reflects its chemical stability. In general, if a drug has an activation energy above 20 Kcal./mole, it is considered to be relatively stable; if it is less than 10 Kcal./mole, the development pharmacist may be involved with a dated product with a short shelf life. Knowledge of the mechanism of decomposition of a drug—i.e., hydrolytic, oxidative, etc.—provides the formulator with additional information in regard to which excipients to avoid, which stabilizing agents might be useful, and what type of protective steps (i.e., packaging) for the dosage form might be most effective.

The *pharmacokinetic studies* in Table 11-6 are initially undertaken in animals, later in man. The arrows between *Pharmacokinetic Characterization,* and *Product Design* go both ways, because preclinical tests in animals and/or man may be undertaken to determine the best drug delivery system approach when a drug poses a bioavailability problem. With solid dosage forms in particular, it is often very useful to carry out preclinical studies in man to verify that the drug delivery system is performing satisfactorily, or to establish which of two or three possible formulation or dosage form design approaches is providing the best drug delivery. No matter how many or how sophisticated the in-vitro tests are, the real test is the performance of the drug product in man.

Preclinical testing of this type is usually done in a small number of normal subjects to reduce the number of variables involved. Verification of the in-vivo performance of a newly designed drug product is good business, because product modifications and product "optimization" should be accomplished before a full-scale clinical study of efficacy is undertaken. The product a drug company has taken into and through clinical trial is the *only* product it may market. If any significant change in formula or processing is made thereafter, the FDA will require further expensive clinical verification, if not another full-scale clinical trial.

Once tablet product design has been properly completed, the first step toward achieving a high quality drug product is completed. The second step is *manufacture and control.* The guiding principle here is that quality cannot be assayed into a product, it must be built in. Hence, great care must be taken in every step of tablet production to ensure reproducible quality from batch to batch. Figure 11-36 shows a modern tablet manufacturing facility in which each tablet manufacturing step is undertaken in a separate isolated room with its own purified air supply, to provide a high order of process control and preclude product mix-ups and cross-contamination. Figure 11-37 shows a tableting operation in such an isolated room. The rooms are used exclusively for a single product at any given time.

Optimization. Optimization of drug action through dosage form design is a relatively new concept in pharmaceutical research. Optimization is a loosely used and much misused word. Many development pharmacists use it when they have simply improved a product, not made it the best possible product from all major standpoints. Optimization is an engineering development of the space age. It involves determining what characteristics of a product are important and whether it is desirable either to maximize or to minimize them (i.e., achieve the highest or the lowest possible value). These characteristics become the *"objectives,"* and they are in actuality *response variables* or *dependent variables* affected by a series of *independent* or *controllable variables.*

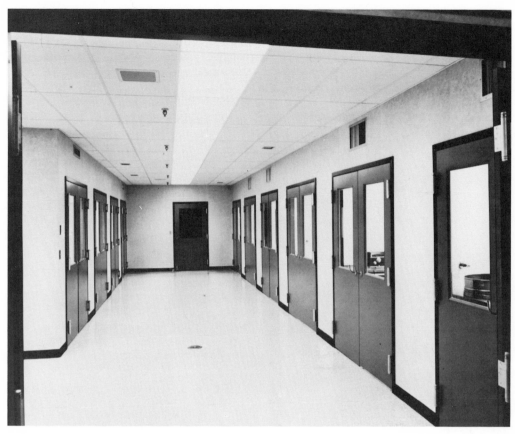

Fig. 11-36. Tablet manufacturing facility with isolated, compartmentalized work areas. (Rowell Laboratories, Baudette, Minn.)

For example, in tablet making, controllable variables might be the concentration of carefully selected binder and disintegrant in the formulation, as well as compression conditions if these are also varied. The dependent or response variables of greatest interest might be tablet hardness, friability, porosity or volume, in-vitro dissolution and release rate, and in-vivo bioavailability.

Once the mathematical relationship between the various dependent and independent variables is known, the pharmaceutical scientist has complete control of his design problem and can optimize his product with mathematical certainty. This does not mean he can make the product the best in all respects. In actuality some objectives will be competing. For example, as distintegrant concentration is increased and binder concentration is decreased, the drug dissolution rate and bioavailability objectives will usually increase and head toward their maximum and optimum values, but tablet friability will probably "degrade," causing this objective to move away from its best value. At this point the pharmacist's judgment comes into play and he or she must decide which is the more important, bioavailability or tablet friability. The pharmacist may then set some maximum value on tablet friability percentage weight loss which serves as a *"constraint"* in the new model to be solved for product optimization. With the friability constraint set, the mathematical model is again solved for the best in-vitro dissolution or in-vivo bioavailability, and the resultant calculated formulation and compression condition specified will be a true solution for a truly optimum product.

Data treatment, known as *sensitivity anal-*

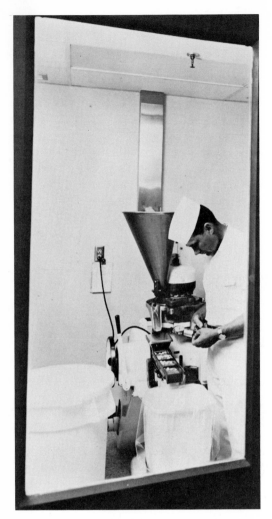

FIG. 11-37.   A tableting operation in an isolated room with complete environmental control. (Rowell Laboratories, Baudette, Minn.)

ysis, may also be applied. In sensitivity analysis, one or more of the secondary objectives are "relaxed" or "tightened," and the effect on the primary objective is calculated. This discloses how critical to the primary objective such alterations in secondary objectives are. If constraints on secondary functions may be tightened (e.g., tablets harder, less friable) with little effect on the primary objective (e.g., bioavailability), constraints on the secondary function(s) would be tightened. If, on the other hand, relaxation of a secondary objective produces a substantial gain in a primary objective, such relaxation

may be in order. Fonner and coworkers in 1970 published the first major paper illustrating the use of mathematical optimization techniques in drug product design and pharmaceutical process analysis,[34] and the reader is referred to that work for illustration of the modeling and mathematics involved.

Optimization may involve more work to define the relationships between dependent and independent variables, compared to standard product development, but the modeling and optimization that follow enable the scientist to design a product with certainty and actually to produce the best (optimum) product. It will increasingly be the preferred method of drug product design in the future.

REFERENCES

1. Albrecht, R.: U.S. Patent 2,645,936, July 21, 1953.
2. Banker, G. S.: J. Pharm. Sci., *55*:81, 1966.
3. ———: U.S. Patent 3,097,144, 1963.
4. Batuyios, N.: J. Pharm. Sci., *55*:727, 1966.
5. Bequette, R. J., and Huyck, C. L.: Drug Cosmetic Ind., *81*:166, 1957.
6. Blythe, R.: U.S. Patent 2,738,303, March 13, 1956.
7. ———: Brit. Patents 742,097 and 765,086.
8. Boger, W. P., and Gavin, J. J.: New Eng. J. Med., *261*:827, 1959.
9. Breunig, H. L., and King, E. P.: J. Pharm. Sci., *51*:1187, 1962.
10. Brochmann-Hanssen, E., and Medina, J. C.: J. Pharm. Sci., *52*:630, 1963.
11. Brodie, B. B., and Hogben, A. M.: J. Pharm. Pharmacol., *9*:345, 1957.
12. Brooke, C., and Boggs, T.: Am. J. Dis. Child., *82*:465, 1951.
13. Caminetsky, S.: Canad. Med. A. J., *88*:950, 1963.
14. Campagna, F. A., Cureton, G., Mirigian, R. A., and Nelson, E.: J. Pharm. Sci., *52*: 605, 1963.
15. Catz, B., Ginsberg, E., and Salenger, S.: New Eng. J. Med., *266*:136, 1962.
16. Cheney, F. L.: Proc. APhA, *59*:85, 1911.
17. Cohn, R., *et al.*: APhA Convention, Ind. Pharm. Sect., Dallas, Tex., Apr., 1966.
18. Coletta, V., and Rubin, H.: J. Pharm. Sci., *53*:953, 1964.
19. Cooper, B. F., and Brecht, J. T.: J. A. Ph. A. (Sci. Ed.), *46*:520, 1957.
20. Cooper, J., and Rees, J. E.: J. Pharm. Sci., *61*:1511, 1972.
21. Costello, R., and Mattocks, A.: J. Pharm. Sci., *51*:106, 1962.
22. Crisati, R. C., and Becker, C. H.: J. A. Ph. A. (Sci. Ed.), *47*:363, 1958.

23. Curlin, L. C.: J. A. Ph. A. (Sci. Ed.), *44*:16, 1955.

24. Daoust, R. G., and Lynch, M. J.: Drug Cosmetic Ind., *93*:26, 1963.

25. Doluisio, J. T. *et al.*: J. Pharm. Sci., *60*: 1160, 1971.

26. Donaghy, L. S.: Drug Cosmetic Ind., *83*: 304, 1958.

27. Duvall, R. N., *et al.*: J. Pharm. Sci., *54*:607, 1965.

28. Eatherton, L. E., *et al.*: Drug Std., *23*:42, 1955.

29. Engle, G. B.: Australasian J. Pharm., *47* (Supp. 39):S22, 1966.

30. Everhard, M. E., and Goodhart, F. W.: J. Pharm. Sci., *52*:281, 1963.

31. Fairchild, H. J., and Michel, F.: J. Pharm. Sci., *50*:966, 1961.

32. Fakouhi, T. A., *et al.*: J. Pharm. Sci., *52*: 700, 1963.

33. Fonner, D. E., Banker, G. S., and Swarbrick, J.: J. Pharm. Sci., *55*:181, 1966.

34. Fonner, D. E., *et al.*: J. Pharm. Sci., *59*: 1587, 1970.

35. Garrett, E. R.: J. Pharm. Sci., *51*:672, 1962.

36. Garrett, E. R., and Olson, E. C.: J. Pharm. Sci., *51*:764, 1962.

37. Gerding, T. G., and Dekay, H. G.: Drug Std., *23*:132, 1955.

38. Gibaldi, M.: *In* Theory and Practice of Industrial Pharmacy. p. 226. Philadelphia, Lea and Febiger, 1970.

39. Glasko, A. J., Kinkel, A. W., Alegnani, W., and Holmes, E. L.: Clin. Pharmacol. Ther., *9*:472, 1968.

40. Goodhart, F. W., *et al.*: J. Pharm. Sci., *56*: 63, 1967.

41. Goodman, H., and Banker, G.: J. Pharm. Sci., *59*:1131, 1970.

42. Goorley, J. T., and Lee, C. O.: J. A. Ph. A., *27*:379, 1938.

43. Granberg, C. B., and Benton, B. E.: J. A. Ph. A. (Sci. Ed.), *48*:648, 1949.

44. Griffin, J. C., and Huyck, C. L.: J. A. Ph. A. (Sci. Ed.), *44*:251, 1955.

45. Gross, H. M., and Becker, C. H.: J. A. Ph. A. (Sci. Ed.), *41*:187, 1952.

46. Gunsel, W. C., *et al.*: *In* Lachman, L., *et al.* (eds.): The Theory and Practice of Industrial Pharmacy. pp. 321–322. Philadelphia, Lea and Febiger, 1970.

47. Gunsel, W. C., and Lachman, L.: J. Pharm. Sci., *52*:178, 1963.

48. Hawkins, D. B., and Thompson, H. D.: J. A. Ph. A. (Sci. Ed.), *42*:424, 1953.

49. Higuchi, T., and Kuramoto, R.: J. A. Ph. A. (Sci. Ed.), *43*:393, 1954.

50. ————: J. A. Ph. A. (Sci. Ed.), *43*:398, 1954.

51. Holstius, E. A., and Dekay, H. G.: J. A. Ph. A. (Sci. Ed.), *41*:505, 1952.

52. Ingram, J. T., and Lowenthal, W.: J. Pharm. Sci., *57*:187, 1968.

53. Kassebaum, H.: Pharm. Ztg. (Frankfurt), *108*:613, 1963.

54. Kavalana, H., and Burlage, H. M.: Am. Profess. Pharmacist, *21*:346, 1965.

55. Kennon, L., and Swintosky, J. V.: J. A. Ph. A. (Sci. Ed.), *47*:396, 1958.

56. Kovac, G. M.: Drug Cosmetic Ind., *91*:171, 1962.

57. ————: Drug Cosmetic Ind., *91*:297, 1962.

58. Kremers, E., and Urdang, G.: History of Pharmacy. pp. 20, 319. Philadelphia, J. B. Lippincott, 1940.

59. Kwan, K. C., and Milosovich, G.: J. Pharm. Sci., *55*:340, 1966.

60. Lachman, L.: Mfg. Chemist Aerosol News, *37*:35, 1966.

61. Lachman, L., *et al.*: J. Pharm. Sci., *51*:321, 1962.

62. ————: J. A. Ph. A. (Sci. Ed.), *49*:165, 1960.

63. ————: J. A. Ph. A. (Sci. Ed.), *49*:163, 1960.

64. Lachman, L., and Cooper, J.: J. Pharm. Sci. *52*:490, 1963.

65. Lehrman, G. P., and Skauen, D. M.: Drug Std., *26*:120, 1958.

66. Levy, G.: J. Pharm. Sci., *50*:388, 1961.

67. Levy, G., and Gumtow, R.: J. A. Ph. A. (Sci. Ed.), *52*:1139, 1963.

68. Levy, G., Hall, N., and Nelson, E.: Am. J. Hosp. Pharm., *21*:402, 1964.

69. Lozinski, E.: Canad. M. A. J., *83*:177, 1960.

70. McAteer, P. J.: APhA Convention, Ind. Pharm. Sec., Las Vegas, Nev., March, 1962.

71. McCallum, A., *et al.*: J. A. Ph. A. (Sci. Ed.), *44*:83, 1955.

72. Macek, T. J.: *In* Remington's Pharmaceutical Sciences. ed. 14, p. 1463. Easton, Pa., Mack Pub. Co., 1970.

73. Maly, J.: Acta fac. pharm. bohemslov., *8*: 81, 1963.

74. Maney, P. V., and Kuever, R. A.: J. A. Ph. A. (Sci. Ed.), *30*:276, 1941.

75. Martin, A. N., *et al.*: Physical Pharmacy. Ed. 2, p. 237. Philadelphia, Lea and Febiger, 1969.

76. Martin, C., Rubin, M., O'Malley, W., Garagusi, V. F., and McCanley, C.: Comparative physiological availability of "brand" and "generic" drugs in man: chloramphenicol, sulfisoxazole and diphenylhydantoin. Presented at the Fall Meeting Am. Soc. Pharmacol. Exp. Ther. Minneapolis, Minn., Aug. 20, 1968.

77. Michel, F.: U.S. Patent 2,975,630, Mar. 21, 1961.

78. Milosovich, G.: Drug Cosmetic Ind., *92*: 557, 1963.

79. Munden, B. J., *et al.*: Drug Std., *28*:12, 1960.

80. Munden, B. J., and Banker, G. S.: Drug Std., *28*:12, 1960.

81. Munzel, K., and Kagi, W.: Pharm. acta helv., *29*:53, 1954.

82. Nazareth, M. R., *et al.*: J. Pharm. Sci., *50*: 564, 1961.

83. Nelson, E., *et al.*: J. A. Ph. A. (Sci. Ed.), *46*:257, 1957.
84. ———: J. A. Ph. A. (Sci. Ed.), *43*:596, 1954.
85. Nielsen, G. N.: Arch. Pharm. Chem., *53*:531, 1946.
86. Patel, B. C., and Guth, E. P.: Drug Std., *23*:37, 1955.
87. Prescott, F.: Drug Cosmetic Ind., *97*:497, 1965.
88. Raff, A. M.: J. Pharm. Sci., *53*:380, 1964.
89. Rankell, A. S., *et al.*: J. Pharm. Sci., *53*:320, 1964.
90. Schroeter, L. C.: *In* Remington's Pharmaceutical Sciences. Ed. 14, p. 1688. Easton, Pa., Mack Pub. Co., 1970.
91. Sciarra, J. J.: J. A. Ph. A. (Pract. Ed.), *19*:494, 1958.
92. Scott, M. W., *et al.*: J. Pharm. Sci., *53*:314, 1964.
93. ———: J. Pharm. Sci., *52*:284, 1963.
94. Searl, R., and Pernarowski, M.: Canad. M. A. J., *96*:1513, 1967.
95. Shafer, E. G. E., *et al.*: J. A. Ph. A. (Sci. Ed.), *40*:114, 1956.
96. Shaheen, R. G.: Diss. Abstr., *17*:868, 1957.
97. Singiser, R. E., and Lowenthal, W.: J. Pharm. Sci., *50*:168, 1961.
98. Smilek, M., *et al.*: Drug Std., *23*:87, 1955.
99. Smith, F. D., and Grosch, D.: U.S. Patent 2,041,869, May 29, 1936.
100. Sperandio, G. J.: J. A. Ph. A. (Pract. Ed.), *10*:572, 1949.
101. Spradling, A. B.: U.S. Patent 2,693,437, 1954.
102. ———: U.S. Patent 2,693,436, 1954.
103. Stecher, P. G., (ed.): The Merck Index. Ed. 8. Rahway, N.J., Merck and Co., 1968.
104. Strickland, W. A., *et al.*: J. A. Ph. A. (Sci. Ed.), *49*:35, 1960.
105. Swartz, C. J., *et al.*: J. Pharm. Sci., *51*:1181, 1962.
106. ———: J. Pharm. Sci., *51*:326, 1962.
107. ———: J. Pharm. Sci., *50*:145, 1961.
108. Sweeny, W. M., *et al.*: Antibiot. Med. Clin. Ther., *4*:642, 1957.
109. Train, D. J.: J. Pharm. Pharmacol., *8*:745, 1956.
110. The United States Pharmacopeia, 18th Revision. pp. 815, 930, 932, 951. Easton, Pa., Mack Pub. Co., 1970.
111. Unna, S.: Pharm. Zentralhalle *25*:577, 1884 (Am. J. Pharm., *57*:338, 1885).
112. Urbanyi, T., *et al.*: J. A. Ph. A. (Sci. Ed.), *49*:163, 1960.
113. Urdang, G.: What's New, *5*:1943 (J. A. Ph. A. *34*:135, 1945).
114. Van Abbe, N. J., and Rees, T. J.: J. A. Ph. A. (Sci. Ed.), *47*:487, 1958.
115. Wagner, J. G.: Biopharmaceutics and Relevant Pharmacokinetics. p. 89. Hamilton, Ill., Drug Intelligence Pubs., 1971.
116. ———: J. Pharm. Sci., *50*:359, 1961.
117. Ward, J. B., and Trachtenberg, A.: Drug Cosmetic Ind., *91*:35, 1962.
118. Warner, W. R., Jr.: Am. J. Pharm., *74*:32, 1902.
119. Webster, A. R.: Brit. Patent 791,281, Feb. 26, 1958.
120. White, R. C.: J. A. Ph. A., *11*:345, 1922.
121. Wiegand, T. S.: Am. J. Pharm., *74*:33, 1902.
122. Wolff, J. E., *et al.*: J. A. Ph. A. (Sci. Ed.), *36*:407, 1947.
123. Wurster, D. E.: U.S. Patent 2,648,609, Aug. 11, 1953.

12

Elmer M. Plein, *Coordinator of Pharmaceutical Services and Professor of Pharmacy, University of Washington*

Gas Dispersions
(Aerosols and Sprays)

The term aerosol is employed in colloid chemistry and has been defined by Whytlaw-Gray and Patterson[44] as a system of finely divided liquid or solid particles dispersed in and surrounded by a gas. Sinclair[40] in his definition limited the size of the particles to less than 50 microns and, usually, less than 10 microns; Avy,[2] in a more recent publication, agreed with Sinclair's definition.

During the 1940's the word aerosol was used to describe pressurized insecticides. The Aerosol Division of the Chemical Specialties Manufacturers Association[8] has defined aerosols as suspensions of fine, solid or liquid particles in air or gas, as smoke, fog, or mist. Their definition further specified that according to the Department of Agriculture the particles in an insecticidal aerosol spray must have diameters of less than 50 microns and 80 percent of the particles must be smaller than 30 microns in diameter. The Chemical Specialties Manufacturers Association further defined aerosol products as self-contained sprayable products in which the propellant force is supplied by a liquefied gas. The term included space, residual, surface-coating, foam and various other types of products but not gas-pressurized products such as whipping cream.

Perhaps a better term than *aerosols* to designate this class of preparations is *pressurized packages,* which would include packages pressurized with compressed gases as well as with liquefied gases. Also, use of the term pressurized package, Herzka and Pickthall[13] state, would avoid confusion of the products with a series of surface-active agents known as Aerosols®, manufactured by the American Cyanamid Company, and with aerosol therapy. Notwithstanding, the term aerosol, with reference to a pressurized package, is commonly used in the United States and will be so used in this chapter.

An aerosol may be defined as a package which contains the product and a propellant capable of expelling that product through an opened valve. Aerosols may be divided into four classifications: space sprays, coating sprays, foams and streams. Space sprays[29] dispense the products as finely divided sprays in which the particles are less than 50 microns in diameter; it is intended that the particles remain suspended in the air for a time. Examples of these aerosols are insecticides and room deodorants. Surface-coating aerosols[29] produce sprays with particles somewhat larger than those produced by space aerosols. Examples of these aerosols are residual insecticides, paints, paint removers and Christmas tree snows. The intention is to deposit the particles directly on a surface rather than to suspend them in the air. In foam aerosols the product is delivered from the valve of the pressurized package in the form of a foam. Foam aerosols are used principally for personal products such as shaving creams, hand creams and lotions. Many medicated creams are formulated to produce foams. In stream aerosols the product is expelled from the pressurized package in the form of a simple stream. Hand lotions and vitamin preparations are examples of this class.

HISTORY

According to Herzka and Pickthall,[13] Root[34] must be given credit for tracing a patent granted in 1862 to Lynde for a valve, complete with dip tube, for dispensing an aerated liquid from a bottle.[18]

The first reference to the use of liquefied

gases appears to be contained in Helbing's and Pertsch's patent of 1899.[12] The inventors used methyl and ethyl chlorides as propellants of fluids in vessels of glass or metal having suitable orifices. In use, the container was heated in the hand and the liquid thus was forced through the orifice in a fine jet or spray. The vessel could be sealed with a tightly fitting cap when not in use, to prevent loss of fluid.[13]

The first of Gebauer's patents was issued in 1901,[9] and the second one the next year.[10] His patents described containers for holding and ejecting a spray or stream. Moore[24] was granted a patent in 1903 for a perfume atomizer in which carbon dioxide was the propellant. In 1921 Mobley[23] obtained a patent in which he described a method for applying liquid antiseptics with carbon dioxide as a propellant. In 1926 Lemoine was granted a patent for atomizing perfumes with carbon dioxide,[13, 16] and in 1931 Riedel and de Haen received a patent for atomizing perfumes with methyl chloride.[33] Rotheim was awarded patents in 1931[35] and 1933[36] in which the aerosol possibilities for perfumes and cosmetics were described. He suggested the use of dimethyl ether, methyl chloride, isobutane, vinyl chloride and other materials as likely propellants and designed containers and spray nozzles for the aerosol packages.

In 1933, Midgley, Henne and McNary[20] were granted a patent for the use of fluorinated hydrocarbons as fire extinguishers. They stated in their patent that the fluorinated hydrocarbons may be useful as pressure devices in which a low-boiling-point compound creates pressure to expel itself. The patent specifically mentioned dichlorodifluoromethane which had been synthesized a short time previously as a result of a project aimed at replacing sulfur dioxide and ammonia in refrigeration machines. Actually, modern propellants for aerosols were developed as refrigerant gases; however, their discovery was a significant contribution to pressurized packaging as it is known today. Bichowsky[4] obtained a patent in 1935 for developing a self-pressurized fire extinguisher in which fluorinated hydrocarbons were used to expel other fire-extinguishing products

(mainly powders) which had no capacity for self-propulsion.

Some of the most significant contributions to modern aerosol technology were the work of Goodhue[11] and Sullivan[41] which led to a patent for metal containers filled with insecticides and dichlorodifluoromethane.[42] These aerosols, known as bug bombs, were of heavy steel construction and were enormously helpful in combating insects which caused disease and discomfort among overseas troops. The bug bombs reached the civilian market in the United States in 1945 and were well accepted. Attention then was turned to the development of less expensive, lighter weight containers to make possible packing of a wide range of products.

It was estimated that approximately 5.5 million units of aerosols, almost entirely insecticides, were produced in the United States in 1947. In 1970 the total number of units produced by 147 companies in their own plants was estimated to be 2,622.8 million.[7] In 1952 less than 500,000 units of pharmaceutical aerosols were produced. Eighteen years later, in 1970, the annual production of pharmaceutical aerosols had increased to slightly more than 48.9 million units.[7] Figure 12-1 illustrates by major product groups the number of units of aerosol and pressurized products produced in the United States in 1970. This figure indicates that 1,380 million units of aerosol and pressurized products for personal use were filled. In addition to the 48.9 million units of pharmaceutical aerosols, the personal use category of products includes shaving lathers, hair sprays and other hair products, colognes and perfumes, deodorants and anti-perspirants, dental products, sun tan preparations, lotions, powders, after shave preparations, breath fresheners, etc.[7]

OPERATION OF AEROSOLS

Liquefied Gas Systems

When a liquefied gas propellant is sealed within an aerosol container, a portion of it vaporizes and the remainder exists as a liquid. When equilibrium is established, the vapor phase occupies the upper portion of the container and the liquid phase occupies

FIG. 12-1. Aerosol and Pressurized Products Survey, United States—1970 Contribution of major groups to the adjusted total production. (Chemical Specialties Manufacturers Association)

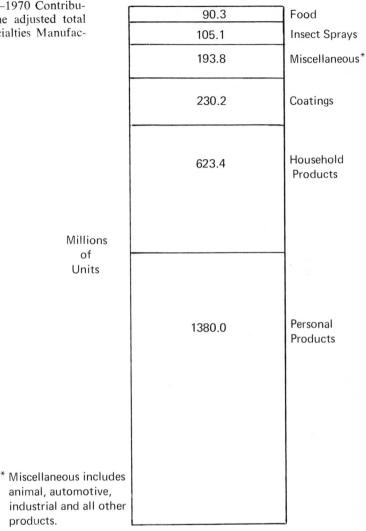

Total—2622.8

90.3	Food
105.1	Insect Sprays
193.8	Miscellaneous*
230.2	Coatings
623.4	Household Products
1380.0	Personal Products

Millions of Units

* Miscellaneous includes animal, automotive, industrial and all other products.

the lower portion of the container. The vapor phase exerts pressure in all directions, and this pressure effect on the surface of the liquid phase forces the liquid up the dip tube. When the valve is opened by operating the actuator button, the liquid passes through the valve into the atmosphere. The boiling point of the propellant is usually considerably below room temperature so the liquefied gas instantly vaporizes. As liquid propellant leaves the container, the space above the surface of the liquid is increased, causing a slight depression in propulsion pressure. Some of the liquid phase now passes into the vapor state, thus quickly restoring equilibrium and the original pressure.

Two-Phase Systems. Aerosols of the two-phase system operate in a manner similar to that described in the preceding paragraph and are shown diagrammatically in Figure 12-2. Many space and surface coating aerosols fall into this classification. The liquid phase may be composed of (1) a solution of active constituent in propellant or in a mixture of a propellant and a solvent if a solvent is necessary to effect solution; (2) a suspension of active constituent in propellant, as in powder aerosols for local application or in epinephrine bitartrate aerosol for oral in-

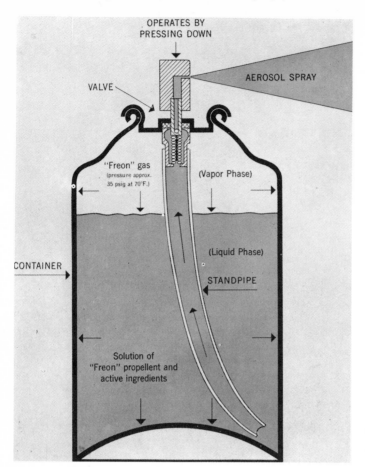

OPERATES BY
PRESSING DOWN

AEROSOL SPRAY

VALVE

"Freon" gas
(pressure approx.
35 psig at 70°F.)

(Vapor Phase)

(Liquid Phase)

STANDPIPE

CONTAINER

Solution of
"Freon" propellent and
active ingredients

Fig. 12-2. Cross section of a typical two-phase aerosol package. (E. I. du Pont de Nemours & Co.)

halation therapy. Technically speaking, the addition of a solid powdered material which exists as such in the aerosol might be interpreted as the addition of another phase; however, for practical purposes, these aerosols are classified as two-phase aerosols. The subclassification *dispersions,* or *suspensions,* would be descriptive of the aerosols that contain powdered medications.

As these space and surface coating materials are expelled from the aerosol unit, rapid expansion of the propellant into vapor form leaves the active constituent suspended in space or deposited on a surface. If the particles are less than 50 microns in size (and some of them may be less than 1 micron in diameter), the aerosol is termed a space aerosol. When the particle size is larger (up to 100 or 200 microns) the aerosol is termed a surface coating or wet spray. Some of the factors that affect particle size are

valve mechanism, proportion of propellant, vapor pressure of the propellant and viscosity of the liquid phase. Space aerosols are less viscous, they contain a greater proportion of propellant and they operate at higher pressure than surface coating aerosols.

Foam aerosols might be considered to operate like a two-phase system. The propellant is emulsified into the aqueous product by agitation just before the valve is opened. As soon as the emulsion is expelled into the atmosphere, propellant globules within it vaporize and produce a thick foam. A dip tube is optional, in which case the aerosol is to be operated in an upright position. Without a dip tube, the aerosol is to be inverted in use.

Three-Phase Systems. Three-phase aerosols contain considerably more water than two-phase aerosols, and, since the aqueous product is not miscible with the propellants, it forms a separate layer. Propellants produce the other two layers, with propellant vapor at the top or head space of the aerosol to force the product up the dip tube and through the opened valve. The third phase or layer is propellant which may float on the aqueous layer or remain on the bottom of the package, depending on the specific gravity of the propellant. The length of the dip tube is such that the tube dips into the aqueous product and not the propellant, should the latter be the bottom layer of the system (Fig. 12-3). The aqueous product is broken up into a spray by mechanical action of the valve system. The vapor phase is replenished by vaporization of the propellant, and, if the propellant forms the bottom layer of the system, boiling chips may be added to promote vaporization of the propellant. Boiling chips minimize the lag phase of pressure build-up during prolonged spraying.[21]

Compressed Gas Systems

Compressed gases can be used in aerosols, and, by controlling the formulations and types of valves, these aerosols will dispense the product as a solid stream, a foam or a fine mist. It is the pressure of the gas in the head space of the aerosol which expels the product from the package. Since there is no reservoir of gas as in the aerosols prepared with liquefied gases, pressure in these aerosols decreases as the products are dispensed.

Solid Stream Aerosols. Nitrogen is used as the propellant in solid stream aerosols. The gas is colorless, odorless, tasteless and prac-

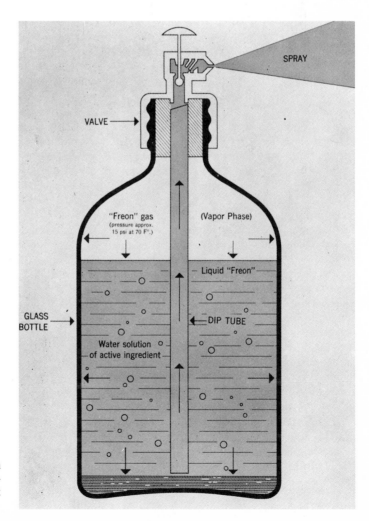

FIG. 12-3. Cross section of a typical three-phase aerosol package. (E. I. du Pont de Nemours & Co.)

tically insoluble in water. Its low solubility makes it possible to dispense only the product without any gas from the aerosol. The gas is suitable for aerosols containing vitamin syrups, cough syrups, ointments, hand lotions, cosmetic creams and toothpaste. These aerosols are designed to operate at initial pressures of 90 to 100 psig* to ensure adequate pressure to expel all the ingredients from the container.

Foam Aerosols. Foam aerosols prepared with compressed gases operate in much the same manner as those made with liquefied gases. The gases employed may be carbon dioxide and nitrous oxide, both of which are slightly soluble in the aqueous product. When the valve is opened and the product is expelled into the atmosphere the gases expand and produce the foam.

Mist Aerosols. Compressed gases do not possess the dispersing power of liquefied gases. Therefore it is necessary to employ a mechanical breakup actuator to produce wet sprays.

Propellants

In addition to serving as the force by which the product is expelled from the aerosol package, propellants may serve as solvents, suspending agents or diluents and may affect the properties of the product as it leaves the package. Propellants used in the preparation of pharmaceutical aerosols are the liquefied gases, principally halogenated hydrocarbons, and compressed gases such as carbon dioxide or nitrogen.

Liquefied Gas Propellants. Liquid gas propellants, mostly chlorinated, fluorinated hydrocarbons, have been used in refrigeration units for a number of years. They are well suited as propellants and as refrigerants due to their low boiling points and low vapor pressures. Since each propellant has a definite vapor pressure at a given temperature, it may be possible to select a propellant to give the desired pressure in an aerosol. Furthermore, if a single propellant does not give the desired pressure, two of these propellants can be blended to obtain a mixture which will produce the desired pressure at a given temperature. In Table 12-1 are listed a

number of liquefied gas propellants and some of their properties.

Since it is awkward to refer to liquefied gases by their chemical names, the refrigeration industry has devised a three-digit numerical system to identify each chemical compound (*see* Table 12-1). The digit on the right refers to the number of fluorine atoms in the molecule. The second digit from the right is one more than the number of hydrogen atoms in the molecule, and the third digit from the right is one less than the number of carbon atoms in the compound. When this number is 0 (as it would be in designating methane derivatives), the third digit is omitted, and a two-digit number is used. The number of chlorine atoms in the molecule can be determined by subtracting the sum of the number of fluorine atoms and the number of hydrogen atoms from the total number of atoms which can be added to the carbon chain. Isomeric compounds are designated by the same three-digit number followed by lower case letters, a, b, c, etc. The most symmetric compound of the group is identified by the three-digit number only, and as the isomers become less symmetrical the small letters are added. A capital letter C immediately preceding the number indicates a cyclic compound.

Dichlorotetrafluoroethane, $CClF_2CClF_2$, is identified as Propellant 114. According to the discussion in the preceding paragraph the first digit on the right is 4 to indicate the presence of four atoms of fluorine in the compound. There are no hydrogen atoms so the number 1 $(0 + 1)$ is used as the second digit from the right. The third digit from the right is 1 since there are two carbon atoms in the chain $(2 - 1)$.

Several commercial concerns supply propellants under the following trade names:

Freon®—Freon Products Division, E. I. du Pont de Nemours and Company.

Genetron®—General Chemical Division, Allied Chemical Corporation.

Isotron®—Industrial Chemicals Division, Pennwalt Chemical Corporation.

Ucon®—Union Carbide Chemicals Company, Union Carbide Corporation.

Boiling Point. The boiling points of the liquefied propellants listed in Table 12-1 vary from $-41.4°$ F. to $117.6°$ F. This informa-

---

* psig = pounds per square inch gauge.

TABLE 12-1. PHYSICAL PROPERTIES OF SOME FLUORINATED HYDROCARBONS

CHEMICAL NAME	CHEMICAL FORMULA	NUMERICAL DESIGNATION	BOILING POINT AT 1 ATM. (° F.)	VAPOR PRESSURE PSIA* 70° F.	LIQUID DENSITY g./ml. 70° F.	SOLUBILITY IN WATER g./100 g. 70° F.
Trichloromonofluoromethane	CCl_3F	11	74.8	13.4	1.485	0.028
Dichlorodifluoromethane	CCl_2F_2	12	−21.6	84.9	1.325	0.040
Monochlorodifluoromethane	$CHClF_2$	22	−41.4	138.0	1.210	0.34
Trichlorotrifluoroethane	CCl_2FCClF_2	113	117.6	5.5	1.580	0.028
Dichlorotetrafluoroethane	$CClF_2CClF_2$	114	38.4	27.6	1.468	0.024 (at 77° F.)
Chloropentafluoroethane	$CClF_2CF_3$	115	−37.7	118.0	—	0.006 (at 77° F.)
Monochlorodifluoroethane	CH_3CClF_2	142b	15.1	43.8	1.119	0.14
Difluoroethane	CH_3CHF_2	152a	−11.2	76.4	0.911	0.32
Octafluorocyclobutane	$CF_2CF_2CF_2CF_2$	C318	21.1	40.1	1.513	0.005 (at 79° F.)

* psia = pounds per square inch absolute (psig + 14.7)

tion is of value in deciding how the propellants should be handled in the filling operations.

Density. Most formulations are written to give the amount of propellant in terms of weight. If, in the filling operation, the propellant is weighed into the container, density of the propellant can be ignored. However, it is often more convenient to measure the propellant by volume in the filling procedure; hence, the density of the propellant in its liquefied form must be taken into consideration.

Vapor Pressure. It has been pointed out that one advantage of liquefied propellants is the fact that as long as there is some liquid propellant in the pressurized package the product will have a constant pressure at a given temperature. The vapor pressure of the propellants listed in Table 12-1 varies from 5.5 psia* to 138 psia at 70° F. These values are as high as 300 psia at 130° F. One can select mixtures of propellants to control the pressure. Several mixtures of propellants which can be used to obtain the gauge pressures indicated are illustrated in Figure 12-4.

Solvent Characteristics. The fluorinated hydrocarbons are nonpolar organic solvents and as such are not miscible with water or with many glycols.[37] There are a number of methods by which one can determine the comparative solubility properties of a sub-

* Psia −14.7 = psig (gauge).

stance with other solvents. One of these procedures is to determine the amount of a solvent necessary to produce a turbidity when added to a standard solution of kaurie resin (copal) in n-butanol. Of the three popularly used propellants, propellant 11 has the best solvent properties (Kauri-Butanol value of 60); but propellant 12 and propellant 114 are relatively poor solvents (Kauri-Butanol values of 18 and 12, respectively).[37] In order to prepare solutions of active constituents in propellants it is frequently necessary to add other liquids as cosolvents in the formulations.

Chemical Properties. Although the fluorinated hydrocarbons generally are considered to be nonreactive, some of them do react with water and alcohol under certain conditions. Propellant 11, for example, cannot be used in packaging some products that contain water or ethyl alcohol. When propellant 11 contacts metal and water the propellant is decomposed, with ultimate formation of hydrochloric and hydrofluoric acids which are corrosive to metals of the container or valve. Some water-in-oil emulsions can be safely packaged with propellant 11 because the propellant is a part of the external phase. The water droplets, being the internal phase, are protected from contacting metal, the catalyst for the chemical reaction.[37]

Propellant 11 is decomposed in the presence of ethyl alcohol to form first acet-

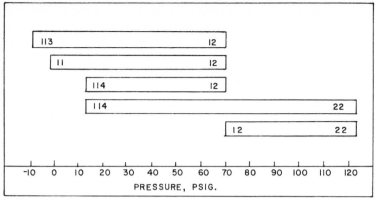

Fig. 12-4. Range of pressures (pounds per square inch) obtainable at 70°F. with various mixtures of fluorinated hydrocarbon propellants.

aldehyde and hydrochloric acid and then acetal and ethyl chloride. Nitromethane has been used as a stabilizer of propellant 11 to prevent corrosion in both the aqueous systems and the alcoholic systems. Nitromethane is fairly effective as a stabilizer in the alcoholic systems containing alcohol of 95 percent strength, but it is ineffective when the alcoholic strength is less than 95 percent.[37]

Propellants 12 and 114 are relatively stable in the presence of water and alcohol, and propellant C 318 possesses extreme chemical stability with these liquids.

Compressed Gas Propellants. The compressed gases that are used most frequently in preparing aerosols are nitrogen, carbon dioxide and nitrous oxide. Nitrogen is practically insoluble in water, whereas the other two gases are slightly soluble. The insolubility of nitrogen makes it possible to prepare aerosols so that the dispensed products have the same consistency that they had when they were placed in the package—an advantage in aerosols of vitamin syrups, tooth pastes and some lotions and ointments in which a foaming product would be objectionable.

The use of nitrogen has additional advantages. Products packaged with nitrogen are not subject to oxidation. The gas is colorless, odorless and tasteless and is readily available at low cost.

Nitrogen as a propellant has one serious disadvantage (as have also nitrous oxide and carbon dioxide, although to a lesser degree). Aerosols using nitrogen as the propellant must be packaged at a higher pressure than aerosols prepared with liquefied gases because there is a considerable pressure drop as the product is dispensed from the container. For example, if three ounces of lotion were packaged in a 4-ounce container and the aerosol pressurized with nitrogen at 80 psia, when 1 ounce of lotion had been dispensed, the pressure, according to Boyle's Law, would be only 40 psia; and when the entire quantity of lotion was just dispensed, the pressure would be only 20 psia. If the valve of the aerosol should be opened accidentally while the package was in an inverted position, the entire quantity of gas would be lost in a short interval of time. The compressed gases which are slightly soluble in water have a slight reserve in pressure because of the dissolved quantity of gas.

Carbon dioxide, nitrous oxide or mixtures of both are used to pressurize aerosols from which it is desired to dispense the product as a foam. When the product emerges from the open valve into the atmosphere, the dissolved gases expand and produce the foamy product.

PACKAGING

Containers

Heavy-walled steel containers were employed to prepare bug bombs for the armed services during World War II. Immediately following the war these containers were made available on the civilian market as refillable containers. Soon thereafter, tin cans modeled after beer cans made their appearance as disposable or nonrefillable containers. Valves are crimped into 1-inch openings of the cans which openings now are standardized and will accommodate valves of various types.

Metal cans for aerosols are made by rolling or extrusion. Those made by the former method usually have a side seam. Containers made by extrusion have a neater appearance and withstand greater pressures. Black plate, tin plate, aluminum and stainless steel are used in making aerosol containers and, except for those made of stainless steel, they may have a protective coating of alkyd, phenolic, vinyl or epoxy resin applied to the inner surface to protect them from the corrosive effect of some aerosol constituents.

Two special container arrangements are now available to keep the propellant from contacting the product. One of these arrangements makes use of a polyethylene piston fitted to the inside of the can. The can is filled with product through the usual opening, the valve is sealed in place, and the propellant, either nitrogen or a liquid propellant, is added through a small opening in the bottom of the can and sealed with a rubber plug called a dart. In use, pressure on the piston by the propellant forces the product out through the valve. Products packaged in this type of container must be viscous, since the product itself must form the seal between the piston and the wall of the can.[37] The other arrangement makes use of a polyethylene bag on the inside of the container to hold the product. As the product is used the bag collapses.

Glass as an aerosol container has advantages over metal in that it is not subject to corrosion and it is capable of being molded into many attractive shapes. Glass containers may be of the unprotected or uncoated kind into which low-pressure aerosols are placed or of the protected kind for moderately high pressures. Glass can be protected with a metal shell or a plastic coating. Plastic coatings serve to cushion impacts if the bottles are dropped on a hard surface, and, should the impact be sufficiently hard to break the

bottle, the plastic will serve as a container for the broken glass and the aerosol contents as well. On breakage of the glass container, the gas causes the plastic to balloon. A small hole in the plastic then allows the gas to escape harmlessly.

Aerosol containers prepared from plastics of several different types also have been developed. Being almost entirely unbreakable, these containers obviously are even safer than plastic-coated glass containers. Since plastics are so variable in many of their properties, much research will be necessary before they will be generally adopted as a material for aerosol containers.

Valves

The purpose of the aerosol valve is to control the flow of the product from the container. It serves to allow the flow of the desired quantity of product from the container when in use, and it serves to prevent the flow of product during storage of the aerosol. The valve also affects the properties of the product as it flows from the container, although the formulation itself plays a part in these properties.

Although valves for aerosols are of many types, depending on the particular use to which the product will be put, the majority fall into the following general classifications:

Standard Valves. The type of valve used most commonly is the standard valve with an ordinary actuator button. These valves are suitable for space and surface sprays in which the liquid propellant is a part of the liquid phase. The actuator button for sprays usually has an external orifice which is about 0.020 inch in diameter, and the size obviously is a factor in rate of spray. Other factors which affect spray rate are the diameters and the number of internal orifices in the valve itself. Valves usually have from 1 to 3 internal orifices.

All spray valves have a series of communicating passages which serve as expansion chambers. As the propellant solution passes through the first orifice into the first expansion chamber, the drop in pressure is sufficient to cause the liquefied propellant to expand and boil. As the material passes through successive orifices into other passages, there are additional expansion and violent boiling which serve to break the product up into small particles as it is forced along in the expanding gas stream.

Dip tubes usually are made of polyethylene or nylon and serve to carry the product from the bottom of the container to the valve mechanism. Some valves are constructed to operate with the aerosol in an inverted position. Such valves have no dip tubes.

Standard valves can be equipped with break-up spray actuators for use with three-phase systems, two-phase systems in which the liquid phase is made up of product only and systems packaged at low pressures. In break-up spray actuators the product is forced through a swirling chamber, thus setting up a turbulent stream which is atomized as it leaves the orifice of the actuator button.

Foam Valves. These valves are designed to deliver foamy or aerated products. They have only one expansion orifice which connects directly into the actuator button without intermediary obstruction. The actuator usually has a large external orifice approximately 0.3 inch in diameter. The relatively large expansion chamber of the valve and the actuator button allows the formation of foam within the button so that the product is forced out in a foamy condition. If one were to put the same formulation in a container equipped with an ordinary valve and actuator button, the product would be forced from the system in a stream and the foamy ball would form on the surface to which applied.

Metering Valves. These valves deliver a measured quantity of aerosol mixture at each actuation. Metering can be accomplished by one of two methods. The dip tube may contain a steel ball which operates between a lower stop (merely a pin through the polyethylene tube) and a ball valve seat at the upper level. When the valve is actuated, the fast-flowing product carries the steel ball up in the tube until the ball seats in the valve, at which time no more product can flow up the dip tube. When the actuator is released, the steel ball returns slowly to its lower position in the tube and is then ready to deliver another quantity.

Metering can be accomplished by the use of 2 valves separated by a metering chamber or reservoir. Product is admitted to the reservoir by opening the valve from the pressure package and simultaneously closing the valve on the dispensing end of the reservoir. When the dose is to be taken, the dispensing valve is opened and the other valve is closed simultaneously. The valves are constructed to operate together on up and down strokes of the valve controls. It might be explained further that the upper valve (dispensing valve) is a sleeve valve which is held in closed position by a spring in the assembly and the lower valve is a plug valve held open by the same spring. In use, as the activator button is pressed, the upper valve opens and the lower valve closes.

The volume of the reservoir determines the quantity of spray per dose. Metering valves prevent overdosage of potent drugs, use of excessive quantities of nonpotent drugs, and discharge of excessive quantities of gas into body cavities.

Powder Valves. Standard valves can be used with many powder formulations, especially if the powder is very fine and the concentration of powder in the pressurized package is not too high. The most serious difficulty experienced in preparing powder aerosols is the accumulation of powder at the valve seat. Valves with a high seating pressure and with the valve seat located close to the orifice seem to be the most effective for powder aerosols. If the valve is operated wide open, there is less accumulation of powder at the valve than if the valve were only partially opened in operation. Wide-open operation may result in the discharge of a large plume of powder.

Compressed Gas Valves. Valves intended for use in systems that employ compressed gases may be provided with large orifices and large-diameter dip tubes to permit the passage of thick, viscous preparations such as syrups and lotions.

Protective Caps

Protective caps are necessary to protect the valve assembly during storage and transport. In addition to being serviceable they are often decorative and add considerably to the appearance of the aerosol. Protective caps usually are made of metal or polyethylene or some other plastic material. Caps for aerosol cans may be made to fit around the outside of the 1-inch aperture holding the valve or they may be made to fit around the periphery of the package. Caps for glass and plastic containers usually are fitted down to the shoulder of the container.

Filling Operations

If a propellant gas is kept at a temperature below its boiling point or at a pressure higher than its vapor pressure, it will remain liquefied. These two conditions are utilized in the packaging of aerosols that contain liquefied gas propellants by either of the general procedures—cold filling or pressure filling.

Cold Filling. In the cold filling process, first the product is chilled and loaded quantitatively into the container, then the propellant, also chilled (below its boiling point), is loaded into the container quantitatively, and immediately afterward the valve is crimped into place. The equipment for this procedure is shown in Figure 12-5. Dry ice or a mixture of dry ice and acetone is placed in the chamber containing the coils through which the propellant is allowed to flow. In large scale production the dry ice bath may

be replaced by a refrigeration system for chilling the propellant. The propellant, being chilled below its boiling point, now flows through the valve as a liquid. Cold filling is an economical procedure and offers little opportunity for entrapment of air in the container. Heavy vapors of propellant displace air from the container prior to installation of the valve. However, there are certain disadvantages involved in the process. Aqueous preparations cannot be filled by this process because the water will freeze. In packages intended to contain no water the moisture content may be considerable because of condensation of atmospheric moisture within the cold containers.

Pressure Filling (Using Liquefied Propellants). In this process the product is placed in the container, the valve crimped in place and then the propellant is metered under pressure at room temperature into the container through the valve. The air in the package might be ignored, although its presence could cause pressure variations and oxidation of the product. However, there are methods of removing air from the container in pressure filling. With the product in the container and the valve in place the air can

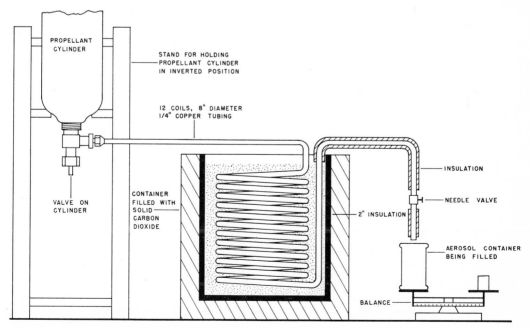

FIG. 12-5. Arrangement for cold-loading aerosol containers in the laboratory (adapted from set-up suggested by E. I. du Pont de Nemours & Co.).

be exhausted from the container by means of a vacuum before addition of the propellant through the valve. This procedure is feasible only if the valve has no dip tube or the container is inverted. Even with the container inverted some product may be drawn through the dip tube. Another procedure is to expel air by displacement from the container before sealing the valve in place. In this procedure, the product is placed in the container at room temperature, a small amount of cold propellant is added which, on striking the warm product, will boil and displace the air, and then the valve is crimped in place. Finally, propellant in proper quantity is forced through the valve.

Pressure filling can be accomplished with a vapor-pressure filling apparatus such as shown in Figure 12-6, or with a pumping system. Although pressure filling is slower than cold filling, it has several advantages. Pro-

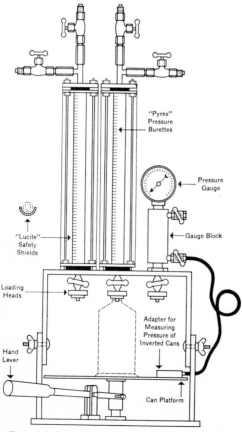

FIG. 12-6. Apparatus for pressure-loading aerosol containers in the laboratory. (E. I. du Pont de Nemours & Co.)

pellant losses are very small, the product and the propellants do not require refrigeration, and anhydrous filling is possible.

Pressure Filling (Using Compressed Gases). When compressed gases are used as propellants, the gas is not metered quantitatively into the container, but, rather, is filled to a predetermined pressure. The product is measured into the container, the valve is crimped in place and the gas is added through the valve. Air can be removed from the container by vacuum at the time the valve is inserted or by flushing with the gas prior to sealing. If an insoluble gas such as nitrogen is employed, filling can be carried out without agitation. However, if soluble gases such as nitrous oxide or carbon dioxide are used, the product should be shaken vigorously during filling to aid solution of the gas in the product.

A pressure regulator on the compressed-gas storage tank controls the amount of gas delivered in the filling process, and a flow meter can be installed in the line to indicate if gas is flowing.

Testing. Packaged aerosols are tested for leaks by immersing them in hot water until they reach a temperature of 55° C. (130° F.). This test is not required for preparations which are damaged by heat. Other tests now recognized by N.F. XIII include delivery rate, pressure, unit spray sampling, container sampling, liquid propellant sampling, and water content.

PHARMACEUTICAL PREPARATIONS

The dispensing of drugs from pressurized packages presents certain advantages over conventional procedures. Aerosols are supplied usually in small, easily portable packages ready for use and are therefore more convenient for the patient, especially when otherwise it might be necessary for him to measure doses and use special equipment for the application of the drug. Aerosols are dispensed as sealed containers. The contents may have been packaged under aseptic conditions and, if so, will remain sterile for the life of the product. Air and water can be excluded from aerosols, thus preventing decomposition of the drug by oxidation of the effects of moisture. Sometimes medications must be applied to highly irritated areas; foamy ointments and wet sprays can be applied to these areas from aerosols without the necessity of touching the area with swabs or other equipment. Uniform, controlled dosage can be obtained from aerosols. Metering valves supply measured quantities of drug for oral inhalation as well as for topical preparations. A number of drugs can be administered by oral inhalation to give prompt systemic response. In fact, drugs so administered are effective almost as rapidly as if they had been injected intravenously.

It has been mentioned that over 48.9 million aerosol units of medicinals and pharmaceuticals were produced during 1970.[7] These preparations included anesthetics, topical antiseptics, antibiotics, burn remedies, fungicides, oral medicinals, room vaporizers, products for vaginal application, etc. These medicinal products may be classified, as previously pointed out, into wet or surface sprays, space sprays, streams and foams.

In the wet or surface spray class are included local anesthetics, antiseptics, burn remedies and protective sprays, thin applications of which can be applied conveniently to injured areas without causing irritation. A typical aerosol formula for a burn remedy is as follows[6]:

BURN REMEDY

p-chloro-m-xylenol	0.50
Chlorobutanol	0.30
Isopropanol	12.11
Dipropylene glycol	17.10
Menthol	0.10
Tyrothricin	0.04
Propellant 12/11 (50:50)	69.85

Local anesthetics such as cyclomethycaine, benzocaine and tetracaine may be used in aerosol formulations. Ethyl chloride or some of the propellants, alone or in combination, may be used for their local anesthetic activity.

Throat sprays are illustrated by the following formula[38]:

THROAT SPRAY

Concentrate	Percent
Cetyldimethylbenzyl ammonium chloride	0.129
Tyrothricin	0.306
Benzocaine	4.595
Ethanol	94.970
Concentrate	33.02
Flavor	0.50
Propellant 12/114 (20:80)	66.48

Throat sprays are supplied usually in small containers equipped with metering valves to prevent overdosage. The valves are constructed so as to simplify directing the spray to the proper areas.

Aerosol powders also are classified as surface sprays. The following formula for athlete's foot medication serves as an example[1]:

ATHLETE'S FOOT MEDICATION

Dichlorophene	0.04
Hexachlorophene	0.02
Dipropylene glycol	0.50
Isopropyl myristate	0.50
Menthol	0.04
Talc (350 mesh)	10.00
Propellant 12/11 (50:50)	88.90

It will be noted from the above formula that the proportion of propellant in aerosol powders is quite high.

Bandage adherents and adhesive tape removers are classified as wet or surface sprays. The former contain rosin, benzoin, or other resinous materials to be used as an application prior to bandaging to keep the dressing in place. Tape removers consist of various solvents dissolved in the propellant to aid in the removal of adhesive tape. Protective film aerosols contain polyvinyl pyrrolidone, vinyl acetate copolymers, and methacrylate resins and, as the name implies, leave a protective film when the solvent evaporates. Some of them are suitable replacements for bandages.

Stream sprays include body rubs, some dermatologic preparations, and oral preparations. Body rubs are made up essentially of alcohol or silicone-containing creams. The dermatologic preparations may be various types of medicated ointments or lotions. Vitamin preparations usually are packaged as a syrup, with nitrogen as the propellant. The usual pressure is 90 psig.

Ointments and lotions can be pressure packed to yield foams on use of the aerosol. Foamy preparations may be of the quick-breaking type, in which the foam after application quickly subsides and leaves a thin layer on the skin, or they may be of a long-lasting type. With the latter, coverage of relatively large areas is possible by spreading the foam before it breaks. The following formula is for a foam type aerosol containing neomycin[26]:

FOAM BASE

Part A	% by weight
Myristic acid	1.33
Stearic acid	5.33
Cetyl alcohol	0.50
Lanolin	0.20
Isopropyl myristate	1.33
Part B	
Triethanolamine	3.34
Glycerin	4.70
Polyvinylpyrrolidone	0.34
Water	82.93

Prepare parts A and B separately and heat each to 80° C. Slowly add part B to part A with constant stirring and continue stirring until the mixture has cooled to room temperature. To complete the formulation add neomycin and propellants to the base in the proportions:

	% by weight
Foam Base	91.24
Neomycin sulfate	0.76
Propellant 12/114a* (40:60)	8.00

Blaug, Slattery and Henderson[5] have devised a special valve arrangement to introduce a medicated aerosol foam into the ear canal for the treatment of infections.

Space aerosols produce particles small enough to remain suspended in the air for some length of time. Insecticides, room deodorizers, and room vaporizers are good examples of this classification. Nasal Relief Spray[25] is an example of a space aerosol formulation:

NASAL RELIEF SPRAY

Thymol	0.10
Menthol	0.50
Camphor	0.50
Eucalyptol	0.15
Triethylene glycol	1.25
Dipropylene glycol	2.50
Propellant 12/11 (50:50)	95.00

This product can be used either as a space spray in confined areas or as a residual spray on a pillow or handkerchief.

If the particles of a spray are small enough, the spray is suitable for oral inhalation. Epinephrine, isoproterenol, octyl nitrite, and some corticosteroids are administered in this manner. Isoproterenol aerosol for oral inhalation may be prepared with a cosolvent

---

* Dichlorotetrafluoroethane (CCl_2FCF_3).

(alcohol), as illustrated in the next formula,[31] or it may be prepared as a suspension[32] without the use of a cosolvent. In the latter case, finely powdered isoproterenol is suspended in the propellant and the aerosol has to be shaken before use.

ISOPROTERENOL ORAL INHALANT

Isoproterenol hydrochloride ...	0.25% by weight
Ascorbic acid	0.10
Alcohol	33.00
Propellants 12/114	qs 100.00

A number of authors have discussed the importance of particle size in aerosols intended for administration by nasal or oral inhalation.[3, 14, 17, 22, 28, 30] The range of acceptable values seems to be from somewhat less than 1 micron to about 10 microns. Suggested values for pulmonary therapy are from 0.5 to 5 microns with an ideal value of 3 microns; aerosols of drugs intended for systemic effects probably should produce particles 2 microns or less in diameter. It is known that particulate matter inhaled in a stream of air may be deposited somewhere in the respiratory system. The larger particles may be trapped in the nasal passages or in the mouth, and the smaller ones will penetrate deeper into the lungs. Some of the very small particles may be deposited on the walls of the alveolar ducts and alveolar sacs, and the extremely small particles may be carried back out of the system by exhaled air. Retention of particulate matter in the respiratory system will also depend on the density of the particles, their shapes (whether spherical or fibrous), their moisture-absorbing properties, and the velocity of the air (rate and depth of breathing). If the particle of drug is soluble in natural secretions, it will dissolve and will be absorbed. Particles of insoluble or slowly soluble drugs, however, will be moved away from the lungs by cilia which may carry the particles upward at a rate of about 16 millimeters a minute into the throat where they are either swallowed or expectorated. Such drugs are not suitable for oral inhalation therapy. Neither are drugs with irritating qualities, because they cause reflex bronchial constriction and coughing.

The alveolar surface of the lungs is an excellent surface for the absorption of drugs. Since the alveolar membrane is thin and highly vascular and since collectively the alveoli present a very large surface area, absorption of drugs reaching the alveoli is rapid. The effects of drugs administered by oral inhalation occur as rapidly as the effects of drugs administered parenterally. Antibiotics, sulfonamides, expectorants, enzymes, anticoagulants, corticosteroids, surfactants, and analgesics are some of the drugs that have been administered by oral inhalation in the form of aerosols. It has been pointed out that aerosols intended to provide systemic effects of drugs should be capable of producing small particles of 2 microns and less. Valves and actuators can be designed to deliver particles in an optimum size range and to measure doses of aerosols accurately. Porush et al.[32] and Young et al.[43] have presented analytical procedures for determining the dosage and particle size of such aerosols.

Inhalants. None is official in the U.S.P. XVIII; and only one, Propylhexedrine Inhalant, is official in the N.F. XIII. Inhalants are defined as drugs or combinations of drugs which, because of their high vapor pressure, can be carried from the dosage form by an air current into the patient's nasal passages as he inhales. The device known as an inhaler makes possible the administration of an inhalant. The volatile drug is absorbed in fibrous material and enclosed in the inhaler which is made of plastic and is fitted with a cap to prevent loss of medicament when not in use. The patient removes the cap, inserts the nasal tip into a nostril, and breathes the air drawn through the inhaler to obtain the drug.

The N.F. XIII includes in the definition of inhalants products consisting of finely powdered or liquid medicaments that are carried into the respiratory passages by means of special devices. These devices include low-pressure aerosols that contain a solution or suspension of the drug in a liquefied propellant. Dosage of the medicament is controlled by means of metering valves. Isoproterenol Inhalant, the formula for which is given above, is an example.

Aerosols. Although aerosols are defined and briefly discussed in the U.S.P. XVIII, none is official in that compendium. The N.F. XIII contains monographs for six aerosol preparations: Dexamethasone, Isopro-terenol Sulfate, Povidone-Iodine, Thimerosal, Triacetin, and Triamcinolone Acetonide. All of these aerosols are intended for topical application except isoproterenol sulfate which is used by oral inhalation. Recognition of aerosols by the *N.F.* has been made possible by the development of standards and test procedures for these products. The tests might include determination of pressure and possible leaks, determination of particle size delivered, and determination of quantity of drug delivered by a metering valve as well as procedures for sampling and analyzing the product. The fact that these products are packaged under pressure complicates to a degree the procedures for testing them. Accurate and complete collection of a dose of a metered aerosol presents a difficult technical problem.

Inhalations. In the U.S.P. XVIII and the N.F. XIII, inhalations are defined as solutions for administration as nebulized mists intended to reach the respiratory tract. The official compendia point out that nebulizers (see Fig. 12-13) are suitable for the administration of inhalations only "if they give a droplet size not exceeding a few microns" (N.F. XIII) or "give droplets sufficiently fine and uniform in size so that the mist reaches the bronchioles" (U.S.P. XVIII). Epinephrine Inhalation, Isoproterenol Hydrochloride Inhalation, and Isoproterenol Sulfate Inhalation are official in the U.S.P. XVIII.

Sprays. Currently no sprays for use in atomizers are recognized by the official compendia. However, there are a number of commercially available nasal decongestants, antihistaminics, and antiinfectives. These include drugs such as ephedrine, hydroxyamphetamine, phenylephrine, naphazoline, tripelennamine, chlorobutanol, sulfonamides, nitrofurazone, oxymetazoline, tetrahydrozoline, tuaminoheptane, cyclopentamine, and cetylpyridium. These nasal solutions are aqueous in nature.

Atomizers, Insufflators, Nebulizers, and Vaporizers

The application of medications in the form of finely divided particles to the mouth, the throat, the nasal passages, and the lower respiratory tract is not new. Atomizers, nebulizers, vaporizers, and inhalators as instruments to apply these products have been known for some time. The first apparatus developed to atomize medicinals was made by Bergson in 1860.[19] His invention was really a combination inhaler and atomizer because steam generated by heating water in a closed vessel carried the medicament to the nostril or the mouth of the patient.

Atomizers. Atomizers are instruments used to reduce liquids or solids to fine particles or sprays. The principle on which atomizers are dependent for their operation is expressed by Bernoulli's theorem.[15] For example, in Figure 12-7 a fluid or, in the case of atomizers, air, which is flowing in the direction of the arrows, will flow more rapidly at B than at A or C. According to Bernoulli's theorem, decreased pressure will exist in an area of increased velocity; hence, the pressure is lower at B than at A or C.

In Figure 12-8 is represented a simplified atomizer.[27] Air is directed through tube A, the open end of which is close to the opening of tube B (dipping into the liquid). In Figure 12-8, air is moving at high velocity over the dip tube, thus producing a pressure (corresponding to position B in Fig. 12-7) lower than that normally present in the surrounding area. Since there is now reduced pressure in tube B, atmospheric pressure on the liquid in the reservoir of the atomizer forces the liquid up the tube where it meets with the air stream and is broken up into a spray. The atomizer shown in Figure 12-9 is constructed on these principles and is known as a vacuum type atomizer. Its operation is

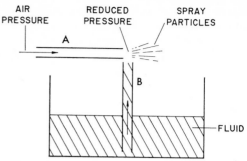

Fig. 12-8.   Operation of a simple vacuum atomizer.

identical with that of the simplified atomizer shown in Figure 12-8. By compressing the bulb, air is forced through the left tube; this creates a lowered pressure at the outlet of the right tube, and atmospheric pressure forces fluid from the reservoir up to the tip of the atomizer. At this point the fluid is broken up into a fine spray by the stream of air. This particular atomizer is shown to have an adjustable tip which allows for directing the spray to a specific area.

In Figure 12-10 is illustrated a simplified pressure atomizer. The operation of this atomizer is similar to that of the vacuum atomizer except that a portion of the air passing through tube A is directed into the closed system reservoir and produces a pressure (greater than atmospheric) on the surface of the liquid. Decreased pressure at the open end of the dip tube (B) now exists, and pressure within the reservoir forces fluid up the dip tube; when it meets the air stream, it is broken up into a spray.

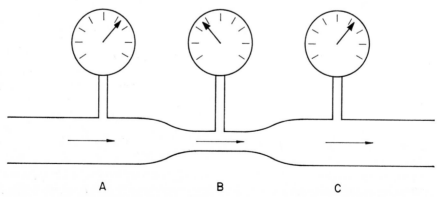

Fig. 12-7.   Illustration of Bernoulli's theorem. The fluid (or gas) flows more rapidly at B than at A or C, and the pressure is less at B than at A or C.

Fig. 12-9. Sketch of a commercially available atomizer which operates on the vacuum principle.

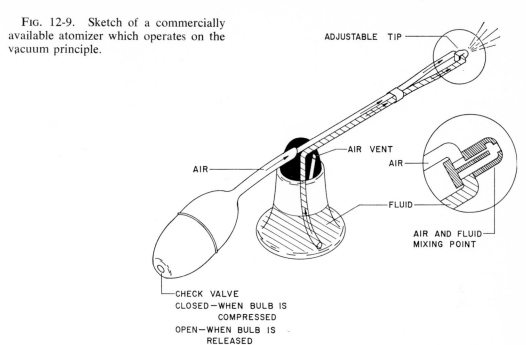

ADJUSTABLE TIP

AIR VENT

AIR

AIR

FLUID

FLUID

AIR AND FLUID MIXING POINT

CHECK VALVE
CLOSED—WHEN BULB IS COMPRESSED
OPEN—WHEN BULB IS RELEASED

The atomizer shown in Figure 12-11 also is a pressure type atomizer. Decreased pressure is created at the tip of the atomizer, and increased pressure within the reservoir forces the liquid through a tube to the tip of the atomizer. As the liquid and the air streams meet, spray is produced.

Powder Blowers. Figure 12-12 is a diagram of a powder blower. The operation of this apparatus is dependent on air turbulence set up in the reservoir of powder as air pressure is applied. Air and powder are then forced through the tip of the blower.

Nebulizers. Nebulizers (Fig. 12-13) are intended to produce very small particles (0.5 to 5 microns). The instrument is constructed to contain a small atomizing unit within a curved chamber. Larger, heavier droplets produced by the atomizing unit drop back into the reservoir to be processed again, whereas the mist or fog of very fine particles floats out in the air stream produced by pressure from the bulb and air drawn through the air vent. Small particles are necessary in oral inhalation therapy to ensure their reaching the alveolar sacs. The patient is directed to place the outlet of the nebulizer well in his mouth above his tongue and to inhale simultaneously as he depresses the bulb of the nebulizer. Controlled dosage can be administered by measuring the quantity of solution added to the reservoir of the nebulizer.

Plastic Bottle Atomizers. Plastic squeeze bottle atomizers can be used to dispense their contents by drops, if they are inverted and squeezed lightly, or to dispense their contents in the form of a spray, if they are held upright and squeezed. When they are used to dispense a spray, the mechanics of operation are similar to a pressure-type atomizer. Liquid is forced up a dip tube to meet a stream of fast moving air which then produces the spray.

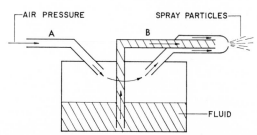

AIR PRESSURE   SPRAY PARTICLES

A   B

FLUID

Fig. 12-10. Operation of a simple pressure-type atomizer.

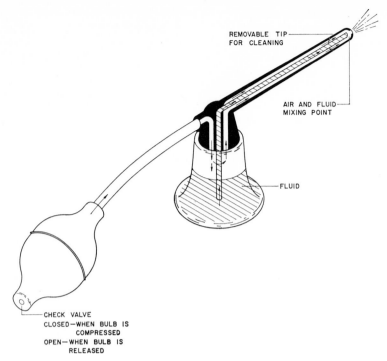

FIG. 12-11.   Sketch of a commercially available atomizer which operates on the pressure principle.

Vaporizers. Vaporizers are devices used to produce water vapor or small droplets of water intended to be inhaled by the patient in the treatment of pulmonary disorders.[28, 30] Moist air in itself is soothing to those suffer-

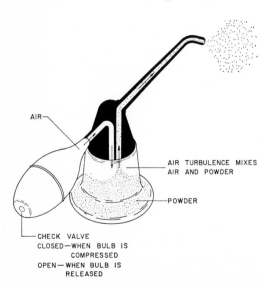

FIG. 12-12.   Sketch of a commercially available powder blower or powder insufflator.

ing from respiratory difficulties, and the intent may be merely to increase the humidity of the air being breathed or to carry medicinal agents into the lungs, or both. Vaporizers may produce vapor by means of heat or by mechanical means. In the electrolytic type of vaporizer the conductivity of the water is responsible for the amount of heat produced and subsequently the amount of steam generated. If distilled water or tap water of low mineral content is used in the vaporizer, it will be necessary to add sodium bicarbonate or borax to increase conductivity of the liquid. Sodium chloride should not be used in the vaporizer because it will increase conductivity excessively and it will cause corrosion of the electrodes. When the water level in the reservoir drops below the electrodes, operation of the unit is interrupted. Volatile medication, usually absorbed on cotton, may be added to the medication cup of the vaporizer to medicate the steam as it passes over the cup.

In one type of cold steam vaporizer, water is pumped up onto a rapidly revolving disc which, by centrifugal force, throws the water

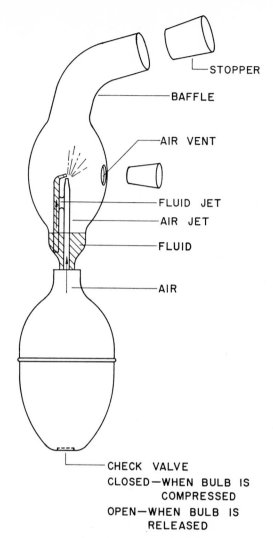

STOPPER

BAFFLE

AIR VENT

FLUID JET

AIR JET

FLUID

AIR

CHECK VALVE
CLOSED—WHEN BULB IS
COMPRESSED
OPEN—WHEN BULB IS
RELEASED

Fig. 12-13.   Sketch of a commercially available nebulizer.

particles against a slit screen surrounding the disc to produce a mist. A baffle removes the larger particles of the mist as it passes through a vent into the atmosphere of the room.

Cool, fine particles of water vapor are also produced by jet nebulizers and by ultrasonic nebulizers.[39] Jet nebulizers, if operated at 7 psig, will produce particles of 1 or 2 microns; and the ultrasonic device will produce very small particles of less than 1 micron. The mist from these nebulizers can be medicated. These units can be used with tents,

face masks, or intermittent positive pressure breathing devices.

REFERENCES

1. Athlete's Foot Medication, A. T. P. Bull. No. 8, New York. Allied Chem. Corp., General Chemical Division, 1957.
2. Avy, A. P.: Les aerosols. p. 2. Paris, Dunod, 1956.
3. Bell, J. H.: Inhalation Aerosols. Mfg. Chemist Aerosol News, *38*:37 1967. (Sept.)
4. Bichowsky, F. R.: U.S. Pat. 2,021,981, 1935.
5. Blaug, S. M., Slattery, T. W., and Henderson, W. M.: A medicated aerosol foam for otitic application. Am. J. Hosp. Pharm., *20*:326, 1963.
6. Burn Remedy: A. T. P. Bull. No. 14. New York, Allied Chem. Corp. General Chemical Division, 1958.
7. Chemical Specialties Manufacturers Association, Aerosol Division: Aerosol and Pressure Products Survey—1970. Presented at the meeting of the Aerosol Division, Chicago, May 17, 1971.
8. ———: Aerosol Guide Glossary of Terms Used in the Aerosol Industry. p. 25. New York, March, 1966.
9. Gebauer, C. L.: U.S. Pat. 668,815, 1901.
10. ———: U.S. Pat. 711,045, 1902.
11. Goodhue, L. D.: Insecticidal aerosol production: spraying solutions in liquefied gases. Industr. Eng. Chem., *34*:1456, 1942.
12. Helbing, H., and Pertsch, G.: U.S. Pat. 628,463, 1899.
13. Herzka, A., and Pickthall, J.: Pressurized Packaging (Aerosols). ed. 2. London, Butterworth, 1961.
14. Idson, B.: Inhalation therapy. Drug Cosmetic Ind., *107*:46, 1970.
15. Kenworthy, R. W.: College Physics. New York, Davis, 1961.
16. Lemoine, R. M. L.: D. R. Pat. 532,194, 1926.
17. Lovejoy, F. W., Jr., Constantine, H., and Dautrebande, L.: Importance of particle size in aerosol therapy. Proc. Soc. Exp. Biol. Med., *103*:836, 1960.
18. Lynde, J. D.: U.S. Pat. 34,894, 1862.
19. Hoover, J. E., Remington's Pharmaceutical Sciences, ed. 14, Easton, Pa., Mack, 1970.
20. Midgley, T., Jr., Henne, A. L., and McNary, R. R.: U.S. Pat. 1,926,396, 1933.
21. Mina, F. A.: Glass aerosols for pharmaceuticals. Drug and Cosmetic Index, *75*:625, 1954.
22. Mitchell, R. I.: Retention of aerosol particles in the respiratory tract. Am. Rev. Resp. Dis., *82*:627, 1960.
23. Mobley, L. K.: U.S. Pat. 1,378,481, 1921.
24. Moore, R. W.: U.S. Pat. 746,866, 1903.
25. Nasal Relief Spray: A. T. P. Bull. No. 15. New York, Allied Chem. Corp., General Chemical Division, 1958.

26. Neomycin Foam: A. T. P. Bull. No. 32. New York, Allied Chem. Corp., General Chemical Division, 1958.

27. Neuroth, M. L.: Am. Prof. Pharm., *26*:233, 1960.

28. Olsen, A. M.: Aerosol therapy in bronchopulmonary disease. Calif. Med., *96*:237, 1962.

29. Package for Profit: Wilmington, Delaware, Freon Products Division, E. I. du Pont de Nemours & Co., 1960.

30. Palmer, K. N. V.: Indications for aerosol treatment in pulmonary disease. Geriatrics, *19*:612, 1964.

31. Physician's Handbook (No. 6592). New York, Winthrop Laboratories Division, Sterling Drug Inc., May 1964.

32. Porush, I., Thiel, C. G., and Young, J. G.: Pressurized pharmaceutical aerosols for inhalation therapy. I. Physical testing methods. J. Am. Pharm. A. (Sci. Ed.), *49*:70, 1960.

33. Riedel-E., J. D., and de Haën, A.-G.: D. R. Pat. 557,259, 1931.

34. Root, M. J.: Package Engineering 3 (No. 5): 28, 1958.

35. Rotheim, E.: U.S. Pat. 1,800,156, 1931.

36. ———: U.S. Pat. 1,892,750, 1933.

37. Sanders, P. A.: Principles of Aerosol Technology. New York, Van Nostrand Reinhold, 1970.

38. Sciarra, J. J.: Aerosol pharmaceuticals. Aerosol Age, *9* (No. 7):49, 1964.

39. Secor, J.: Patient Care in Respiratory Problems. Philadelphia, W. B. Saunders, 1969.

40. Sinclair, D.: Handbook on Aerosols. p. 64. Washington, D.C., 1950.

41. Sullivan, W. N., Goodhue, L. D., and Fales, J. H.: J. Econ. Ent., *35*:48, 1942.

42. U.S.D.A.: U.S. Patent 2,321,023.

43. Young, J. G., Porush, I., Thiel, C. G., Cohen, S., and Stimmel, C. H.: Pressurized pharmaceutical aerosols for inhalation therapy. II. J. Am. Pharm. A. (Sci. Ed.), *49*:72, 1960.

44. Whytlaw-Gray, R. W., and Patterson, H. S.: Smoke. London, Arnold, 1932.

13

Rodney D. Ice, Ph.D., *Director, Radiopharmaceutical Services*
Associate Professor of Pharmacy, College of Pharmacy,
University of Michigan

Radioactive Dosage Forms

Ever since the discovery of x-rays in 1895 by Roentgen[11] and natural radioactivity in 1896 by Becquerel,[1] man has been interested in utilizing radiation in medicine. Within the two months following his discovery of x-rays, Roentgen had investigated and characterized this new radiation. Roentgen's observation that radiation could be used to reveal internal body structures initiated an extensive use of x-rays immediately after their discovery.

The Curies,[5] using a uranium ore called pitchblende, first isolated radium as a specific naturally occurring radionuclide. Their achievement made the first radionuclides available to medicine. The first reported medical use of natural radioactivity involved exposure of a saline solution to radon gas and administration of the radioactive saline solution to man to determine blood circulation.[3] At present, 65 naturally occurring radionuclides are known.

In 1919 Rutherford[12] first described the production of artificial radioactivity when he noted that alpha radiation interacted with nitrogen to form a proton. With the advent of charged particle accelerators—e.g., the cyclotron—during the 1930's, new artificial radionuclides were made available in limited quantities. Polycythemia vera was treated with cyclotron-produced phosphorus-32 soon after its discovery.

The development of the nuclear pile in 1944 made available a source of neutrons so that radionuclides could be produced in abundance. With the establishment of the Atomic Energy Commission and its emphasis on the peaceful use of the atom, radiopharmaceuticals became a well established component of pharmacy.

Manufactured radioactive products for human use are now regulated by the Food and Drug Administration in the same manner as other pharmaceuticals. Pharmacies specializing in radiopharmaceuticals are being located in large hospitals. Over five million patients are examined or treated each year with radioactive drugs.

FUNDAMENTALS

Atomic Structure

The atom is made up of protons and neutrons in the nucleus, with electrons located in discrete energy states around the nucleus. The number of electrons varies from one to over 100 and determines the chemical nature of the atom. The atom has a radius of approximately 10^{-8} cm., with the nucleus having a radius of 10^{-12} cm. The nucleus occupies about 0.0001 of the total atom.

Radiopharmaceuticals are pharmaceuticals that emit particular types of ionizing radiation. *Radiation* refers to particles or waves coming predominantly from the nucleus of the atom, representing discrete energy changes through which the atom attempts to attain a more stable configuration. This radiation, a form of energy, produces ion pairs along the path of the photon or particle emitted. Human senses cannot detect this radiation.

The stability of the atom depends on the neutron to proton (n/z) ratio in the nucleus. Protons are positively charged, with a mass 1,800 times that of an orbital electron. Neutrons have an equivalent mass to the proton but carry no electrical charge. In a stable atom, the number of electrons, which are negatively charged, equals the number of protons. The number of protons in an atom is referred to as the *atomic number* (Z). An element is an atom of specific atomic

423

number. *Isotopes* are atoms of various masses having the same atomic number. The atomic number 11, for example, describes sodium and its isotopes. The number of protons plus the number of neutrons, combined, is the *mass number* (A) of an isotope. The chemical properties of an element are not affected by the number of neutrons in the atom. In sodium, the number of available neutrons varies from 9 to 14. Sodium-23 has 11 protons and 12 neutrons and is stable. Two isotopes of sodium that are widely used in pharmacy are sodium-24, which has 11 protons and 13 neutrons, and sodium-22, which has 11 protons and 11 neutrons. In all elements up to atomic number 83, there are specific neutron to proton ratios which lead to nuclear stability. Above atomic number 83, all elements are radioactive. If additional neutrons or a deficiency of neutrons occurs and upsets the stability of an atom, the atom attempts to regain its stability by giving off either a photon, such as a gamma ray, or a particle from the nucleus to attain a more stable n/z ratio.

Nuclide defines any species of atom characterized by a specific number of neutrons and protons within the atom. There are over 1,675 nuclides, of which 264 are stable.[3] Of all the radionuclides available, 9 radionuclides of 6 elements comprise 70 percent of the radiopharmaceuticals used today. They are ^{131}I, ^{51}Cr, ^{125}I, ^{99m}Tc, ^{132}I, ^{22}Na, ^{85}Kr, ^{197}Hg, and ^{203}Hg.[13]

Production of Radiopharmaceuticals

Radiopharmaceuticals are produced by two methods. Neutron-deficient radionuclides are produced by particle accelerators, e.g., the cyclotron; neutron excess radionuclides are generally produced by nuclear reactors.

For a charged particle to interact with a target atom, the charged particle must have sufficient energy to overcome the repulsive forces produced between the positively charged target nucleus and the positively charged bombarding particle. A number of particle accelerators have been produced through which a charged particle is given kinetic energy via stepwise acceleration. In a *cyclotron,* a *betatron,* or a *synchrotron,* this is done with alternating electrical fields. Within a cyclotron are two flat, hollow ob-

jects called dees because they are shaped like the letter "D." The dees are part of an electrical circuit which oscillates in the radiofrequency range. On either side of the dees are large magnets that steer the injected charged particles in a circular path. The charged particles are accelerated from one dee to the other at the oscillation frequency by high voltages applied to the dees. The charged particle follows a circular path until the particle has such energy that it passes out of the field and interacts with the target nucleus. The most commonly used charged particles include protons (p^+), deuterons (d^+), alphas ($^4_2He^{++}$) and helium ($^3_2He^{++}$).

The majority of radiopharmaceuticals are produced by the process of *nuclear activation* in a *nuclear reactor.* In an operational nuclear reactor there are a large number of excess neutrons. Stable nuclides are placed in the reactor, where the excess neutrons bombard them. Depending on neutron energies, the number of neutrons available, and the size of the stable atom, neutrons are added to the stable atom. The result is an increase in the n/z ratio. In this manner nuclear stability is upset and radioactive nuclides are produced.

Another means by which radioactive nuclides are produced in a reactor is through *byproduct radionuclide recovery.* The core of a reactor consists of uranium or plutonium. The excess neutrons in the reactor cause the uranium or plutonium to fission— i.e., the breaking of the atom in two parts, resulting in materials with lower atomic numbers. The newly formed fission products are called byproducts. Fissioning is accompanied by release of additional neutrons which go on to produce further fissioning of core material and to provide the neutrons necessary for neutron activation. After a reactor has been in operation for some time, the amount of byproduct material in the core increases to such a degree that a decrease in fission efficiency results, necessitating replacement of the core. The segments of core removed from the reactor are highly radioactive and contain a variety of fission products. Through radiochemical reprocessing, it is possible to separate out and utilize these fission products for radiochemical and radiopharmaceutical purposes.

It is for this reason that the Atomic Energy Commission uses the term "byproduct material" license for the type of license required to handle radioactive materials.

Radioactive Decay

Radioactive nuclides attain a more stable configuration through a process known as radioactive decay. Important to the consideration of radioactive decay is the *physical half-life* ($t_{1/2}$) i.e., the amount of time required for a radionuclide to decay to 50 percent of its original activity. Consideration of radioactive decay involves the types of radiation produced, the energy of each radiation, and the nature of the resulting product after radioactive decay. Table 13-1 indicates some radiopharmaceutical physical decay parameters.

Nuclear medicine has been dependent mostly on radiopharmaceuticals that decay by *gamma* (γ) *emission*. Gamma radiation is composed of electromagnetic waves of no mass and no charge traveling at the speed of light. Gamma rays originate from the nucleus

of the atom and are very penetrating because of their short wave length and high energy.

X-rays, while similar to gamma rays in physical properties, originate from changes in orbital electron energy states. Because orbital electron energy states are lower than nuclear energy states, x-rays are emitted with less energy (longer wave length) than gamma rays. X-rays and gamma rays have the same characteristics except for their origin. Gamma rays have proved their usefulness as radiopharmaceutical agents: after they are administered, their radiation emerges from the body and its origin may be selectively localized with a proper detection system. Examples of gamma-emitting radiopharmaceuticals include cyanacobalamin Co-60, sodium iodide I-131, and sodium pertechnetate Tc-99m.

Another way in which the atom can attain a more stable configuration is through the emission of a *beta particle*. Beta particles are either positively charged electrons (positrons, β^+) or negatively charged electrons (negatrons, β^-). Because of the associated

TABLE 13-1.   PHYSICAL PROPERTIES OF COMMONLY USED RADIOPHARMACEUTICALS

RADIONUCLIDE	PRINCIPAL DECAY MODE AND ENERGY	HALF-LIFE	
Hydrogen-3 (Tritium)	β^-, 0.0186.	12.3	y
Carbon-14	β^-, 0.156.	5730	y
Sodium-24	β^-, 1.392; γ_1, 1.369; γ_2, 2.754.	15.0	h
Phosphorus-32	β^-, 1.710.	14.3	d
Potassium-42	18% β^-_1, 2.00; 82% β^-_2, 3.52; 18% γ, 1.52.	12.4	h
Chromium-51	9% EC, 0.432; 91% EC, 0.752; 9% γ, 0.320.	27.8	d
Iron-59	45% β^-_1, 0.273; 53% β^-_2, 0.475; 3% γ_1, 0.192; 56% γ_2, 1.095; 43% γ_3, 1.292.	45	d
Cobalt-57	EC, 0.701; 89% γ_1, 0.014; 89% γ_2, 0.122; 11% γ_3, 0.136.	270	d
Cobalt-60	β^-, 0.313; γ_1, 1.17; γ_2, 1.33.	5.26	y
Technetium-99m	γ, 0.140.	6.0	h
Iodine-125	EC, 0.149; γ, 0.036.	60	d
Iodine-131	7.0% β^-_2, 0.330; 90% β^-_4, 0.606; 5% γ_1, 0.080; 5% γ_4, 0.284; 85% γ_6, 0.364; 7% γ_8, 0.637.	8.05	d
Cesium-137	94% β^-_1, 0.514; 6% β^-_2, 1.176; 94% γ_1, 0.662.	30.0	y
Gold-198	99% β^-_2, 0.962; γ_1, 0.412.	2.7	d
Mercury-197	98% EC_2, 0.34; γ_1, 0.077; 2% γ_2, 0.192.	65	h
Mercury-203	β^-, 0.213; γ, 0.279.	46.9	d
Sodium-22	90% β^+, 0.546; 10% EC, 1.568 γ, 1.275.	2.6	y

All energies in MeV. Where percent is not indicated, it is 100%. Beta energies all E_{max}.
h, hour; d, day; y, year.

mass and charge of the particle, beta particles are not as penetrating as gamma radiation. An example of a widely used radiopharmaceutical that emits a negative electron is phosphorus-32. Examples of radiopharmaceuticals that emit positrons include fluorine-18 and sodium-22.

Negatrons have found limited use in nuclear medicine because of their low penetration. They are useful in therapeutic applications where a large radiation dose is needed to inhibit tissue function. Phosphorus-32 is used to treat polycythemia vera because phosphorus localizes in the bone marrow and delivers a large radiation dose selectively to the bone marrow. The associated beta radiation is not very penetrating and little is lost outside the body. Iodine-131 is preferred for thyroid carcinoma treatment because of its five betas emitted per disintegration. As such, it delivers a large radiation dose localized to the thyroid gland. Iodine-131 also emits gammas and thus can be used selectively to visualize the thyroid gland. Iodine-125 is the radiopharmaceutical of choice for scanning the thyroid gland because it disintegrates with only a single gamma photon and thus results in a low radiation dose to the gland.

There are other types of radioactive decay which are made use of in radiopharmaceuticals. Iodine-125 decays by *electron capture* (EC). In electron capture, the atom attempts to attain a more stable configuration in its nucleus by attracting one of the orbital electrons into the nucleus. The electron added to the nucleus provides the necessary energy required to release a photon. A gamma photon is released immediately on the capture of the orbital electron by the nucleus. Important radiopharmaceuticals that decay by electron capture include chromium-51, cobalt-57, strontium-85, and mercury-197.

Another mode of radionuclidic decay is *isomeric transition*. Isomeric transition results in an emitted gamma ray during the change from one nuclear energy state to another. An excited nuclear isomer representing an elevated energy level in the nucleus releases its excitation energy by the emission of a photon. This type of decay occurs where there is a large difference between the angular momenta of the excited

and ground states and usually results in a relatively low energy gamma photon. Radiopharmaceuticals that decay by isomeric transition include technetium-99m, indium-113m, and strontium-87m. The suffix m indicates a *meta*stable state of an atom that will undergo isomeric transition.

Internal conversion radioactive decay takes place when an excited nucleus interacts with an orbital electron and transfers the excitation energy to the electron, causing the electron to be ejected from its orbit. This electron, called a *conversion electron,* is a monoenergetic electron (unlike beta particles, which are emitted with a spectrum of energies).

A radioactive decay mode seldom used in radiopharmaceuticals is the emission of an *alpha particle,* which consists of the helium nucleus ($^{4}_{2}He^{++}$). Alpha decay occurs in elements (including some naturally occurring elements—e.g., uranium and radium) with atomic numbers greater than 83. Because of the large particle size and the double positive charge, alpha particles deposit their energy very close to the atom emitting them. Thus, alpha particles are not very penetrating and are difficult to detect, but they are easily shielded.

Units of Energy

The unit of energy used to describe radiation is the *electron volt*. An electron volt is the work done when one electron is accelerated by a potential difference of one volt. In chemical reactions, the magnitude of energy involved is roughly ten electron volts per atom. In nuclear reactions, the energy of the photons or particles emitted are generally in the *keV* (1,000 electron volts) or the *MeV* (1,000,000 electron volts) range. Gamma rays are emitted from an atom at discrete energy levels, i.e., each photon from a particular radionuclide has a definite associated energy. Thus, gamma rays are *monoenergetic*. During cobalt-60 decay two photons are emitted, having energies of 1.33 MeV and 1.17 MeV.

Beta particles, however, are emitted with a full spectrum of energies. A beta particle is described by its *maximum energy* (E_{max}). In general, the beta particles most often emitted during beta decay of an atom have an energy approximately $\frac{1}{3}$ the maximum energy. This is an important consideration in evaluating potential detection systems for beta emitters. For example, carbon-14 has an E_{max} of 156 keV; but there are few particles with this energy. Thus, the detection system utilized for the beta particles emitted by carbon-14 must be most sensitive to those particles having an energy occurring in the range of 50 to 55 keV.

Beta particles are often characterized by the energy of the particle emitted. *Soft betas* are particles with a maximum energy (E_{max}) of less than 250 keV. Typical soft beta emitters include sulfur-35 (168 keV), carbon-14 (156 keV), and hydrogen-3 (tritium, 18 keV). Beta particles with an energy greater than 250 keV, such as those emitted by phosphorus-32 (E_{max} 1.8 MeV), are known as *hard betas*. Soft betas readily interact with the medium they are traversing and thus are easily shielded. In tracer quantities, the shipping vial generally provides the necessary shielding. Hard betas, because of their higher energy, are more penetrating and require additional shielding for protection.

Measurement of Radiation

Radiation exposure is measured in roentgens. A *roentgen* (r) is a specific quantity of X- or gamma-radiation such that the number of ion pairs produced in one cc. of air will produce one electrostatic unit of electrical charge (2.58×10^{-4} Coulomb/kg). One roentgen in air represents the absorption of 87.7 ergs of energy per gram of air. The *rad* is a unit of absorbed radiation dose. The rad is specifically reserved for the amount of energy that has been *absorbed*. The rad represents 100 ergs of energy absorbed per gram of tissue. Different types of radiation may have different relative toxicities. By multiplying the rad dose by a qualifying factor (QF), such as a distribution factor or a specific toxicity factor, the *rem* dose is obtained. The rem dose, sometimes called the dose equivalent, is used to equate the differences in biological responses produced by different radiations such as gamma, beta, neutron, and alpha.

In addition to the units of exposure and absorbed dose, the units of radioactive disintegration are often used in nuclear pharmacy. The output of all radiation detection instruments is measured in *relative units,* such as counts per minute (cpm) or counts per some other time interval. These units indicate the number of interactions that have taken place in the detector, but they do not describe the total number of atoms that have decayed in the sample unless the efficiency of the detector is known. The conversion of relative units by an efficiency factor yields an *absolute unit* known as the Curie (Ci). The Curie, by definition, refers only to the rate of disintegration; thus, there is no simple method for relating activities in curies to resulting exposure or absorbed dose. The *curie* is 3.7×10^{10} disintegrations per second (dps). (The Curie is a large quantity of radioactivity; smaller units, the millicurie (mCi) or microcurie (μCi), are commonly used.) The *millicurie* is 10^{-3} Curie, and the *microcurie* is 10^{-6} Curie. There are 2.2×10^6 dpm/μCi—a useful conversion factor in calculating absolute units.

Definitions

Specific Activity is the ratio of the total number of radioactive atoms present in a sample to the total number of atoms present. Specific activity has a theoretical limit of 0 to 1. A more common definition of specific activity is the ratio of any quantity of radioactive material per some unit quantity of total material. With this practical definition, specific activity can be measured as μCi/mg., dpm/g., or any such combination of units.

Specific concentration, i.e., radioactivity per unit volume, can be utilized in some radiation measurements—e.g., blood volume determination. In blood volume determinations, the administered I.V. dose in cpm/ml. is related to the radioactivity after dilution by the patient's blood. When relative units are used for measurement, instrumental conditions and units of specific activity must remain constant. The blood volume is calculated from the change in specific activity resulting from dilution of the administered dose by the blood.

Carrier-free material is material in which all of the atoms present are radioactive. Carrier-free material has a specific activity of one. Carrier-free radiopharmaceuticals result in physically very small quantities of material. Radiopharmaceuticals are usually diluted with carrier solutions, i.e., solutions containing molecules of the same chemical nature. For example, carrier-free carbon-14 labeled ethanol would be diluted with stable ethanol.

Carrier solutions are often used for decontamination purposes, because a rapid exchange of similar chemical ions occurs.[4] The washing of a contaminated area with carrier will reduce the amount of remaining radioactivity. Use of carrier-free radiopharmaceuticals presents special problems that must be carefully considered, because a large amount of radioactivity may represent a very small quantity of drug, and that small amount of drug may be absorbed by the container.

As nuclear radiation passes through matter, ion pairs are produced. The number of ion pairs produced per specific length of path traveled is known as the *specific ionization* of the radiation. This specific ionization is related to the kinetic energy, the molecular charge, and the physical mass of the particle. About 32 to 35 electron volts of energy are required for the formation of a primary ion pair in air. The energy transferred to a system will also depend on the atomic number of the absorbing material. *Linear Energy Transfer* (LET) is the amount of energy transferred to the interacting system per centimeter of path traveled by the ionizing particle or photon.

Health Physics

Nuclear pharmacy and medical health physics are closely allied. *Health physics* is a profession devoted to the protection of man and his environment from unwarranted radiation exposure. Health physicists work with pharmacists in the hospital in the determination of radiation dosimetry and establishment of safe work procedures for the handling of radioactive materials.

In addition to standard pharmacy equipment, each nuclear pharmacy must have adequate equipment and facilities for radiation safety. "Adequacy" depends on the radionuclides used, the quantity of the radiopharmaceuticals to be prepared, and the chemical form(s) involved. For licensure by the Atomic Energy Commission, minimum training requirements must be met prior to the handling of radioactive materials. This can be obtained through formal course work or through experience. Pharmacists must be aware of handling procedures for each of the radionuclides, with its particular hazards. Nuclear pharmacy requires the art of handling microliter (μl) and picogram (pg) quantities of materials. The pharmacist must be well versed in the handling of monitoring instruments and must be adequately trained to handle medical radiation accidents.

Radiation, because of its ability to produce ion pairs, can destroy living tissue, form toxic products, and affect kinetic processes in the body. Thus, it is important that the nuclear pharmacist, in addition to his pharmacy training, be aware of the physics, biology, and chemistry of nuclear radiation.

Radiopharmaceuticals or Radiochemicals

Radiopharmaceuticals are radiochemicals, but radiochemicals are not always radiopharmaceuticals. The Atomic Energy Commission, along with the Food and Drug Administration, require that the pharmaceutical quality of radioactive materials be ascertained before use in humans. A *radiopharmaceutical* is a chemical containing a radionuclide suitable for us in humans and is used for the diagnosis, mitigation, or therapy of a disease. Nuclear pharmacy requires a thorough knowledge of each pharmacy specialty and an expertise in the handling of radioactive materials. The utilization of a radiopharmaceutical requires the following considerations: radionuclidic purity, radiochemical purity, chemical purity, sterility, nonpyrogenicity, assay, stability, formulation, efficacy, and drug interaction.

Nuclear medicine is using radionuclides with shorter and shorter half-lives because the radiation dose received by the patient is a function of the physical half-life. The use of short half-life radiopharmaceuticals offers the pharmacist an opportunity to prepare and compound pharmaceuticals on an individual basis for the patient. The nuclear pharmacist is involved with preparing a product which not only is suitable for human usage but also can be individually calibrated for a patient at a specific time.

Quality control has always been a predominant concern of the manufacturer; however, the nuclear pharmacist, because of the short half-lives of the drugs, must establish his own quality control procedures for the use of radiopharmaceuticals. Whereas formulation, compounding, and quality control are only a small fraction of the duties of a community pharmacist, the nuclear pharmacist devotes the greater part of his time to formulation, compounding, and quality control of unidose radiopharmaceuticals.

Sterility and Nonpyrogenicity

Radiopharmaceuticals present special problems in regard to sterility and nonpyrogenicity. Tests for both are time consuming and cannot always be done prior to the utilization of the radiopharmaceutical because of the short physical half-life of the radiopharmaceutical.

In most nuclear pharmacies, a *systems approach* is used for the production of parenteral products. The systems approach depends on assurance of sterility and nonpyrogenicity throughout the product formulation, compounding, and dispensing processes. This technique requires continual evaluation to determine whether or not sterility and nonpyrogenicity are maintained throughout the preparation process. All stable ingredients are tested prior to use. The radiopharmaceutical dispensed is actually used without sterility and pyrogenicity testing, but an aliquot of each dispensed product is tested, to ensure that the system has been maintained sterile and pyrogen-free. The ionizing radiation associated with the radiopharmaceutical is, in itself, insufficient to provide a sterile product.

Terminal sterilization of radiopharmaceuticals by autoclaving is acceptable if the products are heat stable. However, many radiopharmaceuticals are heat labile (e.g., radioiodinated human serum albumin).

Another commonly used technique is *sterilization by filtration* through 0.22 μ cellulose filters. This technique may be used for solutions, but it does not lend itself to large molecules such as those of aggregated albumin or colloids. The integrity of the filter should be assessed after each usage to ensure freedom from bacterial contamination.[7]

Pyrogens are thought to be metabolic products formed during the growth of various bacteria, yeasts, and molds. Pyrogens are not removed through sterilization and may be adsorbed onto glassware and equipment. Pyrogens are destroyed by strong oxidizing acids or highly alcoholic solutions. Pyrogen-free glassware is obtained by heating glassware in a hot-air oven at 175° for 2 hours.

Regulations

There are a number of organizations—e.g., the National Council on Radiation Protection (NCRP), the International Council on Radiation Protection (ICRP), and the Federal Radiation Council (FRC)—which make recommendations in regard to the utilization of ionizing radiation. Recommendations per se are not legally binding. The recommendations, however, have been used in establishing standard working procedures with radioactive material and are often used to define safe and accepted professional practices.

Three governmental agencies are concerned with radiopharmaceutical regulations: the Atomic Energy Commission, the Food and Drug Administration, and the individual State Boards of Health.

If a *State Board of Health* has proved to the AEC its ability to regulate radionuclide usage, the AEC transfers licensing responsibility to the State Board of Health. States that have assumed this responsibility are called *agreement states*. Nuclear pharmacists located in agreement states apply to their own State Department of Public Health for licensure and not to the Atomic Energy Commission. If the state is not an agreement state, the pharmacy must have an Atomic Energy Commission License for the handling of radioactive materials. The Atomic Energy Commission controls byproduct material only—i.e., material produced in a nuclear reactor. Thus, a pharmacy that is using cyclotron-produced radioactive materials as well as reactor-produced materials may require licensure from both the individual State Board of Health and the Atomic Energy Commission.

The *Atomic Energy Commission* provides a variety of license structures, depending on the extent of radionuclide utilization. The

AEC permits exempt concentrations and quantities of some radiopharmaceuticals, such as in-vitro triiodothyronine (T-3) and tetraiodothyronine (T-4) kits. The AEC also issues a general license to manufacturers of exempt quantities or of sealed sources that are utilized on a regular basis either in photographic devices or in static eliminators. A third category of AEC licensure is the specific license issued to a person for specific radionuclides, in specific chemical forms, at a specific location, for a specific use and for a specific period of time. Each specific license application is reviewed by the Atomic Energy Commission in terms of the applicant's experience and facilities.

Large users of radioactivity may obtain a broad specific license which requires a full-time radiation safety officer available for health physics considerations. This license also requires the appointment of a medical radiation committee for the evaluation of individual users and proposed uses. The AEC uses the broad specific license to assign radiation responsibility from the AEC to an expert committee within an institution. Broad specific licenses are generally used at universities or very large institutions. Agreement states follow closely the same pattern of licensure established by the Atomic Energy Commission.

The *Food and Drug Administration (FDA)* in 1963 recognized the need for regulations regarding radiopharmaceuticals; however, an exemption to FDA regulations was given for investigational new radiopharmaceuticals if a license was obtained from the Atomic Energy Commission. In January of 1971, however, notice of intent to withdraw this exemption was published. Since the AEC controls by-product material only, any user of cyclotron or accelerator produced material has always been under the jurisdiction of the FDA. At present, the FDA publishes a list of well established radiopharmaceuticals (see Table 13-2). Anyone desiring to distribute these radiopharmaceuticals commercially must submit a new drug application (NDA). Utilization of radiopharmaceuticals that are not on the well established list requires submission of an investigational new drug (IND) application by both the manufacturer and the physician. The pharmacist must be cognizant of the current status of radiopharmaceuticals used so as to be in full conformance with the legal requirements of the AEC and the FDA as well as his respective State Board of Health.

RADIOPHARMACEUTICAL DOSAGE FORMS

Choice of Radionuclide

The selection of the optimum radionuclide in a pharmaceutical depends on a number of parameters including detector response, radiation dose, chemical properties, physical half-life, and type of radiation emitted. One of the most important parameters is *detector response* to the radiation. Most nuclear medicine facilities use scintillation scanning equipment that is optimized for detecting gamma photons with energies of 100 to 200 keV. Gamma photons with energies less than 100 keV will not penetrate the detector completely to utilize the full efficiency of the detector. Photons with energies over 200 keV may pass through the detector without interacting. Thus, the detector to be utilized is an important consideration in determining which radionuclide is to be used in the radiopharmaceutical.

A second consideration in selecting a radionuclide for a pharmaceutical is the *radiation dose* produced from the radionuclide. For example, I-131 has five beta particles which contribute extensively to the absorbed radiation dose, whereas I-125 has no beta emission and only a single gamma photon of 55 keV. Thus, for scanning or measuring iodine uptake in the thyroid, I-125 is the radionuclide of choice. I-131 would be the radionuclide of choice, however, to give a large radiation dose to the thyroid gland as an antineoplastic.

The *chemical properties* of the radionuclide and the compound into which it is incorporated must also be considered. The chemical properties may be modified by incorporating the radionuclide into an organic compound. Labeled organic compounds may allow specific localization by the molecule. For example, chlormerodrin labeled with mercury-197 localizes in the cortex of the kidney. Specific localization may also result from the radionuclide's passing the blood

TABLE 13-2. WELL ESTABLISHED RADIOPHARMACEUTICALS

RADIONUCLIDE	CHEMICAL FORM	TRADE NAMES	USE	DOSE RANGE
137Cs	Encased in needles and/or applicator cells		Interstitial or intracavitary treatment of cancer	Variable
51Cr	Sodium Chromate	Rachromate (A)	Spleen scans Placental localization RBC labeling and survival studies	150–300 μCi (I.V.) 10 μCi (I.V.) 75–150 μCi (I.V.)
	Labeled Human Serum Albumin	Chromalbin (S)	G-I protein loss studies Placental localization	75–150 μCi (I.V.) 10 μCi (I.V.)
58Co	Cyanocobalamin	Racobalamin (A) Rubratope-58 (S)	Intestinal absorption studies	0.25–1.0 μCi (I.V.)
60Co	Encased in needles and/or applicator cells		Interstitial or intracavitary treatment of cancer	Variable
198Au	Seeds		Interstitial treatment of cancer	Variable
131I	Sodium Iodide	Radiocap (A) Iodotope (S)	Thyroid scans Hyperthyroidism and/or cardiac dysfunction	50–100 μCi (Os) 50–100 μCi to be retained per g. of gland (Os)
131I	Iodinated Human Serum Albumin	RISA (A) Albumotope (S)	Brain tumor Placenta localization Cardiac scan	300–500 μCi (I.V.) 3–20 μCi (I.V.) 300–400 μCi (I.V.)
131I or 125I	Sodium Rose Bengal	Robengatope (S)	Liver scans	50–300 μCi (I.V.)
131I or 125I	Labeled Triolein	Trioleotope (S) Raolein (A)	Fat absorption studies	5–100 μCi (Os)
131I	Cholografin		Cardiac scans	50–100 μCi (I.V.)
131I or 125I	Sodium Iothalamate	Glofil (A)	Renal function	50–100 μCi (I.V.)
131I or 125I	Macroaggregated Iodinated Human Serum Albumin	Macroscan (A) Albumotope-LS (S)	Lung scans	200–250 μCi (I.V.)
131I or 125I	Microaggregated Iodinated Human Serum Albumin (Colloidal)	Albumotope-H (S)	Liver scans	150–300 μCi (I.V.)
59Fe	Chloride Citrate or Sulfate	Ferrutope (S) (Citrate)	Iron turnover studies	1–10 μCi (I.V.)

(continued on page 432)

TABLE 13-2. (*Continued*)

Radionuclide	Chemical Form	Trade Names	Use	Dose Range
^{192}Ir	Seeds encased in nylon ribbon		Interstitial treatment of cancer	Variable
^{85}Kr	Gas		Diagnosis of cardiac abnormalities	5 mCi (Intra-arterial; carotid)
^{32}P	Colloidal Chromic Phosphate	Chromphosphotope (S) Phosphocal (M)	Interstitial or intracavitary treatment of cancer	6–40 mCi (i.s.)
^{42}K	Potassium Chloride		Potassium space studies	50–150 μCi
^{75}Se	Labeled Methionine	Sethotope (S)	Pancreas scans	250 μCi (I.V.)
^{85}Sr	Strontium Nitrate or Chloride	Strotope (NO$_3$) (S)	Bone scans	50–100 μCi
^{90}Sr	Medical Applicator		Treatment of superficial eye conditions	Variable
^{99m}Tc	Sodium Pertechnetate	Pertscan (A)	Brain scans	8–15 mCi (I.V.)
^{99m}Tc	Sodium Pertechnetate		Thyroid scans	1 mCi (I.V.)
^{99m}Tc	Labeled Human Serum Albumin		Placenta localization Blood pool scans	2 mCi (I.V.) 2–10 mCi (I.V.)
^{99m}Tc	Sulfur Colloid		Liver and spleen scans	1–3 mCi (I.V.)
^{133}Xe	Gas		Study of cardiac abnormalities, cerebral flow, pulmonary function, or muscle blood flow	5 mCi (Inhalation)
^{99m}Tc	Sodium Pertechnetate Generator	Technetope II (S) Pertgen-99m (A) Ultra-Technekow (M) Neimotec (M)	Brain scans	8–15 mCi (I.V.)

A, Abbott; S, Squibb; M, Mallinckrodt.

brain barrier, as does technetium-99m in localizing brain tumors.

Another consideration in selecting a radionuclide is its *physical half-life*. The half-life of a radiopharmaceutical is directly related to the radiation dose to the patient; thus, the pharmacist should use the shortest half-life material available, bearing in mind the other radionuclidic considerations. This presents problems when the delivery and dispensing of the radiopharmaceutical takes a long time. Technetium-99m has been found to be a nearly ideal radiopharmaceutical because of its chemical characteristics, its energy range, and its 6-hour half-life which allows utilization the same day of preparation. This short half-life, however, requires special handling of technetium-99m by the pharmacist (see below).

A final consideration in the choice of the radionuclide involves the selection of the proper *radiation decay mode*. Beta and alpha radiopharmaceuticals contribute little to the detector response after administration in the body. Alpha radiopharmaceuticals are rarely used in nuclear medicine and even beta radiopharmaceuticals have limited use because of their limited penetrating capabilities. However, beta emitting radionuclides are frequently used in studying the metabolic pathways of a drug in both animals and man. If the drug is labeled with carbon-14 or tritium, very low concentrations of the drug and its metabolites can be measured in the blood, tissues, and excreta of animals and humans with little danger of exposing them to excessive doses of radiation.

Generators

One of the most significant advances in radiopharmaceuticals is the use of generators for the production of short half-life radiopharmaceuticals. *Generators* (*"cows"*) are either ion exchange resins or alumina columns which contain a parent radionuclide. With time, the parent radionuclide decays to a daughter radionuclide that is not specifically adsorbed on the column. An example is technetium-99m, which is obtained from a generator constructed of molybdenum-99 adsorbed to an alumina column. Molybdenum-99 decays with a 66 hour half-life to technetium-99m, and the technetium-99m is eluted from the column with normal saline solution. The 66 hour half-life of molybdenum-99 provides sufficient manufacturing time for once weekly preparation. Elution of the generator on a daily basis, by the nuclear pharmacist, provides technetium-99m for the preparation of radiopharmaceuticals. Other generators in use today include tin-indium and strontium-yttrium.

Product Types

Radiopharmaceuticals may be divided into several specific types. *Inorganic radionuclides* have received the widest use because of their ease of production and availability from nuclear reactors. Examples of inorganic radionuclides used in medicine include technetium-99m, iodine-131, and phosphorus-32.

The newest area of radiopharmaceutical research is organic compounds containing labeled radionuclides. Examples of *organic radiopharmaceuticals* include iodine-131 labeled insulin, mercury-197 labeled chlormerodrin, carbon-11 labeled dopamine, and iodine-131 labeled rose bengal. In each moiety, the radionuclide is covalently bonded to the organic compound.

A third type of radiopharmaceutical consists of *analogues* of compounds well known for their specific tissue localization capability. For instance, the iodine-131 iodopropamide analogue of chloropropamide shows promise as a pancreas-specific radioscanning agent. Other radiopharmaceutical analogues include iodine-131 iodocholesterol for adrenal scanning and iodine-131 iodochloroquine for eye tumor scanning. The development of labeled analogues assumes that the molecular integrity and the specific localization capability of the drug will remain intact after labeling with a radionuclide.

A fourth category of radiopharmaceuticals consists of those in which the *physical state* of the molecule has been changed. This is accomplished through preparation of the radionuclide in the form of a solid with a specific particle size, such as microspheres or colloids. Radiopharmaceuticals having a colloidal size of 500 mμ to 1,000 mμ localize in the liver, and a widely used liver scanning agent using this principle is technetium sulfur colloid. Radioiodinated macroaggregated albumin has a size of 50 to 70 μ; thus, a lung scanning agent is produced, since this size colloid is trapped in the capillary beds of the lungs.

The last radiopharmaceutical category to be considered includes *sealed sources* such as cesium, radium, and cobalt. Sealed sources are used as inplants within the patient for the treatment of specific malignancies. The sources are removed from the patient after the calculated radiation dose has been absorbed by the tissue.

Kits

A complete quality control test of a radiopharmaceutical requires time in excess of the usable physical half-life of a radionuclide. To improve quality control, radiopharmaceutical kits are being utilized (see Table 13-3). Each in-vivo kit contains all the necessary components required to make a radiopharmaceutical except the radionuclide. All kit components undergo the same rigorous quality control as stable pharmaceuticals. The kit is available through regular pharmaceutical distribution channels and has a shelf-life of 6 months to one year. The pharmacist compounds the radiopharmaceutical, using the kit in combination with the radionuclide.

The most widely used kit is *technetium sulfur colloid*. This kit consists of a reaction vial and two prefilled syringes. The pharmacist adds the radionuclide and the contents of the first syringe (hydrochloric acid) to the reaction vial containing sodium thiosulfate. The acid reduces the solution pH, causing the technetium to react with the sodium thiosulfate. The solution is then heated to form the colloid product, and the second syringe containing buffer is injected into the reaction vial to reconstitute the radiopharmaceutical in a physiologically compatible solution. Since technetium sulfur colloid is administered I.V., aseptic preparation of the radiopharmaceutical is required.

Another radiopharmaceutical kit in common use is the in-vitro *radioimmunoassay kit*. Radioimmunoassay is an analytical technique used for measuring nanogram (10^{-9} g) quantities of enzymes and hormones. Since the amount of radioactivity in each test is

TABLE 13-3.   RADIOPHARMACEUTICAL KITS

KIT	TRADE NAME	USE	DOSE RANGE
Protein Bound Iodide Conversion Ratio Kit	Ioresin (A)	Used with I-131 to determine thyroid function	25–100 μCi (I.V. or Os)
^{59}Fe Sponge-Resin Kit	Irosorb (A)	Measurement of iron binding capacity of serum	In Vitro
Preparation Kit for ^{99m}Tc$_2$S$_7$ for injection	Collokit (A) Tesuloid (S) Technecoll (M)	Used with ^{99m}TcO$_4$ to produce sulfur colloid for liver scans	1–3 mCi (I.V.)
^{131}I or ^{125}I T-4 Kit	Tetrasorb (A) Res-o-Mat T-3 (M) Tetralute (Am)	Used to measure total serum thyroxine	In Vitro
^{131}I or ^{125}I T-3 Kit	Res-o-Mat T-4 (M) Triosorb (A) Tresitope (S) Trilute (Am) Thyopac (Am/S)	Used to measure L-Triiodothyronine	In Vitro
Diethylenetriamine Pentacetic Acid Kit	Renotec (S)	Used with ^{99m}TcO$_4$ to produce labeled chelate for kidney scans	2–5 mCi (I.V.)
Ferrous Ascorbate Complex	Labelaid (D)	Labeled with ^{99m}TcO$_4$ for kidney scans	2–5 mCi (I.V.)
Digoxin, Renin, HGH Insulin, Digitoxin, Gastrin, Angiotensin, B-12, Cyclic Amp		Radioimmunoassay	In Vitro
Human Growth Hormone	HGH-125 Imusay (A)	HGH radioimmunoassay	In Vitro

A, Abbott; S, Squibb; M, Mallinckrodt; D, Duphar; Am, Ames; Am/S, Amersham/Searle.

small, the radioactivity is generally exempt from licensure. Longer half-life radionuclides, such as iodine-125 or tritium, are often used so that the kits may be prepared commercially. The assay depends on the fact that a known amount of labeled hormone or enzyme, when mixed with a hormone or enzyme in a test sample, will compete for available sites on the corresponding antibody or selected adsorbent. The amount of radioactivity remaining on the antibody or selected adsorbent is inversely proportional to the amount of hormone or enzyme contained in the test sample. Radioimmunoassay kits are available for quantitating triiodothyronine (T-3), thyroxine (T-4), renin, human growth hormone (HGH), insulin, parathyroid hormone, adrenocorticotropic hormone (ACTH), chorionic gonadotropin, follicle stimulating hormone (FSH), and digoxin.

OFFICIAL RADIOPHARMACEUTICALS

The official radiopharmaceuticals are listed in Table 13-4.

Unless otherwise stated, radiopharmaceuticals must contain not less than 90.0 percent or more than 110.0 percent of the labeled quantity (radionuclidic purity) expressed in microcuries (μCi) or millicuries (mCi) at the time indicated on the label. Radiochemical impurities cannot exceed 5 percent of the total radioactivity.

Upon standing, the radiopharmaceutical as well as the container may darken from radiation effects. Thus, all radiopharmaceuticals possess an expiration date. Since radiation contributes to product decomposition, the greater the specific activity of the product the greater the rate of decomposition. With all radiopharmaceuticals, radioactive decay must be taken into account in making absorbed dose calculations.

Each of the products must meet applicable official requirements, such as those required for biologicals, injections, and solutions and for sterility, nonpyrogenicity, etc. Radiopharmaceuticals are exempt from official recommendations in regard to the volume in the container.

The First Supplement to N.F. XIII notes the need for release of some radiopharma-ceutical products prior to sterility testing. In such cases the manufacturer must have evidence that sterility is maintained throughout the manufacturing process, and he must complete a sterility test ipso facto as additional evidence of the adequacy of the methods of manufacture and sterilization.

New admissions to U.S.P. XVIII include Iodinated I 125 Serum Albumin, Chlormerodrin Hg 197 (and 203) Injection, Gold Au 198 Injection, and Sodium Iodide I 125 Solution. Cyanocobalamin Co 60 Capsules (and Solution) were included in U.S.P. XVII but were not admitted to U.S.P. XVIII. Cyanocobalamin Co 60 Capsules (and Solution) are official in N.F. XIII.

Iodinated I 125 Serum Albumin, U.S.P. XVIII

Iodinated I 125 Serum Albumin is a sterile, buffered, isotonic solution containing at least 10 mg. of radio-iodinated normal human serum albumin per ml. and providing not more than 1 mCi per ml. The solution is prepared by incorporating one gram-atom of iodine (as ^{125}I) for each gram-molecule (60,000 g.) of albumin. Radionuclidic purity is not less than 95.0 percent nor more than 105.0 percent and radiochemical impurity is not to exceed 3 percent of the total radioactivity at the time of labeling. The expiration date is not later than 120 days after completion of iodination.

The solution is clear and colorless to slightly yellow when freshly prepared. Bacteriostatic activity is normally provided by 0.9 percent benzyl alcohol. Both single-dose and multiple-dose containers are available. The product should be kept cool (2° to 8°) and protected from freezing.

Radioiodinated serum albumins are used for the determination of blood volumes and plasma volumes by quantitating the dilution of the administered radiopharmaceutical. Labeled albumins are also used for measuring cardiac output and localizing brain tumors.

Iodinated I 131 Serum Albumin, U.S.P. XVIII

Iodinated I 131 Serum Albumin is similar to Iodinated I 125 Serum Albumin in regard to standards, tolerances, and method of pro-

TABLE 13-4. OFFICIAL RADIOPHARMACEUTICALS

RADIONUCLIDE	CHEMICAL FORM	OFFICIAL IN	TRADE NAMES	USE	DOSE RANGE
^{51}Cr	Sodium Chromate Cr 51 Injection	*U.S.P.*	Rachromate (A) Chromitope (S)	Blood volume determination	10–200 μCi (I.V.)
^{57}Co	Cyanocobalamin Co 57 Capsules	*U.S.P.*	Racobalamin (A) Rubratope-57 (S)	Pernicious anemia determination	0.5–1.0 μCi (Os)
^{57}Co	Cyanocobalamin Co 57 Solution	*U.S.P.*	Racobalamin (A) Rubratope-57 (S)	Pernicious anemia determination	0.5–1.0 μCi (Os)
^{60}Co	Cyanocobalamin Co 60 Capsules	*N.F.*	Racobalamin (A) Rubratope-60 (S)	Pernicious anemia determination	0.5–1.0 μCi (Os)
^{60}Co	Cyanocobalamin Co 60 Solution	*N.F.*	Racobalamin (A) Rubratope-60 (S)	Pernicious anemia determination	0.5–1.0 μCi (Os)
^{198}Au	Gold Au 198 Injection (Colloid)	*U.S.P.*	Aurcoloid (A) Auretope (S)	Antineoplastic	35–150 mCi (i.c.)
^{198}Au	Gold Au 198 Injection (Colloid)	*U.S.P.*	Aureoscan (A) Auretope Diagnostic (S)	Liver scan	1–5 μCi (I.V.)
^{125}I	Iodinated I 125 Serum Albumin (Human)	*U.S.P.*	RISA (A) Volemetron (Am)	Blood volume and cardiac output determinations	5–60 μCi (I.V.)
^{131}I	Iodinated I 131 Serum Albumin (Human)	*U.S.P.*	RISA (A)	Blood volume and cardiac output determinations	5–60 μCi (I.V.)
^{131}I	Sodium Iodohippurate I 131 Injection	*U.S.P.*	Hippuran I 131 (A, M) Hipputope (S)	Renal function determination	2–35 μCi (I.V.)
^{125}I	Sodium Iodide I 125 Solution	*U.S.P.*	Iodotope (S)	Thyroid function determination	50–100 μCi (Os)
^{131}I	Sodium Iodide I 131 Capsules	*U.S.P.*	Radiocaps (A) Iodotope (S)	Thyroid function determination	1–100 μCi (I.V. or Os)
^{131}I	Sodium Iodide I 131 Capsules	*U.S.P.*	Theriodide (A) Iodotope (S)	Antineoplastic	1–200 mCi (I.V. or Os)
^{131}I	Sodium Iodide I 131 Solution	*U.S.P.*	Tracervial (A) Iodotope (S)	Thyroid function determination	1–100 μCi (I.V. or Os)
^{131}I	Sodium Iodide I 131 Solution	*U.S.P.*	Oriodide (A) Iodotope (S)	Antineoplastic	1–200 mCi (I.V. or Os)

TABLE 13-4. (*Continued*)

RADIONUCLIDE	CHEMICAL FORM	OFFICIAL IN	TRADE NAMES	USE	DOSE RANGE
131I	Sodium Rose Bengal I 131 Injection	U.S.P.	Robengatope (S)	Hepatic function determination	10–200 μCi (I.V.)
197Hg	Chlormerodrin Hg 197 Injection	U.S.P.	Neohydrin (A)	Kidney and brain scans	10 μCi/Kg (I.V.)
203Hg	Chlormerodrin Hg 203 Injection	U.S.P.	Neohydrin (A)	Kidney and brain scans	10 μCi/Kg (I.V.)
32P	Sodium Phosphate P 32 Solution	U.S.P.	Phosphotope (S)	Tumor localization	250 μCi–1 mCi (I.V. or Os)
32P	Sodium Phosphate P 32 Solution	U.S.P.	Phosphotope (S).	Antineoplastic Antipolycythemic	1–12 mCi (I.V. or Os)

A, Abbott; Am, Ames; M, Mallinckrodt; S, Squibb.

[437]

duction, except that the ^{131}I radionuclide is used for iodination rather than ^{125}I. The change in radionuclides changes the physical decay route and rate, thus changing radiation dosimetry, stability, and safe handling procedure.

Since ^{131}I gives off 5 betas and 9 gammas during decay and ^{125}I decays by electron capture and a single gamma, ^{131}I delivers a much larger radiation dose to the patient than does ^{125}I. The energies of the emitted gammas also indicate ^{125}I to be the safest of the two isotopes to handle. Because ^{131}I has a shorter physical half-life than ^{125}I, the expiration date for Iodinated I 131 Serum Albumin is not later than 30 days after the date of completion of iodination.

Chlormerodrin Hg 197 Injection, U.S.P. XVIII

Chlormerodrin Hg 197 Injection is a sterile solution of [3-(chloromercuri)-2-methoxypropyl]urea in which a portion of the molecules contain the ^{197}Hg radionuclide in the structure.

$$NH_2\!-\!\overset{\overset{\displaystyle O}{\|}}{C}\!-\!NH\!-\!CH_2\!-\!\underset{\underset{\displaystyle O\!-\!CH_3}{|}}{CH}\!-\!CH_2\!-\!HgCl;$$

$$C_5H_{11}Cl^{197}HgN_2O_2; \text{ MW, } 367.20$$

The solution is clear and colorless. It is available in single and multiple-dose containers. The expiration date is not later than 8 days after date of standardization.

Because chlormerodrin localizes in the renal cortex, it is used as a renal scanning agent. Chlormerodrin is also used as a tumor localization agent because it concentrates in brain tumors.

An I.V. dose of 150 μCi chlormerodrin delivers a radiation dose of 1 to 2 rads to the kidney and about 10 millirads to the total body.

Chlormerodrin Hg 203 Injection, U.S.P. XVIII

Hg 203 Injection Chlormerodrin is similar to Chlormerodrin Hg 197 Injection in regard to standards, tolerances, and method of production, except that the radionuclide ^{203}Hg is utilized in this product's preparation. The

change in radionuclide changes the physical decay route and rate, thus changing radiation dosimetry and stability. The expiration date is not later than 45 days after the date of standardization.

Mercury-203 decays with the emission of a single beta particle and a single gamma photon, whereas mercury-197 decays by 2 electron captures and with the emission of 3 gamma photons. Chlormerodrin Hg 203 delivers about ten times the radiation dose of Chlormerodrin Hg 197 to the kidneys.

Cysteine may be used as an adjunct with chlormerodrin, because cysteine inhibits binding of chlormerodrin more to other tissues than to renal tissue and thus increases renal radioisotope concentration. This reduces the dose required to produce a good scan and ultimately reduces the radiation dose.

Cyanocobalamin Co 57 Capsules, U.S.P. XVIII

Cyanocobalamin Co 57 Capsules contain cyanocobalamin in which a portion of the molecules contain cobalt-57 in the molecular structure. The capsules may contain a small amount of solids or may appear empty. The specific activity is not less than 0.5 μCi/mcg. of cyanocobalamin.

The capsules are orally administered in doses of 0.5 to 1.0 μCi as part of the Schilling test for pernicious anemia. In this test, the patient is fasted for 24 hours, after which 1 μCi of cyanocobalamin Co 57 and a 1,000-mcg. dose of vitamin B-12 are administered. Urine is collected for 24 hours and tested for radioactivity; in normal patients about 10 to 40 percent of the radioactivity is excreted. If percent excretion is low, the study is repeated and a capsule of intrinsic factor also is given orally. If the 24-hour urine excretion becomes normal, the patient has pernicious anemia.

The capsules should be kept in well-closed, light resistant containers. The expiration date is not later than 6 months after the date of standardization.

Cyanocobalamin Co 57 Solution, U.S.P. XVIII

Cyanocobalamin Co 57 Solution has the same requirements, usage and expiration date as Cyanocobalamin Co 57 Capsules. The solution generally contains a bacteriostatic agent and is clear and colorless to pink. It comes in single and multiple-dose containers.

Cyanocobalamin Co 60 Capsules, N.F. XIII

Cyanocobalamin Co 60 Capsules are similar to Cyanocobalamin Co 57 Capsules in regard to requirements, except that the ^{60}Co radionuclide is used during the microbial synthesis rather than ^{57}Co. The change in radionuclides changes the physical decay route and rate, thus changing the radiation dosimetry of the product. The administered dose (0.5 to 1.0 μCi) remains the same regardless of the radionuclide.

Cyanocobalamin labeled with ^{57}Co is the pharmaceutical of choice, owing to an increased counting efficiency and decreased radiation dose when compared with cyanocobalamin labeled with ^{60}Co.

Cyanocobalamin Co 60 Solution, N.F. XIII

Cyanocobalamin Co 60 Solution is similar to Cyanocobalamin Co 57 Solution in regard to requirements, except that the ^{60}Co radionuclide is used during the microbial synthesis rather than ^{57}Co. The parameters affected by the change in radionuclide are the same as with Cyanocobalamin Co 60 Capsules.

Sodium Chromate Cr 51 Injection, U.S.P. XVIII

Sodium Chromate Cr 51 Injection is a sterile, clear to slightly yellow solution containing a bacteriostatic agent. For certain uses, the solution may be made isotonic by adding sodium chloride.

The specific activity of the pharmaceutical is not less than 10 mCi per mg. of sodium chromate at the end of the expiration period. The expiration date is not later than 3 months after the standardization date. Radiochemical impurities must not exceed 10.0 percent of the total radioactivity. The pH must be between 7.5 and 8.5 to maintain the hexavalent chromium ion necessary for labeling red blood cells. The product is available in single and multiple-dose containers.

Sodium Chromate Cr 51 Injection is ad-ministered in a dose of μCi (range of 10 to 200 μCi) for the determination of blood volume. Red blood cells are often tagged with sodium radiochromate in vitro and the labeled red blood cells readministered to the patient. Ascorbic acid may be added to the ^{51}Cr erythrocyte solution to prevent further erythrocyte labeling in vivo when the solution is injected. The ascorbic acid reduces the hexavalent chromium to the trivalent form.

Sodium Iodide I 125 Solution, U.S.P. XVIII

Sodium Iodide I 125 Solution is an essentially carrier-free sodium iodide solution containing radioactive iodine and is suitable for oral or intravenous administration. Radionuclidic purity is not less than 85.0 percent nor more than 115.0 percent at the time of labeling. The expiration date is not later than 6 months after date of standardization.

The product is a clear, colorless solution having a pH between 7.5 and 9.0. It is packaged in single and multiple-dose containers that have been pretreated with a solution containing 0.8 percent NaHSO$_3$ and 0.25 percent NaI followed by water rinsings until the last rinsing is neutral to litmus.

Sodium Iodide I 125 Solution is used as a diagnostic aid (thyroid function and thyroid scanning) and for preparing Radioiodinated I 125 Serum Albumin.

Sodium Iodide I 131 Capsules, U.S.P. XVIII

Sodium Iodide I 131 Capsules contain essentially carrier-free radioactive iodine. The capsules are formulated by evaporating a solution of radioactive sodium iodide I 131 on the interior wall of a gelatin capsule or by pipetting the radioactive solution onto a small absorbent pellet within the capsule. In either case, the capsule is sealed to prevent leakage and consequent radioactive contamination of the product and the environment. Capsules provide a relatively safe and convenient method of dispensing radioactive iodine. The capsules may contain a small amount of solids or may appear to be empty.

The expiration date is not later than 1 month after date of standardization.

Sodium Iodide I 131 is the most widely

used radiopharmaceutical in the world. This is due to the simplicity and reliability of in-vivo thyroid tests and the ease of production of ^{131}I from uranium fission or neutron bombardment of tellurium. The thyroid gland uses radioiodine for catabolism of hormones in the same way that it uses stable iodine. Thus, administration of 5 to 10 μCi of radioiodine and its subsequent measurement in the thyroid gland (from 4 to 48 hours) can be used to measure percent thyroid uptake and aid in the diagnosis of hyperthyroidism or hypothyroidism. A large number of drugs interact with the thyroid gland or the body's iodide ion pool; therefore, the patient's drug profile is essential prior to utilization of radioiodine.

Sodium Iodide I 131 is also used for scanning the thyroid gland because the thyroid rapidly concentrates the radioiodine for a sufficient period of time to allow a scan of the gland. The administered dose is 50 to 100 μCi, and this results in a radiation dose of 50 to 150 rads to the thyroid gland and 20 to 50 rads to the whole body. The thyroid scan is used to evaluate nodule localization and iodine uptake within a nodule. Nodules that do not take up radioiodine (cold nodules) are frequently cancerous and may be surgically removed. Nodules that take up radioiodine (hot nodules) more than adjacent thyroid tissue uptake are usually benign.

Sodium Iodide I 131 is also used therapeutically in millicurie doses for the treatment of thyrotoxicosis and as an antineoplastic.

Sodium Iodide I 131 Solution, U.S.P. XVIII

Sodium Iodide I 131 Solution is a solution containing radioactive sodium iodide (^{131}I) suitable for oral or intravenous administration. The solution is essentially carrier-free and contains only minute amounts of naturally occurring iodine-127.

Sodium Iodide I 131 Solution is a clear, colorless solution having a pH between 7.5 and 9.0. The product is packaged in single and multiple-dose containers that have been pretreated to prevent adsorption (see Sodium Iodide I 125 Solution). On standing, both the solution and the glass container may darken as the result of the effects of the radiation. This product has the same uses and doses as indicated under Sodium Iodide I 131 Capsules. The expiration date is not later than 1 month after date of standardization.

The ^{131}I solution provides a convenient method of obtaining exact doses for patient administration, but it requires additional dose quantitation by the pharmacist. This increases product handling and the probability of contamination and radiation exposure.

Sodium Iodohippurate I 131 Injection, U.S.P. XVIII

Sodium Iodohippurate I 131 Injection is a clear, colorless, sterile solution of sodium o-iodohippurate-^{131}I in which a portion of the molecules contain the ^{131}I radionuclide in the molecular structure.

$$C_9H_7{}^{131}INNaO_3 , \ MW = 331.05$$

The solution is available in single and multiple-dose containers. The expiration date is not later than 1 month after date of standardization. Radiochemical impurities may not exceed 3 percent of the total radioactivity.

Sodium Iodohippurate I 131 is administered intravenously to determine kidney function. Renograms are readily obtained because the product is excreted mainly (90%) by tubular secretion. The administered dose of 15 to 20 μCi produces a radiation dose of 20 mrads to the kidney and about 0.6 mrads to the whole body.

Sodium Phosphate P 32 Solution, U.S.P. XVIII

Sodium Phosphate P 32 Solution is a sterile, buffered, isotonic clear, colorless solution suitable for oral or intravenous administration. Carrier sodium phosphate is generally added during processing to minimize the loss of radioactive phosphate by adsorption on the glass container.

Radioactive phosphorus solution is the only official radiopharmaceutical that is a pure beta particle emitter. Radionuclidic purity is determined by calculating the absorption of the beta particles by increasing thicknesses of aluminum absorbers or by liquid scintillation spectrometry.[6] The official product is free of radiochemical impurities. Unlike gamma-emitting radiopharmaceuticals, phosphorus-32 should be shielded with materials with low atomic numbers to prevent production of bremsstrahlung ("collision radiation").

Radioactive phosphorus solution is available in single and multiple-dose containers. The expiration date is not later than 2 months from date of standardization.

Sodium radiophosphate is used most frequently for treatment of polycythemia vera. Treatment consists of 3 to 5 mCi of $Na_2H^{32}PO_3$. A repeat dose may be indicated after 3 months. Normally, no more than two treatments are necessary, with remissions in 85 percent of cases lasting over 2 years.

Sodium Phosphate P 32 Solution has been used occasionally for diagnosis of brain lesions, because all growing cells need phosphorus. However, $Na^{99m}TcO_4$ is now the radiopharmaceutical of choice for brain tumors. Sodium Phosphate P 32 Solution is also used in chronic myelocytic leukemia in a dose of 1 to 2 mCi per week over a 4- to 8-week period.

Sodium Rose Bengal I 131 Injection, U.S.P. XVIII

Sodium Rose Bengal I 131 Injection is a sterile, buffered solution of 4,5,6,7-tetrachloro-2′,4′,5′,7′-tetraiodofluorescein disodium salt-^{131}I in which a portion of the molecules contain radioactive iodine (^{131}I) in the molecular structure. Radiochemical impurities may not exceed 10 percent of the total radioactivity.

$C_{20}H_2Cl_4{}^{131}I_4Na_2O_5$ MW = 1,033.65

Sodium Rose Bengal I 131 Injection is a clear, deep red, sterile solution available in single dose and multiple dose containers, intended for intravenous administration. The expiration date is not later than 1 month from date of standardization.

Rose bengal is removed from the blood rapidly by the polygonal cells of the liver and is excreted with the bile into the gastrointestinal tract. The administration of 150 μCi of Sodium Rose Bengal I 131 Injection thus provides a scan of the liver within 10 to 15 minutes after administration. Lugol's solution is generally administered prior to rose bengal (^{131}I) to reduce the radiation dose to the thyroid. With prior administration of Lugol's solution, the radiation dose to the liver is 0.2 to 0.7 rads and about 0.22 rads to the whole body.

PHYSICAL NUCLEAR PHARMACY

Physical and Mathematical Fundamentals

In addition to the mode of radioactive decay of radiopharmaceuticals, an understanding of radiation mathematics is essential to radiopharmaceutical dosimetry. Radioactive decay is described by *first-order kinetics,* i.e., the quantity of decay (decomposition) occurring is proportional to the remaining quantity of product at any time. The constant of proportionality (disintegration constant) is indicated by lambda (λ). Radioactive decay is a fixed parameter for each radionuclide and there are no known physical or chemical agents that influence the decay rate.

The *disintegration constant* is that fraction of the remaining radioactive atoms that will decay in some unit time. The units of time can vary, e.g., $\sec^{-1}$, $\min^{-1}$, hr^{-1}. Thus, the rate of change is a function of the remaining radioactive atoms times the disintegration constant as shown in Equation 1.

$$-\frac{dN}{dt} = -\lambda N \qquad \text{Eq. 1}$$

Where N is the number of atoms remaining,
t is the time elapsed, and
"—" indicates that the number of atoms is decreasing with time.

The basic decay law can be derived by rearranging and integrating Equation 1 as follows:

TABLE 13-5.   MISCELLANEOUS RADIOPHARMACEUTICALS

RADIONUCLIDE	CHEMICAL FORM	TRADE NAME	USE	DOSE RANGE
^{131}Cs	Cesium Chloride	Cescan (A)	Myocardial scanning	1–2 mCi (I.V.)
^{64}Cu	Cupric Acetate		Copper metabolism studies, diagnosis of Wilson's disease	100 μCi–1 mCi (I.V. or Os)
^{131}I or ^{125}I	Sodium Iothalamate	Glofil (A)	Measurement of glomerular filtration rate	50–100 μCi (I.V.)
^{131}I	Insulin		Insulin studies	25–200 μCi (I.V.)
^{22}Na	Sodium Chloride		Measurement of sodium space and exchangeable sodium	10–25 μCi (I.V.)
^{131}I	Ethiodized Oil	Ethiodol (A)	Lymph node carcinoma	10–25 mCi (intralymphatic into the foot)
^{113m}In	Indium Chloride		Blood volume, placental localization	1–4 mCi
^{18}F	Sodium Fluoride		Bone scans	1–2 mCi (I.V.)

A, Abbott.

$$-\frac{dN}{N} = -\lambda dt \qquad \text{Eq. 2}$$

$$\int_{N_0}^{N_t} \frac{dN}{N} = -\lambda \int_0^t dt \qquad \text{Eq. 3}$$

or

$$\ln N_t - \ln N_0 = -\lambda t \qquad \text{Eq. 4}$$

where

$$\ln = \text{natural logarithm.}$$

Changing to the base e,

$$\frac{N_t}{N_0} = e^{-\lambda t} \qquad \text{Eq. 5}$$

or

$$N_t = N_0 e^{-\lambda t} \qquad \text{Eq. 6}$$

Equation 6 states that the number of atoms (N_t) remaining after time (t) is equal to the number of atoms originally present (N_0) multiplied by $e^{-\lambda t}$ where lambda (λ) is the disintegration constant.

The pharmacist generally works with activity (A) in μCi or mCi rather than the number of atoms in a sample. The activity of a sample is the product of the number of atoms in the sample multiplied by the disintegration constant.

$$\lambda N = A \qquad \text{Eq. 7}$$

Therefore, by substituting A into Equation 6, the equation becomes

$$A_t = A_0 e^{-\lambda t} \qquad \text{Eq. 8}$$

Equation 8 describes the basic decay law in terms of activity.

The basic decay law can also be described using common, base 10 logarithms (log). Natural logarithms (ln) can be converted to base 10 logarithms (log) by dividing the natural logarithm by 2.303. Therefore Equation 4 can be rewritten as

$$\log N_t - \log N_0 = \frac{-\lambda t}{2.303} \qquad \text{Eq. 9}$$

The reciprocal of 2.303 may be used to simplify the mathematics.

$$\log N_t - \log N_0 = 0.434 \, (-\lambda t) \quad \text{Eq. 10}$$

Rearranging equation 10 gives

$$\log N_t = \log N_0 + 0.434 \, (-\lambda t) \quad \text{Eq. 11}$$

or

$$\log N_t = \log N_0 - 0.434\lambda t \qquad \text{Eq. 12}$$

When the radioactive decay of a radionuclide is plotted on semilogarithmic paper (activity on ordinate and time on abscissa), a straight line results when sufficient radioactivity is present. This is illustrated in Figure 13-1. The reason for the straight line in Figure 13-1 is evident from a rearrangement of equation 9 to

FIGURE 13-1

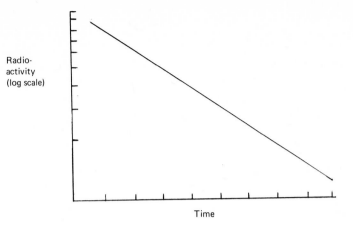

Radio-
activity
(log scale)

Time

$$\log N_t = \log N_o - \left(\frac{\lambda}{2.303}\right)t \qquad \text{Eq. 13}$$

Where in the straight line equation $Y = a + bX$

$Y = \log N_t$,

$a = \log N_o = Y$ intercept,

$b = -\dfrac{\lambda}{2.303} = $ slope,

and $x = t = $ time.

Radioactive decay is also described by the term *physical half-life* $(t_{1/2}$ or $t_p)$. *Physical half-life* is the length of time required for one half of the original number of atoms (N_o) or the original amount of radioactivity (A_o) to decay or disintegrate. Half-life can be related to the disintegration constant by defining the ratio of N_t/N_o or A_t/A_o as 0.5 when $t = t_{1/2}$. Then, using natural logarithms,

$$\frac{N_t}{N_o} = \frac{A_t}{A_o} = 0.5 = e^{-\lambda t_{1/2}} \qquad \text{Eq. 14}$$

or

$$\ln 0.5 = -\lambda t_{1/2} \qquad \text{Eq. 15}$$

Since the natural logarithm of 0.5 is —0.693, then

$$0.693 = \lambda t_{1/2} \qquad \text{Eq. 16}$$

or

$$\frac{0.693}{\lambda} = t_{1/2} \qquad \text{Eq. 17}$$

or

$$\frac{0.693}{t_{1/2}} = \lambda \qquad \text{Eq. 18}$$

The amount of radioactivity associated with a product after any elapsed time can be calculated using the aforementioned equations or can be determined graphically as illustrated in Figures 13-1, 13-2 and 13-3. When the amount of remaining radioactivity of a specific radionuclide is plotted against time on linear paper, as in Figure 13-2, an asymptotic exponential curve results. The same decay curve can be plotted on semilogarithmic paper as shown previously in Figure 13-1. The amount of remaining radioactivity can be obtained from either plot by drawing a perpendicular from the amount of time elapsed on the abscissa to the curve, and then from the point of intersection on the curve to the ordinate. The point of intersection with the ordinate indicates the remaining radioactivity. This is more conveniently done using semilogarithmic plots such as that shown in Figure 13-1, since straight line plots are easier to construct.

An even more simplified curve can be obtained by using percent radioactivity as the ordinate and time, in units of physical half-life, on the abscissa as shown in Figure 13-3. Such curves are often supplied by radiopharmaceutical manufacturers. By determining the number of elapsed half-lives since the radiopharmaceutical was assayed, and using the same procedure as in Figure 13-1, the intercept at the ordinate will indi-

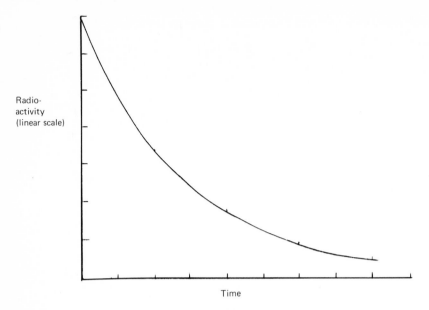

FIGURE 13-2

Radio-
activity
(linear scale)

Time

cate the percent remaining radioactivity at the elapsed time.

Two widely used "rules of thumb" are (1) after seven half-lives of a radionuclide, approximately 1 percent of the radioactivity remains and (2) after 10 half-lives, approximately 0.1% remains. This is indicated by the following:

Half Life	Percent Remaining Radioactivity
$1 = (1/2)^1$	50
$2 = (1/2)^2$	25.0
$3 = (1/2)^3$	12.5
$4 = (1/2)^4$	6.25
$5 = (1/2)^5$	3.12
$6 = (1/2)^6$	1.56
$7 = (1/2)^7$	0.78
$8 = (1/2)^8$	0.39
$9 = (1/2)^9$	0.20
$10 = (1/2)^{10}$	0.1

There are other mathematical manipulations available to the pharmacist for simplifying the calculations in regard to the amount of remaining radioactivity. Equation 18 may be substituted into equation 8 replacing λ, thus giving

$$A_t = A_o e^{-\left(\frac{0.693}{t_{1/2}}\right)t} \qquad \text{Eq. 19}$$

knowing that

$$e^{0.693} = 2 \qquad \text{Eq. 20}$$

then

$$A_t = A_o 2^{-t/t_{1/2}} \qquad \text{Eq. 21}$$

Rearranging equation 21 provides the useful equation

$$A_t = \frac{A_o}{2^{t/t_{1/2}}} \qquad \text{Eq. 22}$$

or

$$A_t = \frac{A_o}{\text{antilog}\,(0.3)\,(t/t_{1/2})} \qquad \text{Eq. 23}$$

An example of the usefulness of this equation can be given by answering the question, how much ^{131}I is left after 12 days starting with 5 mCi?

$$A_t = \frac{5}{\text{antilog}\,(0.3)\left(\dfrac{12}{8}\right)} = \frac{5}{\text{antilog}\,0.45} =$$

$$\frac{5}{2.83} = 1.75 \text{ mCi}$$

The answer may be verified by using equation 19:

$$A_t = A_o e^{-\left(\frac{0.693}{t_{1/2}}\right)t} = 5e^{-0.693\frac{12}{8}} = 5e^{-1.05}$$

$$A_t = 5(0.35) = 1.75 \text{ mCi}$$

Because of the many mathematical mistakes that occur in the handling of logarithms, the pharmacist should always try to appraise the amount of remaining radio-

FIGURE 13-3

% Radio-activity remaining (log scale)

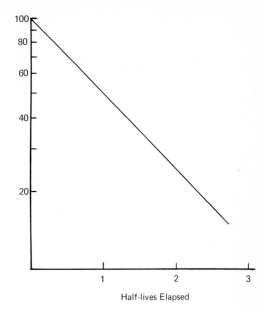

Half-lives Elapsed

activity of a sample by the "rules of thumb" method first and then calculate the specific quantity of remaining radioactivity. The calculation of the dose by more than one of the pathways mentioned assures the patient of the proper quantity of radioactive material. Decay calculations are simplified if elapsed time is expressed in terms of whole numbers of half-lives. For example, after 16.1 days, how many mCi of ^{131}I remain of an original shipment of 10 mCi? Iodine has a physical half-life of 8.05 days, thus two half-lives have passed. Since one half-life reduces the radioactivity to 50 percent, two half-lives must reduce the radioactivity to 25 percent or 2.5 mCi. The approximation can be checked with a variety of the previous equations.

1. $\log A_t = \log A_o - \dfrac{\lambda}{2.303} t$ Eq. 24

(This is equation 13 converted to activity).

$\log A_t = \log 10 - \dfrac{0.693/8}{2.303} 16 = 1.0 - 0.6$

$\log A_t = 0.4$

$A_t = \text{antilog } 0.4 = 2.5 \text{ mCi}$

2. $A_t = A_o 2^{-t/t_{1/2}}$ (Eq. 21)

$A_t = (10)(2^{-16/8}) = (10)(2^{-2})$

$A_t = \dfrac{10}{2^2} = \dfrac{10}{4} = 2.5 \text{ mCi}$

3. $\text{Log } A_t = \log A_o - 0.3 t/t_{1/2}$ Eq. 25

$\text{Log } A_t = \log 10 - 0.3(16/8)$

$\text{Log } A_t = 1 - 0.6 = 0.4$

$A_t = \text{antilog } 0.4 = 2.5 \text{ mCi}$

Example: On Friday noon an order is placed for sodium-22 to contain 2 mCi of radioactivity at noon the following Monday. Since sodium-22 has a 15-hour physical half-life, how much sodium-22 should be ordered on Friday at noon? (Fortunately for some, radiopharmaceutical manufacturers do this calculation.)

1. First estimate the approximate answer. Noon Friday to noon Monday is 3 days or 72 hours, which is greater than four half-lives, but less than five half-lives. Since four half-lives equals 2^4 and five half-lives equals 2^5, the answer should be $> (2)(2^4) = > 32$ but $< (2)(2^5) = < 64$ mCi.

2. Next, use the basic equations:

$A_t = A_o e^{-\lambda t}$

or

$\log 2 \text{ mCi} = \log A_o - 0.3 t/t_{1/2}$

$0.3 = \log A_o - 0.3 (72/15)$

$0.3 = \log A_o - 1.42$

$\log A_o = 1.72$

$A_o = \text{antilog } 1.72 = 5.25 \times 10^1 \text{ or } 52.5 \text{ mCi}$

3. Check your answer.

$$A_t = \frac{A_o}{\text{antilog} (0.3)(t/t_{1/2})}$$

$$A_o = [2 \text{ mCi}][\text{antilog} (0.3)\left(\frac{72}{15}\right)]$$

$$A_o = 2(\text{antilog of } 1.42) = 2(26.25) = 52.5 \text{ mCi.}$$

Methods of Radiation Detection

Ion pairs produced by radiation are the basis of all detector systems. Detectors may be classified according to their function: direct measurement of ions, measurement of the fluorescence induced by the ions, or measurement of chemical products produced by the ion pairs.

Detectors that use *gas ionization* as their basis of detection include Geiger-Müller (GM) counters, proportional counters, and ionization chambers. The detectors differ in the physical size of the detector, the type of gas used as interacting medium, and the amount of applied voltage across the detector.

Each of the detectors contains a central anode, an outer wall serving as a cathode, and a gaseous interphase. As voltage is applied across the anode and cathode, the electrons produced from the formation of ion pairs by the radiation are attracted to the anode, and the resulting electrical current is measured. Detectors using this principle are called *ionization chamber detectors.*

As the voltage applied across the electrodes of a detector is increased, the electrons will not only be attracted to the anode but will also be accelerated. The electrons, in their haste toward the anode, undergo additional collisions with the molecules of the gaseous interphase, producing additional ion pairs. The new secondary electrons are also accelerated toward the anode. The number of secondary electrons produced is known as the *gas multiplication factor* (*GMF*). With a GMF of 10^3 to 10^5, the detector response is proportional to the number of primary ion pairs produced. Consequently, this sensitive detector system is called a *proportional detector.*

With a further increase in the voltage applied across the electrodes, a maximum GMF of 10^6 to 10^8 may be realized. Above this limit, the ion chamber continuously discharges. With a GMF of 10^6 to 10^8, the secondary ions form an electron cloud around the anode. When the electron cloud is of sufficient size, it is released all at once, producing a pulse of electricity. The pulse is of sufficient size to trigger a counting mechanism. Radiation detectors that use this principle are called *Geiger-Müller* (*GM*) *counters.*

Radiation detectors that measure the amount of fluorescence induced in a chemical are called *scintillation detectors.* The ion pairs produced by the radiation cause the orbital electrons of the interacting fluor to assume new, excited, metastable energy states. When the higher (excited) energy electrons drop back to the ground energy state of the fluor, a photon is released in the visible region. This photon can be detected and amplified by a photomultiplier tube (PMT). The electrical signal from the PMT can be totalized with auxiliary electronics. The combination of crystal, PMT, and associated electronics is called a *scintillation counter.* A specially fabricated sodium iodide crystal is generally used as a fluor for gamma radiation detection. Fluorescent chemicals may be dissolved in aromatic solvents and serve as high efficiency beta detectors.

Radiation is also detected by the *photographic process.* Ionizing radiation interacts with film in the same manner as visible light. The amount of darkening on the film (density), (i.e., the amount of *chemical product* formed) is directly proportional to the quantity and energy of radiation. This principle is used by health physicists to assess radiation exposure of personnel working with radiopharmaceuticals. By wearing a film badge, each pharmacist who handles radiopharmaceuticals is monitored for radiation exposure.

BIOPHARMACEUTICS

Radiation Biology

Pharmacists who handle radioactive drugs should be aware of the biological effects of radiation. These effects have been extensively studied and documented. Radiation is a recognized treatment for certain types of cancer, and as a result, dose versus effect has been established.

Since World War II, a large number of people have become occupationally exposed to radiation—e.g., employees of nuclear power plants and technicians in the fields of medical radiation and nuclear physics. Each occupational group has been extensively studied for radiation effects. Our understanding of radiation biology has been enlarged by studies of the survivors of the bombs dropped on Japan during World War II at Hiroshima and Nagasaki. The effects of radiation on large numbers of animals and the parameters that influence the effects of radiation have been studied. Thus, radiation biology is probably one of the better understood biological sciences today.

Biological effects produced by radiation are of two broad types—*somatic,* and *genetic. Somatic effects* are those effects of radiation on the somatic (non-reproductive) cells and therefore are not passed on to progeny. They include, for example, epilation, life shortening, cancer, etc. Somatic effects are observable in the person exposed to the radiation. With such effects there appears to be a threshold of radiation below which no effect is observed. However, above the threshold, the effect is linear with dose. An extrapolation of the dose-effect curve does pass through zero.

Genetic effects are produced upon the reproductive cells of the person exposed and therefore on his progeny. Such effects are difficult to measure. Because of the difficulty in assessing the genetic effects of radiation and the limited knowledge of radiation genetics, it is assumed that all radiation is harmful and that no threshold exists between the observed effect and the amount of radiation exposure. Thus, all radiation exposure is harmful, and increased radiation exposure increases the probability of genetic effect.

All radiation effects are modified by the person's age, general health, the extent of the body irradiated, the critical organs (the organs most susceptible to the radiation), total radiation dose, dose rate, and type of radiation.

Radiation effects may be observed from acute and chronic exposures. A larger total radiation dose can be tolerated from chronic exposure because the somatic cells have a chance to recover between exposures.

The acute $LD_{50/30}$ for radiation in humans is 450 rems. This means that, without medical treatment, 50 percent of the population will die within 30 days after an exposure of 450 rems. In practice, no fatalities have occurred with less than 1,000 rems because of extensive medical treatment.

With acute radiation exposure, there are no observable effects with less than 25 rems. As the radiation dose is increased above 25 rems, there are observable effects on the hematopoietic system and the gastrointestinal tract. Large acute doses of radiation produce a rapid fall in white blood cell count plus the acute radiation syndrome of nausea, vomiting, and diarrhea.

A person who is occupationally exposed to radiation as part of his employment is allowed to receive five rems per year. A safety factor of 10 is required for people who are not occupationally employed, i.e., 0.5 rem per year.

Radiometabolism

The retention, distribution, routes and rates of excretion, and metabolic fate are important pharmacological factors of a drug. A procedure often used for studying these factors is the *radioactive tracer method*. The drug is labeled with a radioactive nuclide and traced in a biological sample by the radiation emitted. A basic assumption of the technique is that the tagged material will act quantitatively and qualitatively like its stable counterpart. Since the chemical activity of a compound is dictated by its orbital electrons and the added radiation only changes the nucleus of the atom, the labeled material should react like its stable counterpart. A small change in mass does occur with a tracer labeled drug. However, this change in mass generally represents no significant change in the total mass of the compound. Thus, the assumption of chemical equivalence is generally accepted except where the mass change is significant (e.g., water versus tritiated water) or where the radiation effect would vary the experimental results (e.g., enzyme kinetic or genetic studies).

Labeled pharmaceuticals can be administered and metabolic routes and rates of excretion can be determined in humans and experimental animals. Examination of metabolic products in excreta serves to indicate the probable metabolic pathways. The technique is also used clinically to diagnose disease states that effect metabolism. The technique is generally used on all new pharmaceuticals prior to their clinical trials to elucidate their normal metabolic pathways.

The tracer technique involves labeling the drug and conducting the pharmacological investigation by evaluation of the emitted radiation. The most important advantage of the technique is its sensitivity. Since each disintegration represents an atom, it is possible to measure quantitatively 10^{-14} to 10^{-16} g. of the drug, depending upon the instrumentation and radionuclide used.

Other advantages of the technique include the labeling of specific atoms or specific functional groups on a molecule, as well as the capability of carrying out the experiment under normal physiological conditions. In addition, because of the radiation emitted, sample preparation is usually quite simple, compared to other analytical techniques.

There are a number of disadvantages with the tracer technique. The main disadvantage is the synthesis of the radiolabeled compound. Since most metabolic studies are on new products, the labeled compound is not likely to be available commercially. Synthesis of radioactive compounds requires facilities and capabilities for handling intermediate to large quantities of radioactive materials. Radiochemical synthesis employs miniaturization techniques and remote handling. Special considerations must be given to carrier-free chemistry, procedures for adding radioactivity, and health physics.

The tracer technique is a specialized technique requiring specialized equipment and qualified users. A specific license from the AEC is required. Each licensee must have training or experience prior to licensure. Evidence of suitable equipment and facilities must be included as part of a license application.

The tracer technique has other disadvantages: Because the tracer method only follows the label, the amount of radioactivity in tissue is not always a true measurement of the labeled material originally administered. The measured radioactivity may be a reaction or decomposition product of the administered material. Loose radioactive contamination in a laboratory as a result of poor technique may negate the tracer technique, present a health hazard, or disrupt instrument sensitivity.

Finally, output data from limited tracer studies do not follow a normal statistical distribution. Researchers who use radioactivity measurements should be acquainted with nuclear counting statistics.

Radiopharmaceutical Dosimetry

Radiopharmaceuticals are unique in that the physical quantity of radioactive material required is so small that no pharmacological effect is produced. Thus, the physical dose of an administered radiopharmaceutical is of minimal significance. The observed biological effects are due to the formation of ion pairs by the radiation and not to the pharmaceutical per se.

Of primary importance, however, is the amount of radiation absorbed by the body, its organs, or molecules as the radiopharmaceutical passes through the organism. Factors that affect internal radiation absorption include physical half-life ($t_{1/2}$) of the radionuclide, the energy and type of radiation emitted by the radionuclide, the volume and homogeneity of the tissue in which the radionuclide is distributed, the biological half-life (t_b) of the radiopharmaceutical, the quantity of radiation to which the organ is exposed, the mean duration exposure, and the fraction of energy absorbed by the target.

In the body, both the physical decay ($t_{1/2}$) and biological elimination (t_b) take place. The sum of the two rate processes is the *effective elimination constant* (λ_{eff}).

$$\lambda_{eff} = \lambda_{1/2} + \lambda_B \qquad \text{Eq. 26}$$

Substituting equation 17 for each λ gives

$$\frac{0.693}{T_{eff}} = \frac{0.693}{T_{1/2}} + \frac{0.693}{T_B} \qquad \text{Eq. 27}$$

or

$$\frac{1}{T_{eff}} = \frac{1}{T_{1/2}} + \frac{1}{T_B} \qquad \text{Eq. 28}$$

Rearranging:

$$T_{eff} = \frac{(T_B)(T_{1/2})}{T_B + T_{1/2}} \qquad \text{Eq. 29}$$

Since the unit of absorbed dose is the rad and is defined as the absorption of 100 ergs of energy per gram of tissue, the particular radiation dose in rads per second is obtained from the equation

$$\text{Rads/sec} = \frac{(3.7 \times 10^4 \text{d/s/}\mu\text{Ci})(\mu\text{Ci/g.})(\text{Mev/d})(1.6 \times 10^{-6} \text{ergs/Mev})}{100 \text{ ergs/g.}} \qquad \text{Eq. 30}$$

or

$$\text{Rads/day} = 51.2(E)(C), \qquad \text{Eq. 31}$$

where E is the energy in Mev (all absorbed) and C is the concentration of radionuclide uniformly distributed in the organ in μCi/g.

The absorbed dose over the time course of the radionuclide is the rad/day dose, times 1.44 (the *mean life*) times the *effective half-life,* or

$$\text{Rads}_{total} = 73.8(E)(C)(T_{eff}). \qquad \text{Eq. 32}$$

For gamma radiation, the emitted photons are not completely absorbed by the body. Thus, gamma dosimetry must include either a source strength, Γ, and correction for geometry, $\bar{g}$,[8] or the energy emitted by the radionuclide in g.-Rads per μCi-hr, Δ, and the fraction of the emitted energy which is absorbed in the target, ϕ.[9]

The units of Γ are rads per hour per mCi at 1 cm.; thus the absorbed dose is

$$\text{Rads/hr} = (10^{-3}\Gamma)(C)(g) \qquad \text{Eq. 33}$$

or

$$\text{Rads}_{total} = (0.0346)(\Gamma)(C)(g)(T_{eff}) \qquad \text{Eq. 34}$$

The absorbed dose may be calculated using Δ, ϕ, and the following equation:

$$\text{Rads}_{total} = \hat{c}\Sigma_i\Delta_i\phi_i \qquad \text{Eq. 35}$$

where the cumulative concentration ($\hat{c}$) is obtained from the applicable physical and biological half-lives, Δ_i is obtained from standardized decay schemes for each radio-nuclide, the specific absorbed fraction is obtained from tables,[9] and the individual photons are summed (Σ_i) for all emissions with due consideration for multiple effective half-life components. Standard organ weights are available in the Radiological Health Handbook.[10]

REFERENCES

1. Becquerel, H.: Sur les radiations emises par phosphorescence. Compt. Rend., *122*:420, 1896.
2. Blumgart, H. L., and Yens, O. C.: Studies on the velocity of blood flow. J. Clin. Invest., *4*:1, 1927.
3. Chart of the Nuclides. 10th Edition. General Electric Company, Schenectady, N.Y. 12305, Dec. 1968.
4. Chase, G. D., and Rabinowitz, J. L.: Principles of Radioisotope Methodology. Ed. 3. pp. 415–419. Burgess Publishing Co., Minneapolis, Minn., 1968.
5. Curie, E.: Madame Curie. A Biography. New York, Doubleday Doran, 1937.
6. Ice, R. D., and Dugan, M. A.: Beta radio-pharmaceutical identification by quench analysis. J. Nucl. Med., *12*:552, 1971.
7. Leach, K. G.: Sterilization by filtration. J. Nucl. Med., *12*:140, 1971.
8. Marinelli, L. D.: Dosage determinations with radioactive isotopes. Am. J. Roentgenol., *47*: 210, 1942.
9. Medical Internal Radiation Dose Committee, Supplement to the Journal of Nuclear Medicine, Feb. 1968.
10. Radiological Health Handbook. Bureau of Radiological Health, USDHEW, PHS, Consumer Prot. and Env. Health Service, Rockville, Maryland 20852, Revised Edition, January 1970.
11. Roentgen, W.: Ueber sine neus Art von Strahlen (vor laufige Mitteilung). Sitzungs Berichte der Physikalisch-Medicinschen Gesellschaft Zu Wurzburg, *9*:132, 1895.
12. Rutherford, E.: Collision of alpha particles with light atoms: I. Hydrogen. Phil. Mag., *37*:537, 1919.
13. Wagner, H. N., Jr.: Nuclear medicine: present and future. Radiology, *86*:601, 1966.

BIBLIOGRAPHY

Andrews, G., Kniseley, R. M., and Wagner, H. N. Jr. (eds.): Radioactive Pharmaceuticals. AEC Symposium Series No. 6. Oak Ridge, Tenn., U.S. Atomic Energy Commission, 1966.

Blahd, W. H.: Nuclear Medicine. New York, McGraw Hill, 1965.

Cember, H.: Introduction to Health Physics. New York, Pergamon Press, 1969.

Christian, J. E.: Radioisotopes in the pharmaceutical sciences and industry. J. Pharm. Sci., *50*:1, 1961.

Cloutier, R. J., Edwards, C. L., and Snyder, W. S. (eds.): Medical Radionuclides: Radiation Dose and Effects. AEC Symposium Series No. 20. Oak Ridge, Tenn., U.S. Atomic Energy Commission, 1970.

IAEA Panel Proceedings: Analytical Control of Radionuclides. Vienna, IAEA, 1970.

Lapp, R. E., and Andrews, H. L.: Nuclear Radiation Physics. Ed. 3. Englewood Cliffs, N.J., Prentice-Hall, 1963.

Maynard, C. D.: Clinical Nuclear Medicine. Philadelphia, Lea and Febiger, 1969.

National Academy of Sciences: Source Material for Radiochemistry. Nuclear Science Series Report No. 42. Washington, D.C., National Academy of Sciences, 1970.

The National Formulary. Thirteenth Edition. Easton, Pa., Mack Publishing Co., 1970.

The Pharmacopeia of the United States of America. Eighteenth Revision. Easton, Pa., Mack Publishing Company, 1970.

Silver, S.: Radioactive Nuclides in Medicine and Biology. Philadelphia, Lea and Febiger, 1969.

Wolf, W., and Tubis, M.: Radiopharmaceuticals. J. Pharm. Sci., *56*:1, 1967.

14

Patrick P. DeLuca, PH. D., *Assistant Dean
and Associate Professor of Pharmacy,
College of Pharmacy, University of Kentucky Medical Center*

Sterile Products

INTRODUCTION

A sterile product can properly be defined as a preparation or device that either is introduced into or comes in contact with internal body compartments. Consequently, because the body's most protective barriers —the skin and mucous membranes—have been circumvented, purity, freedom from toxicity, and freedom from contamination become essential requirements. These characteristics are the principal qualities that distinguish parenteral products from other types of pharmaceutical dosage forms.

Types of sterile products include:

1. Parenteral Products
2. Ophthalmic Preparations
3. Irrigating Solutions

Parenterals are those sterile drugs, solutions, or suspensions that are packaged in a manner suitable for administration by hypodermic injection, either in the form in which they are prepared or after the addition of a suitable solvent or suspending agent (Fig. 14-1). Although the term parenteral may be interpreted literally as meaning administration by any means other than through the intestine (from *para,* "beside," and *enteron,* "bowel"), common usage has limited it to those methods of administration that involve the use of the hypodermic needle, i.e., intracutaneous, subcutaneous, intravenous, etc. These avenues of drug administration have become so widely accepted that numerous preparations for such purposes are now included in the official compendia.

Ophthalmic preparations are intended for instillation in the eye, and though not introduced into internal body cavities, are placed in contact with tissues that are very sensitive to contamination. Therefore, freedom from microbial contamination and toxic components as well as a high level of purity are required for ophthalmic preparations.

Irrigating solutions also are required to meet the same standards as parenteral solutions because, during an irrigation procedure, substantial amounts of these solutions can be absorbed directly into the bloodstream through the open blood vessels of wounds or abraded mucous membranes.

HISTORY

Compared with other routes of administration, the use of the parenteral route is in its infancy. Prior to 1926, the official compendia did not include one official injectable preparation. In 1926, the National Formulary included 6 injectable preparations under the official classification of "Ampuls."

The idea of injecting various substances, including blood, into the bloodstream had been in the mind of man for several centuries, and it was the discovery of the circulation of the blood by William Harvey in 1628 that stimulated increased experimentation. The first experimental injection of drugs has been credited to Sir Christopher Wren who, in 1657, successfully administered opium intravenously to dogs, using a quill and bladder. Six years later, J. D. Major gave the first successful injection to man.[45]

The earliest record of a blood transfusion is from 1665, when an animal near death from loss of blood was restored by infusion of blood from another animal. In 1667, the first successful transfusion of blood to a human being was performed by Jean Baptiste Denis, physician to Louis XIV, who administered lamb's blood directly into the circulation of a 15-year-old boy. The success

451

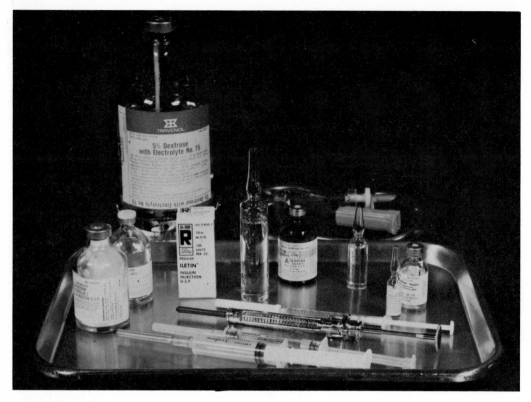

Fig. 14-1.   Representative samples of sterile products. (University of Kentucky College of Pharmacy)

of this transfusion generated enthusiasm which led to promiscuous transfusion of blood from animals to man. In 1687, after a number of fatalities, animal-to-man transfusions were prohibited. It wasn't until 1834 that attempts were again made to inject blood into man. James Blundell, an English obstetrician, infused blood into many women who were threatened by hemorrhage during childbirth. He saved many lives and proved that only human blood was safe to inject into man.

In 1855, the first subcutaneous injection of drugs, using a true hypodermic syringe, was described by Dr. Alexander Wood of Edinburgh. However, complications persisted. It was not until the latter part of the 19th century and the early 20th century that technological developments provided the basis for an increasing use of parenteral routes of administration. The successful utilization of such routes resulted primarily from the following significant developments:

1. Proof of the germ theory of disease and the discovery of the principles of antisepsis and methods of producing sterility by Pasteur, Koch, Lister, et al. in the latter half of the 19th century.

2. Introduction of the hypodermic syringe (invented by C. G. Pravez in 1853, popularized by Wood and Hunter in 1855, and improved by Luer in 1894*).

3. Invention of the sealed-glass container (ampul) for injections by Limousin in 1886.

4. Development of air and steam sterilization techniques.

5. Use of bacteria-retentive filters.

In 1867, a committee of the Royal Medical and Chirurgical Society of London gave approval to hypodermic injections. It issued the following statements in its report concerning parenteral solutions:

1. Only clear neutral solutions should be injected.

* Clendenning, L.: Source Book of Medical History. New York, Paul B. Hoeber, 1942.

2. Physiologic and therapeutic effects are the same regardless of route used (rectal, oral, parenteral).

3. Certain unpleasant symptoms of some drugs are avoided when the parenteral route is used.

4. More rapid absorption and increased intensity of action are observed when the parenteral route is used.

5. Nearness of, or distance from the affected part to the site of injection has no noticeable effect.

The British Pharmacopoeia of 1867 contained the first official injection—morphine. In 1885, apomorphine and ergotin injections were added, but there was still no attempt made to sterilize them, although camphor water was used probably as a preservative. In 1898, when cocaine was added, an attempt at sterilization was made: distilled water was boiled for a few minutes and cooled; 0.15 percent of salicylic acid and 1.5 percent of phenol were used as preservatives.

In 1900, Landsteiner proved that not all human blood is alike, and subsequently the well-known classifications were developed. Early in the 20th century, physicians began to complain of undesirable reactions which were often observed following use of the then crudely prepared injections. The following statement is abstracted from an article appearing in the British Medical Journal in 1911:

Hort and Peafold of the Lister Institute have shown that distilled water which is allowed to stand in sealed sterile containers and subsequently used as an infusion gives rise to toxic symptoms the cause of which has not been fully explained. Similar symptoms are not observed if recently freshly distilled water is employed.[21]

This is an early observation of the existence of *pyrogens,* or fever-producing substances, which are carefully guarded against in modern preparations. In the last decade, considerable research was undertaken to learn more about the pyrogens, and it is now commonly accepted that pyrogens result from bacterial growth and may remain in a solution after the bacteria have been filtered off. However, any material, chemical or biological, which produces a rise in body temperature, chills, body aches, increased arterial blood pressure, and cutaneous vasoconstriction may be classified as a pyrogen.

Most bacteria and many molds and viruses have been reported as producing pyrogens. The gram-negative bacteria produce the most potent of the pyrogenic substances. Chemically, pyrogens are lipid substances associated with a carrier molecule which is usually a polysaccharide but may be a protein. Antipyretics eliminate the fever but not the systemic effects of pyrogens. Generally, a product is maintained pyrogen-free by exercising good manufacturing practices and proper control procedures.

The use of preservatives in injectable products began at an early date. Dr. E. R. Squibb recommended in 1873 that parenteral solutions be preserved by the addition of up to 1 percent of carbolic acid. Others suggested the use of salicylic acid or chloroform. The latter was to be included by substituting chloroform water for distilled water as the solvent.[7]

In 1914, sodium citrate was found to prevent blood from clotting. This discovery contributed to rapid advances in the use of whole blood fractions.

Research and development over the last three decades have been of such magnitude that the technology of preparing and administering sterile products has advanced significantly. The use of parenteral fluids for the critically ill or fasting patient during this period has contributed to the advancement. Parenteral preparations first received official acceptance in this country in the National Formulary, Fifth Edition (1926). Monographs were included in that standard for 7 ampuls (*ampullae*) which were described as *"hermetically sealed containers which are filled with a medicinal liquid in a sterile condition, intended for parenteral use."* The Tenth Revision of the United States Pharmacopoeia of the same date included a chapter on sterilization but no monographs for individual ampuls. The monograph for Physiological Saline Solution in the same revision required that the product be sterilized by autoclaving. Obviously, the preparation was intended for parenteral use even though its title does not suggest such purpose.

Presently, the U.S.P. and the N.F. contain a combined total of 256 monographs under the category of injections, emphasizing the growing importance of parenteral products among therapeutic dosage forms. It is anticipated that the nineteenth revision of the U.S.P. will contain nearly 400 sterile forms.

UTILITY OF INJECTABLES

The expanding use of parenteral products is a reflection of true *therapeutic need* in patient care. For example, it is often necessary to produce drug response in a patient immediately in cases of critical illness, and administration by injection can provide immediate physiological action. Additionally, since the inconsistencies of intestinal absorption are not involved, the therapeutic response can be more easily controlled. Another important advantage of injectables is that they may be used when no other route of administration is available—for example, when the patient is unconscious or uncooperative, when he cannot swallow, or when the drug is not absorbed orally or is destroyed enzymatically in the gastrointestinal tract.

Our knowledge of fluid and electrolyte balance has increased and we now recognize that an imbalance in these parameters is a threat to life. This understanding has brought about an increase in the use of intravenous fluids. Today the patient who has been seriously injured or has undergone surgery recently commonly receives plasma or other physiologic fluid by intravenous drip or hypodermoclysis (Fig. 14-2). These procedures are used to restore to the bloodstream fluid, glucose, and electrolytes which have been lost as a result of shock or severe bleeding. Injections such as dextrose, dextrose and sodium chloride, and Ringer's solution are only a few of the many preparations of this type which are official.

Since very little or no time is needed for absorption when intravenous or subcutaneous injections are involved, these routes are generally selected for emergency drugs. Injections such as levarteranol bitartrate, epinephrine, and sodium bicarbonate are a few examples of this group of drugs. On the other hand, the routes of administration are so flexible that it is possible to use the parenteral route for long-acting medication. In such a case, oil solutions or suspensions may be given by deep intramuscular injection. Thickening or emulsifying agents may be added to further prolong the time of action. Examples of such preparations are Repository Corticotropin Injection, Sterile Procaine Penicillin Suspension, and Procaine Penicillin in Oil Injection.

It is possible, in some instances, to localize the action of a drug by injecting it adjacent to the tissue with which it is expected to react. This is the principle which is used in producing a nerve block by use of a local anesthetic drug, for example, in dental surgery.

Injection procedures lend themselves to exact regulation of dosage because essentially all of the drug enters the circulatory system before it is eliminated. This procedure provides an avenue for the administration of diagnostic agents such as those used in the estimation of blood volume, kidney function, or other physiologic "rates."

Parenteral forms are not without disadvantages. Perhaps the greatest disadvantage is the fear which many people have of the hypodermic needle. Increased cost of medication is another factor. It is considerably more expensive to market a drug in an injectable form rather than as a tablet or a capsule. Obviously, injectables require much more care in handling than do the simpler dosage forms. Finally, they may not be administered without the use of specialized equipment, and the methods of administration require specialized training.

PRINCIPLES AND TERMS PERTINENT TO BACTERIOLOGY AND STERILE TECHNIQUES

Sterility is the absence of life or the absolute freedom from biological contamination. Therefore, a product or device is either sterile or it is contaminated. It may be moderately contaminated or grossly contaminated, but it can only be sterile or not sterile. There is no compromise with sterility. *Asepsis* is a condition of freedom from organisms which produce sepsis; therefore, an aseptic

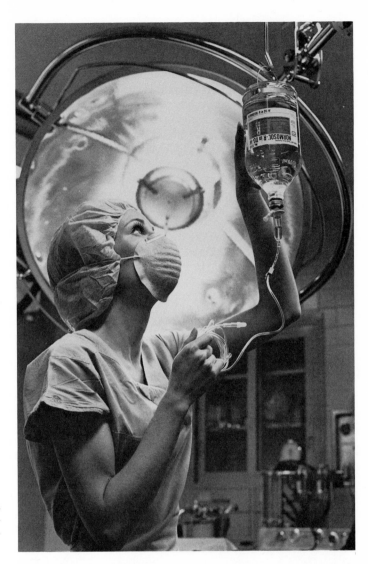

Fig. 14-2. A nurse in a hospital emergency ward setting up intravenous fluid therapy for an injured patient.

technique does not necessarily imply a sterile technique.

In order to have a better understanding of sterility, the following terms are presented and defined:

Sterilization—Inactivation or elimination of all viable organisms.

Disinfectant—A substance used on nonliving objects to render them noninfectious; kills vegetative bacteria, fungi, and viruses but not spores.

Bactericide—A substance that kills vegetative bacteria and some spores; synonymous with germicide.

Antiseptic—A substance used to prevent the multiplication of microorganisms when applied to living systems. An antiseptic is bacteriostatic in action but not necessarily bactericidal.

Bacteriostat—A substance which stops the growth and multiplication of bacteria but does not necessarily kill them. Usually growth resumes when the bacteriostat is removed.

Vegetative Cell—A bacterial cell capable of multiplication, as opposed to the spore form, which cannot multiply. A vegetative cell is less resistant than the spore form.

Spore—A body which some species of bacteria form within their cells which is considerably more resistant than the vegetative cell.

STERILIZATION

Pharmaceutical materials may be rendered sterile by a number of physical or chemical means. These include exposure to heat, ultraviolet light, ionizing radiation, or gases (such as ethylene oxide, propylene oxide, or formaldehyde); addition of sterile chemicals; or passage through one of a number of types of filters to remove bacteria. When full treatment with one method causes deterioration, combinations of sterilization methods are often employed.

In the sterilization and subsequent use of a pharmaceutical product or device, there are 5 important requirements:

1. An adequate sterilization treatment must be effected.

2. Adequate test procedures must be performed to ensure sterility.

3. The sterile product must be adequately protected during storage to maintain sterility.

4. The preparation for administration and the ultimate use of the product or device must be accomplished without the entrance of contamination.

5. The process must not have a deleterious effect on the material.

Some fundamental facts about microorganisms are of help in understanding and fulfilling the above requirements. In general, most pathogenic bacteria have rather specific environmental requirements, with optimum temperatures between 30° and 37° and neutral pH. Nevertheless, some bacteria survive and even multiply at refrigerator temperatures and at temperatures as high as 60°C. Oxygen requirements vary considerably. Some bacteria, called *aerobes,* demand oxygen; others, called *anaerobes,* cannot tolerate oxygen. Some microorganisms have the ability to utilize nitrogen and carbon dioxide from the air and can multiply in distilled water. Many bacteria can grow in concentrated pharmaceutical preparations, but a large number of drugs act as bactericidal or bacteriostatic agents and, in sufficient concentrations, are often self-sterilizing.

Slightly alkaline media support the multiplication of many microorganisms; acid conditions are favorable to a host of other organisms. Contaminating yeasts and molds can flourish in dextrose and other sugar solutions.

Most of the active bacteria are vegetative and sensitive to heat and bactericidal agents, but those bacteria that form a *spore* or *hibernation state* are very resistant to heat and bactericidal agents. Although some of the spore-forming bacteria are extremely pathogenic, most are not disease-producing. However, even the nonpathogenic forms can give rise to pyrogenic reactions.

Sterilization methods. Microorganisms are destroyed by heat, ultraviolet light, ionizing radiations, and many chemical agents, and these processes serve as the basis for several methods of sterilization. Most popular are the *thermal methods,* and the greater part of the literature on sterilization is on these methods. The lethal effectiveness of heat is dependent upon the degree of heat, the duration of exposure, and the humidity. Naturally, the higher the temperature, the shorter the required period of exposure, but the relationship between time and temperature is not linear. For example, for a particular microorganism, sterilization may be achieved at 170°C. in 15 minutes, whereas at 120°C. 2 hours are required.[32] Table 14-1 shows the times required for lethal effect on bacterial spores by thermal exposure.

The mechanism by which microorganisms

TABLE 14-1.   EFFECT OF THERMAL EXPOSURE ON BACTERIAL SPORES

	KILLING TIME (MIN.)					
	MOIST HEAT			DRY HEAT		
	100°C.	110°C.	121°C.	120°C.	140°C.	170°C.
B. Anthracis	5–15	—	—	—	180	—
Cl. botulinum	330	90	10	120	60	15
Cl. welchii	5–10	—	—	50	5	7
Cl. tetani	5–15	—	—	—	15	—
Soil Bacilli	> 1020	120	6	—	—	15

are killed by heat is thought to depend on the presence of moisture. According to Perkins,[33] in the presence of moisture death is due to the coagulation of the protein of the living cell whereas, in the absence of water, oxidation is the primary process. In Table 14-2, this principle is demonstrated by listing the effect of moisture and heat on the coagulation of albumin. From the information listed in the table, it is obvious that moist heat is a more effective means of killing microorganisms than dry heat. This is attributed to the ability of moist heat to coagulate the cell protein at a much lower temperature than dry heat. Additionally, steam has a much greater thermal capacity than hot air. For example, when steam condenses, the amount of thermal energy liberated is equal to its heat of vaporization. This amounts to approximately 540 calories per gram at 100°C. and about 524 calories per gram at 121°C. The heat liberated by hot air is approximately 1 calorie per gram per degree centigrade of cooling. Thus, steam at 100°C. striking a cold object will liberate 500 times more heat than hot air at the same temperature striking a similar object.

Substances that are not heat labile and can tolerate temperatures greater than 120°C. may be rendered sterile by means of *dry heat.* Both the vegetative cells and spores of all microorganisms can be killed by exposure to a temperature of 180°C. (356° F.) for 2 hours or to a temperature of 260°C. (500° F.) for about 45 minutes. The total sterilizing cycle time for *hot air sterilization* normally includes the time it requires for the substance to reach the sterilizing temperature of the oven chamber, an appropriate dwell period to achieve sterilization, and a cooling period to allow the material to return to room temperature. Because of the high temperature required for effective sterilization with dry heat, many substances may be adversely affected. Many chemicals and drugs can undergo decomposition between 120 and 260°C. Container components are destroyed or deformed; at around 160°C., rubber rapidly oxidizes, thermoplastics melt, and wrapping material containing cellulose, such as paper and cloth, begin to char. Dry heat sterilization is particularly suitable for glassware, metalware and anhydrous oils, since these materials can withstand elevated temperatures without degradation.

Since the most reliable means for killing microorganisms is the use of moist heat under pressure, this method of sterilization, commonly referred to as *autoclaving,* is employed whenever possible. Aqueous pharmaceutical preparations in hermetically sealed containers can be sterilized by autoclaving and sterility will be maintained indefinitely as long as the seal is not disturbed. It is not possible to sterilize nonaqueous preparations in this manner because water must be present within the container to generate steam and thereby produce a lethal action.

Supplies such as rubber closures, glassware, and other equipment with rubber attachments as well as filters of various types and sterile room garments have been sterilized by autoclaving. To be effective, however, air pockets must be eliminated and sufficient moisture must be present on the materials in the autoclave. Consequently, the material will be wet at the end of the sterilizing cycle. When containers and other equipment are to be used shortly after autoclaving, care must be taken not to allow water to dilute the product. Such a situation can be avoided by rinsing the equipment with a small portion of the sterilized product. This problem can be avoided or minimized by drying the materials in a vacuum oven following autoclaving.

It is preferable to sterilize glass containers and metal equipment by dry heat because of the advantage of attaining sterile and dry materials; however, care must be taken to avoid breakage or distortion due to uneven thermal expansion. Certain chemicals and oleaginous vehicles are sometimes sterilized with dry heat at temperatures as low as 120°C. When these marginal methods are

TABLE 14-2. EFFECT OF MOISTURE AND HEAT ON EGG ALBUMIN

WATER (PERCENT)	TEMPERATURE (°C.)	EFFECT
50	56	Coagulation
25	80	Coagulation
6	145	Coagulation
0	170	Coagulation and Oxidation

employed, it is essential to allow adequate time to ensure sterilization. Additionally, it must be validated that the prolonged heating cycle has no deleterious effects on the efficacy and safety of the product.

Ultraviolet light radiation in the region of 2,537 angstrom units is commonly used to reduce the level of airborne contamination and maintain sterility of work surfaces and equipment. Generally, penetration of ultraviolet light is negligible; therefore, its bactericidal effectiveness is limited to exposed surfaces.

When ultraviolet light passes through matter, energy is absorbed by specific electrons within molecules. This absorbed energy makes the molecules more reactive. When such electronic excitation occurs among essential molecules within microorganisms, the reproductive system of the organism is destroyed or the organism dies.[34] The effectiveness of ultraviolet radiation depends on its ability to penetrate. Unfortunately, the 2,537-Å wavelength radiation is screened out by most materials. Clumps of organisms and organisms covered with a film of dirt or dust can escape the lethal effect of ultraviolet, owing to its limited ability to penetrate. Therefore, the application of ultraviolet radiation is restricted to surface sterilization and sterilization of clean air and water. Ultraviolet lamps are frequently installed in clean rooms, air ducts, laminar flow hoods and large equipment where exposed surfaces and air can be irradiated. Water supplies may be equipped with ultraviolet lamps to either maintain the water in a sterile condition or reduce the level of bacterial contamination of incoming water. The bactericidal effectiveness of ultraviolet light is principally a function of the intensity of radiation and duration of exposure. It also varies with the susceptibility of the organism. Vegetative bacteria are most susceptible; bacteria spores appear to be from 3 to 10 times as resistant to inactivation and fungal spores may be from 100 to 1,000 times more resistant to ultraviolet light.[30] Cellular nucleic acids are capable of absorbing light radiation in the ultraviolet wavelength range and it is believed that the lethal mechanism associated with the absorption of ultraviolet energy involves these molecules.

The use of higher energy ionizing radiations for sterilization has been growing. These are radiations emitted from radioactive isotopes, such as cobalt 60 which produces gamma rays, or are generated by mechanical acceleration of electrons to very high velocities, which gives rise to cathode or beta rays. The ionizing radiation produced directly from charged electrons and indirectly from gamma rays can penetrate matter to a significantly greater degree than ultraviolet radiation. The degree of penetrability, of course, depends on the type and energy of the specific radiation and the density of the material being irradiated. *Gamma rays* from isotopes have the advantage of being absolutely reliable, since there is no possibility of interruption in their production due to a mechanical breakdown. However, gamma ray sources are not readily available, and the radioactive emission cannot be controlled or stopped, as is possible with a mechanical source.

Electron accelerators have been designed which are theoretically capable of unlimited energy generation. Figure 14-3 illustrates the operating principle of microwave accelerator. In this system, the electrons hitch a ride on a microwave traveling down a column. The electrons continue to gain speed and by the time they exit from the vacuum tube, they are traveling at the speed of light.

Ionizing radiations interfere with the reproductive process of microorganisms by causing lethal mutations resulting in the ultimate death of the organism. Mutations are believed to be brought about by two methods.[17] One is by direct contact and the transfer of radiation energy to receptive bacterial molecules, as illustrated in Figure 14-4. Highly accelerated electron particles bombard nucleoproteins within the cell and rupture the molecules. The second method is by indirect action, whereby hydrogen and hydroxyl ions are formed which then react with nucleic acids and other bacterial molecules, eliminating their availability for the metabolism of the bacterial cell. A suggested scheme for the formation of hydrogen and hydroxyl ions is as follows:

$$H_2O \longrightarrow H + OH$$
$$3H + 3OH \longrightarrow H_2O_2 + H_2 + H_2O$$
$$H + H_2O_2 \longrightarrow H_2O + OH$$
$$OH + H_2 \longrightarrow H_2O + H$$

Electron Supply

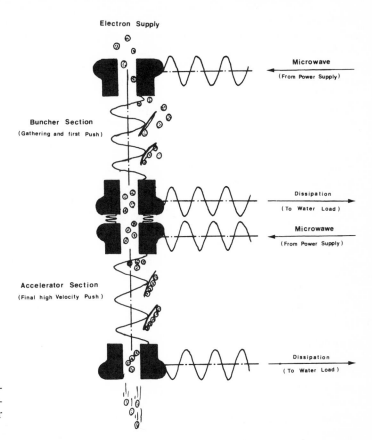

Microwave
(From Power Supply)

Buncher Section
(Gathering and first Push)

Dissipation
(To Water Load)

Microwawe
(From Power Supply)

Accelerator Section
(Final high Velocity Push)

Dissipation
(To Water Load)

FIG. 14-3. A diagram, illustrating the operating principles of a microwave linear accelerator.

In comparison to ultraviolet light, ionizing radiation has much higher energy levels and actually causes ionization of molecules, and survival of microorganisms after exposure to ionizing radiation has not been shown to occur. Bacterial spores and viruses are more resistant than vegetative cells, requiring 4 to 5 times the dose to ensure complete destruction of the microorganism.[35]

Some of the materials that have been successfully sterilized by the use of linear accelerators include surgical sutures, plastic intravenous administration sets, and a number of vitamins, antibiotics and hormones in the dry state.[3] There has been limited application to liquid pharmaceuticals because of the degradation of the drug and other excipients in the product, owing to the ionizing effect on the vehicle system.

Gas sterilization is a chemical method of sterilization which has been used for many years. *Formaldehyde* and *sulfur dioxide* have

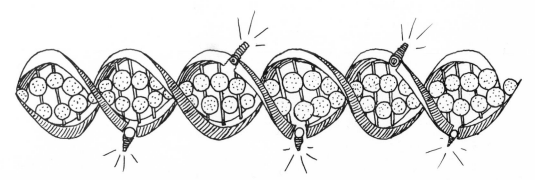

FIG. 14-4. Diagram presenting the direct hit theory of sterilization by ionizing radiation.

long been used for this purpose, but both are very reactive and difficult to remove after exposure. *Ethylene oxide* and *betapropiolactone* are two newer gases which are less reactive chemically and more easily removed.[6] They have gained popularity and presently occupy an important place in the area of sterilization. These gases exert a lethal effect on microorganisms by reacting with bacterial proteins. The altered metabolites are no longer available to the microorganism and so it dies without reproducing.

There are many occasions when solid materials may not be sterilized by either moist or dry heat because of damage or destruction to the material or product. The use of chemical sterilization with gaseous agents frequently avoids these problems and, since gases by nature dissipate when unconfined, the problem of removal is readily solved. Use of these gaseous agents has solved many difficulties encountered in the sterilization of certain biologicals, foodstuffs, cotton, wool, laboratory equipment, and more recently a large number of plastic disposable syringes, needles, and intravenous administration sets.

Filtration is a nonthermal, nonchemical method for sterilization which is generally employed for solutions that cannot be heated. Sterile filtration must remove all microorganisms while allowing passage of all desired components of the solution (Fig. 14-5). To be effective in removing microorganisms, the pore size of the filter must be small enough to prevent microorganisms from moving through the filter. The smallest viable bacterial particles are spores, which may have a diameter of 0.5 micron or, occasionally, slightly less. Vegetative bacteria rarely are found smaller than 1 micron in at least one dimension. Therefore, for a filter that functions primarily by sieving, such as a cellulose ester membrane filter, the pore size must be small enough to prevent the bacterial spore from entering the pore. The diameter of the pores used for dependable sterilization of a solution by a membrane filter is approximately 0.2 micron. Figure 14-6 illustrates the size relationships among some microorganisms and commercially available membrane filters.

GENERAL REQUIREMENTS

In the processing of any pharmaceutical preparation, high standards must be imposed to assure a preparation of the highest quality.

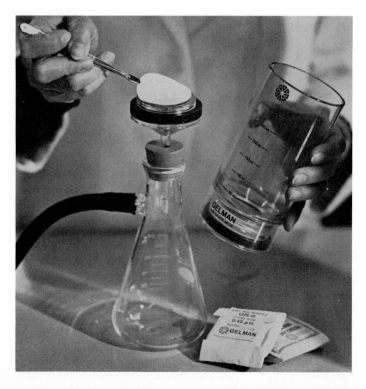

Fig. 14-5. Assembly of a membrane filter for small volume sterilization. (Courtesy of Gelman Instruments)

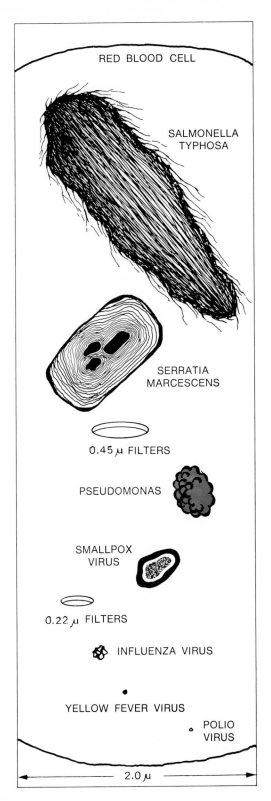

RED BLOOD CELL

SALMONELLA
TYPHOSA

SERRATIA
MARCESCENS

0.45 μ FILTERS

PSEUDOMONAS

SMALLPOX
VIRUS

0.22 μ FILTERS

INFLUENZA VIRUS

YELLOW FEVER VIRUS

POLIO
VIRUS

2.0 μ

FIG. 14-6. Relative sizes of some micro-organisms and commercially available filters.

With parenteral products, maintenance of the standards and adherence to specifications are so essential that the personnel associated with the manufacture of such products not only must be competent and properly trained, but also must possess a highly developed sense of moral and professional responsibility.

Specialized techniques are required for the manufacture of sterile preparations, and these techniques must be subjected to a continuous critical review, for faults, omissions, and improvements. Ingredients of the highest quality must be used—even if additional purification beyond that of the commercial supply is required.

The effectiveness and safety of the final product must be established. Once effectiveness and safety have been established, standard operating procedures for preparing the product should be implemented to ensure that no alterations in techniques or ingredients are permitted. Since changes or deviations from the established procedures might alter the physical or chemical integrity of the product, all proposed changes in either ingredients or procedures must be thoroughly investigated before they are instituted.

An efficient quality control program must also be instituted to ensure the integrity of the product. Not only is it required that the finished product meet all the specifications, but it is essential that valid manufacturing procedures be employed throughout the production operation. In addition to containing the required amount of drug and other ingredients, a parenteral dosage form must fulfill the following mandatory requirements:

Safety. The dosage form must not cause tissue irritation nor give rise to toxic responses. The solvent system and other additives must be thoroughly tested in animals to assure adequate safety in humans. Container components should not release materials that could result in an undesirable reaction.

Sterility. The dosage form must be free of any bacteriological contamination as tested by known methods. In addition, the delivery system must be designed in a manner to provide assurance that contamination will not occur upon administration.

Freedom from Pyrogens. Although only the metabolic products of microorganisms are classified as pyrogens, any material, chemical or biological, that produces a rise in body temperature must be eliminated from parenteral products.

Clarity. Introduction of particulate matter into the bloodstream can be extremely harmful to the patient. A product containing visible particles should never be used intravenously, since this constitutes a particle size of approximately 50 microns and the average size of blood cells is 7.5 microns. Limits below 50 microns should be established and controlled by electronic counting devices.

Stability. The dosage form must be physically and chemically stable in the selected container to assure effectiveness and safety throughout the storage life of the product.

PARENTERAL ROUTES OF ADMINISTRATION

Parenteral preparations are introduced directly into the body fluid systems comprising the intra- or extracellular fluid compartments, the lymphatic system, or the blood. Therefore, in addition to purity, freedom from toxicity, and freedom from contamination, isotonicity and absence of hemolytic properties are essential. The following routes are used to administer parenteral preparations:

Intravenous (I.V.)—directly into the blood via a major peripheral vein.

Intramuscular (I.M.)—directly into a skeletal muscle.

Subcutaneous (S.C.)—directly into the alveolar region beneath the layers of the skin.

Intradermal (I.D.)—directly between the layers of the skin.

Intraspinal—directly into the spinal canal.

Intracisternal—directly in the caudal part between the cerebellum and the medulla oblongata.

Intrathecal—directly into the cerebral spinal fluid via the subarachnoid space at the base of the spine.

Intra-arterial (I.A.)—directly into an artery.

The nature of the product and the desired pharmacological action are factors determining the particular route of administration to be employed. The desired route of administration in turn, places certain requirements and limitations on the formulation as well as the devices used for administering the dosage form. The advantages, requirements and limitations of the various routes will be discussed.

Intravenous Route. The intravenous route is employed when an instantaneous systemic response and moment-by-moment control of dosage are required. There is no delay due to a need for absorption before the drug can reach the circulation, and therapeutic blood levels are attained as rapidly as the time required to empty the syringe allows. Additionally, greater predictability of peak plasma levels is possible. The greater intensity of response affords another advantage, in that drugs given by the intravenous route can be given in smaller doses than are required with other routes of administration. Drugs that are relatively irritating when given orally, intramuscularly, and subcutaneously can often be tolerated intravenously.

Large volumes of fluids containing essential electrolytes and nutrient substances can be administered only by the intravenous route. Generally, this prolonged form of intravenous therapy is restricted to hospitalized patients who are unable to eat and take medication via the oral route.

The intravenous route is generally restricted to solutions because of the danger of insoluble particles blocking fine capillaries. The vein used must not be occluded by a clot, constriction, or collapse. Administration of the solution must be over a sufficient period to allow the drug to mix freely with the blood. Two minutes is usually considered a minimum safety time for an I.V. injection. Damage can occur to the blood vessel if irritant drugs are injected too rapidly or if proper techniques are not employed. Additionally, if an injection is administered too rapidly, a bolus of drug can circulate and reach the brain or the heart in high concentration, causing a dramatic and undesirable response. A common occurrence during prolonged I.V. fluid administration is *phlebitis,* a red swollen area at the site of the venipuncture. A *thromboembolism* may occur from a needle breaking off during injection or during an infusion. Drugs that cause *hemolysis* of red blood cells or precipitation of protein must not be given intravenously.

Intramuscular Route.   Solutions, suspensions, and emulsions can all be administered by the intramuscular route, provided that special consideration is given to the osmolality of the preparations. In many instances, if the solution is not isotonic or nearly so, severe pain may result, owing to irritation of the nerve endings exposed to the preparation. A solution injected intramuscularly will elicit a slower onset and a more prolonged action than if it were administered intravenously. Thus, intramuscular deposition may be used to provide a *repository effect.* An even slower onset and more prolonged action can be achieved by formulating the drug in an oily solution or an aqueous or oily suspension with a thickening agent. Such formulations can either solubilize the drug directly or otherwise influence its rate of release. In general, intramuscular administration is easier and less dangerous than I.V. administration.

Subcutaneous Route.   Subcutaneous injection is frequently employed for small-volume injections when it is desired to spread the drug action out over an extended period. Such an approach avoids too intense a response, a short response, and frequent injection. Next after oral administration, this is the method of choice for patient self-administration because it is the simplest of the parenteral routes. It is possible to teach the patient to routinely inject insulin or certain mercurial diuretics, for example, and a large body area is available for injection. When the skin is pulled away from the body, the pocket formed under the fold of the skin is called the *alveolar space* and is the site of subcutaneous injection. As illustrated in Figure 14-7, the injected drug diffuses from the alveolar space into the blood capillaries which carry it away. Absorption is controlled by lipid solubility; the drug must diffuse to the capillaries, then it must diffuse across the capillary membrane into the blood.

A snake bite closely approximates a subcutaneous injection. The poison is contained at the site of injection, and the rate of blood flow through the capillaries determines the rate of absorption. To minimize the effect of snake poison, i.e., decrease the rate of absorption, it is recommended to:

1.   Immobilize the affected limb in order to relax the muscles in that limb.

2.   Apply ice or vasoconstrictors.

3.   Apply a tourniquet proximally, between the wound and the center of the body. If, in the case of a subcutaneous injection, the above three conditions were reversed, the rate of absorption would increase.

Intradermal Route.   This route is not used for drug administration for systemic action. It is generally reserved for diagnostic agents where localization is desired. An in-

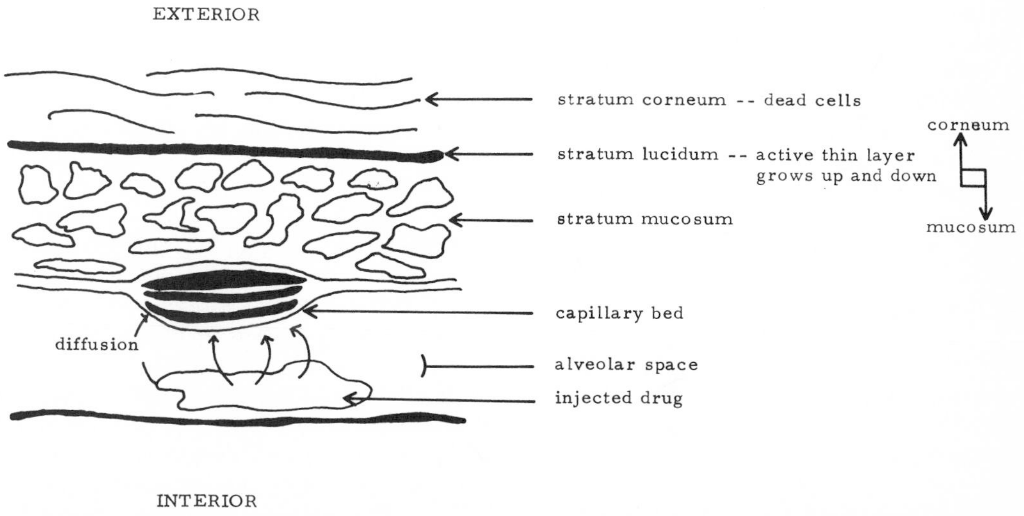

EXTERIOR

INTERIOR

FIG. 14-7.   Representation of the layers of skin and the location of a subcutaneous injection of a parenteral during administration.

tradermal injection is in or between the layers of the epidermis, i.e., the *stratum corneum,* the *stratum lucidum,* the *stratum mucosum* (see Fig. 14-7).

Intra-arterial Route. The drug is injected directly into an artery instead of a vein. Great care must be employed with intra-arterial administration, since it is easy to miss an artery and cause serious damage to nerves which often lie close to them. This parenteral route may be used for: (1) administration of diagnostic agents such as radiopaque media to view an organ such as the kidney or heart, and (2) perfusion of an antineoplastic drug so that the highest possible concentration reaches only the target organ. A disadvantage of the intra-arterial route is that a surgical procedure may be required to reach the artery. Additionally, special care must be exercised to administer minimal doses, since once the drug is injected the effect cannot be counteracted.

Other Routes of Injection. In some cases, it is not possible to achieve high enough plasma levels to cause the drug to penetrate the cerebrospinal fluid. Consequently, the *intrathecal route* may be employed to administer the drug directly into the cerebrospinal fluid at any level of the cerebrospinal axis, including injection into the cerebral ventricles. Preparations administered via the *intrathecal, intraspinal,* and *intracisternal* routes must be of the highest purity because of the sensitivity of the nerve tissues.

Influence of Route of Administration on Formulation. During the formulation of a parenteral product, the route of administration must be taken into consideration. One of the most important factors is incorporating the drug into the appropriate volume. The intravenous route is the only route by which large volumes, i.e., greater than 10 ml., can be administered, although this must be done with great care with regard to the rate of administration. Volumes up to 10 ml. can be administered intraspinally while the intramuscular route is limited to 2 ml., subcutaneous to 2 ml., and intradermal to 0.2 ml.

The choice of the solvent system is directly related to the intended route of administration of the product. Intravenous and intra-

spinal injections are generally restricted to dilute aqueous solutions, whereas oily solutions, emulsions, and suspensions can be injected intramuscularly and subcutaneously.

Isotonicity is another factor which must be taken into consideration. Although isotonic solutions are less irritating, cause fewer toxicities, and eliminate the possibility of hemolysis, it is not essential that all injectables be strictly isotonic. Subcutaneous and intramuscular injections, for example, need not be isotonic, and in some cases a hypertonic solution will facilitate absorption of drug, owing to local effusion of tissue fluids. Intravenous solutions need not be isotonic so long as administration is slow enough to permit dilution and adjustment of tonicity by the blood. On the other hand, intraspinal injections must be isotonic because of the slow circulation of the cerebrospinal fluid in which abrupt changes of osmotic pressure can give rise to many side effects.

Hypodermic Needles for Various Routes of Administration. The construction of the hypodermic needle (also referred to as a cannula) often is dictated by the route of administration. Figure 14-8 illustrates the various parts of a hypodermic needle.

Needles are generally described in terms of length, gauge, and the geometry of the bevel at the point. Lengths range from ¼ inch to 6 inches and gauges from 13 gauge (approximately ⅛ inch) to 27 gauge (approximately 0.01 inch). Regular needles are measured for length from the point at which the cannula joins the hub to the tip of the needle point.

Hypodermic needles are characterized by beveled cutting edges of varying degree and are available with regular, short, long and intradermal bevels. The regular bevel is used primarily for intravenous, intramuscular, subcutaneous, and spinal administration in gauges ranging from 17 to 27 gauge and in lengths from ⅝ inch to 6 inches. For subcutaneous injection a 25 gauge, ⅝-inch needle is generally employed. Intramuscular and intravenous needles vary from 18 to 23 gauge and from 1 to 1½ inches. For injection deep into the cardiothoracic area a 20-gauge, 6-inch needle is used, and for spinal injections lengths vary from 2 to 4 inches. A short bevel needle is used for infusions and trans-

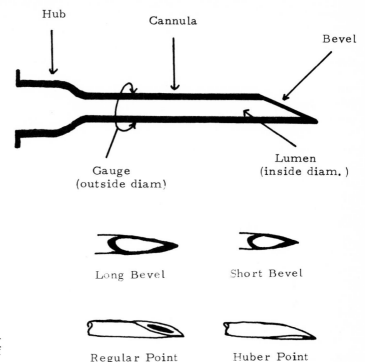

Fig. 14-8. Parts of hypodermic syringe and types of
bevel.

fusions, or when there is a risk of puncturing the posterior wall of a vein after insertion of the needle. The intradermal or special short bevel or long taper needle is used for local anesthesia, aspirating, hypodermoclysis, and subcutaneous administration. Needles for long-term intravenous use are often coated with a blunt plastic tubing which may be left in the vein as a cannula after the needle has been removed.

Needles are also available in standard wall and thin wall types. A thin-wall needle has a lumen one size larger than its gauge. For example, a 19-gauge thin-wall needle has the same lumen as an 18-gauge standard wall. This allows use of a thinner needle without sacrificing flow rate through the lumen.

TYPES OF PARENTERAL PRODUCTS

Classification

Parenteral preparations are classified by the U.S.P. and N.F. according to the following five classifications:

1. Solutions of medicaments suitable for injection, referred to by titles of the form, _____ *Injection*. (Example: Morphine Injection).

2. Dry solids which, upon the addition of suitable solvents, yield solutions conforming in all respects to the requirements for injections and which are distinguished by titles of the form, _____ *for Injection*, or *Sterile* _____. (Examples: Sodium Thiopental for Injection; Sterile Chloramphenicol Sodium Succinate).

3. Solids which are suspended in a suitable fluid medium and which are **not** to be injected intravenously or into the spinal canal, distinguished by titles of the form, *Sterile* _____ *Suspensions*. (Example: Sterile Epinephrine Suspension).

4. Dry solids which, upon the addition of suitable vehicles, yield preparations conforming in all respects to the requirements for sterile suspensions, and which are distinguished by titles of the form, *Sterile* _____ *for Suspension:* (Example: Sterile Chloramphenicol for Suspension).

5. Emulsions of fluids in fluid media, suitable for parenteral administration, which are **not** to be injected into the spinal canal,

and which are distinguished by titles of the form, *Sterile _____ Emulsion.* (Example: Sterile Phytonadione Emulsion).

SOLUTIONS

The majority of parenteral products are aqueous solutions which are preferred because of their physiologic inertness and their versatility with regard to route of administration. The commonly used solvent for aqueous injections is Water for Injection, U.S.P. This highly purified water should not be confused with Sterile Water for Injection, U.S.P., which is in a separate monograph. Whereas only sterile water for injection must meet the requirements of sterility, both forms must be pyrogen free.

Because of the pyrogen-free requirement, it is essential that Water for Injection, U.S.P., be free from bacterial contamination at the time of collection and be used in a product that is sterilized within a relatively short time after collection. This procedure will prevent bacterial growth and the ultimate presence of pyrogens. It is often impractical economically to use freshly prepared water for injection. If storage becomes necessary, the proper storage conditions are required. Large quantities of water for injection can be stored for extended periods of time at temperatures above or below that which will support bacterial growth. Generally, the water is warm at the time of collection and can be conveniently stored in heated tanks at about 80°C. For the storage of relatively small quantities of water, the water is collected in clean sterile bottles, preferably pyrex or type I glass, and stored either at 80°C. or in a refrigerator. Storage in tanks under ultraviolet irradiation has also been employed.

Another important requirement which Water for Injection, U.S.P., must meet is that of total solids. The monograph permits a maximum in total solids of 10 parts per million, including both ionic and nonionic substances. It is important to note that there are several limits, depending upon container size, for total solids for Sterile Water for Injection, U.S.P., all of which are higher than for Water for Injection, U.S.P., because the sterilization process will cause some dissolution of the container surface.

Sodium chloride may be added to Water for Injection to render the resulting solution isotonic, or Sodium Chloride Injection may be substituted in whole or in part for Water for Injection unless otherwise directed by the individual monograph.

SUSPENSIONS

A parenteral suspension can be defined as a sterile heterogeneous system in which insoluble solid particles are dispersed in a liquid medium. Boylan[5] cited the following criteria for electing to formulate a parenteral suspension:

1. To achieve a prolonged or "depot" drug action upon injection.

2. To suspend an insoluble form of a drug when solubility is a problem and there are few pharmaceutically acceptable parenteral solvents.

3. To improve the chemical and physical stability by reducing the interfacial contact between the drug and the surrounding environment.

An acceptable suspension possesses certain desirable qualities, among which are the following:

The suspended material should not settle rapidly.

Particles which do settle should not form a hard cake and should be easily redispersed upon shaking the container.

The viscosity should be such as to permit ready passage through a hypodermic needle.

Generally speaking, suspensions are administered by deep intramuscular injection so that the material may be absorbed gradually. Therefore, an important requirement for parenteral suspensions is a small and uniform particle size. Small, uniform particles give rise to slow, uniform sedimentation rates and in most cases allow for predictable rates of drug dissolution and release. A wide distribution range of particle sizes can result in caking and nonuniformity of a suspension, owing to nonuniform settling, difficult syringeability due to the large particles, and changes in dissolution and drug release rates due to the nonuniformity and possible crystal growth.

Syringeability is one of the most important properties of a good parenteral suspension. This is an important factor because it is a measure of the ability of the product to pass in and out of a syringe through a hypodermic needle. Factors that tend to reduce syringeability or make material transfer through the needle more difficult are: (a) a high viscosity of the vehicle; (b) a high density of the vehicle; (c) large particle size of suspended particulate matter, and (d) a high concentration of suspended drug.

Probably the most important of these factors is *viscosity*. The amount and particle size of the solids, the nature of the vehicle, and the method of preparation determine the viscosity of the product. At times it is desirable to make a formulation which will gel during storage in order to increase the stability of the drug suspension. Materials such as partially hydrolyzed gelatin, lecithin, and nonionic surfactants have been used for this purpose. A commercial preparation containing phytonadione in a sterile dosage form (Mephyton, Merck Sharp & Dohme) is reported to contain 1 percent of lecithin as a suspending agent. In such cases, the product must be thixotropic so that the gelled product can be made fluid at the time of administration by simple shaking.

The *sedimentation* of a suspension can be improved by the use of surfactants which aid in the stabilization and preparation of suspensions by reducing the interfacial tension between the particles and the vehicle. The most commonly used types of surfactants are the Tweens and Pluronics.[8] The addition of a hydrocolloid or a protective colloid, such as sodium carboxymethylcellulose, may enhance the effect of the surfactant by reducing the surface charge on the dispersed particles which, in turn, reduces the tendency for agglomeration and facilitates associations with the water molecules. Among other protective colloids that have been employed are acacia, gelatin, methylcellulose, and polyvinylpyrrolidone.

Oil suspensions may have a thickening agent added. An example is found in Sterile Procaine Penicillin with Aluminum Stearate Suspension, U.S.P., in which aluminum monostearate is used to gel the oil suspension. Procedures for formulating suspensions have been suggested by several researchers.[5,9,31]

EMULSIONS

Injectable emulsions are of the oil-in-water type to permit easy mixing with water, blood, or aqueous fluids, since water is the continuous phase. The major problem in the preparation of emulsions for intravenous administration is to provide and maintain uniform oil droplets measuring less than 5 microns as the dispersed internal phase. A rigid requirement is the control of particle size to prevent emboli in the blood.

Emulsions are generally sterilized by autoclaving; consequently, the preparation must be able to tolerate elevated temperatures. Elevated temperatures tend to cause coalescence of the dispersed phase, and a stabilizing agent is often required. A major problem is that the number of emulsifiers and stabilizers with sufficiently low toxicity for this purpose is limited.

FREEZE-DRIED PRODUCTS

A freeze-dried injectable consists of a dry solid cake which is dissolved in water or a suitable diluent to provide a sterile dose of a specific drug for parenteral administration. The process of freeze drying, also referred to as *lyophilization,* encompasses dissolving the solids in water, filtering the solution through a sterile bacteria-retentive membrane filter, filling individual containers with the filtered solution under aseptic conditions, and removing the water from the frozen solution by sublimation. Freeze drying is usually employed for products that are thermolabile or unstable in aqueous solution.

The design of a freeze-drying cycle depends largely on the nature of the product, the amount of solids, and the volume or thickness of the resulting dry cake. The temperature to which a product must be frozen depends upon the *eutectic temperature* and the supercooling characteristics of the solution.[13] The eutectic temperature is that at which liquid solution and solid mixture exist in equilibrium. Below the eutectic temperature there is no liquid present. Therefore, during the freezing phase, the frozen mass must be kept below the eutectic temperature. How far below the eutectic temperature depends on the supercooling tendency of the solution.

Drying must be carried out at a temperature which is sufficient to cause as rapid a removal of moisture as possible and still maintain the product in the frozen state at a temperature below the eutectic point. Should the temperature of the product rise above the eutectic point before all the moisture is removed, the product will melt and the high internal pressure of the solution will cause "frothing" or "boiling." The rate of drying is dependent on the thermal conductivity of the frozen material. A highly conductive material will allow for more rapid heat transfer and faster drying, while a poorly conductive material will retain more heat. In the latter case, drying temperatures, i.e., the amount of heat applied, must be kept lower.

After completion of the drying cycle, the vials must be sealed immediately under low humidity conditions to prevent reabsorption of moisture. Care must be exercised during the freeze drying process because of the length of time the product must be exposed to an environment in which the chances for particle and bacterial contamination are great. The main reason for freeze drying is simply for stability and maintenance of product integrity and quality. With these goals in mind, in addition to processing pharmaceuticals and biologicals, freeze drying has been used in the preservation of *blood plasma* and *blood products, foodstuffs, viruses, bacteria* and *tissues.*

Dry Solids

Sterile solids are often packaged in the dry form in containers suitable for reconstitution with sterile solvents. In many cases, this is done because the drug is extremely unstable in aqueous solution and its aqueous solubility is not sufficient to permit freeze drying without the addition of a solubilizing agent or a cosolvent.

Sterile solids are more difficult than liquids to subdivide accurately and precisely into individual dose containers on automated manufacturing equipment. The rate of flow of solid materials tends to be irregular, particularly if the material is in a finely powdered state. Humidity conditions generally must

be rigidly controlled in order to effect accurate filling. If the material is hygroscopic, high humidity can cause *"caking and sticking."* On the other hand, low humidity can cause electrostatic charges to build up, especially if the material is finely ground.

Sterile powders are usually prepared by *aseptic crystallization* because terminal sterilization, for example with ethylene oxide, may not adequately contact the internal portion of the powder mass. Aseptic crystallization involves dissolving the drug in a solvent and sterilizing the solution by passing it through a bacteria-retentive filter. To the sterile drug solution, a sterile solvent is added which causes precipitation of the drug. The drug is then removed by filtration, washed with sterile solvent, and dried, all under aseptic conditions.

Radiopharmaceuticals

Many pharmaceuticals are prepared as sterile intravenous solutions for diagnostic purposes. Generally, these are solutions of short-lived radionuclides which are used clinically in nuclear medicine to diagnose disease or lesions in various organs or tissues. For example, radiopharmaceuticals are used to study blood flow or localization of the agent within an organ or body system through the use of various scanning procedures. Following intravenous injection, a scintillation counter can follow a radiopharmaceutical as it enters or leaves an organ or body region. Such a procedure for scanning the brain offers safe and reasonably reliable detection of cerebral disease. A thorough discussion of the theory and fundamentals of producing radioactive dosage forms has been presented in Chapter 13. Suffice it to point out here that intravenous radiopharmaceuticals must meet all of the requirements for sterile injectables and, in addition, must adhere to more stringent requirements of packaging, labeling, storage, shipment and administration.

PRODUCT DEVELOPMENT

The formulation of an injectable preparation presents many technical problems. Some drugs are chemically unstable, and this property is magnified when the drug is in solution. The solubilization of poorly soluble drugs is a problem which requires the use of special techniques or the addition of solubilizing agents or cosolvents. The extent to which a substance dissolves in a solvent depends on the nature of the interaction and the forces present in the solute, in the solvent, and between the solute and solvent. The solubility of many poorly soluble compounds has been increased by utilizing one of the following approaches: cosolvency, complexation, solubilization, pH control, and chemical modification of the drug. Control of bacterial contamination is another problem, and often preservative agents must be added to injectable products. In the past decade, the interaction between the vial stopper and the vial contents of injections, especially interaction between the stopper and preservative(s) in multiple-dose vials, is a problem that has been investigated extensively.[25,26,37,47] Since rubber seems to be the most satisfactory closure for such vials, consideration must be given to its chemical makeup. Thus, the chemical reactivity of the closure and the container as well as the inherent stability of the injectable solution must be considered in the formulation of a parenteral to be supplied in multidose vials.

Selection of a Vehicle. Although water is always the solvent of choice for an injectable preparation, cosolvents are often used. In these systems, some of the water in the preparation is replaced by a water-miscible vehicle, such as ethyl alcohol, glycerin, dimethylacetamide, propylene glycol, or polyethylene glycol. Cosolvents may be used either to increase the solubility of the drug or to reduce its rate of hyrolytic degradation.

In selecting a vehicle for parenterals, there are three requirements: *solubility, stability,* and *safety.* It is generally understood that the vehicle should afford adequate solubility of the active ingredient and stability of the product, but it must also be pharmacologically acceptable. The chosen solvent must be nontoxic, nonirritating, and nonsensitizing and must not exert any pharmacological activity of its own, nor adversely affect the action of the active medicament. Additionally, the solvent must not cause hemolysis of the red blood cells.

Spiegel and Noseworthy[41] have published a rather extensive discussion of the use of nonaqueous solvents in parenteral products, particularly in cases where the drug is unstable in a wholly aqueous solution. For example, hydrolytic instability is a problem with barbiturate injections for which the solvent is not specified. Sixty percent propylene glycol is the solvent generally used because this delays hydrolysis of the barbiturate. However, the glycols are avoided whenever possible because of their undesirable side-reactions on injection.

Often, limited solubility and poor stability necessitate complete elimination of water from the dosage form and dictate the use of *nonaqueous hydrophobic solvents.* The group of compounds classified as fixed oils have been most commonly used for this purpose. The fixed oils must be of vegetable origin in order to undergo metabolism in the body following administration. Additionally, the fixed oils must be fluid at room temperature and possess sufficient chemical stability. The U.S.P. lists specifications for the fixed oils. Especially important is the requirement with regard to degree of unsaturation, an excess of which will produce tissue irritation. Standards for saponification value, iodine number, free fatty acids, and unsaponifiable matter have also been established. Even though the fixed oils employed for parenterals are of vegetable origin, it is required that the specific oil be listed on the label of a product, since some patients have exhibited allergic responses to certain vegetable oils. The oils most commonly employed are peanut, sesame, corn, and cottonseed. The steroids are often incorporated into an oil because the restricted diffusion of the drug from this hydrophobic solvent into the aqueous body fluids provides a prolonged type of action.

Oil solutions for parenteral injection require the same care in regard to providing clarity as do aqueous solutions. Since they are produced by expression, they invariably contain fragmentary cellular matter and bacteria. They may be clarified by repeated filtration through hard filter paper or very conveniently by the use of a membrane filter.

Selection of Added Substances. The same general principles apply to the formulation of parenterals, as apply in the preparation of ordinary dosage forms, with the following additional considerations:

1. Added substances must not be used in such quantity that they produce irritation or excessive toxicity.

2. Many substances which could be added with safety to an oral preparation would be too toxic or irritating for hypodermic use.

The official compendia place limitations upon added substances as follows:

Suitable substances may be added to preparations for injection to increase stability or usefulness unless proscribed in the individual monograph, provided that they are harmless in the amounts administered and do not interfere with the therapeutic efficacy or with responses to the specified assays and tests. No coloring agent may be added solely for the purpose of coloring the finished preparation, to a solution intended for parenteral administration.

Additives are generally employed in a parenteral preparation to enhance its chemical or physical stability, i.e., shelf life or esthetic appearance. Such additives include *buffering agents, antioxidants, solubilizers, tonicity contributors, antibacterial agents, chelating agents,* and numerous other substances. The requirements that these agents be nontoxic in the quantity administered to the patient and that they not interfere with the therapeutic efficacy or with the assay of the active substances makes selection of added substances a very crucial task. Specific limits are placed on certain additives. For example, agents containing mercury and cationic surface-active compounds are limited to a maximum concentration of 0.01 percent. For chlorobutanol, cresol, and phenol type preservatives, the limit is 0.5 percent, and for sulfur dioxide or an equivalent amount of sodium bisulfite or sodium sulfite, 0.2 percent. Additives which are routinely used in parenteral preparations are listed in Table 14-3.

Buffers. Changes in the pH of a preparation may occur during storage because of degradative reactions in the product, interaction of the product with container components (i.e., glass or rubber) and dissolution or loss of gases and vapors. To avoid

TABLE 14-3. ADDED SUBSTANCES IN PARENTERAL PRODUCTS

	USUAL CONCENTRATIONS
Preservatives	
Benzalkonium Chloride	0.01
Benzethonium Chloride	0.01
Benzyl Alcohol	2.0
Chlorobutanol	0.5
Phenylethyl Alcohol	0.5
Chlorocresol	0.1–0.3
Cresol	0.3–0.5
Methyl *p*-hydroxybenzoate	0.18
Propyl *p*-hydroxybenzoate	0.02
Phenol	0.5
Phenylmercuric Nitrate & Acetate	0.002
Thimerosal	0.01
*Antioxidants**	
Ascorbic Acid	0.1
Ascorbic Acid Esters	0.015
Butylhydroxy anisole (BHA)	0.02
Butylhydroxy voluene (BHT)	0.02
Cysteine	0.5
Sodium bisulfite	0.15
Sodium metabisulfite	0.2
Sodium formaldehyde sulfoxylate	0.1
Acetone sodium bisulfite	0.2
Tocopherols	0.5
Nordihydroguaiaretic acid (NDGA)	0.01
Chelating Agent	
Ethylenediaminetetraacetic acid (salt)	0.01–0.075
Buffers	
Acetic Acid and a salt	1–2
Citric Acid and a salt	1–3
Phosphoric Acid Salts	0.8–2
Tonicity Adjustment	
Dextrose	5.5
Sodium Chloride	0.9
Sodium sulfate	1.6

* Concentrations represent the maximum concentrations in parenterals.

these problems, buffers are added to many products to suppress changes in pH. A suitable buffer system should have a buffer capacity sufficient to maintain the pH of the product at a stable value during storage while permitting the body fluids to easily adjust the pH of the product to that of the blood following administration.

Buffer systems consist of either a combination of a weak acid and a salt of a weak acid or a weak base and the salt of a weak base. An example of the former is acetic acid and sodium acetate. In the acetic acid–sodium acetate system, the acid which exists largely in molecular (nonionized) form, combines with hydroxyl ions that may be added to form more acetate ion and water,

$$CH_3COOH + OH^- \rightarrow CH_3COO^- + H_2O$$

The acetate ion, which is a base, combines with hydronium ions that may be added to form more nonionized acetic acid and water.

$$CH_3COO^- + H_3O^+ \rightarrow CH_3COOH + H_2O$$

The change in pH is slight as long as the buffer capacity of the system is not exceeded. The principal buffer systems employed for parenterals are acetate, citrate, and phosphate. The effect of buffers on parenteral preparations has been studied by many workers[11,28,40,42,46] who have emphasized the importance of *buffer capacity* and *buffer effect* on both the stability and activity of the product.

Antioxidants. Many therapeutic agents are sensitive to oxygen. Even small amounts of air entrapped in a vial or ampul can cause oxidative degradation, particularly if the product is sterilized by a thermal method. Antioxidants can protect the product by acting as a reducing agent and being preferentially oxidized or by blocking an oxidative chain reaction.[38] Those that act as reducing agents include ascorbic acid, sodium bisulfite, and thiourea.[43] Those that block an oxidative chain reaction include the ascorbic acid esters, butylhydroxy anisole, and the tocopherols.[1]

Some substances act as synergists by increasing the effectiveness of the blocking agents. These include ascorbic acid, citric acid, and tartaric acid. A fourth group are the chelating agents such as the ethylenediaminetetraacetate salts. These salts complex with metal ions which can catalyze oxidative reactions.[4,18,39]

Another approach to the problem of oxidative instability is to reduce the oxygen content of solutions by flushing them prior to and during filling with an inert gas such as nitrogen or carbon dioxide.

Preservatives. Suitable antibacterial or preservative agents must be added to preparations packaged in multi-dose containers, regardless of the method of sterilization, unless prohibited by the monograph or unless the active agent is itself bacteriostatic. Such substances, when added, must be in sufficient concentration to prevent the growth of, or kill, microorganisms. Sterilization procedures are employed even though such agents are present. Antibacterial agents are specifically excluded in the large-volume injections which are used to replace fluid, nutrients, or electrolytes, such as Dextrose and Sodium Chloride Injection, U.S.P., Dextrose Injection, U.S.P., Ringer's Injection, U.S.P., Lactated Ringer's Injection, U.S.P., and Sodium Chloride Injection, U.S.P. Bacteriostatic agents may be added to Dextrose and Sodium Chloride Injection, U.S.P., when it is labeled for use as a sclerosing agent, because the amount of injection used for such purpose is small, and the quantity of bactericide present would not be harmful to the patient.

Antibacterial agents are often included in formulations packaged in ampuls and unit dose containers especially if the products are sterilized by marginal processes or filtration. The effectiveness of the antibacterial agent in a specific product must be demonstrated as stipulated by the compendia under antimicrobial effectiveness tests. In order for the antibacterial agent to be considered effective, a static effect against spores and a cidal effect against nonsporulating organisms is required when the product is challenged with inoculums of vegetative bacteria, yeasts, and bacterial spores. The effectiveness and stability of preservatives has been discussed in several publications.[15,23,24] Some commonly used antibacterial agents are listed in Table 14-3.

Tonicity Contributors. Red blood cells (erythrocytes), when introduced into water or sodium chloride solutions containing less than 0.9 grams of solute per 100 ml., will swell and often burst because of the diffusion of water into the cell and the fact that the cell wall is not sufficiently strong to resist the pressure. This phenomenon is referred to as *hemolysis*. Isotonicity is important for parenteral preparations because the possibility that the product may penetrate red blood cells and cause hemolysis is greatly reduced if the solution is isotonic with blood, i.e., the cells maintain their "tone." Also, compounds contributing to the isotonicity of a product often reduce pain at the site of injection in areas with nerve endings. A 0.9 percent sodium chloride solution is isotonic with the blood.

The isotonicity of a solution depends not only upon its *colligative properties,* but also upon the permeability of mammalian cell membranes. Even though a solution may have the same freezing point as blood, i.e., it is iso-osmotic, penetration of the cell membrane by components of the solution can cause the cell to rupture. For example, a 1.8 percent solution of urea has the same osmotic pressure as 0.9 percent sodium chloride, but the urea solution produces hemolysis. Therefore, a preparation cannot be considered to be isotonic until it has been tested in a biological system. Hemolytic methods using red blood cells have been described.[2,19]

Containers and Container Components. Although the use of plastic containers has been increasing for nonsterile pharmaceutical products, parenteral preparations are generally packaged in glass containers (Fig. 14-9). In many cases the glass containers are sealed or closed with rubber stoppers. The fact that the product is in intimate contact with glass and rubber surfaces makes the selection of the container and container components as important as selection of the product ingredient and added substances.

Glass containers are preferred because of their relative chemical inertness compared to plastic materials. However, no container can be shown to be totally nonreactive. Aqueous solutions, especially at alkaline pH's, can react at glass surfaces. Adsorption of ingredients has occurred on glass surfaces, and often materials are leached from the glass and deposited as fine swirls or flakes in the solution. These reactions are generally accelerated by the elevated temperature required for autoclaving.

Glass compounds are classified into four types by the U.S.P., and each type must meet specific test limits for chemical resistance. Table 14-4 lists the types of glass and gives a description and general use for each type. Type I glass offers the greatest chemical resistance and is preferred for most sterile products; however, Types II and III may be used as long as suitable testing has shown that the product is stable in contact with these glass types.

The glass container should be of sufficient strength to withstand the abuse of washing, processing, sterilization, shipping and storage, it should be uniform in physical dimensions, to allow mechanical handling, and should be transparent, to permit inspection of the solution for particulate matter. Containers for injectable preparations range from 1,000 ml. for intravenous fluids to 0.5 ml, for some highly potent therapeutic agents. Multi-dose containers are limited to 30 ml. in size by the U.S.P. This limitation is intended to limit the number of doses in a single container, since each entry into the vial increases the risk of

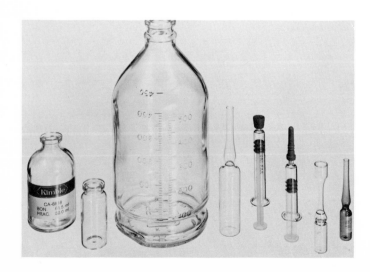

FIG. 14-9. Various types of containers used for parenteral products. (Courtesy of Kimble, Owens, Illinois)

TABLE 14-4.   U.S.P. XVIII CLASSIFICATION OF GLASS TYPES

TYPE	DESCRIPTION	GENERAL USE
I	Highly resistant borosilicate glass	All uses.
II	Treated soda-lime glass	Buffered aqueous solutions with pH below 7.0. Dry powders, oil solutions.
III	Soda-lime glass	Dry powders, oil solutions.
NP	General purpose soda-lime glass	Not for parenterals.

microbial contamination. Glass cartridges are used to contain the drug solution in disposable syringes.

The application of a thin film of silicone (referred to as *siliconization*) to coat the inside of vials and ampuls has been employed to prevent interaction of the preparation with the glass surface. Siliconization of glass containers minimizes adsorption of active ingredient from homogenous solutions, prevents aggregation at the glass surface in colloidal preparations, and prevents adsorption of solids from suspensions. Siliconization of glass and rubber components is essential in prefilled disposable syringes in order to provide the lubrication required for ease of administration. The methods for siliconizing glass containers include application of the silicone by spraying (*atomization*), rinsing or swabbing, followed by curing at elevated temperatures.

Rubber closures and plastic materials are considered part of the container when they serve to contain the product and are in direct contact with it. The compendia describe biological and physicochemical tests on extracts from rubber closures and plastics. Such tests are used to determine acute toxicity and control the quality of subsequent supplies of materials.

Safety Testing. All parenteral products must be subjected to rigid evaluations of *toxicity, tissue tolerance, pyrogenicity,* and *tonicity* in order to assess their safety. *Pyrogenicity,* i.e., the ability to produce a rise in body temperature, and *tonicity* have been discussed previously in this chapter. For determination of toxicity and tissue tolerance it is necessary that the product be in the final container so that all the factors that might contribute to an unsafe product will be present.

Toxicity is determined by *behavior stud-ies* in animals, which are conducted to observe functions such as *motor activity, respiration rate, righting reflex, loss of consciousness,* etc. An assessment of *acute toxicity* is made by determining both the LD_{50}, i.e., the dose which causes death in 50 percent of the animals, and the cause of death. *Chronic toxicity* is evaluated by administering a fraction of the LD_{50} for extended periods of time and observing the cumulative effects of the product.

Tissue tolerance is evaluated by administering the product, generally to rabbits, by the subcutaneous and intramuscular routes for extended periods. The animals are sacrificed at varying time intervals and tissues are fixed for histological examination. The effect of repeated injections, pH, and volume are evaluated.

PRODUCTION OF PARENTERALS

A product that is developed utilizing the best methods and with ingredients of the highest quality can be rendered unacceptable if the manufacturing process or facilities are not adequate. Therefore, strict controls to ensure adherence to standard operating procedures and the maintenance of a clean environment are essential in order to produce a quality product. As with other pharmaceutical dosage forms, the production operation encompasses a multitude of functions, from the weighing of the ingredients of the formula to the final packaging of the product for distribution. The major elements in carrying out these varied functions are the personnel and the facilities.

DESIGN OF FACILITIES

Maximum cleanliness is required for the manufacture of sterile products. Therefore, the facilities must be designed to assure low

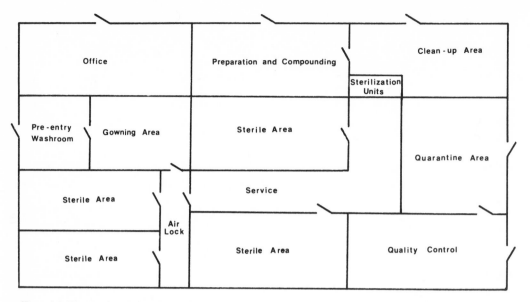

FIG. 14-10.   A hypothetical floor plan of a sterile products area with its services.

levels of biological and particulate contamination under actual operating conditions. Knowledge of the purpose of the facilities is essential in the layout of an operation and the selection of construction materials. Additionally, it is extremely important that the design of the facilities and selection of materials be approached with the goal of effecting optimum control. Last but not least is the need to create an attractive operation and one that permits maximum comfort to the personnel.

Although the design for the manufacture of disposable syringes varies in detail from that for the manufacture of ampuls and vials, in both cases the production operation is normally divided into five distinct areas. These include the *clean-up area,* the *preparation area,* the *aseptic area,* the *quarantine area,* and the *finishing* or *packaging area* (Fig. 14-10). The flow of materials is generally in the order given above and can be illustrated by the following process flow scheme:

The *aseptic area* is the heart of the sterile products operation. It is where the product begins to take on an identity. The environment in which the product is born must be ultra-clean and, to achieve optimum control of cleanliness, clean rooms are used. In order to permit an efficient flow of materials, the aseptic area should be located adjacent to the other areas. However, to maintain an aseptic environment, adequate isolation is required. The ceilings, walls, and floors must be of a construction which permits easy cleaning. Partitions should be properly sealed to prevent the accumulation of dirt and moisture and to prevent the exchange of air with other areas. Glass panels are generally built into the walls to permit greater visibility and facilitate supervision from a nonsterile area. Additionally, the glass partitions bring comfort to the personnel by providing less confining surroundings. The floors can be a particular problem in clean rooms because they are subject to shear forces when people walk across them,

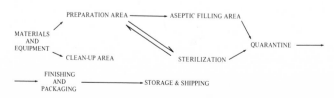

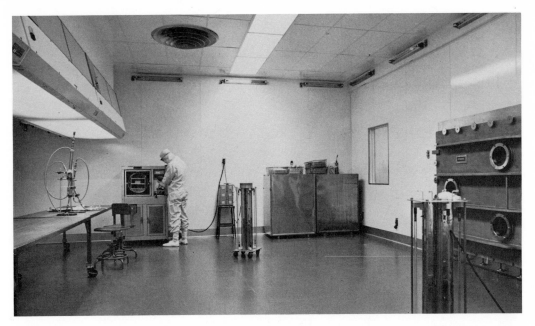

Fig. 14-11.   An aseptic area demonstrating typical construction features. (Courtesy of Ben Venue Laboratories)

resulting in the generation of particles. A resilient vinyl which resists breakdown is generally used in clean rooms (Fig. 14-11).

The aseptic area should be equipped with ports and services to permit the passage of solution from one area to another, thereby eliminating the need for transferring tanks of material to the area. Items of equipment that are difficult or impossible to sterilize should be kept out of the aseptic areas, if possible. If they must be used in the aseptic area, they should remain there and be continuously exposed to disinfecting processes (Fig. 14-12). Whenever possible, operating machinery parts should be enclosed in stainless steel housings.

Entry of personnel to the aseptic area should be through airlocks, in accordance with rigidly established procedures. Such procedures include removal of street clothing, washing of hands, and donning of the appropriate attire, i.e., gowns, hats, shoes, face masks, and gloves (Fig. 14-13). During an aseptic operation, personnel movement within the room should be minimal, and unauthorized personnel and personnel assigned to other areas should be prohibited from the aseptic area.

The *clean-up area* does not need to be aseptic but it must be easily cleaned and kept clean. Since this area is subjected to considerable moisture and heat, the construction must be able to withstand such rigors. An adequate exhaust system should be provided for employee comfort and to minimize the risk of contamination entering the sterile room from this area.

Compounding of the formula is generally carried out in the *preparation area,* and it is here that the materials and items are prepared for sterile processing. Therefore, adequate space and services are required. Although the preparation room need not be sterile, it should be maintained in a cleaner state than the clean-up area.

Sterilization equipment should be provided with access from both a sterile and a nonsterile environment. Double door units with one door in the sterile area are most desirable. A *gowning room* should be located next to the aseptic area but separated from it by an airlock. It is most desirable that sinks and drying units be kept out of the gowning area and be located in a pre-entry room next to the gowning area. A pre-entry room prevents personnel from

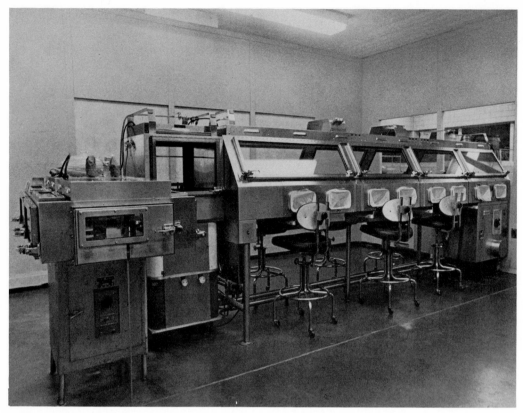

Fig. 14-12.   A clean room, showing an enclosed cabinet in which filling and sealing operations are performed. (Courtesy of Schering-Plough Corporation)

entering the gowning area directly from a hallway and permits them to remove street shoes, jewelry, head covers, lab coats, etc., and "scrub-up" before entering the gowning area. The doors on these rooms should be electronically controlled to permit the opening of only one door at a time in any one room.

Environmental Control. The cleanliness achieved by a clean room is dependent on the air-handling system's ability to purge the room of contaminants. This includes not only effectiveness of the filters and the number of air changes per hour but also the distribution of the air within the room.

The air in the sterile production operation must be exchanged at frequent intervals. Fresh outside air must be filtered through a prefilter to remove large particles. It then passes through filters of various capabilities, depending on the area the air is entering. In the aseptic area, a *high efficiency particulate air filter* is used. This filter has the capability of removing particles of 0.5 microns or greater with an efficiency of 99.97 percent. In most clean rooms, the air then passes through an electrostatic filter which removes virtually all foreign matter. A further precaution is to install ultraviolet lights in the air ducts downstream from the filters.

The air handling system should be designed to change the room air approximately 20 times per hour. The room's ability to rid itself of contaminants is a function of air changes; however, at some point the increased velocities stir up more dust than they purge. Clean, aseptic air enters the room under positive pressure and this positive pressure should be maintained in the aseptic area and adjacent rooms which enter into the aseptic area. The pressure should be greatest in the aseptic area and progressively decrease in going from the aseptic area to the airlock to the gowning area to the pre-

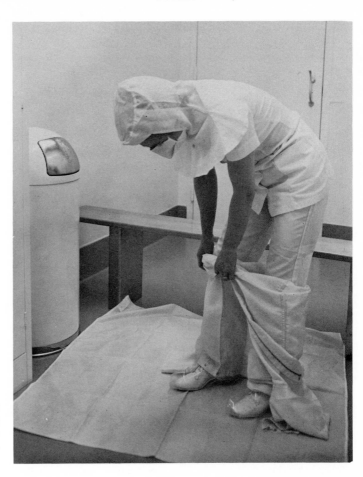

Fig. 14-13. An operator in the process of gowning prior to entry into an aseptic area. (Courtesy of Ciba-Geigy)

entry room. Positive pressure prevents outside air from rushing into the aseptic area through cracks, temporarily open doors, or other openings. Mercury gauges should be clearly visible, showing the pressures in these areas at all times, or a recording device should be installed to monitor pressure at all times and provide a permanent record.

Technological advances in the last decade have significantly improved environmental control of aseptic areas. The development of *laminar air flow enclosures* is an example. In laminar air flow the air passes through high efficiency particulate air filters and is blown at a uniform velocity in one direction (Fig. 14-14). Contamination is prevented in the enclosure because it is continually swept clean with the air flow. Laminar flow stratifies the air so that minimum cross-stream contamination occurs. There is little or no transfer of energy from one streamline to another. Suspended particulate matter or microorganisms in one streamline tend to stay in that streamline until they are captured or collide.

Laminar flow rooms are second generation clean rooms. In the pharmaceutical industry, such rooms are still in their infancy, mainly because the majority of clean rooms in use today are of the conventional type and were designed and built prior to the introduction of the laminar-flow principle. These first generation rooms represent a substantial investment. However, it would be safe to say that all pharmaceutical operations utilize laminar flow to some extent. Hoods and cabinets, available at reasonable cost, are being used in filling and assembling operations, and these have been found to be as good as if the entire room were laminar flow. Hoods, which can be positioned over filling machines without taking up any floor

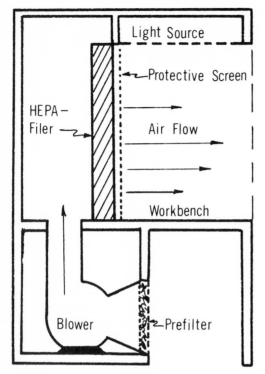

FIG. 14-14. A cut-away view of a horizontal laminar air flow console.

space, and cabinets, which provide either vertical or horizontal flow, are being used for specific assembly, filling, and filtration operations. Additionally, specially built units are used to control the environment in staging areas.

Classification of Clean Rooms. The need for classifying clean rooms and establishing standards was demonstrated by the aerospace industry long before the pharmaceutical industry began using such rooms. With the development of laminar flow rooms, several standards from different agencies resulted. The standard accepted by the pharmaceutical industry is one that classifies clean rooms according to the level of particulate matter. The three classes of clean rooms defined by this standard are shown in Table 14-5.

Clean room classifications are based on particle count per cubic foot of air and are defined in terms of the maximum number of particles in the 0.5 micron or larger and 5.0 microns or larger size ranges. These limits are established as operational levels. All clean rooms and work stations as desig-

TABLE 14-5.   CLEAN ROOM CLASSES

CLASS	MAXIMUM NUMBER OF PARTICLES PER CUBIC FOOT 0.5 MICRON AND LARGER	MAXIMUM NUMBER OF PARTICLES PER CUBIC FOOT 5.0 MICRON AND LARGER
100	100	—
10,000	10,000	65
100,000	100,000	700

nated by this standard must be capable of meeting at least one of the following performance classes:

Class 100: particle count not to exceed a total of 100 particles per cu. ft. 0.5 micron and larger.

Class 10,000: particle count not to exceed a total of 10,000 particles per cu. ft. 0.5 micron and larger, or 65 particles per cu. ft. 5.0 microns and larger.

Class 100,000: particle count not to exceed a total of 100,000 particles per cu. ft. 0.5 micron and larger or 700 particles per cu. ft. 5.0 microns and larger.

The pressure in all clean rooms shall be above that of surrounding areas to assure that all leakage shall be outward.

Personnel.   Staffing requirements for preparing sterile products vary, depending on the nature of the operation and the products prepared. Common to all operations is the fact that nonprofessional persons are required, and these people are generally supervised by persons with professional training. Supervisors must be individuals who understand the particular requirements of aseptic procedures and who are able to obtain the full cooperation of other employees in fulfilling these exacting requirements.

Where a pharmaceutical product is involved, it is desirable to have pharmacists supervising the development and manufacturing operations. Although his training and formal education in manufacturing sterile products are often limited, his knowledge and appreciation for drugs and drug systems makes him readily adaptable to this type of undertaking. In those operations in which a pharmaceutical product is not involved, i.e., empty syringes, surgical gloves, I.V. administration sets, a person with a strong background in the biological sciences is desirable to supervise the sterile operations. Quality Control supervisors should have a good science background with particular expertise in analytical chemistry or microbiology. All operations should have the services of a professional engineer, an accountant, and a personnel (labor relations) expert.

In any sterile products operation, nonprofessional personnel are used in all its aspects, and it is important that they appreciate the vital role they play in determining the quality of the final product. Intensive instruction in the principles of aseptic processes is required. Personnel involved with the preparation of sterile products must be neat, orderly, reliable, and mentally alert. They should be in good health and should receive physical examinations at regular intervals to be sure that they are not carriers of a disease or are not in a weakened condition so that they themselves may be vulnerable to a disease state. Personnel assigned to the aseptic area should be cognizant of the necessity to report

the symptoms of a head cold or other communicable illness.

STEPS IN PROCESSING

In the processing of a sterile product there are five essential elements to be considered— the *facility,* the *ingredients,* the *equipment,* the *container components,* and the *personnel.* To facilitate a clear comprehension of the passage of materials through the various phases of processing in the preparation of sterile products, flow diagrams for aseptic and nonaseptic processing operations are represented in Figures 14-15 and 14-16.

The *facility* must be properly prepared for each type of operation. Generally, the clean room or aseptic area is prepared in the same manner whether an aseptic or a nonaseptic run is planned, because the requirements for particulate matter are the same in each case. However, for an aseptic run, after cleaning the room is usually left idle and exposed to ultraviolet irradiation for a period of 2 to 8 hours. This provides

ASEPTIC   PROCESSING

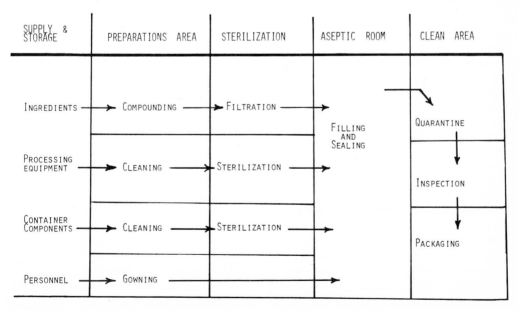

FIG. 14-15.   A typical flow diagram for the processing of a product to be sterilized by filtration.

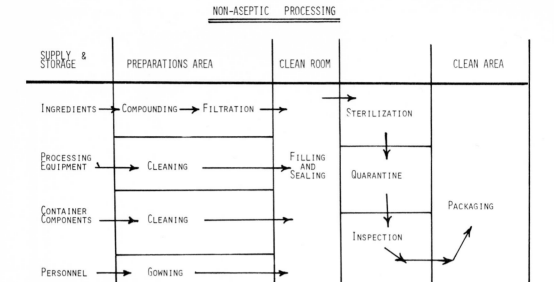

FIG. 14-16.   A typical flow diagram for the processing of a product to be terminally sterilized.

greater assurance of asepsis should the cleaning procedure have failed to destroy all microbial contamination. As much as possible of the equipment and components needed for the run should be in the room during the idle period to permit maximum exposure to ultraviolet light and, more important, to limit movement just before or during the run.

The *ingredients* are compounded according to the master formula in a clean area. For a solution, the product is filtered and transferred to the clean room for filling into individual containers. *Equipment* is processed in a clean area and transferred to the clean room. *Container components,* i.e., vials, ampuls, closures, are processed in a clean environment in an area designed for a low particulate level. They are then depyrogenated and transferred to the clean room. *Personnel* enter the clean room through the gowning area after donning the required garments. After filling and sealing, the product is subjected to sterilization by the appropriate method and placed in quarantine until the quality control tests are conducted. If the product specifications are met, the product is 100 percent inspected for visual defects and transferred to the packaging area.

In an *aseptic process,* the sterilization step

occurs prior to the filling step. It is very important in an aseptic operation that the facilities undergo bacteriological monitoring prior to and during the filling operation. This is done by placing culture plates at predetermined locations to determine the microbial contamination levels in those areas.[22] It is also appropriate to follow an aseptic filling operation with filling of sterile nutrient media to determine if an effective aseptic operation was conducted. Such control procedures help in locating problems and enable corrective action to be taken.

All equipment and supplies introduced into the aseptic area should be sterile and should have entered the aseptic area directly from the sterilizers, preferably through double-ended chambers (Fig. 14-17). The solution should enter the aseptic area during the sterile filtration process through small ports in the wall. This eliminates transfer of bulk material manually from nonsterile to sterile areas. Small equipment, supplies, and glassware should be wrapped with easily sterilized paper. While a product is undergoing processing, all supplies must be introduced into the aseptic filling rooms in a manner that maintains the environment in an aesptic state. Once the product containers have been sealed, the risk of contamination

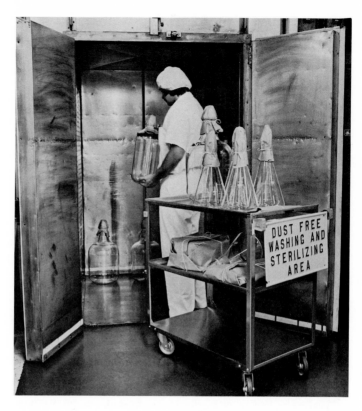

FIG. 14-17. Double door sterilizing chambers in the process of being loaded. Following sterilization the contents will exit directly to the sterile area. (Courtesy of Schering Corporation)

of the contents is greatly minimized or eliminated.

Cleaning of Container Components. Containers of all types and all container components should be cleaned before filling. This is accomplished by washing with a detergent solution, rinsing with freshly distilled water and drying. For glassware, it is convenient to dry, sterilize, and depyrogenate in a single operation by using dry heat at 225°C. Detergents that leave a residue during washing should be avoided. In many cases it is possible to eliminate the use of detergents by using alternate treatments of hot and cold water. Machines are available that mechanically inject the washing and rinsing needles through the neck of the containers and partially dry them by blowing in filtered compressed air (Fig. 14-18). Another method for cleaning glassware is by ultrasonics. This is a more expensive method and involves special equipment to transfer electrical energy into physical energy. Whatever method is used for cleaning containers, it is important that the wet, clean containers be handled in such a way that contamination

will not be reintroduced. A wet surface collects contaminants more readily than a dry surface.

Rubber Closures. Rubber closures as received from the supplier require careful cleaning because they are generally coated with lubricants from the molding operation as well as other debris which may have adhered to the surface. The recommended procedure for cleaning rubber closures calls for gentle mechanical agitation in a hot solution of a water softener such as 0.5 percent sodium pyrophosphate. The gentle motion of the liquid aids in the removal of the contaminants. Excessive agitation or tumbling, especially during the drying cycle, should be avoided, because it can result in the abrasion of the closures with formation of particles of rubber.

Filling. When the bulk liquid has been compounded and filtered or the suspension properly dispersed, the liquid is ready for filling of the containers. In the case of suspensions, provision must be made to keep the liquid agitated in order to ensure uniform distribution of the active constituent.

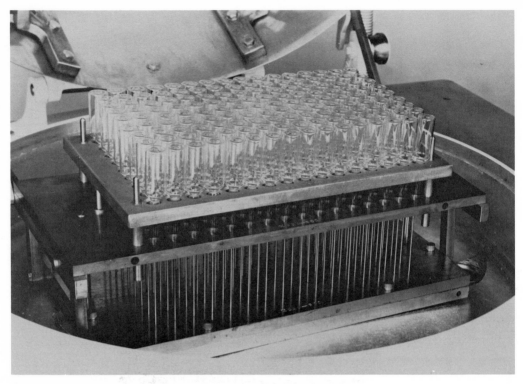

Fig. 14-18. Cleaning of glass vials by intermittent washing with hot and cold water and then final rinsing with distilled water. (Courtesy of Cozzoli Machine Company)

Normally, the liquid is fed directly from the collecting vessel to the filling machine by means of sterile tubing.

The filling machine is equipped with glass or stainless steel syringes and plungers to accurately dispense small volumes into individual containers. The stroke of the syringe plunger forces the liquid from a reservoir through a valve before delivery into the container. The parts of the filling machine that come into contact with the liquid should be easily demounted for cleaning and sterilization. Additionally, these parts should be of a nonreactive composition and should withstand the rigors of processing, cleaning, and sterilization. More sophisticated machinery has provision for flushing containers with an inert gas, such as nitrogen or carbon dioxide, prior to introducing the liquid and sealing. The ideal equipment is a fully automated system to wash, dry, sterilize, flush, fill, and seal the containers in one continuous operation (Fig.14-19).

Because it is practically impossible to withdraw the entire content of a container into a hypodermic syringe, a slight excess is placed in the container. The excess amount necessary varies with the size of the container and the viscosity of the liquid; hence, the official compendia present tables indicating the excess volumes which are usually sufficient. For mobile liquids, the recommended excess varies from 20 percent for a volume of 0.5 ml. to 2 percent for a volume of 50 ml. For viscous liquids the variation is from 24 to 30 percent for the same volumes.

The filling of *sterile solids* such as the antibiotics into individual containers is a more difficult matter, since many factors can influence the flow properties of the material. Powders are usually filled by weighing or volumetric measurement. Weighing the quantity of powder into the container is a manual operation and is very slow. Consequently, volumetric measuring is employed on automatic filling machines. One type of machine utilizes an auger which rotates in the stem of a funnel containing the powder. The size

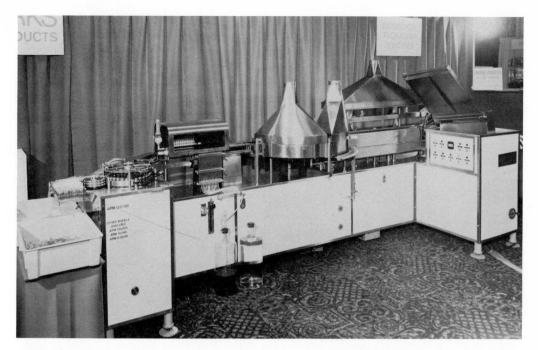

Fig. 14-19.   High-speed processing machine for ampuls. Starting from the right, the equipment will feed ampuls directly from the suppliers package, and wash, dry and sterilize the ampuls prior to filling and sealing. (Courtesy of Corning Glass Works)

and rotation of the auger regulates the amount of powder dispensed. Another type of filling machine operates on a vacuum principle in which a vacuum is pulled on a cavity into which the powder flows before being discharged into the container. The fill weights on either type of powder-filling equipment must be monitored continually. Regardless of the accuracy claimed by the manufacturer, the accuracy of the quantity delivered cannot be controlled as well with powder as with liquids; therefore, the tolerances permitted for the content of containers may be relatively large. Allowable tolerances generally run as high as ±10 percent, calculated from the average labeled net weight of contents.

Sealing.   The sealing operation constitutes a critical step in the processing of a sterile product, because generally it represents the final aseptic procedure. Once the container is sealed, the chances for contamination are greatly minimized or completely eliminated (Fig. 14-20). Ampuls may be closed by melting a portion of the glass of the neck with a fine jet of flame. The fine string of glass which results when the tip is pulled away melts down to a round bead and forms a seal. In some cases, the very tip of the open end of the ampul is heated to form a bead-seal. In all cases, however, there should be no droplets of liquid remaining from the filling step in the neck of the ampul during sealing. Such materials would carbonize and discolor the ampul at the point of sealing and may also cause the seal to crack as it cools.

In the sealing of *vials with rubber closures,* the closures must fit snugly into the opening to produce an airtight seal. Generally, the closures are coated with silicone or Teflon in order to facilitate introduction into the vial opening. Aluminum caps are placed over the stopper and crimped around and under the lip of the vial. The caps possess a covered center hold which can be exposed at the time of use (Fig. 14-21).

OPHTHALMIC PRODUCTS

Sterile ophthalmic products may be relatively uncomplicated over-the-counter products, such as ocular decongestants and con-

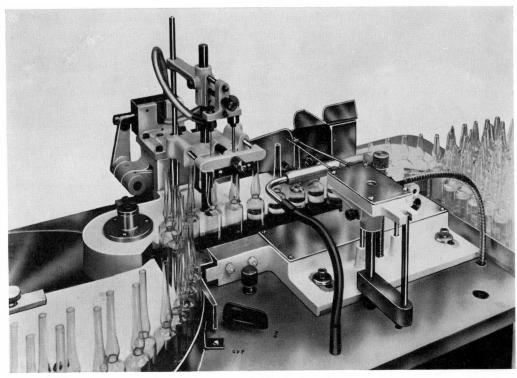

FIG. 14-20. Automatic ampul-filling and sealing machines which mechanically flushes with an inert gas, fills, pull-seals and ejects the ampuls. (From Cozzoli Machine Company)

tact lens solutions, or relatively complex corticosteroid suspension products prescribed for various inflammatory conditions of the eye, or specialized parenteral-type products for use intraocularly in various surgical procedures, such as foreign body removal, corneal transplant, or cataract removal.

Although the unabraded cornea is relatively resistant to infection from various environmental microorganisms, predisposition of the eye to infection due to minor abrasion or other factors contributing to the reduction of corneal or conjunctival integrity requires that products designed for instillation onto the exterior surfaces of the eye, especially an injured eye, must be free from microorganisms which could cause infection. Even under ideal circumstances, microorganisms ordinarily considered to be nonpathogens can cause an infection in the eye. The most dangerous of the microorganisms is the pathogen *Pseudomonas aeruginosa.* Fulminant corneal infection caused by this microorganism can result in total corneal destruction with loss of sight within 24 to 48 hours.

Staphylococcus aureus and *albus* infections, while less fulminating in their course, can be equally as dangerous. In addition to these, various fungal and viral infections are of increasing concern to the ophthalmologist.

Because of these factors, ophthalmic medication must be manufactured using the latest aseptic methodology to produce sterile products. Moreover, highly efficient microbiological preservative systems are included in products designed for instillation onto the exterior surface of the eye to ensure the microbiological cleanliness of ophthalmic products while in the hands of the patient. The effectiveness of these preservative systems must be verified by challenging the product with large concentrations of up to 20 different microorganisms representing gram-negative and gram-positive varieties plus molds, yeasts, and fungi.

In considering the formulation of ophthalmic products, the site of application of the product determines, to a large extent, the formulation design criteria. Products designed for introduction into the anterior or

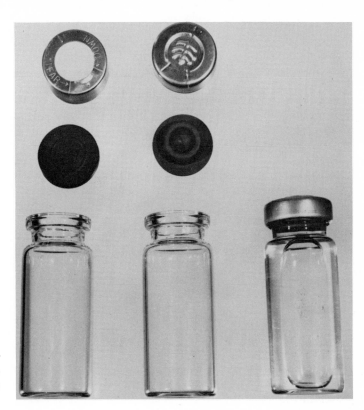

Fig. 14-21. Various components of a multidose vial. (Courtesy of Kimble, Owens, Illinois)

posterior chambers, such as alpha chymotrypsin, carbachol, acetylcholine, and various balanced salt solutions, should contain no preservative substances, because these have been shown to be incompatible with the tissues of the anterior chamber of the eye.[20] Additionally, the proper balance of various ionic species in such a solution is necessary for the viability of various tissues of the anterior chamber of the eye.[12,16] Products designed for this use should be adjusted to the physiologic range of pH 7.0 to 7.4, if possible. If pH values outside the physiologic range are required—for instance, to maintain optimal drug stability—these solutions should be as lightly buffered as possible.

Particulate contamination in ophthalmic products must be avoided. While it is not completely known what the *total* effect of particle inclusion in the anterior chamber might be, possible results include iritis, uveitis, granulomas, and, due to blockage of the aqueous humor outflow mechanism, increased intraocular pressure and the onset of glaucoma.

For products designed for instillation into the cul-de-sac, ocular irritation, discomfort, and the propensity to induce pathology are important considerations. Comfortable use can be achieved with many products simply by adjusting the solution to isotonicity and, if outside the physiologic pH range, providing for minimal buffer capacity. In general, comfort is directly related to buffer capacity at pH values outside of the physiologic range. In other instances, however, a component (or components) of the composition may contribute to discomfort. If this happens to be the active ingredient or some unexpendable component, the problem becomes more difficult.

Ocular irritation and propensity to induce pathology must be evaluated by a discrete and highly specialized methodology and evaluated by methods similar to those described by Daize et al.[12] As an example, some manufacturers require a product to show a low "Daize" score when 20 doses are administered to rabbits in a single day at dosing intervals of 20 minutes. Preservative systems must be chosen for optimal performance in balance with minimal irritation.

When suspension products are a uniformly small particle size will ensure absence of particle generated discomfort and irritation, especially at concentrations of greater than 0.5 percent of suspended solid. Cosolvents such as glycols and surfactants must be used with caution, taking into consideration their propensity to cause ocular irritation and to diminish the efficacy of included preservative systems.

Vehicles, in general, play an important role in ophthalmic products designed for instillation into the cul-de-sac. Cellulosic viscosity-imparting agents such as hydroxypropylmethylcellulose, methylcellulose, and hydroxyethylcellulose as well as the noncellulosic agent polyvinyl alcohol have been shown to increase the residence time of a drop of solution on the eye. This increased residence time has been shown to increase the efficacy of certain drugs when incorporated with these viscosity-imparting agents.[27,44]

After the final formulation has been developed with careful attention to the problems of patient discomfort and pharmaceutical stability, it must be determined, by close cooperation with the preclinical pharmacologist, that no component of the total formula diminishes the activity or increases the toxicity of the active component.

New concepts in drug delivery to the eye are continuously evolving through vigorous study of various liquid, semisolid, and solid drug delivery systems. The next decade should witness improvements in the delivery of drug products to the eye never before thought feasible. This will enable the medical practitioner to treat various disorders of the eye with concentrations of drug greatly reduced from those in use today, thus eliminating some of the discomforting side effects accompanying today's therapy.

QUALITY CONTROL

The principles of quality control and quality assurance are basically the same for the manufacture of any pharmaceutical product, and the responsibility for supervising these tasks is an enormous one, requiring strict adherence to procedural requirements and specifications. For the manufacture of parenteral products, this grave responsibility is especially critical. *Quality control cannot begin with the finished product; it is important to accept the concept that it is a stepwise control of the product during all phases of the manufacturing process.* Thus, the overall quality of the product is directly related to and influenced by its design during research and development. Total drug quality depends on the interrelationship of many factors besides just the placing of the active substance in a dosage form. The design of a new product must provide for appropriate physical-chemical characteristics of the material in the dosage form and the appropriate manufacturing process for the product. Consideration of these factors allow specifications to be established which assure product uniformity.

Most organizations involved in producing sterile products appreciate the value of *good manufacturing practices.*[14] Therefore, it has become necessary that buildings, facilities, and equipment used in the production of sterile products be specially designed for their purpose. Contamination of a product is minimized by maintaining a clean environment. All components and materials are identified and examined to assure that they are of the highest standards and devoid of contamination. Proper storage of the materials further aids the production of clean products.

Rules and regulations published in the Federal Register, Section 133.11, call for the establishment of scientifically sound and appropriate specifications, standards, and test procedures to assure that components in processed drugs and finished products conform to appropriate standards of identity, strength, quality, and purity. It is stated that laboratory controls should be developed to assure adherence to these regulations.

For sterile products, incoming stock control encompasses routine analytical tests on all ingredients to assure adherence to established raw material specifications. Special tests include pyrogen tests on water for injection, glass tests on containers, and identity tests on rubber closures. *In-process control* involves a multitude of tests, check points, and observations during the manufacturing process. Some of these in-process controls include conductivity measurements during the distillation of water for injection, volume fill checks during the filling operations, bacteriological plate monitoring of the processing areas, visual inspection of the product, and confirmation of the suitability of processing equipment and the identity of labels for the product. Sterilization procedures are often monitored continually with biological indicators. This involves samples of the product which contain an inoculum of specific microorganisms. In this way, the efficiency of the equipment and the process can be assured, since sterility tests can be performed on only a relatively small number of samples from a batch. Controls on the finished product involve a number of final tests. These include chemical and biological analysis, sterility evaluation, clarity testing, and leak and pyrogen testing where applicable. Further discussion of quality control of sterile products will be limited to specific finished product tests required by the official compendia.

Sterility Testing. Present methods of sterilization, with the exception of aseptic filtration, depend on the destruction rather than removal of microorganisms from products. Therefore, microscopic examination for the determination of sterility is of little value. Sterility test methods for pharmaceutical and other sterile products are dependent on the presence of viable microorganisms in the product. The tests are designed to detect the presence of bacteria, yeasts, and fungi. Unfortunately, specific tests for viruses require cumbersome cultivation, and for practical purposes the absence of bacteria, yeasts, and fungi is regarded as the absence of all viable organisms.

The only sure method for guaranteeing absolute sterility of a batch is to test every unit. However, this is not possible, since the sterility test is a destructive test. The U.S.P. lists the procedural details for sterility testing and the sample sizes to be employed. The type of culture media employed and the time and temperature of incubation are important considerations in sterility testing. Of main concern is the detection of microorganisms capable of growing at body temperatures. Therefore, present methods employ temperatures of 30 to 35°C., which are suitable for a wide variety of microorganisms. Fluid thioglycollate is the culture medium generally selected for this purpose; the incubation time varies, depending on the nature of the product and the type of sterilization employed. For a liquid product sterilized in the final container by steam under pressure, a 7-day incubation period is sufficient. However, for the same product sterilized by other means, a 14-day incubation period is required. For a product that is a solid and is sterilized by steam under pressure, a 10-day incubation period is required.

Molds and fungi grow readily at room temperature and, for this reason, the accepted temperature of incubation is 20 to 25°C. Soybean-Casein Digest is the medium selected for this purpose and incubation periods are the same as for the thioglycollate fluid.

Since many products possess bacteriostatic properties or contain preservatives, false negatives can often occur. It is necessary, therefore, to treat such products with a suitable inactivating agent, such as Tween 80 or lecithin, prior to culturing on the medium. A better method of overcoming the inherent inhibitory properties of the product involves the use of *membrane* filters (Fig. 14-22). The filtration method involves the passage of the product through a sterile bacteria-retentive membrane filter and washing of the filter with suitable nutrient fluid. The filter is then removed and subjected to the sterility test. The membrane method is not restricted to products possessing bacteriostatic and fungistatic activity but is also used for the testing of oils and ointments.

Since the current sampling plans for the official sterility test procedures cannot guarantee the detection of low levels of contamination (i.e., if the contamination level in a large batch is below 5 percent), the probability of detecting contamination in the 10 or 20 samples is very small. In such cases, if the sterilization process should fail, it is quite possible that the discrepancy would go unnoticed. Therefore, it is advantageous to challenge the process with a known live bacterial culture. These *inoculated controls* are called *biological indicators* and consist of resistant microorganisms on various materials. The indicators are sealed in envelopes to

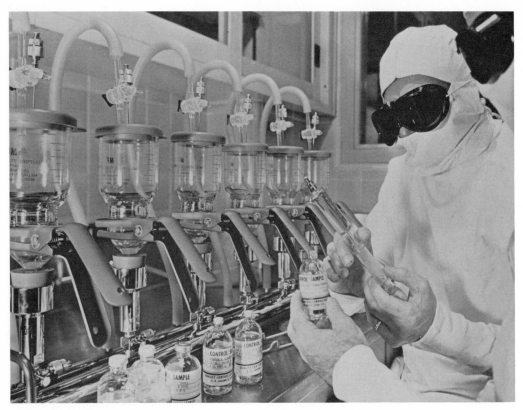

FIG. 14-22. Apparatus for sterility test by membrane filtration. Solutions are added to flasks and passed through 0.22-micron filters. The filters are then transferred to sterile culture media to determine if microorganisms are present on the filters. (Courtesy of Millipore Corp.)

prevent contamination of equipment and product. By inserting these indicators into the sterilizing chamber with the product, they serve to demonstrate the efficacy of the sterilization process and in so doing assure sterility in the product.

Pyrogen Testing. The U.S.P. test is a qualitative test which evaluates the fever response in mature rabbits. Rabbits are employed because of their sensitivity to pyrogenic material and the reliability of the response obtained. It is important that all materials and glassware to be used in the performance of the pyrogen test be rendered pyrogen free. This is done by heating at 250°C. for 30 minutes. The test involves injection of the test solution into the ear vein of each of 3 rabbits. At no time during a 3-hour period following injection must the temperature of any individual rabbit rise more than 0.6°C. or the sum of the rise for the three rabbits exceed 1.4°C. in order for the sample to pass.

Not all parenteral products may be subjected to a pyrogen test, since the medicinal substance itself may elicit a temperature effect in the rabbit. Consequently, pyrogen tests are generally performed only on the vehicle used in the product.

Another method for the detection of pyrogenic endotoxins is the *limulus test*.[10] Although this test is not recognized as an official test by the compendia, it is growing in popularity as an in-process control test. The test involves combining the test solution with a cell lysate from the amebocytes (blood cells) of the horseshoe crab. The protein fraction of the amebocytes will coagulate with any endotoxin that might be present and result in the formation of a gel. The limulus test is particularly of value for assuring that short-lived radiopharmaceuticals are pyrogen free.

Clarity Test. Presently, the U.S.P. does not list specifications for particulate matter contamination in injectables, but it does require that each final container be subjected individually to a physical inspection. Pressure is growing for the establishment of such standards for injectables because of the adverse effects foreign particles can have on the patient (e.g., the obstruction of vital organs or the formation of emboli in the circulatory system). Particulate matter that can be found in injectables includes glass, metal, rubber, paper or cellulose fibers, dirt, microcrystalline particles, and fragments of biological matter. These particles can range in size from less than 1 micron to as large as 500 microns. The capillaries in the human lung are approximately 15 microns in diameter, and many of the vessels supplying the brain, liver, and heart are smaller. Consequently, particles that are not filtered out in the lung can be entrapped in one of these vital organs.

Unfortunately, visual counting of particles is limited to approximately 50 microns even with the best illumination. Magnification and tyndallizing procedures can extend the capability of experienced inspectors down to the 15- to 20-micron range. Electronic counting of particles has extended the capability down to the 3 to 5 micron range. However, present methods only permit such counting on selected samples and in most cases only on solutions.

The *Coulter Counter* has been employed for in-process monitoring of particulate matter in solutions. This instrument detects the change in resistance when a particle in the solution is passed through a small orifice separating two electrodes. The magnitude of the change is then related to the size of the particle. Another instrument that has gained popularity for monitoring of particulate matter is the *HIAC counter* (Fig. 14-23). This unit works on the principle

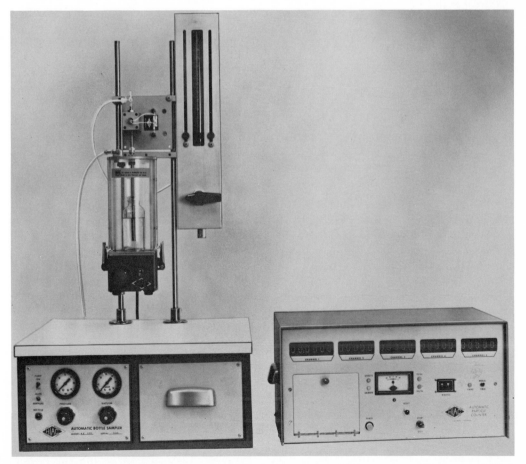

Fɪɢ. 14-23. An electronic counter used for monitoring particulate matter. (Courtesy of High Accuracy Products Corporation)

of interference of a light beam and does not require an electrolytic solution as is the case with the Coulter Counter. The light source is focused on a photocell and the particles obstruct the beam and cause a decrease in transmission of light. The HIAC also separates the particles into various sizes and counts the distribution in the various sizes. Particles may be counted and examined microscopically by collection on the surface of a membrane filter, a method that permits identification of particles as well as count. The ΠMC instrument can be utilized to project the microscopic field on a screen and its computer system can give distribution and particle size analysis.

Although efforts continue to both evaluate the clinical significance of particulate matter in injectables and develop standard methodology for the determination of particles, there has been increased interest in eliminating particles by final filtration of solutions during intravenous fluid administration. In this way, contamination introduced in the hospital can also be removed. A recent study showed that the use of filters almost eliminated the incidence of phlebitis in surgical patients receiving I.V. therapy.[36]

Leak Testing.   During the sealing of ampuls by fusion, an incomplete seal may result. This leaves an open passageway between the solution and a nonsterile environment. Since it is not always possible to detect faulty seals during visual inspection, a leak test is employed.

The leak test is performed by producing a negative pressure in the ampuls while they are submerged in a bath of dye solution. The dye solution rushes into the ampuls, coloring those that are incompletely sealed. The leak test is limited to ampuls, since vials, bottles, and disposable syringes are not designed to withstand such treatment.

REFERENCES

1. Alemany, P., and DelPozo, A.: Galenica acta, *16*:335, 1963.
2. Ansel, H. C.: Am. J. Hosp. Pharm., *21*(1): 25, 1964.
3. Artandi, C., and Van Winkle, W., Jr.: Nucleonics, *17*:86, 1959.
4. Behringwerke, A. G.: German patent DAS 1,178,170, Sept. 17, 1964. Drugs Made in Germany, *7*:201, 1964.
5. Boylan, J. C.: Bull. P.D.A., *19*:98, 1965.
6. Bruch, C. W.: Ann. Rev. Microbiol., *15*:245, 1961.
7. Bull. Nat. Inst. Nutrition: The Nion Corp., July 1953.
8. Charnicki, W. F.: Am. J. Pharm., *130*:409, 1958.
9. Chong, C. W.: J. Soc. Cosmet. Chem., *14*: 123, 1963.
10. Cooper, J. F., Levin, J., and Wagner, H. N.: J. Lab. Clin. Med., *78*:138, 1971.
11. Crevar, G. E., and Slotnick, I. J.: J. Pharm. Pharmacol., *16*:429, 1964.
12. Daize, J. H.: Food, Drug, Cosmetic Law J., *10*:722, 1959.
13. DeLuca, P., and Lachman, L.: J. Pharm. Sci., *54*:617, 1965.
14. Drugs: Current Good Manufacturing Practice Code of Federal Regulations, Part 133, Title 21. Food and Drug Administration, Washington, D. C., Jan. 1971.
15. Eisman, P. C., Ebersold, E., Weerts, J., and Lachman, L.: J. Pharm. Sci., *52*:183, 1963.
16. Girard, L. J., Dukes, C. D., and Fleming, T. C.: Presented at International Congress on Ophthalmology, Brussels, September 1958.
17. Gordon, L. E.: New Horizons in Sterilization. The Becton, Dickinson Lectures on Sterilization. p. 98. Given at Seton Hall, College of Medicine and Dentistry, Jersey City, N. J., Feb. 27, 1959.
18. Griffith, D. E.: J. Pharm. Sci., *56*:1197, 1967.
19. Grosicki, T. S., and Husa, W. J.: J. Am. Pharm. A. (Sci. Ed.), *43*:632, 1954.
20. Herrell, W. E., and Heilman, D.: Am. J. Med. Sci., *206*:221, 1943.
21. Hort and Peafold: Brit. Med. J.. No. 2659, 1911.
22. Howarth, W. R.: Bull. Parenteral Drug A., *26*:147, 1972.
23. Kenney, D. S., Grunoy, W. E., and Otto, R. H.: Bull. Parenteral Drug A., *18*(5):10, 1964.
24. Lachman, L.: Bull. Parenteral Drug A., *22*: 127, 1968.
25. Lachman, L., Pauli, W. A., Sheth, P. B., and Pagliery, M.: J. Pharm. Sci., *55*:962, 1966.
26. Lachman, L., Urbanyi, T., and Weinstein, S.: J. Pharm. Sci., *52*:244, 1963.
27. Linn, M. L., and Jones, L. T.: Am. J. Ophthalmol., *65*:76, 1968.
28. Marcus, A. D., and Stanley, J. L.: J. Pharm. Sci., *53*:91, 1964.
29. Merrill, D. L., Fleming, T. C., and Girard, L. J.: Am. J. Ophthalmol., *49*:895, 1960.
30. Nagy, R.: Research paper BL-P-8-0089-6G6-3, Oct. 9, 1958. Westinghouse Electric Corporation, Bloomfield, N. J.
31. Nash, R. A.: Drug Cosmetic Ind., *97*:843, 1965; *98*:39, 1966.
32. Perkins, J. J.: Principles and Methods of Sterilization, p. 42. Springfield, Illinois, Charles C Thomas, 1956.

33. ———: *In* Reddish, G. F. (ed.): Antiseptics, Disinfectants, Fungicides and Sterilization. p. 656. Philadelphia, Lea and Febiger, 1954.

34. Phillips, G. V., and Havel, E., Jr.: Use of Ultraviolet Radiation in Microbiological Laboratories. (P.B. 147043). U.S. Library of Congress, Washington, D. C. U.S. Govt. Res. Rept., *34* (2):122, Aug. 19, 1960.

35. Powell, D. B.: Pharm. J., *186*:321, 1961.

36. Rapp, R. P., Ryan, P., DeLuca, P., Griffen, W. O., Cloys, D., and Clark, J.: Bull. Parenteral Drug A., *27*:1, 1973.

37. Rowles, B., Sperandio, G. L., and Shaw, S. M.: Bull. Parenteral Drug A., *25*:1, 1971.

38. Schroeter, L. C.: J. Pharm. Sci., *50*:891, 1961.

39. ———: J. Pharm. Sci., *52*:888, 1963.

40. Schwartz, M. A., Bard, E., Rubycz, I., and Granatek, A. P.: J. Pharm. Sci., *54*:149, 1965.

41. Spiegel, A. J., and Noseworthy, M. M.: J. Pharm. Sci., *52*:917, 1963.

42. Suess, W.: Pharmazie, *20*:34, 1965.

43. Volkovinskaya, L. P., and Poyharskaya, A. M.: Med. Prom. SSSR, *15*(12):48, 1962.

44. Waltman, S. R., and Patrowicz, T. C.: Invest. Ophthalmol., *9*:966, 1970.

45. Williams, J. R., and Moravec, D. F.: Intra-venous Therapy, pp. 41–42. Hammond, Ind., Clissold Publishing Co., 1967.

46. Windheuser, J. J.: Bull. Parenteral Drug A., *17*:1, 1963.

47. Yanchik, W. A., and Sperandia, G. J.: Bull. Parenteral Drug A., *23*:53, 1969.

BIBLIOGRAPHY

Austin, P. R., and Timmerman, S. W.: Design and Operation of Clean Rooms. Detroit, Business News Publishing Company, 1965.

Avis, K. E.: Parenteral Preparations. *In* Remington's Pharmaceutical Sciences, ed. 14, pp. 1519–1544. Easton, Pa., Mack, 1970.

———: Sterile Products. *In* The Theory and Practice of Industrial Pharmacy, pp. 563–604. Philadelphia, Lea & Febiger, 1970.

Boenigk, J. W.: Parenteral Products. *In* Husa's Pharmaceutical Dispensing. ed. 6, pp. 398–419. Easton, Pa., Mack, 1966.

Maynard, C. D.: Clinical Nuclear Medicine. Philadelphia, Lea & Febiger, 1969.

Sykes, G.: Disinfection and Sterilization. ed. 2. Philadelphia, J. B. Lippincott, 1965.

Appendix

TABLES OF WEIGHTS AND MEASURES

| METRIC SYSTEM | ENGLISH SYSTEM |

Metric Table of Lengths

10 millimeters (mm) = 1 centimeter (cm)
10 centimeters (cm) = 1 decimeter (dm)
10 decimeters (dm) = 1 meter (m)
10 meters (m) = 1 dekameter (dam)
10 dekameters (dam) = 1 hectometer (hm)
10 hectometers (hm) = 1 kilometer (km)

1,000 micrometers = 1,000 microns (μ)
(μm)
= 1 millimeter (mm)

Metric Table of Volumes

10 milliliters (ml) = 1 centiliter (cl)
10 centiliters (cl) = 1 deciliter (dl)
10 deciliters (dl) = 1 liter (l)
10 liters (l) = 1 dekaliter (dal)
10 dekaliters (dal) = 1 hectoliter (hl)
10 hectoliters (hl) = 1 kiloliter (kl)

1 liter (l) = 1 cubic decimeter
(dm^3)

1 milliliter (ml) = 1 cubic centimeter
(cc) or (cm^3)*

Metric Table of Weights

10 milligrams (mg) = 1 centigram (cg)
10 centigrams (cg) = 1 decigram (dg)
10 decigrams (dg) = 1 gram (g)
10 grams (g) = 1 dekagram (dag)
10 dekagrams (dag) = 1 hectogram (hg)
10 hectograms (hg) = 1 kilogram (kg)

1,000 micrograms = 1 milligram (mg)
(mcg)
1,000 nanograms = 1 microgram (mcg)
(ng)

1 microgram (mcg) = 1 gamma (γ) (in
biochemistry)

= 1 microgram (μg)
(in physics and
physical chemis-
try)

* By statements in the U.S.P. and N.F.

English Table of Lengths

12 inches (in.) = 1 foot (ft.)
3 feet (ft.) = 1 yard (yd.)

Apothecaries' Fluid Measure

60 minims (♏) = 1 fluidram (f℥)
(or fluid drachm)
8 fluidrams (f℥) = 1 fluidounce (f℥)
(or fluid ounce)
16 fluidounces (f℥) = 1 pint (O.)
8 pints (O.) = 1 gallon (Cong. or C.)

Imperial Volume (British)

60 minims (min.) = 1 fluid drachms (fl. dr.)
8 fluid drachms = 1 fluid ounce (fl. oz.)
20 fluid ounces = 1 pint (O. or pt.)
8 pints = 1 gallon (C. or gal.)

Apothecaries' Weight

20 grains (gr.) = 1 scruple (℈)
3 scruples (℈) = 1 dram (℥) (or drachm)
8 drams (℥) = 1 ounce (℥)
12 ounces (℥) = 1 pound (℔.)

Troy Weight

24 grains (gr.) = 1 pennyweight (dwt.)
20 pennyweights = 1 ounce (oz. t.)
12 ounces = 1 pound (lb. t.)

Avoirdupois Weight

437½ grains (gr.) = 1 ounce (oz.)
16 ounces (oz.) = 1 pound (lb.)

Index

Numerals in italics indicates a figure; "t" following a page number indicates a table.